W9-BHV-341

This "Handbook of Clinical Drug Data" is presented
to you by Merrell Dow Pharmaceuticals Inc. We hope
that it will serve you as a ready reference of important
clinically useful drug information.

Your Merrell Dow
Hospital Representative

MERRELL DOW PHARMACEUTICALS INC.
Subsidiary of The Dow Chemical Company
Cincinnati, Ohio 45215, U.S.A.

Merrell Dow

handbook of
CLINICAL
DRUG
DATA

handbook of CLINICAL DRUG DATA

FIFTH EDITION

Editors
James E. Knoben, Pharm.D.
Philip O. Anderson, Pharm.D.

Assistant Editor
Larry Jay Davis, Pharm.D.

Contributing Editors
William D. Ball, Pharm.D.
William G. Troutman, Pharm.D.

DRUG INTELLIGENCE PUBLICATIONS, INC., HAMILTON, ILLINOIS 62341

Library of Congress Cataloging in Publication Data

Knoben, James E.
  Handbook of clinical drug data.

  Includes bibliographies and index.
  1. Pharmacology — Handbooks, manuals, etc.   2. Drugs —
Handbooks, manuals, etc.   I. Anderson, Philip O.
II. Title.   [DNLM: 1. Drugs.   QV 55 H2464]
RM300.K5   1983   615′.1   82-22145
ISBN 0-914768-41-7 (pbk.)

First Printing, January 1983
Second Printing, August 1983
Third Printing, April 1984

PRINTED IN THE UNITED STATES OF AMERICA BY HAMILTON PRESS, INC.

PREFACE TO THE FIFTH EDITION

WITH THE INTRODUCTION OF EVER-INCREASING NUMBERS OF DRUGS and the concomitant growth in the drug literature, the need for a concise, yet comprehensive, compilation of clinically useful drug information is essential. The *Handbook of Clinical Drug Data* was developed to meet this need.

The Fourth Edition was especially well received, reflecting the utility of a new format and an expanded scope of information. Those familiar with the Fourth Edition will therefore be pleased with the even greater attention to clinically relevant data and extensive documentation (over 2300 cited references) in this edition. The addition of expert contributors, each of whom wrote within his or her area of clinical specialty, is largely responsible for this improved perspective.

Other major improvements are the inclusion of new areas achieving recent clinical advancements, such as nutritional assessment, parenteral nutrition and cancer chemotherapy. The drug monograph format has also been enhanced by the addition of new headings dealing with pharmacologic action and individualization of drug dosage. New topics have been added to both the Drug-Induced Diseases and Medical Emergencies chapters. All other chapters in the book have been completely revised and updated.

This revision could not have been accomplished without the assistance of many people. Larry Davis, Bill Ball and Bill Troutman have been instrumental in the development of the book over the years and have helped greatly in the preparation of this edition. The contributions of Dr. Art Watanabe to the development of previous editions of the book are also appreciated. We owe a real debt of gratitude to the many Contributors who spent countless hours researching and distilling the current literature and to Dr. Dianne Tobias who compiled the index. And to our distinguished medical and pharmacy colleagues for their invaluable review and critique of the manuscript, we are most appreciative: David N. Bailey, M.D., Steven L. Barriere, Pharm.D., Robert A. Bauernfeind, M.D., C.H. Beck, Jr., M.D., Kanu Chatterjee, M.D., Gerald F. Chernoff, Ph.D., Unamarie Clibon, Pharm.D., Martin G. Cogan, M.D., R. Dennis Collins, M.D., Robert A. Curtis, Pharm.D., Alexander M. Gilderman, Pharm.D., Mark R. Green, M.D., Leslie Hendeles, Pharm.D., Jon I. Isenberg, M.D., H. William Kelly, Pharm.D., Mary Anne Koda-Kimble, Pharm.D., James R. Lane, Pharm.D., Anthony S. Manoguerra, Pharm.D., Arnold S. Milstein, M.D., Robert J. Michocki, Pharm.D., Katherine L. Sheehan, M.D., Carol A. Stoner, Pharm.D., John F. Thompson, Pharm.D., and Helmuth Vorherr, M.D. Finally, Mary Ann Jaske of Drug Intelligence Publications deserves special thanks for her exceptional efforts in preparing the manuscript for publication.

JAMES E. KNOBEN
PHILIP O. ANDERSON

NOTICE

THE INDICATIONS, DOSAGES, and other drug information presented in this *Handbook* conform to that found in the medical literature or in the manufacturer's product literature. However, this *Handbook* provides only the more important elements of prescribing data, and is *not* a comprehensive drug information source. The manufacturer's current product information or other standard references should always be consulted for more detailed information, especially before prescribing is undertaken.

EDITORS AND CONTRIBUTORS

Editors

James E. Knoben, Pharm.D., M.P.H.
Chief, Drug Information Analysis Branch
Division of Drug Information Resources
National Center for Drugs and Biologics
Food and Drug Administration
Rockville, Maryland

Philip O. Anderson, Pharm.D.
Director, Drug Information Service
University of California Medical Center
Assistant Clinical Professor of Pharmacy
University of California, San Francisco,
San Diego Program
San Diego, California

Assistant Editor

Larry Jay Davis, Pharm.D.
Clinical Pharmacist, Moffitt Hospital
University of California Medical Center
Assistant Clinical Professor of Pharmacy
University of California, San Francisco
San Francisco, California

Contributing Editors

William D. Ball, Pharm.D.
Clinical Pharmacist
Department of Pharmacy Services
University Hospitals of Cleveland
Cleveland, Ohio

William G. Troutman, Pharm.D.
Director, New Mexico Poison, Drug
Information and Medical Crisis Center
Associate Professor of Pharmacy
University of New Mexico
Albuquerque, New Mexico

CONTRIBUTORS

Richard C. Andersen, Pharm.D.
  Clinical Pharmacist, San Francisco Poison Control Center
  Assistant Clinical Professor of Pharmacy, School of Pharmacy,
    University of California, San Francisco
  San Francisco, California

Jerry L. Bauman, Pharm.D.
  Clinical Pharmacist/Cardiology, Department of Pharmacy,
    University of Illinois Hospital
  Assistant Professor of Pharmacy Practice, College of Pharmacy,
    University of Illinois
  Chicago, Illinois

Lawrence R. Borgsdorf, Pharm.D.
  Clinical Pharmacist, Department of Medicine, Kern Medical Center
  Assistant Professor of Medicine, School of Medicine,
    University of California, Los Angeles,
    Kern Medical Center Program
  Bakersfield, California

Ronald R. Conte, Pharm.D.
  Clinical Pharmacist, Outpatient Department,
    San Francisco General Hospital
  Associate Clinical Professor of Pharmacy, School of Pharmacy,
    University of California, San Francisco
  San Francisco, California

Betty Jean Dong, Pharm.D.
  Clinical Pharmacist, Family Practice, San Francisco General Hospital
  Associate Clinical Professor of Pharmacy, School of Pharmacy,
    University of California, San Francisco
  San Francisco, California

Robert T. Dorr, M.S.
  Chief, Cancer Research Pharmacy Service, Cancer Center Division, and
    Research Associate, Department of Internal Medicine,
    University of Arizona
  Tucson, Arizona

Robert C. Eschbach, Pharm.D.
  Assistant Professor of Clinical Pharmacy, College of Pharmacy,
    University of New Mexico
  Albuquerque, New Mexico

John G. Gambertoglio, Pharm.D.
  Clinical Pharmacist, Kidney Transplant Service, and
    Adjunct Associate Professor of Pharmacy, School of Pharmacy,
    University of California, San Francisco
  San Francisco, California

Philip D. Hansten, Pharm.D.
  Associate Professor of Clinical Pharmacy, College of Pharmacy,
    Washington State University
  Pullman, Washington

George M. Lasezkay, Pharm.D.
Assistant Professor, Clinical Pharmacokinetics Laboratory, Department
of Pharmacy, Millard Fillmore Hospital,
State University of New York at Buffalo
Buffalo, New York

Tara K. Mochizuki, Pharm.D.
Clinical Pharmacist, Department of Pharmacy,
University of California Medical Center
Assistant Clinical Professor of Pharmacy, School of Pharmacy,
University of California, San Francisco, San Diego Program
San Diego, California

Robert E. Pachorek, Pharm.D.
Clinical Pharmacist, Department of Pharmacy,
Mercy Hospital and Medical Center
San Diego, California

Fred Shatsky, B.S. Pharm.
Coordinator, Nutritional and Metabolic Support,
University of California Medical Center
Assistant Clinical Professor of Pharmacy, School of Pharmacy,
University of California, San Francisco, San Diego Program
San Diego, California

Sam K. Shimomura, Pharm.D.
Vice Chairman, Division of Clinical Pharmacy, and Associate Clinical
Professor of Pharmacy, School of Pharmacy,
University of California, San Francisco, U.C. Irvine/Long Beach
Memorial Hospital Program
Irvine, California

John K. Siepler, Pharm.D.
Clinical Pharmacist, Department of Pharmacy,
University of California Medical Center
Davis, California

Raymond E. Smith, Pharm.D.
Clinical Pharmacist, Department of Pharmacy,
University of California Medical Center
Assistant Clinical Professor of Pharmacy, School of Pharmacy,
University of California, San Francisco, San Diego Program
San Diego, California

Glen L. Stimmel, Pharm.D.
Associate Professor of Clinical Pharmacy, Psychiatry and the
Behavioral Sciences, Schools of Pharmacy and Medicine,
University of Southern California
Los Angeles, California

Dianne E. Tobias, Pharm.D.
Consultant Pharmacist, Long Term Care Practice
Assistant Clinical Professor of Pharmacy, School of Pharmacy,
University of California, San Francisco, U.C. Irvine Program
Irvine, California

Lai J. Wong, Pharm.D.
Pharmacist Specialist, Inpatient Pharmacy,
Kaiser Foundation Hospital
Los Angeles, California

CONTENTS

DRUG REVIEWS

1 ABBREVIATIONS AND CONVERSION FACTORS

THE FOLLOWING medical record and prescription abbreviations are in common usage, but variations will occur by institution or geographic area.

Medical Record Abbreviations

A	Apical; Artery; Assessment (POMR)	ASHD	Arteriosclerotic heart disease
A₂	Aortic second sound	ASO	Arteriosclerosis obliterans
AAL	Anterior axillary line	ATN	Acute tubular necrosis
Ab	Abort; Abortion; Antibody	AV	Arteriovenous; Atrioventricular
Abd	Abdomen; Abdominal	A & W	Alive and well
ABE	Acute bacterial endocarditis	Ax	Axillary
ABG	Arterial blood gases	BaE	Barium enema
ACD	Acid citrate dextrose; Anterior chest diameter	BBB	Bundle branch block
		BBT	Basal body temperature
ACT	Activated clotting time	BCG	Bacille Calmette-Guerin
ACTH	Adrenocorticotropic hormone	BE	Bacterial endocarditis; Barium enema
ADH	Antidiuretic hormone	BEI	Butanol-extractable iodine
ADL	Activities of daily living	BJ	Biceps jerk; Bone and joint
ADR	Adverse drug reaction	BK	Below knee
AF	Atrial fibrillation	Bl Obs	Bladder observation
AFB	Acid fast bacillus	BLS	Basic life support
Ag	Antigen	BM	Bone marrow; Bowel movement
A/G	Albumin/globulin ratio	BMR	Basal metabolic rate
AGL	Acute granulocytic leukemia	BP	Blood pressure
AGN	Acute glomerular nephritis	BPH	Benign prostatic hypertrophy
AHF	Antihemophilic factor	BR	Bathroom; Bedrest
AHG	Antihemophilic globulin	BRP	Bathroom privileges
AI	Aortic insufficiency	BS	Blood sugar; Bowel sounds; Breath sounds
AJ	Ankle jerk		
AK	Above knee	BSA	Body surface area
ALL	Acute lymphocytic leukemia	BSO	Bilateral salpingo-oophorectomy
AMA	Against medical advice	BT	Bedtime; Brain tumor; Breast tumor
AML	Acute myelocytic leukemia	BTFS	Breast tumor frozen section
ANA	Antinuclear antibodies	BTL	Bilateral tubal ligation
AODM	Adult onset diabetes mellitus	BU	Bodansky unit
AP	Antepartum; Anteroposterior; Apical pulse	BUN	Blood urea nitrogen
		BVL	Bilateral vas ligation
A & P	Anterior and posterior; Auscultation and percussion	BW	Body weight
		Bx	Biopsy
Appy	Appendectomy	C₂	Second cervical vertebra
APTT	Activated partial thromboplastin time	CA	Cancer; Carcinoma; Chronologic age
ARD	Acute respiratory disease; Acute respiratory distress	CABG	Coronary artery bypass graft
		CAD	Coronary artery disease
ARF	Acute renal failure	CAPD	Chronic ambulatory peritoneal dialysis
AS	Anal sphincter; Aortic stenosis; Arteriosclerosis	CAT	Computerized axial tomography
		CBC	Complete blood count
ASCVD	Arteriosclerotic cardiovascular disease	CBS	Chronic brain syndrome
ASD	Atrial septal defect	CC	Chief complaint

CCU	Coronary care unit	EKG	Electrocardiogram
CF	Complement fixation; Cystic fibrosis	EMG	Electromyogram
CGH	Chorionic gonadotropic hormone	ENT	Ears, nose and throat
CGL	Chronic granulocytic leukemia	ER	Emergency room
CHD	Congenital heart disease; Coronary heart disease	ESR	Erythrocyte sedimentation rate
		EST	Electroshock therapy
CHF	Congestive heart failure	EUA	Examine under anesthesia
CHO	Carbohydrate	FAS	Fetal alcohol syndrome
CI	Cardiac index; Color index	FB	Finger breadths; Foreign bodies
CLL	Chronic lymphocytic leukemia	FBS	Fasting blood sugar
CML	Chronic myelocytic leukemia	F Cath	Foley catheter
CNS	Central nervous system	FEV₁	Forced expiratory volume in one second
CO	Cardiac output		
C/O	Complaint of	FF	Filtration fraction
COLD	Chronic obstructive lung disease	FFA	Free fatty acids
COPD	Chronic obstructive pulmonary disease	FH	Family history; Fetal heart
		FHR	Fetal heart rate
C & P	Cystoscopy and pyelogram	FHS	Fetal heart sounds
CPAP	Continuous positive airway pressure	FP	Family planning
CPK	Creatine phosphokinase	FRC	Functional residual capacity
CPP	Cerebral perfusion pressure	FSH	Follicle stimulating hormone
CPR	Cardiopulmonary resuscitation	FTA	Fluorescent titer antibody; Fluorescent treponema antibody
CRF	Chronic renal failure; Corticotropin releasing factor		
		FTND	Full-term normal delivery
CRP	C-reactive protein	FUO	Fever of undetermined origin
CS	Cesarean section; Coronary sclerosis	FVC	Forced vital capacity
C & S	Culture and sensitivity	Fx	Fracture
CS & CC	Culture, sensitivity and colony count	GA	Gastric analysis; General appearance
CSF	Cerebrospinal fluid	GB	Gallbladder
CT	Circulation time; Clotting time; Computerized tomography	GC	Gonococcal; Gonococcus
		GFR	Glomerular filtration rate
CUC	Chronic ulcerative colitis	GH	Growth hormone
CV	Cardiovascular; Conjugata vera	GI	Gastrointestinal
CVA	Cerebral vascular accident; Costovertebral angle	GMP	General medical problem(s)
		G-P-	Gravida-, para-
CVI	Cerebral vascular insufficiency	G6PD	Glucose-6-phosphate dehydrogenase
CVP	Central venous pressure	GTT	Glucose tolerance test
CVS	Clean voided specimen	GU	Genitourinary
Cx	Cervical; Cervix	Gyn	Gynecology
CXR	Chest x-ray	HA	Headache; Hyperalimentation
DC or	Discharge; Discontinue	HAA	Hepatitis-associated antigen
D/C		HBAg	Hepatitis B antigen
D & C	Dilatation and curettage	HB/BW	Hold breakfast for blood work
DD or	Differential diagnosis	HBP	High blood pressure
DDX		HCG	Human chorionic gonadotropin
DDD	Degenerative disc disease	Hct	Hematocrit
DHL	Diffuse histiocytic lymphoma	HCVD	Hypertensive cardiovascular disease
Diff	Differential blood count	HDL	High-density lipoproteins
DJD	Degenerative joint disease	HEENT	Head, eyes, ears, nose, throat
DM	Diabetes mellitus; Diastolic murmur	Hgb	Hemoglobin
DOA	Date of admission; Dead on arrival	HHD	Hypertensive heart disease
DOE	Dyspnea on exertion	HNV	Has not voided
DPT	Diphtheria-pertussis-tetanus	HO	House officer
DSD	Dry sterile dressing	H/O	History of
DTR	Deep tendon reflex	HPF	High power field
DTs	Delirium tremens	HPI	History of present illness
DU	Duodenal ulcer	HPLC	High pressure liquid chromatography
DW	Dextrose in water; Distilled water	HR	Heart rate
D5W	Dextrose 5% in water	HT	Hypertension; Hypodermic tablet
Dx	Diagnosis	HTN	Hypertension
EBL	Estimated blood loss	HTVD	Hypertensive vascular disease
ECF	Extracellular fluid	Hx	History
ECG	Electrocardiogram	I	Impression (POMR)
ECT	Electroconvulsive therapy	IA	Intra-amniotically
EDTA	Ethylenediaminetetraacetate	IASD	Interatrial septal defect
EEG	Electroencephalogram	IBC	Iron binding capacity
EENT	Eyes, ears, nose, throat	IBI	Intermittent bladder irrigation
EFA	Essential fatty acids	ICF	Intracellular fluid

ICG	Indocyanine green
ICM	Intercostal margin
ICS	Intercostal space
ICSH	Interstitial cell-stimulating hormone
ICU	Intensive care unit
ID	Initial dose; Intradermal(ly)
I & D	Incision and drainage
IF	Inspiratory force; Interstitial fluid; Intrinsic factor
Ig	Immunoglobulin
IHD	Ischemic heart disease
ILDL	Intermediate low-density lipoproteins
IM	Intramuscular(ly)
IMP	Impression
IMV	Intermittent mechanical ventilation
I & O	Intake and output
IOP	Intraocular pressure
IP	Intraperitoneal(ly)
IPPB	Intermittent positive pressure breathing
IT	Inhalation therapy; Intrathecal(ly)
IU	International unit
IUCD or	Intrauterine (contraceptive) device
IUD	
IUP	Intrauterine pregnancy
IV	Intravenous(ly)
IVP	Intravenous push; Intravenous pyelogram
IVPB	Intravenous piggyback
IVSD	Interventricular septal defect
JVD	Jugular-venous distention
JVP	Jugular-venous pulse
KJ	Knee jerk
KO	Keep open
KUB	Kidneys, ureters, bladder
KVO	Keep vein open
KW	Keith-Wagener (ophthalmoscopic findings)
L	Left
L₂	Second lumbar vertebra
LA	Left atrium
Lap	Laparotomy
LATS	Long-acting thyroid stimulator
LBBB	Left bundle branch block
LCM	Left costal margin
LD	Lethal dose; Liver disease; Longitudinal diameter (of heart)
LDH	Lactic dehydrogenase
LDL	Low-density lipoproteins
LE	Lower extremities; Lupus erythematosus
LFS	Liver function series
LFT	Liver function test(s)
LH	Luteinizing hormone
LKS	Liver, kidneys, spleen
LLD	Left lateral decubitus
LLL	Left lower lobe
LLQ	Left lower quadrant
LMP	Last menstrual period
LOA	Left occipital anterior
LOM	Limitation of motion
LOP	Left occipital posterior
LP	Light perception; Lumbar puncture
LPF	Low power field
LT	Levine tube; Luken's trap
LTC	Long term care
LUL	Left upper lobe
LUQ	Left upper quadrant

LVH	Left ventricular hypertrophy
L & W	Living and well
Lytes	Electrolytes
M	Meter; Molar; Murmur
M₁	Mitral first sound
MA	Mental age
M/A	Mood and/or affect
MAP	Mean arterial pressure
MBC	Maximum breathing capacity; Minimum bactericidal concentration
MCH	Mean corpuscular hemoglobin
MCHC	Mean corpuscular hemoglobin concentration
MCL	Midclavicular line; Midcostal line
MCV	Mean corpuscular volume
MDV	Multiple dose vial
MF	Myocardial fibrosis
MH	Marital history; Menstrual history
MI	Mitral insufficiency; Myocardial infarction
MIC	Minimum inhibitory concentration
ML	Midline
MLD	Minimum lethal dose
MS	Mitral stenosis; Morphine sulfate; Multiple sclerosis
MSL	Midsternal line
N or NL	Normal
NAD	No acute distress
NAS	No added salt
NG	Nasogastric
NGU	Nongonococcal urethritis
NKA	No known allergies
NPN	Nonprotein nitrogen
NPO	Nothing by mouth
NS	Normal saline
NSFTD	Normal spontaneous full-term delivery
NSR	Normal sinus rhythm
NSU	Nonspecific urethritis
N & T	Nose and throat
N & V	Nausea and vomiting
NVD	Nausea, vomiting, diarrhea
NYD	Not yet diagnosed
O	Objective data (POMR)
Ob	Obstetrics
OB	Occult blood
OBS	Organic brain syndrome
O/E	On examination
OOB	Out of bed
OPV	Outpatient visit; Oral polio vaccine
OR	Operating room
OT	Occupational therapy; Old tuberculin
P	Plan (POMR); Pulse
PA	Pernicious anemia; Posteroanterior; Pulmonary artery
P & A	Percussion and auscultation
PABA	Para-aminobenzoic acid
PAT	Paroxysmal atrial tachycardia
PBI	Protein bound iodine
PC	Porto-caval; Present complaint
PCS	Porto-caval shunt
PCV	Packed cell volume
PE	Physical examination; Pulmonary embolism
PEEP	Positive end-expiratory pressure
PEG	Pneumoencephalogram; Polyethylene glycol
PERLA	Pupils equal, react to light and accommodation

PFT	Pulmonary function test(s)	RTC	Return to clinic
PGH	Pituitary growth hormone	RUL	Right upper lobe
pHa	Arterial blood pH	RUQ	Right upper quadrant
PH	Patient history	RVH	Right ventricular hypertrophy
PI	Present illness	S	Subjective data (POMR)
PID	Pelvic inflammatory disease	S_1	First heart sound
PIE	Pulmonary infiltration with eosinophilia	S_2	Second heart sound
PKU	Phenylketonuria	S-A	Sino-atrial
PMH	Past medical history	SBE	Subacute bacterial endocarditis
PMI	Point of maximal impulse; Point of maximal intensity	SBO	Small bowel obstruction
		SC	Sickle cell; Static compliance; Subclavian; Subcutaneous(ly)
PMN	Polymorphonuclear leukocytes		
PMP	Past menstrual period	SGOT	Serum glutamic oxaloacetic transaminase
PM & R	Physical medicine and rehabilitation		
PMT	Premenstrual tension	SGPT	Serum glutamic pyruvic transaminase
PND	Paroxysmal nocturnal dyspnea; Post-nasal drip	SH	Serum hepatitis; Social history
		SIADH	Syndrome of inappropriate ADH (secretion)
Pnx	Pneumothorax		
PO	By mouth	SL	Sublingual(ly)
POLYS	Polymorphonuclear leukocytes	SLE	Systemic lupus erythematosus
POMR	Problem oriented medical record	SMA	Serial multiple analysis
POR	Problem oriented record	SMR	Somnolent metabolic rate
PP	Postpartum; Postprandial	SOAP	Subjective, objective, assessment and plans (POMR)
PPBS	Postprandial blood sugar		
PPD	Purified protein derivative	SOB	Shortness of breath
ppm	Parts per million	S/P	Status post
PR	Per rectum	SQ	Subcutaneous(ly)
P & R	Pulse and respiration	SR	Sedimentation rate; Systems review
PSP	Phenolsulfonphthalein	SSE	Saline solution enema; Soap solution enema
Pt	Patient		
PT	Physical therapy; Prothrombin time	STD	Sexually transmitted disease; Skin test dose
PTA	Plasma thromboplastic antecedent; Prior to admission; Prothrombin activity		
		STS	Serologic test for syphilis
		Sx	Symptom(s)
PTC	Plasma thromboplastin component	T	Temperature
PTT	Partial thromboplastin time	T & A	Tonsillectomy and adenoidectomy
PU	Peptic ulcer	TAb	Therapeutic abortion
PUD	Peptic ulcer disease	TAH	Total abdominal hysterectomy
PVC	Premature ventricular contraction	TAO	Thromboangiitis obliterans
PVT	Paroxysmal ventricular tachycardia	TAT	Tetanus antitoxin
Px	Physical examination; Pneumothorax	TB	Tuberculosis
R	Respiration; Right	TBA	To be administered; To be arranged
RA	Rheumatoid arthritis; Right atrium	TBG	Thyroxine binding globulin
RAI	Radioactive iodine	TBW	Total body water
RBBB	Right bundle branch block	T & C	Type and crossmatch
RBC	Red blood cell; Red blood count	TD	Transverse diameter (of heart)
RBF	Renal blood flow	TEA	Thromboendartectomy
RCM	Right costal margin	TIA	Transient ischemic attack
RDS	Respiratory distress syndrome	TIBC	Total iron-binding capacity
REM	Rapid eye movement	TKO	To keep open
RF	Renal failure; Rheumatic fever; Rheumatoid factor	TL	Tubal ligation
		TLA	Trans-lumbar aortogram
Rh	Rhesus factor	TLC	Tender loving care; Thin layer chromatography
RHD	Rheumatic heart disease		
RIA	Radioimmunoassay	Tm	Maximal renal tubular clearance
RLD	Right lateral decubitus	TM	Tympanic membrane
RLL	Right lower lobe	TOPV	Trivalent oral polio vaccine
RLQ	Right lower quadrant	TP	Thrombophlebitis; Total protein
R/O	Rule out	TPI	Treponema pallidium immobilization
ROM	Range of motion	TPN	Total parenteral nutrition
ROS	Review of symptoms; Review of systems	TPR	Temperature, pulse, respiration
		T-set	Tracheotomy set
ROT	Right occipital transverse	TSH	Thyroid stimulating hormone
RPF	Renal plasma flow	TURP	Transurethral resection of prostate
RQ	Respiratory quotient	TV	Trichomonas vaginalis
RR	Recovery room; Respiratory rate	TVC	Triple voiding cystogram
RSR	Regular sinus rhythm	TWE	Tap water enema
RTA	Renal tubular acidosis	Tx	Treatment

T & X	Type and crossmatch	**VLDL**	Very low-density lipoproteins
UA	Uric acid; Urinalysis	**VP**	Venous pressure
UCG	Urine chorionic gonadotropin	**VS**	Vital signs
UGI	Upper gastrointestinal	**VSD**	Ventricular septal defect
URI	Upper respiratory infection	**VSS**	Vital signs stable
UTI	Urinary tract infection	**VT**	Ventricular tachycardia
VC	Vena cava; Vital capacity	**WB**	Whole blood
VCT	Venous clotting time	**WBC**	White blood cell; White blood count
VCU	Voiding cysto-urethrogram	**WD**	Well developed
VD	Venereal disease	**WF**	White female
VDRL	Venereal disease research laboratory	**WM**	White male
VF	Ventricular fibrillation	**WN**	Well nourished
VI	Volume index	**WNL**	Within normal limits

Prescription Abbreviations

aa	Of each (ana)	**os**	Left eye (oculus sinister)
ac	Before meals (ante cibum)	**ou**	Each eye (oculus uterque)
ad	Right ear (auris dextra)	**pc**	After meals (post cibum)
ad	Up to (ad)	**po**	By mouth (per os)
ad lib	As desired (ad libitum)	**prn**	As needed (pro re nata)
aq	Water (aqua)	**q**	Each (quaque)
as	Left ear (auris sinistra)	**qd**	Every day (quaque die)
au	Each ear (auris utro)	**q h** *or*	Every hour (quaque hora)
bid	Twice a day (bis in die)	**q hr**	
c	With (cum)	**qid**	Four times a day (quarter in die)
dos	Dose (dosis)	**qs**	Sufficient quantity (quantum sufficiat)
dtd	Let such doses be given (dentur tales doses)	**qs ad**	Sufficient quantity to make (quantum sufficiat ad)
et	And (et)	**repet**	To be repeated (repetatur)
ft	Make (fiat, fiant)	**s**	Without (sine)
gtt(s)	Drop(s) (gutta)	**ss**	One-half (semis)
h *or* **hr**	Hour (hora)	**Sig**	Mark, write (signa)
hs	At bedtime (hora somni)	**stat**	At once (statim)
M	Mix (misce)	**tid**	Three times a day (ter in die)
mt	Send of such (mitte talis)	**ud** *or*	As directed (ut dictum)
nr	Do not repeat (non repetatur)	**ut dict**	
od	Right eye (oculus dexter)		

For abbreviations related to prescription dosages (volume, weight), see "Conversion Factors" below.

Conversion Factors

Milliequivalents
Temperature
Weights and Measures

MILLIEQUIVALENTS

An equivalent weight of a substance is that weight which will combine with or replace one gram of hydrogen; a milliequivalent is 1/1000 of an equivalent weight.

Approximate Milliequivalents-Weights of Selected Ions

SALT	MEQ/GRAM SALT	MG SALT/MEQ
Calcium Carbonate [$CaCO_3$]	20	50
Calcium Chloride [$CaCl_2 \cdot 2H_2O$]	14	73
Calcium Gluconate [Ca Gluconate$_2 \cdot 1H_2O$]	4	224
Calcium Lactate [Ca Lactate$_2 \cdot 5H_2O$]	6	154
Magnesium Sulfate [$MgSO_4$]	16	60
Magnesium Sulfate [$MgSO_4 \cdot 7H_2O$]	8	123
Potassium Acetate [K Acetate]	10	98
Potassium Chloride [KCl]	13	75
Potassium Citrate [K_3 Citrate $\cdot 1H_2O$]	9	108
Potassium Iodide [KI]	6	166
Sodium Bicarbonate [$NaHCO_3$]	12	84
Sodium Chloride [NaCl]	17	58
Sodium Citrate [Na_3 Citrate $\cdot 2H_2O$]	10	98
Sodium Iodide [NaI]	7	150
Sodium Lactate (Na Lactate)	9	112

Valences and Atomic Weights of Selected Ions

SUBSTANCE	ELECTROLYTE	VALENCE	MOLECULAR WEIGHT
Calcium	Ca^{++}	2	40
Chloride	Cl^-	1	35.5
Magnesium	Mg^{++}	2	24
Phosphate	HPO_4^{--} (80%)	1.8	96*
pH = 7.4	$H_2PO_4^-$ (20%)		
Potassium	K^+	1	39
Sodium	Na^+	1	23
Sulfate	SO_4^{--}	2	96*

*The molecular weight of phosphorus only is 31, and sulfur only is 32.

TEMPERATURE

Fahrenheit to Centigrade: $5(°F - 32)/9 = °C$

Centigrade to Fahrenheit: $(°C \times 9)/5 + 32 = °F$

Centigrade to Kelvin: $°C + 273 = °K$

WEIGHTS AND MEASURES

Metric Weight Equivalents

1 kilogram (kg)	= 1,000 grams
1 gram (g)	= 1,000 milligrams
1 milligram (mg)	= 0.001 gram
1 microgram (mcg, μg)	= 0.001 milligram
1 nanogram (ng)	= 0.001 microgram
1 picogram (pg)	= 0.001 nanogram

Metric Volume Equivalents

1 liter (L) = 1,000 milliliters (ml)
1 deciliter (dl) = 100 milliliters

Apothecary Weight Equivalents

1 scruple (℈)	= 20 grains (gr)
60 grains	= 1 dram (ʒ)
8 drams	= 1 ounce (ℨ)
1 ounce	= 480 grains (gr)
12 ounces	= 1 pound (℔)

Apothecary Volume Equivalents

60 minims (♏)	= 1 fluidram (flʒ)
8 fluidrams	= 1 fluidounce (flℨ)
1 fluidounce	= 480 minims (♏)
16 fluidounces	= 1 pint (pt)

Avoirdupois Weight Equivalents

1 ounce (oz) = 437.5 grains
1 pound (lb) = 16 ounces

Weight/Volume Equivalents

1 mg/dl = 10 mcg/ml
1 mg/dl = 1 mg%
1 ppm = 1 mg/L

Conversion Equivalents

1 gram	(g)	= 15.43 grains	0.1 mg	= 1/600 gr
1 milliliter	(ml)	= 16.23 minims	0.12 mg	= 1/500 gr
1 minim	(♏)	= 0.06 milliliter	0.15 mg	= 1/400 gr
1 grain	(gr)	= 64.8 milligrams	0.2 mg	= 1/300 gr
1 ounce	(ℨ)	= 31.1 grams	0.3 mg	= 1/200 gr
1 fluidounce	(flℨ)	= 29.57 ml	0.4 mg	= 1/150 gr
1 pint	(pt)	= 473.2 ml	0.5 mg	= 1/120 gr
1 ounce	(oz)	= 28.35 grams	0.6 mg	= 1/100 gr
1 pound	(lb)	= 453.6 grams	0.8 mg	= 1/80 gr
1 kilogram	(kg)	= 2.2 pounds	1.0 mg	= 1/65 gr

2 BIOPHARMACEUTICS AND PHARMACOKINETICS

General Principles

BIOPHARMACEUTICS IS THE STUDY of the relationship between physicochemical properties of a drug in a dosage form and the therapeutic response observed after its administration. Pharmacokinetics is concerned with the characterization of the time course of drug absorption, distribution, elimination, the relationship among these processes and the observed therapeutic or adverse effects.

The purpose of this section is to provide a brief review of the more important biopharmaceutical factors that influence drug delivery, the pharmacokinetic concepts used to describe drug disposition in the body and their application to the design of drug dosage regimens. More extensive discussions of these topics are available for less experienced[1-6] as well as advanced practitioners.[7,8]

Familiarity with this information is essential for those individuals involved in clinical practice, but its usefulness must be kept in perspective. The goal of drug therapy is more than just the attainment of desired plasma drug concentrations. It is the successful control or eradication of a disease state through the appropriate selection, proper administration and efficient distribution of drugs. The concepts presented in this section, when used in conjunction with these objectives, will make a useful contribution to rational drug therapy.

Pharmacokinetic Model Systems. The most common method used to describe the pharmacokinetic behavior of a drug in the body is by the use of models depicting the body as a single compartment or series of compartments. These compartments do not necessarily have any anatomic or physiologic reality. However, visualization of the body in this fashion helps explain the observed disposition characteristics of various drugs and allows prediction of drug concentrations in the body as a function of time, dose and route of administration.

The single compartment model assumes that a drug is instantly absorbed and uniformly distributed throughout the entire body (Figure 1). This model can be most readily applied to drugs that rapidly distribute between plasma and other body fluids and tissues after reaching the systemic circulation. The rate of drug elimination from the body is assumed to follow first-order or linear

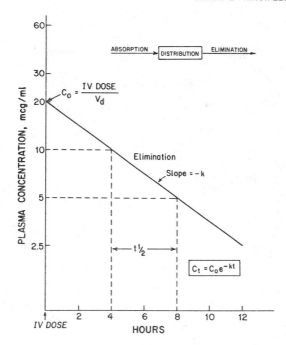

Figure 1. Plasma concentration-time decline after intravenous administration for a drug best characterized by a one-
compartment model.

pharmacokinetics. In other words, the rate of elimination is proportional to the amount (or concentration) of drug present in the
body at any given time.

The two-compartment model separates the body into a central
compartment, usually with a small volume, and a peripheral compartment with a larger volume (Figure 2). Initial distribution of a
drug occurs within the central compartment which is assumed to
consist of the blood and the extracellular fluid of highly perfused
organs such as heart, liver, kidneys and brain. Drug distribution into the peripheral compartment (assumed to consist of less highly
perfused organs and tissues such as skin, muscle and fat) from
the central compartment takes place more slowly. A distribution
equilibrium is eventually established between these two compartments, with drug elimination taking place solely from the central
compartment. Both the transfer of drug between compartments
and drug elimination from the central compartment are again
assumed to obey first-order pharmacokinetics.

Multi-compartment models may be necessary to fully
characterize the observed pharmacokinetic behavior of a drug;

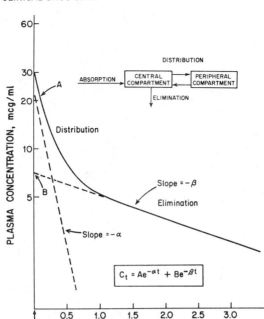

Figure 2. Plasma concentration-time decline after intravenous administration for a drug best characterized by a two-compartment model.

however, the increased complexity of these models may reduce their clinical usefulness. Simpler models, that describe drug disposition in a less complex, but adequate fashion, may prove more useful. For example, while the disposition of gentamicin is more accurately characterized by a two-compartment model,[9] the use of a one-compartment model to predict plasma concentrations and individualize dosing regimens for gentamicin has proven successful clinically.[10]

A more realistic approach to pharmacokinetic modeling is the use of physiologic models to describe drug disposition in the body.[11,12] All pharmacokinetic parameters in such a model are defined in terms of physiologic parameters such as tissue and organ perfusion, plasma protein binding and the intrinsic capacity of the eliminating organs to remove drug from the body. Because of its physiologic relevance, this approach may be more helpful than compartment modeling in explaining the effects of changes in body hemodynamics on drug disposition.

Drug Absorption and Bioavailability. Bioavailability (F) can be defined as the extent to which a drug is absorbed from a particular formulation and reaches the systemic circulation. For routes of administration other than intravenous, the bioavailability of a drug may be less than 100% (F< 1) due to incomplete absorption or metabolism that occurs before the drug can reach the systemic circulation. Therefore, it is important to briefly review some of the factors involved in these processes and how they may affect bioavailability.

In order for a drug to be absorbed from the gastrointestinal (GI) tract or an injection site, it must be in solution. This process of dissolution is most often of concern when dealing with compressed oral dosage forms such as tablets and capsules. After administration, these dosage forms must first undergo disintegration before the drug can dissolve sufficiently to be absorbed. Disintegrating agents (eg, starch, methylcellulose) are used in these formulations to promote swelling and break-up into smaller granules which eventually reduce to fine particles. As the size of these particles decrease, the surface area of drug exposed to GI fluids increases, thus enhancing drug dissolution. The water solubility of drugs also plays an important role in dissolution. It is difficult for a drug with a very low water solubility to dissolve and remain in solution long enough to have significant absorption. This problem can often be overcome by administering these drugs as a more soluble salt form instead of the free acid or base.

Disintegration does not ensure dissolution nor does dissolution guarantee absorption. The process of absorption is dependent on many factors including the extent of surface area available for absorption, existence of a drug concentration gradient, adequate blood flow to and from the absorption site and the physicochemical properties of a drug (eg, lipid solubility and degree of ionization).[1,4] The more lipid soluble a drug, the faster it will be absorbed. For drugs that are weak acids or bases, an increase in the proportion of unionized drug usually increases their ability to cross lipid membranes. Thus, weakly acidic drugs should be more rapidly absorbed in the stomach due to low pH of gastric fluids. However, the absorption of these compounds is actually much faster and more complete in the more basic environment of the small intestine. This is explained by the greater blood flow to the intestines and the tremendous increase in surface area available compared to the stomach. It should be evident that the rate of gastric emptying also influences the rate of drug absorption. The presence of food in the stomach may delay gastric emptying, thereby decreasing the rate of absorption for most drugs.[13] Other conditions that may affect GI drug absorption include malabsorption (due to disease or surgical resection of the intestine), faster GI transit time (due to diarrhea) and chemical reactions in the GI tract such as drug complexation and acid hydrolysis.

When drugs are administered by parenteral or sublingual routes, they directly enter the systemic circulation before significant metabolism can occur. After oral administration, drugs are absorbed from the GI tract, enter the portal circulation and pass through the liver before reaching the systemic circulation. Some drugs (eg, propranolol, nitroglycerin, lidocaine, methyltestosterone) may undergo extensive metabolism either in the wall of the GI tract during absorption or during this initial exposure to the liver immediately after absorption. This "first-pass effect" may considerably reduce the effectiveness of the oral route of administration for these drugs by limiting the amount of unchanged drug reaching the site of action, even if actual absorption of the compound is complete.[7,14]

Bioavailability can be expressed in two ways that have different clinical applications. Absolute bioavailability is measured by comparing the area under the plasma concentration versus time curves (AUC), or the cumulative amount of unchanged drug eventually excreted in the urine after a single oral (or other route of administration) dose and an IV dose of a drug. The bioavailability for the drug product in question can then be calculated by considering the IV dose to be completely available ($F = 1$). If the IV product is a salt of the drug, the F value must be adjusted to reflect the actual amount of drug in the preparation. Absolute bioavailability can also be determined upon multiple dosing by comparison of the AUC or the amount of drug excreted during a dosing interval under steady-state conditions. These estimates of bioavailability may be helpful in determining what dosage adjustment would be required for a patient being switched from IV to the oral route of administration or vice versa.

Relative bioavailability is determined when the intravenous route is not used for comparison either by design or because an IV dosage form is not available. The most common application of this type of bioavailability determination is the comparison of a new oral dosage form of a generic drug to a similar oral product of established efficacy (usually the original product on the market). This type of bioavailability study may also be referred to as a "bioequivalency" study.[15] When evaluating bioequivalency studies, three characteristics of the plasma concentration versus time curve for each of the two products should be examined (Figure 3). Comparison of the *peak concentration* (C_{max}) and time required to achieve this peak (t_{max}) provides an estimate of the rate of absorption of each product. Generally, the faster the rate of absorption, the greater the peak concentration that is attained. At t_{max}, the rate of absorption is equal to the rate of elimination. Absorption continues past t_{max}, but at a rate exceeded by the rate of elimination. Comparison of the *rate of absorption* is important for drugs with a narrow therapeutic index where very rapid absorption may increase the likelihood of toxicity occurring after administration or for drugs that require rapid achievement of a certain peak concentration to produce the desired therapeutic effect. Measurement of the AUC provides an estimate of the total amount of drug absorbed for each product. Determination of this *extent of absorption* is usually more important than the rate of absorption when evaluating the bioequivalence of two products. Proper interpretation of study data is essential to ensure the selection of a generic product that is bioequivalent as well as chemically equivalent to an established product. It should be remembered that when bioequivalency studies are conducted in normal healthy volunteers rather than patients, their results may not always be extrapolated to the clinical setting. The reader is referred to other more detailed discussions of the principles of bioavailability testing[7,8,16] and lists of drugs that may experience bioavailability problems.[15,17]

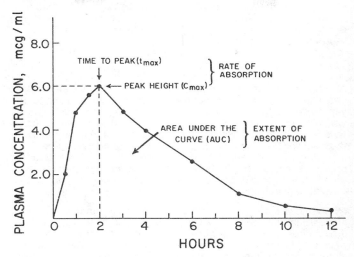

Figure 3. The most important characteristics of the plasma concentration-time curve for determining bioequivalence after oral administration of a drug.

Drug Distribution. The apparent volume of distribution (V_d) is a proportionality constant that correlates the plasma concentration of a drug at a given time (C) to the total amount of drug in the body at the same time (A) as follows:

$$V_d = \frac{A}{C} \qquad (1)$$

This relationship can reasonably predict the dose of a drug required to achieve a desired plasma concentration. The magnitude of V_d for any drug is determined by the extent of tissue and plasma protein binding and the lipid versus water solubility of the drug. Drugs that are more water soluble, extensively bound to plasma proteins or demonstrate little tissue binding may have a V_d as small as the plasma volume (approximately 3 L). A larger V_d (up to several thousand liters) may be observed with drugs (eg, tricyclic antidepressants) that are very lipid soluble or exhibit a large amount of tissue binding. The fact that V_d only represents an *apparent* volume allows for the existence of such large values for many drugs. Even if the value of V_d approximates the volume of an actual body space such as plasma volume, it should not be assumed that distribution of the drug is restricted solely to that space. Great intra- and inter-patient variability in V_d can occur as a result of changes or differences in factors such as age, body weight and surface area, obesity, renal function, metabolic activity, cardiac output and protein binding.

There are several methods for calculating V_d. Due to its simplicity, a common method for estimating V_d in clinical practice is to obtain the difference between the peak concentration (C_{max}) and trough concentration (C_{min}) after multiple administrations of a drug dose (D), such that:[18]

$$V_d = \frac{FD}{C_{max} - C_{min}} \qquad (2)$$

Another method involves extrapolation of the terminal elimination phase of the plasma concentration decline curve back to the y-intercept to obtain the concentration (C_0) that theoretically would have existed if absorption and distribution were instantaneous (Figure 1).[19] Dividing C_0 into the dose administered (D) as in equation (1) would then give V_d. Either method usually provides a usable approximation of V_d for use in dosage calculations, unless absorption is greatly delayed. Other reviews provide more detailed discussions of methods for determining V_d and factors that influence V_d.[20,21]

Protein Binding. The effects of protein binding on drug disposition have been reviewed extensively.[22-26] Acidic drugs are bound largely to albumin while basic drugs are bound primarily to α_1-acid glycoprotein, lipoproteins and also to some degree, albumin. Most often when laboratories report a plasma drug concentration, it is a total concentration (including both bound and unbound drug). The drug bound to proteins is unavailable to the site of action and considered pharmacologically inactive. The unbound (free) drug is considered the active form of the drug, because it has unrestricted access to the site of action. Clinically significant problems with protein binding alterations occur with drugs that have a small V_d, a narrow therapeutic index and are greater than 90% bound to albumin. One of the most common and potentially dangerous problems is partial displacement from albumin binding sites of one highly albumin-bound drug by another. This interaction results in a transient increase in the pharmacologic activity of the displaced drug due to an increase in circulating free drug.[23] With this increase in free drug plasma concentration, more drug is available for distribution, metabolism and elimination, thereby eventually returning the free drug plasma concentration and pharmacologic effect to their previous levels. The free concentration now constitutes an increased percentage (increased free fraction) of the total drug plasma concentration, which is now lower than before displacement. This protein binding interaction is of most importance when a displacing drug is started in a patient already receiving chronic therapy with a highly albumin-bound drug. However, it is also important to note that the displacing agent need not be a drug, but can also be an endogenous compound. Increases in plasma free fatty acids (due to bacterial infection, hyperthyroidism, renal failure, fasting, etc) can cause displacement of highly albumin bound drugs with similar results.

Conditions that result in decreased albumin concentrations due to altered production or excretion (eg, liver disease, nephrotic syndrome) and/or albumin binding capacity (renal disease) also alter the dose-response curve of drugs that are highly albumin-bound. This occurs because of a decrease in the fraction of total plasma drug concentration bound to albumin, increasing the free fraction. Some drugs (eg, lidocaine, valproic acid) demonstrate concentration-dependent protein binding. As the total plasma concentration of these drugs increases, proportionately less drug is bound to plasma proteins. This results in a curvilinear dose-plasma concentration relationship in which the increase in total plasma drug concentration is less than expected from an increase in dose.

Increased concentrations of α_1-acid glycoprotein (due to acute physiologic stress as in myocardial infarction or surgery) and lipoproteins (due to primary or secondary causes of hyperlipoproteinemia) may increase the protein binding of basic drugs, potentially decreasing their therapeutic effectiveness.[27]

Drug Elimination. The two most important eliminating organs for most drugs are the kidneys and the liver. Prediction of creatinine clearance from serum creatinine provides a reasonable estimation of renal function and some indication of the ability of the kidney to eliminate drugs (see the following section Dosing in Renal Impairment).[28,29] No liver function test consistently provides an accurate indication of the metabolic ability of the liver; therefore, the effect of impaired liver function on the metabolism of different drugs is often difficult or impossible to predict. The effects of renal, hepatic, and other disease states on drug pharmacokinetics have been reviewed extensively.[12,25,30-34]

The elimination half-life ($t_{1/2}$) is the time required for the plasma drug concentration to decrease by one-half (Figure 1). The apparent first-order elimination rate constant (k) is a proportionality constant that relates the rate of elimination to A as follows:

$$\frac{dA}{dt} = -kA \qquad (3)$$

and represents the fraction of drug removed from plasma per unit time. The relationship between k and $t_{1/2}$ is:

$$k = \frac{0.693}{t_{1/2}} \qquad (4)$$

The decline of the plasma drug concentration during the elimination phase when using logarithms to the base 10 can be described by:

$$\log C_t = \log C_o - \frac{kt}{2.3} \qquad (5)$$

or

$$C_t = C_o e^{-kt} \qquad (6)$$

where, C_o = drug concentration at time 0

C_t = drug concentration at time t

e^{-kt} = fraction of dose remaining at time t (e is the base of the natural logarithm)

The $t_{1/2}$ and k are often inappropriate expressions of the elimination characteristics of a drug, because they only describe the rate of removal of drug from the plasma and not necessarily from the body. Therefore, the half-life of a drug may reflect the rate of drug distribution into body tissues from plasma as well as elimination from the body. The pharmacokinetic parameter, clearance (Cl), defined as the volume of body fluid (eg, plasma) totally cleared of drug per unit time, is a physiologically more appropriate term than half-life to describe drug elimination from the body.[35] It is a measure of the ability of the eliminating organs (eg, liver, kidneys) to remove drug from the body and is not influenced by drug distribution outside of these organs; this is expressed as:

$$Cl = \frac{\text{Rate of drug removal from body}}{\text{Concentration}} \quad (7)$$

Based on this relationship and equations (1) and (3), Cl can be described in a simple, but clinically useful form:

$$Cl = k\,V_d \quad (8)$$

for those drugs adequately described by a one-compartment model. It is inappropriate to consider that Cl is dependent on k and V_d simply because of equation (8). Rather, the values for k and $t_{1/2}$ are dependent on Cl and V_d. The V_d or Cl may change independent of one another resulting in a change in k and $t_{1/2}$. A drug may have a long $t_{1/2}$, because either it has a large V_d or it is slowly removed from the body by the eliminating organs, or both. Clearance can also be calculated experimentally by:

$$Cl = \frac{\text{Dose}}{\text{AUC}} \quad (9)$$

using AUC after a single dose or AUC of a dosing interval (τ) during multiple dosing.

Clearance values most often cited in the literature refer to the total body clearance (Cl_t) of a drug. Total body clearance is the sum of all clearance processes in the body and thus, the entire body is considered to be a single drug elimination system. Since the kidneys and liver are the major eliminating organs for most drugs, then:

$$Cl_t = Cl_r + Cl_m \quad (10)$$

where Cl_r is the renal clearance and Cl_m is the metabolic (hepatic) clearance. Renal drug excretion occurs by a combination of three distinct processes: filtration, active tubular secretion and tubular reabsorption. The plasma drug concentration, degree of plasma protein binding, urine flow rate and pH, and the overall functional state of the kidneys therefore influence renal clearance.

Hepatic clearance is influenced by blood flow to the liver, drug plasma protein binding and the intrinsic metabolic capacity of liver enzymes (intrinsic metabolic clearance, Cl_{int}).[36] Classifying drugs by hepatic extraction ratio (the fraction of drug removed from the blood in a single pass through the liver) helps predict which of these factors will be the primary determinant of Cl_m for a given drug. For drugs with high (greater than 70%) extraction ratios (eg, lidocaine, propranolol), the Cl_m is considered flow-limited and is directly related to changes in hepatic blood flow. Any condition that decreases blood flow to the liver would reduce Cl_m for these drugs. The Cl_m for drugs with low (less than 20%) extraction ratios (eg, theophylline, phenytoin) is capacity-limited and is more dependent on Cl_{int} of the drug than on hepatic blood flow. Alterations in protein binding or changes in the Cl_{int} due to enzyme induction or liver disease may more greatly affect the Cl_m for this latter group of drugs.[25]

The Cl_{int} is considered to be the actual clearance of a drug if the Cl_m were not limited by protein binding or hepatic blood flow.[36] For most drugs, this clearance is an apparent first-order (linear) process; therefore, any change in dose results in a proportional change in plasma drug concentration (ie, doubling the dose doubles the plasma concentration). However, if the drug metabolizing capacity of the hepatic enzymes is limited (saturable), the clearance may follow nonlinear pharmacokinetics. In this case, Cl_m would then proceed at a constant or fixed rate regardless of the dose administered. Therefore, larger doses of a drug are cleared from the body at a slower rate (and have a longer $t_{1/2}$) when compared to smaller doses. This results in a disproportionate increase in plasma drug concentration with increased doses and the decline in these plasma concentrations can no longer be predicted by equation (6). Phenytoin, salicylates and ethanol are drugs that exhibit significant dose-dependent elimination.

Accumulation with Repetitive Drug Administration. Upon repetitive dosing, the plasma drug concentration will gradually increase until a plateau or steady-state concentration (C_{ss}) is achieved, where the rate of drug administration equals the rate of elimination. The major determinants of the C_{ss} are the maintenance dose of a drug and the patient's clearance. Approximately 95% of the eventual C_{ss} is attained after administration of a fixed drug dose at a given rate for four times the drug's $t_{1/2}$. Equations (11)-(15) are valid only for drugs that obey linear pharmacokinetics and are adequately described by a one-compartment model. Appropriate dosing regimen equations for drugs that exhibit multi-compartment or nonlinear characteristics can be found elsewhere.[7,8]

If a drug is administered by a constant intravenous infusion, then the plasma drug concentration at steady-state is:

$$C_{ss} = \frac{R_o}{kV_d} = \frac{R_o}{Cl} \qquad (11)$$

where R_o is the amount of drug infused per unit time. Therefore, the steady-state concentration is directly proportional to the infusion rate.

If the drug is administered intermittently, the average plasma drug concentration at steady-state ($C_{ss\ av}$) is expressed as:

$$C_{ss\ av} = \frac{F\ D}{k\ V_d\ \tau} = \frac{F\ D}{Cl\ \tau} \tag{12}$$

where, τ = dosing interval

With intermittent drug administration, fluctuations in plasma drug concentrations around $C_{ss\ av}$ will occur throughout the dosing interval (Figure 4). The maximum ($C_{ss\ max}$) and minimum concentrations ($C_{ss\ min}$) during a dosing interval at steady-state are calculated by:

$$C_{ss\ max} = \frac{F\ D}{V_d\ (1 - e^{-k\tau})} \tag{13}$$

and

$$C_{ss\ min} = \frac{F\ D\ e^{-k\tau}}{V_d\ (1 - e^{-k\tau})} \tag{14}$$

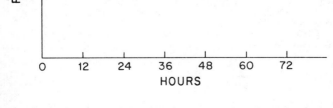

Figure 4. Fluctuations in plasma drug concentrations with intermittent administration of a drug with a $t_{1/2}$ = 7 hours.

The extent of these fluctuations can therefore be minimized by decreasing each dose and the dosing interval or reducing the rate of absorption. Adaptation of equations (12)-(14) for use after oral administration requires the inclusion of absorption rate constants and increases their complexity.[7,8]

In certain clinical situations, it may be necessary to quickly attain the plasma drug concentrations that will produce the desired therapeutic effect. This can be accomplished by the administration of a loading dose (LD):

$$LD = C_{ss} V_d \qquad (15)$$

While administration of this loading dose should produce the desired concentration, the condition of steady-state is not achieved because the rate of drug administration does not equal the rate of drug elimination. Maintenance of this desired plasma drug concentration requires the selection of an appropriate drug dose and rate of administration. The importance of the maintenance dose, rather than the loading dose, in determining the eventual C_{ss} is readily apparent in Figure 5, where the same loading and maintenance doses were administered to three patients with markedly different clearances. Several methods that rapidly predict the maintenance dose required to achieve and sustain a desired steady-state plasma concentration have been proposed for both continuous infusion[37,38] and intermittent drug administration.[39,40]

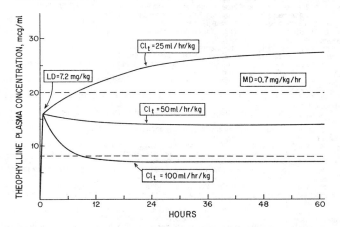

Figure 5. Resultant plasma theophylline concentrations after the administration of a loading dose (LD) = 7.2 mg/kg and a maintenance dose (MD) = 0.7 mg/kg/hr to three patients with differing total body clearances of theophylline.

Plasma Drug Concentrations. Plasma drug concentrations can improve the ability of the clinician to maximize efficacy and minimize the toxicity of certain drugs by allowing a more precise adjustment of dosing regimens through the calculation of individual patient pharmacokinetic parameters. However, poor correlation between plasma concentrations and therapeutic or toxic effects as well as the restricted availability of accurate assays, limits the clinical application of plasma concentrations for most drugs. Therefore, it is essential that one fully understand the pharmacologic and pharmacokinetic properties of each drug in order to determine whether obtaining plasma concentrations is justified, and if so, how to properly obtain and interpret these concentrations.

Individual drug monographs should be consulted for information that will be helpful in making these decisions. The following section discusses using plasma drug concentrations to determine pharmacokinetic parameters for dosing regimen adjustment in patients with altered drug distribution and/or elimination.

References

1. Gibaldi M. Biopharmaceutics and clinical pharmacokinetics. 2nd ed. Philadelphia: Lea and Febiger, 1977.
2. Benet LZ, Sheiner LB. Design and optimization of dosage regimens; pharmacokinetic data. In: Gilman AG, Goodman LS, Gilman A, eds. The pharmacological basis of therapeutics. 6th ed. New York: MacMillan, 1980:1675-737.
3. Winter ME. Basic clinical pharmacokinetics. San Francisco: Applied Therapeutics, 1980.
4. Rowland M, Tozer TN. Clinical pharmacokinetics: concepts and applications. Philadelphia: Lea and Febiger, 1980.
5. Greenblatt DJ, Koch-Weser J. Clinical pharmacokinetics. N Engl J Med 1975; 294:702-5, 964-70.
6. Atkinson AJ, Kushner W. Clinical pharmacokinetics. Ann Rev Pharmacol Toxicol 1979;19:105-27.
7. Gibaldi M, Perrier D. Pharmacokinetics. New York: Marcel Dekker, 1975.
8. Wagner JG. Fundamentals of clinical pharmacokinetics. Hamilton, IL: Drug Intelligence Publications, 1975.
9. Schentag JJ, Jusko WJ, Vance JW et al. Gentamicin disposition and tissue accumulation on multiple dosing. J Pharmacokinet Biopharm 1977;5:559-77.
10. Sawchuk RJ, Zaske DE. Pharmacokinetics of dosing regimens which utilize multiple intravenous infusions: gentamicin in burn patients. J Pharmacokinet Biopharm 1976;4:183-95.
11. Himmelstein KJ, Lutz RJ. A review of the applications of physiologically based pharmacokinetic modeling. J Pharmacokinet Biopharm 1979;7:127-45.
12. Williams RL, Benet LZ. Drug pharmacokinetics in cardiac and hepatic disease. Ann Rev Pharmacol Toxicol 1980;20:389-413.
13. Toothaker RD, Welling PG. The effect of food on drug bioavailability. Ann Rev Pharmacol Toxicol 1980;20:173-99.
14. Riegelman S, Rowland M. Effect of route of administration on drug disposition. J Pharmacokinet Biopharm 1973;1:419-34.
15. Chodos DJ, DiSanto AR. Basics of bioavailability and description of Upjohn single-dose study design. Kalamazoo, MI: The Upjohn Company, 1974.
16. Deasy PB, Timoney RF, eds. The quality control of medicines. Amsterdam: Elsevier Scientific, 1976.
17. Anon. Holders of approved new drug applications for drugs presenting actual or potential bioequivalence problems. (HEW Publication No. (FDA) 76-3009, June 1976, Revised).
18. Bonora MR, Guaglio R, Terzoni PA. Clinical pharmacokinetics: the pharmacological monitoring of plasmatic levels in therapy. Int J Clin Pharmacol Ther Toxicol 1980;18:73-87.
19. Chiou WL, Huang SM, Huang YC. Mid point back-extrapolation method for the rapid estimation of drugs' volume of distribution and dosage adjustment exhibiting multicompartmental characteristics. Int J Clin Pharmacol Ther Toxicol 1980;18:1-4.
20. Perrier D, Gibaldi M. Relationship between plasma or serum drug concentration and amount of drug in the body at steady state upon multiple dosing. J Pharmacokinet Biopharm 1973;1:17-22.
21. Klotz U. Pathophysiological and disease-induced changes in drug distribution volume: pharmacokinetic implications. Clin Pharmacokinet 1976;1:204-18.
22. Jusko WJ, Gretch M. Plasma and tissue protein binding of drugs in pharmacokinetics. Drug Metab Rev 1976;5:43-140.
23. Koch-Weser J, Sellers EM. Binding of drugs to serum albumin. N Engl J Med 1976;294:311-6, 526-31.
24. Gibaldi M. Drug distribution in renal failure. Am J Med 1977;62:471-4.
25. Blaschke TF. Protein binding and kinetics of drugs in liver diseases. Clin Pharmacokinet 1977;2:32-44.
26. Tillement JP, Lhoste F, Giudicelli JF. Diseases and drug protein binding. Clin Pharmacokinet 1978;3:144-54.
27. Piafsky KM. Disease-induced changes in the plasma binding of basic drugs. Clin Pharmacokinet 1980;5:246-62.
28. Kampmann J, Siersbaek-Nielsen K, Kristensen M et al. Rapid evaluation of creatinine clearance. Acta Med Scand 1974;196:517-20.

29. Cockcroft DW, Gault MH. Prediction of creatinine clearance from serum creatinine. Nephron 1976;16:31-41.

30. Pagliaro LA, Benet LZ. Critical compilation of terminal half-lives, percent excreted unchanged, and changes of half-life in renal and hepatic dysfunction for studies in humans with references. J Pharmacokinet Biopharm 1975;3:333-83.

31. Benowitz NL, Meister W. Pharmacokinetics in patients with cardiac failure. Clin Pharmacokinet 1976;1:389-405.

32. Fabre J, Balant L. Renal failure, drug pharmacokinetics and drug action. Clin Pharmacokinet 1976;1:99-120.

33. du Souich P, McLean AJ, Lalka D et al. Pulmonary disease and drug kinetics. Clin Pharmacokinet 1978;3:257-66.

34. Williams RL, Mamelok RD. Hepatic disease and drug pharmacokinetics. Clin Pharmacokinet 1980;5:528-47.

35. Rowland M, Benet LZ, Graham GG. Clearance concepts in pharmacokinetics. J Pharmacokinet Biopharm 1973;1:123-36.

36. Wilkinson GR, Shand DG. A physiological approach to hepatic drug clearance. Clin Pharmacol Ther 1975;18:377-90.

37. Wagner JG. A safe method for rapidly achieving plasma concentration plateaus. Clin Pharmacol Ther 1974;16:691-700.

38. Zimmerman JJ. Rapid attainment of successively higher steady-state plasma levels using the Wagner two-step infusion method. J Pharm Sci 1978;67:1651-6.

39. Ritschel WA, Erni W. Pharmacokinetic comparison of the one-point method with other methods in predicting steady state drug concentrations in multiple dosing. Int J Clin Pharmacol 1977;15:279-87.

40. Slattery JT, Gibaldi M, Koup JR. Prediction of maintenance dose required to attain a desired drug concentration at steady-state from a single determination of concentration after an initial dose. Clin Pharmacokinet 1980;5:377-85.

Dosing in Renal Impairment

Introduction. Epidemiologic evidence indicates that impaired renal function is a major risk factor in predisposing patients to drug toxicity.[1,2] The primary reason for this relationship is the dependence of many drugs on the kidney for their elimination, with the consequent potential for toxic drug accumulation in the presence of impaired renal function. Careful dosage adjustment can prevent much of this toxicity. Therefore, it is important that practitioners possess a basic understanding of the relationship between drug elimination and renal function, and that they have an ability to make appropriate drug dosage adjustments when managing patients with impaired renal function. This section presents general principles and guidelines which can be applied to drug dosage adjustment in specific patient situations. A general understanding of pharmacokinetic principles is requisite to this discussion—see the preceding section entitled General Principles.

Basic Relationships. The renal clearance (Cl_r) of most drugs closely parallels the glomerular filtration rate (GFR).[3] For drugs that depend solely on the kidneys for elimination, the relationship between drug clearance and measures of GFR, such as creatinine clearance (Cl_{cr}), should, in theory, be unity.[4] For drugs eliminated by nonrenal and renal mechanisms, Cl_r should be a product of the fraction of the systemically available dose which is excreted unchanged (f_e) and the Cl_{cr}:

$$Cl_r = f_e \times Cl_{cr} \tag{1}$$

The contribution of Cl_r to the total body clearance (Cl_t) of a drug is:

$$Cl_t = Cl_m + f_e \times Cl_{cr} \tag{2}$$

where Cl_m is the nonrenal metabolic clearance of the drug. The effect of a change in renal function, as reflected in a change in Cl_{cr}, on the Cl_t of a drug can be estimated from equation (2). In general, proper dosage adjustment in renal impairment should be to reduce the rate of drug administration in proportion to the decrease in Cl_t from normal. This would maintain the usual average plasma drug level, assuming that bioavailability and Cl_m are unchanged.

These basic concepts have been explored by many investigators in an attempt to develop guidelines for drug dosing in renal impairment. Work in this area has produced three basic approaches: (1) general drug nomograms, (2) drug-specific nomograms and (3) individualized pharmacokinetic analyses. The dosage modification schemes that have been derived from each of these approaches have distinct advantages and disadvantages which must be considered in applying them to specific patients.

General Nomograms. The simplest approach to dosage adjustment in renal impairment utilizes the basic relationship between drug elimination and renal function shown in equation (2). Tozer,[4,27] Dettli[5] and others[28] have used this relationship to develop methods which may be applied to drugs for which there is appropriate basic pharmacokinetic information. If f_e for a given drug and the fraction of normal renal function in a given patient are known, modification of the dosage regimen to produce normal plasma levels in renal impairment can be made using the nomogram and equations at the end of the section (Figure 1). The accuracy and usefulness of general nomograms is limited, however, because of the stringent assumptions upon which they are based.[24]

Drug-Specific Nomograms. In recent years, a growing number of drug-specific nomograms have become available. These nomograms are based on studies of the elimination of a particular drug in subjects with varying degrees of renal function. They attempt to describe the relationship between drug elimination in the study population and measures of renal function by means of a mathematical equation or graphical representation. For many drugs, a wide variety of dosage modification schemes have been proposed, and considerable debate exists with regard to their relative merits. Some of the differences can be attributed to methodologic variables and errors in study design and implementation; others are the result of limitations inherent in using nomograms for drug dosing. These factors, which should be considered when evaluating or applying dosing nomograms, are discussed below.

Methodologic Variables and Errors.
1. *Patients of varying age, sex, body build and underlying disease state are commonly used as subjects.* These variables produce wide fluctuations in drug elimination which are not necessarily due to changes in renal function. Also, some measures of renal function (especially Cr_s and BUN) are significantly affected by these nonrenal variables, and many studies using serum creatinine (Cr_s) or BUN do not note or attempt to compensate for this variability. The net result is that the predictive accuracy of these nomograms is greatly reduced.

2. *Some study populations are largely composed of people with essentially normal renal function.* Relationships derived from these populations predict most accurately in patients with near normal renal function. Application of such relationships should not, however, be overextended to patients with severely impaired renal function.

3. *Pharmacokinetic parameters may be determined unscientifically.* Frequently, methods used to determine parameters such as the elimination rate constant (k) or $t_{1/2}$ are not adequately documented (eg, time of obtaining blood samples relative to dosing) or are incorrect and inaccurate (eg, poor assay, improper timing of plasma level determinations, oversimplification of compartmental kinetics).

4. *Statistical evaluations of the significance of the results do not adequately reflect clinical implications.* Despite "significant" correlation between measured drug concentrations and those predicted by a nomogram, close examination of data (if available) frequently reveals some potentially serious discrepancies between the individual values and those which the nomogram would predict.

Limitations of Nomograms.

1. *They are only gross estimates.* Even with drugs that are nearly 100% renally eliminated by glomerular filtration (eg, gentamicin, vancomycin), the half-life in individuals with apparently identical renal function can still vary greatly. Also, some subgroups of patients (eg, burn patients) may vary greatly from the relationships found in the nomogram population.[6] Even with the most precise pharmacokinetic estimates, the expected relationship between renal function and drug elimination is not always adequate. Therefore, predictability is not good enough to prevent occasional important errors.

2. *The errors involved in using nomograms are cumulative.* The use of a nomogram for a day or two while waiting for specific plasma drug concentration results is not likely to cause complications, despite some expected errors in prediction. An estimated half-life of 48 hr for a drug which actually has a 60 hr half-life would ultimately result in a 20% overdosage. However, the full expression of this error would not occur for 10–12 days (4–5 half-lives). Errors involving drugs with shorter half-lives would become manifest much sooner.

3. *They should not be used in patients with variable renal function.* Nomograms based on Cr_s as the measure of renal function are especially susceptible to errors, because Cr_s continues to rise for many days following an acute, drastic decrease in renal function.[7] Frequent plasma drug level determinations are the safest guide to drug dosing in patients with variable renal function.[8]

4. *They cannot be used accurately in patients undergoing dialysis.* The dialysis of most drugs has not been studied extensively enough to predict the amount of drug which must be given to replace that removed by dialysis. With hemodialysis, the

amount of drug removed may vary greatly, depending on the particular dialysis apparatus and techniques used—see the following section entitled Dialysis of Drugs. Consequently, great care should be taken in interpreting published recommendations in this area.

5. *Dosage recommendations vary widely for the same drug.* Few prospective clinical evaluations of nomograms have been published (see references 9 and 10). However, theoretical interpretations have been conducted which demonstrate clinically important differences between nomogram dosage recommendations for some agents.[11,24]

6. *In some cases their dosage recommendations may not be suitable.* This is most likely to be the case when intermittently dosed drugs with narrow therapeutic indices (eg, gentamicin) are used in patients with severely impaired renal function. Nomograms which recommend dosage reductions by dosing interval extension only may result in dangerously prolonged periods of subtherapeutic plasma concentrations. Nomograms which recommend dosage reductions by individual dose reduction only may result in such minute peak plasma drug levels that optimal therapeutic concentrations may not be reached or maintained long enough.[11,24,27]

7. *Generally, there has been little or no development of nomograms for use in women or children.*

Compiled Dosing Guidelines. Several authors have developed extensive compilations of guidelines for dosing a wide variety of drugs in patients with renal impairment.[13,14] These recommendations are usually derived from drug-specific nomograms or other general data regarding the elimination of the particular drugs. Usually, the guidelines are presented in tabular form with the specific dosage adjustments classified by broad ranges of renal function. Because of the breadth of these categories, these guidelines may not be as accurate as the nomograms from which they are derived. Also, the data on which these guidelines are based should be examined to determine if they were collected in patients or subjects with physical characteristics similar to those of the patient in question.[24]

Developing Individual Pharmacokinetic Parameters. Specific pharmacokinetic parameters can be determined for individual patients using properly drawn blood samples, accurate and specific assay techniques and general pharmacokinetic principles. These parameters can then be used to calculate dosage adjustments. There are many methods by which this could be accomplished. A relatively simple method is suggested for intermittently administered drugs:

1. Give initial dose(s) as suggested by the best available data.

2. Following any dose, draw one sample at the estimated time of peak plasma concentration (C_{max}).

3. Draw a second sample immediately before the next dose (C_{min}) *(if not at steady-state,* a sample immediately *before* the previous

dose must be used as the C_{min} for the calculation of V_d). Note: if C_{min} is less than the lower limits of assay sensitivity, an alternative procedure must be used (see reference 12).

4. Calculate V_d from the equation:

$$V_d = \frac{F D}{C_{max} - C_{min}} \qquad (3)$$

where $C_{max} - C_{min}$ equals the change in plasma levels due to the dose administered, D and F, the fraction absorbed (bioavailability). If V_d is being calculated from the first dose, $C_{min} = 0$.

5. Calculate k from the equation:

$$k = \frac{\ln C_{max} - \ln C_{min}}{t} \qquad (4)$$

where, t = time interval between C_{max} and C_{min}

6. Select the desired maximum and minimum plasma drug concentrations. Select a reasonable dosing interval, τ. For instance, if the desired minimum plasma concentration is one-half of the maximum, then select an interval equal to $t_{1/2}$, as calculated from k. Calculate the new maintenance dose, D, from the following:

$$D = V_d (C_{max} - C_{min}) \qquad (5)$$

Note that these calculations are suitable only for rapidly and completely absorbed parenteral or oral drugs exhibiting first-order kinetics which can be described satisfactorily by a one-compartment model (or, at most, a short distribution phase), given rapidly relative to elimination. More complex kinetic models should be used when indicated (see reference 12).

Unified Approach. Based on the foregoing discussion, a unified, stepwise approach to the dosing of drugs in patients with impaired renal function can be synthesized.

STEP I. CONSIDER THE PATIENT

1. *To what extent is renal function impaired?* Accurately assessing renal function can be very difficult. Potential inaccuracies exist with all measures of renal function. An accurately timed and collected Cl_{cr} is probably the best available assessment of renal function. However, the use of nomograms can *approximate* Cl_{cr} from Cr_s. A nomogram to rapidly estimate the Cl_{cr} is presented in Chapter 3—"Nomogram for Evaluation of the Endogenous Creatinine Clearance." This, and other such nomograms, should be applied with careful consideration of their limitations.[24]

2. *Is renal function unstable?* Cr_s and Cl_{cr} determinations are not reliable indicators during drastic fluctuations in renal function.[7] In this case, plasma drug concentrations should be measured, if possible, to accurately guide dosing.

3. *Is the patient to be dialyzed? If so, by what method, for what duration and at what intervals?* (See the following section Dialysis of Drugs).

4. *Are there any other patient factors which may alter the absorption, distribution, elimination or response to the drug?* For exam-

ple, it is well known that the status of the cardiovascular system and liver may greatly alter the absorption, distribution or elimination of many drugs.[16-18] Also, patients with renal failure may be unusually sensitive to some agents.[19]

STEP II. CONSIDER THE DRUG

1. *Are specific and accurate dosing recommendations available?* If such recommendations are available and appear to be soundly developed (see *Methodologic Variables and Errors*), they should be used with due regard for their inherent limitations (see *Limitations of Nomograms*).

2. *If no such recommendations are available, what are the known relevant pharmacokinetic characteristics of the drug?*

   a. *To what extent is absorbed drug excreted unchanged in the urine (f_e)?* From this data and the patient's renal function, the nomogram (Figure 1) may be used to calculate an approximate adjustment. However, the points below must also be considered.

   b. *What is the therapeutic index of the drug?* Drugs which have a very low toxic potential or wide therapeutic index (eg, penicillin G) may require little or no dosage adjustment despite expected accumulation with impaired renal function. Conversely, drugs possessing a high potential for toxicity or a narrow therapeutic index (eg, gentamicin) must be adjusted carefully if they are largely excreted by the kidneys.

   c. *Are any active or toxic metabolites renally eliminated? If so, what are their therapeutic indices?* For most drugs this information is not available. However, for some drugs (eg, procainamide) this is an important consideration.[20]

   d. *What is the site of action of the drug? Does impaired renal function change the ability of the drug to reach this site?* As an example, methenamine salts and nitrofurantoin are therapeutically active only in the urinary tract. In the presence of moderate to severe renal impairment they do not achieve therapeutic levels at this site and are ineffective. Also, extrarenal toxicity may occur due to accumulation of such drugs in the body. Dosage adjustments may prevent the latter occurrence, but further decrease urinary tract levels. Consequently, these drugs are contraindicated in moderate to severe renal impairment.

   e. *If the patient is to undergo dialysis, to what extent is the drug removed by this procedure?* See previous comments under *Limitations of Nomograms* and the following section Dialysis of Drugs.

   f. *Does the elimination of the drug obey first order kinetics? Does absorption, distribution, protein binding and metabolism remain generally constant with changing renal function?* If these questions cannot be answered affirmatively, the Figure 1 dosing nomogram cannot be used with confidence, and other nomograms should be examined to determine if these kinetic parameters have been taken into account. There are many drugs which do not exhibit simple, first-order kinetic behavior and whose distribution and metabolism are altered in patients with renal function impairment (eg, phenytoin).[15,17,19,21] When using such drugs, plasma level determinations are the only safe guide to accurate dosing. Without plasma level determinations, such drugs can only be used with careful monitoring for signs of toxicity or subtherapeutic response.

STEP III. CONSIDER THE ADJUSTMENT

1. Consider the loading dose. For most agents, a change in loading dose is unnecessary in the presence of renal impairment. However, for some agents renal impairment may alter the apparent volume of distribution, requiring a change in the loading and maintenance dosages.[22] Also, some drugs with normally short half-lives, which are usually administered without a loading dose, may require a loading dose in the presence of severe renal impairment in order to quickly attain therapeutic levels (eg, carbenicillin). With carbenicillin, reduced elimination necessitates the use of smaller maintenance doses to avoid toxic drug accumulation; however, a loading dose equal to the usual therapeutic dose may be advisable to achieve more rapid therapeutic levels.[23]

2. Choose practical, convenient doses and administration schedules. Consider available dosage form sizes (especially with capsules) and usual administration schedules for drugs. Odd doses and schedules may lead to errors in administration and unnecessary inconvenience. Round-off adjustments within reasonable limits (eg, give 60 mg instead of 58 or 62 mg of gentamicin, every 24 hr instead of 23 or 25 hr).

3. Use available nomograms in a flexible way to suit the situation. For intermittently dosed drugs, the choice between decreasing the individual dose or increasing the dosing interval is largely a theoretical one. However, with severely impaired renal function it may be wise to use some combination of these adjustments to achieve the same decrease in administration rate (D / τ) without the potential risks involved in making either adjustment alone.[11] Thus, a nomogram which adjusts a dosage regimen by recommending a decrease in individual dose can be reinterpreted to increase the dosing interval, or to alter the combined administration rate, in order to achieve the same adjustment factor.

4. Measure plasma drug concentrations when indicated. Plasma level determinations are indicated when they are known to be reliable indicators of potential subtherapeutic or toxic effects and when:
   a. Patients have fluctuating renal function.
   b. Patients are to undergo dialysis.
   c. Suitable specific dosage nomograms are being used for extended periods, especially with more toxic agents.
   d. Suitable specific nomograms are not available and a general pharmacokinetic nomogram is being used (eg, Figure 1), especially for drugs having poorly characterized kinetics.
   e. The drug has nonlinear or unpredictable kinetics.

5. Above all, closely monitor the clinical status of the patient with

renal impairment. Even the best nomograms and pharmacokinetics calculations occasionally produce serious errors in
dosing, due to inherent limitations in predictability and changes
in patient status. Careful observation for signs of drug toxicity or
suboptimal response is imperative.

Summary. To use drugs safely in patients with impaired renal
function, the following approach should be considered:

1. Evaluate the patient carefully, characterizing renal function accurately and noting any other patient factors which may affect absorption, distribution, elimination or efficacy.

2. Choose the best available drug dosing guidelines and use them
within their known limitations.
   a. Carefully prepared drug-specific nomograms should be used
      as initial guides to dosing, if available.
   b. A general nomogram (eg, see Figure 1 and reference 5)
      should be used if a specific nomogram is not available and
      the drug in question meets the restrictions imposed on the
      use of such nomograms.

3. Plasma drug levels should be measured when indicated, to
guide dosing.

4. The patient should be closely monitored for any signs of toxicity or subtherapeutic response.

The references for this section follow on page 30.

Figure 1. Estimation of Dosage Regimens in Patients with Renal Function Impairment[a]

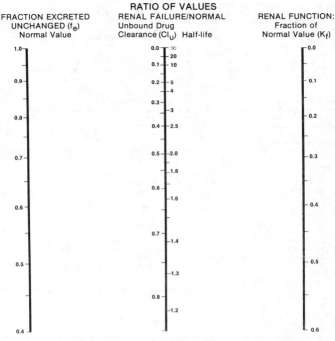

a. From Rowland M, Tozer TN. Clinical pharmacokinetics: concepts and applications. Philadelphia: Lea & Febiger, 1980, reproduced with permission. To be used to determine how to change a normal dosage regimen. The normal dosage regimen depends upon age, weight, and condition being treated. Activity and toxicity of metabolites are not taken into consideration.

How to use nomogram: *With a ruler, connect the fraction of drug normally excreted unchanged and the patient's kidney function, expressed as a fraction of normal value in a person of the same age. Read off from the center line the clearance of unbound drug (Cl$_u$) and the half-life relative to their normal values in a patient of the same age.*

Modification of Dosage Regimen

I. Initial dose–no change (see text)

II. Adjustment of rate of administration for maintenance of drug in body.

A. Change in dosing interval, τ, only

$$\tau \text{ (failure)} = \frac{t_{1/2} \text{ (failure)}}{t_{1/2} \text{ (normal)}} \times \tau \text{ (normal)}$$

B. Change in maintenance dose, D, only.

$$D \text{ (failure)} = \frac{Cl_u \text{ (failure)}}{Cl_u \text{ (normal)}} \times D \text{ (normal)}$$

C. Change in rate of administration D / τ

$$(D / \tau) \text{ (failure)} = \frac{Cl_u \text{ (failure)}}{Cl_u \text{ (normal)}} \times [(D / \tau) \text{ (normal)}]$$

References

1. Smith JW, Seidl LG, Cluff LE. Studies on the epidemiology of adverse drug reactions: V. clinical factors affecting susceptibility. Ann Intern Med 1966;65:629-40.

2. Jick H. Adverse drug effects in relation to renal function. Am J Med 1977;62:514-7.

3. Rowland M. Drug administration and regimens. In: Melmon KL, Morrelli HF, eds. Clinical pharmacology: basic principles in therapeutics. New York: Macmillan, 1978:25-70.

4. Tozer TN. Nomogram for modification of dosage regimens in patients with chronic renal function impairment. J Pharmacol Biopharm 1974;2:13-28.

5. Dettli L. Drug dosage in renal disease. Clin Pharmacokinet 1976;1:126-34.

6. Sawchuk RJ, Rector TS. Drug kinetics in burn patients. Clin Pharmacokinet 1980;5:548-56.

7. Chiou WL, Hsu FH. Pharmacokinetics of creatinine in man and its implications in the monitoring of renal function and in dosage regimen modifications in patients with renal insufficiency. J Clin Pharmacol 1975;15:427-34.

8. Koch-Weser J. Serum drug concentrations in clinical perspective. Ther Drug Monit 1981;3:3-16.

9. Michelson PA, Miller WA, Warner JF et al. Multiple dose pharmacokinetics of gentamicin in man: evaluation of the Jelliffe nomogram and the adjustment of dosage in patients with renal impairment. In: Benet LZ, ed. The effect of disease states on drug pharmacokinetics. Washington: APhA Academy of Pharmaceutical Sciences, 1976, 207-43.

10. Chow M, Deglin J, Harralson A et al. Prediction of gentamicin serum levels using a 1-compartment open linear pharmacokinetic model. Am J Hosp Pharm 1978;35:1078-81.

11. Schumacher GE. Pharmacokinetic analysis of gentamicin dosage regimens recommended for renal impairment. J Clin Pharmacol 1975;15:656-65.

12. Wagner JG. Fundamentals of clinical pharmacokinetics. Hamilton, IL: Drug Intelligence Publications, 1976.

13. Bennett WM, Muther RS, Parker RA et al. Drug therapy in renal failure: guidelines for adults (Parts I, II). Ann Intern Med 1980;93:62-89, 286-325.

14. Cheigh JS. Drug administration in renal failure. Am J Med 1977;62:555-63.

15. Bennett WM, Porter GA, Bagby SP et al. Drugs and renal disease. New York: Churchill Livingstone, 1978

16. Williams RL, Benet LZ. Drug pharmacokinetics in cardiac and hepatic disease. Annual Rev Pharmacol Toxicol 1980;20:389-413.

17. Piafsky KM. Disease-induced changes in the plasma binding of basic drugs. Clin Pharmacokinet 1980;5:246-62.

18. Williams RL, Mamelok RD. Hepatic disease and drug pharmacokinetics. Clin Pharmacokinet 1980;5:528-47.

19. Bennett WM. Drug prescribing in renal failure. Drugs 1979;17:111-23.

20. Drayer DE. Active drug metabolites and renal failure. Am J Med 1977;62:486-9.

21. Reidenberg MM, Drayer DE. Drug therapy in renal failure. Annual Rev Pharmacol Toxicol 1980;20:45-54.

22. Gibaldi M. Drug distribution in renal failure. Am J Med 1977;62:471-4.

23. Latos DL, Bryan CS, Stone WJ. Carbenicillin therapy in patients with normal and impaired renal function. Clin Pharmacol Ther 1975;17:692-700.

24. Chennavasin P, Brater DC. Nomograms for drug use in renal disease. Clin Pharmacokinet 1981;6:193-214.

25. Kampmann J, Siersbaek-Nielsen K, Kristensen M et al. Rapid evaluation of creatinine clearance. Acta Med Scand 1974;196:517-20.

26. Sarubbi FA, Hull JH. Amikacin serum concentrations: prediction of levels and dosage guidelines. Ann Intern Med 1978;89(Part 1):612-8.

27. Rowland M, Tozer TN. Clinical pharmacokinetics: concepts and applications. Philadelphia: Lea & Febiger, 1980.

28. Bryan CS, Stone WJ. Antimicrobial dosage in renal failure: a unifying nomogram. Clin Nephrol 1977;7:81-4.

Dialysis of Drugs

OVER THE PAST SEVERAL YEARS, dialysis has become an important therapeutic approach in the treatment of renal failure. It is estimated that approximately 50,000 patients with chronic renal failure are undergoing dialysis. This is primarily in the form of hemodialysis, although an increasing number are now receiving chronic peritoneal dialysis. It has been shown that patients on chronic dialysis receive an average of 8 drugs for a variety of medical indications.[1] Although the purpose of dialysis is to remove unwanted toxic waste products from the body, it also has the effect of removing drugs as well. Thus, it is important to know to what extent drugs administered for therapeutic purposes are removed, as it may affect the patient's therapy. Supplemental doses or a revised dosage regimen may be required under these circumstances. Dialysis procedures, including hemoperfusion, have also been used in the drug overdose situation as a means of eliminating drug from the body. It is, therefore, important to know how effective these procedures are and whether they offer any substantial advantage over conventional means of treating drug overdoses.

The purpose of this chapter is first, to review various factors involved in assessing the removal of drugs by dialysis and second, to illustrate how the use of pharmacokinetic information can help predict the extent of this removal. This information can be especially useful for drugs whose dialyzability has not been determined. Additionally, the table lists the effect of hemodialysis, peritoneal dialysis and hemoperfusion on the removal of specific drugs for which information is available.

Methodologic Problems. Several problems are encountered in attempting to assess the dialysis removal of drugs. The literature is generally anecdotal for many drugs. This is primarily true in the overdose setting in which the effect of dialysis on drug removal is determined by clinical response alone. For example, a comatose patient awakens during or shortly after dialysis and it is assumed that dialysis removed the drug, accounting for the improved clinical status. The amount of drug ingested and/or the amount of drug recovered in the dialysate are often unknown. The type of dialysis system employed is frequently not specified; this is of importance when comparing the system you are using with published data. Also, there is a general lack of patient data, such as weight, hematocrit, renal and liver function. The method used to calculate drug clearance is commonly unspecified. For example, was it determined from the amount of drug recovered in the dialysate or from differences in arterial and venous plasma concentrations across the dialyzer? A more detailed discussion of the proper method for clearance calculations in hemodialysis is described in reference 2.

A common error is misinterpretation of plasma drug concentrations obtained before and after dialysis. A declining plasma level during dialysis is often believed to be the result of the dialysis procedure. However, a declining level could be due to drug elimination by metabolism or renal excretion, and the contribution of dialysis to this decline may be very small. The situation in which drug concentrations are relatively unchanged during dialysis usually means that little or no drug is being removed by dialysis. However, it is possible that the drug is continually being absorbed from the GI tract, as in the delayed and prolonged absorption of drugs observed in overdose cases. Another problem is that of interpreting drug removal rate by dialysis. It has been assumed by some that if 200 mg of a drug were removed in the first hour of dialysis, that five hours of dialysis would remove five times as much (ie, 1000 mg). This is incorrect, because drug removal by dialysis occurs by a first-order process, so that as the amount of drug in the body declines, so does its removal rate. Thus, the total amount removed is less than that calculated from the initial estimates.

For many drugs, there is a lack of correlation between plasma drug concentrations and clinical response. Some drugs have been found to have active or toxic metabolites which correlate well with the toxic effects of the drug. For example, the toxicity of glutethimide is primarily due to an active metabolite, 4-hydroxy-2-ethyl-2-phenylglutarimide. Thus, in attempting to collect information on the dialysis removal of drugs, attention must be given to metabolites as well. A final point relative to the overdose situation is that the pharmacokinetic disposition of a drug may be altered. In making predictions of drug dialyzability, kinetic data are usually derived from healthy subjects. However, during an overdose there may be changes in drug metabolism, apparent volume of distribution (V_d) or protein binding. For example, with large amounts of drug in the body, saturation of plasma protein binding may occur, which could alter drug distribution and metabolism. The potential for these changes must be considered.

Pharmacokinetic Factors. There are certain properties of a drug which can be used to make some predictions about drug dialyzability.[3,4] Drugs with a small molecular weight, usually less than 500, cross dialysis membranes readily. Large molecular weight drugs, such as vancomycin (MW 1800) and amphotericin B (MW 960) cross membranes only with difficulty, and thus are not effectively removed by hemodialysis or peritoneal dialysis. However, molecular weight is not a limitation for hemoperfusion techniques where the drug is absorbed onto a high surface area material.

Drugs with greater water solubility are more easily removed to the aqueous dialysate than more lipid-soluble compounds. In addition, the latter usually have larger volumes of distribution compared to more water-soluble drugs. A large V_d, such as that of digoxin (approximately 500 L), impairs the ability of dialysis to remove a drug from the body. Because the majority of drug is contained in tissue compartments rather than in the blood, it is not accessible for removal. The effect of a large V_d limits the use of hemoperfusion as well.[5] Hemoperfusion may rapidly clear the blood compartment of a drug (evidenced by a dramatic decrease in plasma level); however, once hemoperfusion has ended, plasma drug concentrations can increase as a result of re-equilibration of drug from tissue stores.

Plasma protein binding of a drug also determines how effectively it can be dialyzed. Drugs with a high degree of protein binding, for example propranolol (90-94%) and warfarin (99%), are not significantly removed by dialysis, because the drug-protein complex is too large to cross the dialysis membrane. This is not a limitation of hemoperfusion, since the drug is removed from plasma proteins as the complex passes through the high surface area adsorbent material.[5]

The clearance of a drug by dialysis can be compared to the clearance of the drug by the body. Clearance terms are additive; therefore, the following equation applies:

$$Cl_{TD} = Cl_t + Cl_D$$

where, Cl_{TD} = total body clearance of drug during dialysis
$\quad\quad\quad Cl_t$ = total body clearance of drug
$\quad\quad\quad Cl_D$ = dialysis clearance of drug

Thus, if dialysis clearance adds substantially to body clearance, forming a much larger total clearance, then the drug will be eliminated that much faster. For example, if the dialysis clearance of a drug was 50 ml/min and the body clearance was 50 ml/min, then the drug would be eliminated from the body twice as fast during the dialysis period. In order to relate clearance to drug half-life ($t_{1/2}$), the following equations are useful:

$$t_{1/2} = \frac{0.693}{Cl_t} \times V_d \quad\quad \text{(off dialysis)}$$

and
$$t_{1/2} = \frac{0.693}{Cl_t + Cl_D} \times V_d \quad\quad \text{(on dialysis)}$$

Thus, the greater the dialysis clearance adds to the body's clearance, the shorter the drug $t_{1/2}$ will be on dialysis (assuming V_d remains constant). A further extension of this gives the following equation:

$$\text{Fraction Lost During a Dialysis Period} = 1 - e^{-(Cl_t + Cl_D)\,(\tau/V_d)}$$

where, τ = duration of the dialysis

This allows calculation of the fraction of drug in the body that is lost during a dialysis period by all routes of elimination (ie, dialysis, metabolism and renal excretion). Thus, it is necessary to acquire from literature sources (keeping in mind the limitations discussed previously) values for V_d, Cl_t and Cl_D. If renal or liver function are diminished, this must be taken into consideration. In addition, changes in V_d in certain disease states (eg, the decreased V_d of digoxin in renal failure) must also be taken into account.

Two examples illustrate the use of these equations. Phenobarbital has a volume of distribution of approximately 50 L, a body clearance of 5 ml/min and a hemodialysis clearance of 70 ml/min. The half-life off dialysis is 115 hours and would decrease to 8 hours with dialysis. Thus, approximately 50% of the drug would be removed from the body during 8 hours of dialysis. As another example, digoxin has a V_d of about 300 L and a Cl_t of 40 ml/min in an anephric patient. The hemodialysis clearance of digoxin is 20 ml/min. Therefore, the half-life of digoxin in this patient off dialysis is 86 hours, while on dialysis it declines to 58 hours. Although this appears to be a substantial decrease in half-life, it means that the patient would have to be dialyzed 58 hours continuously in order to remove half the digoxin in the body. The fraction of drug lost during a routine hemodialysis period of 4 hours would be only 5%. Thus, a supplemental dose of digoxin following hemodialysis is not warranted.

Use of the Table. The table which follows should be consulted for data on specific drugs. For each drug, a qualitative statement of the range of drug removal by dialysis was derived using pharmacokinetic parameters taken from the literature. The ranges used include: "not dialyzed, 0-5% removed;" "slightly dialyzed, 5-20% removed;" "moderately dialyzed, 20-50% removed;" or "dialyzed, 50-100% removed," which describes the extent of removal using the three techniques. Drug removal is intentionally described in a qualitative fashion for a number of reasons. First, much of this information changes quite rapidly (eg, as new dialysis and hemoperfusion techniques are developed). Secondly, a given value for the amount of drug removed or the dialysis clearance determined in one study may be different from that found in another study, due to differences in dialysate or blood flow during dialysis, or the length of the dialysis. The usual duration of dialysis has changed since earlier studies. Most hemodialysis runs are 4 to 5 hours as opposed to 6 hour runs used previously. Also, data on the amount of drug removed by peritoneal dialysis vary, since estimates of removal were determined from the literature in which both constant dialysis for long periods of time (such as in an overdose situation) or by intermittent dialysis for shorter periods each day were used. Data on hemoperfusion varies depending on such factors as the type of adsorbent material, blood flow through the adsorbent and duration of perfusion. This technique for drug removal is generally recommended and used after conservative management of drug overdose has failed. In addition, the table contains comments for clarification of certain points and selected references are provided for more specific information.

The following abbreviations are used in the table:

D — Dialyzed (50-100%)	ND — Not Dialyzed (0-5%)
HD — Hemodialysis	PD — Peritoneal Dialysis
MD — Moderately	SD — Slightly Dialyzed
Dialyzed (20-50%)	(5-20%)

Dialysis of Drugs

DRUG	HEMO-DIALYSIS	PERITONEAL DIALYSIS	HEMO-PERFUSION	COMMENTS	REFERENCES
Acetaminophen	MD	ND	MD	No studies demonstrate HD or hemoperfusion (charcoal) decrease or prevent hepatic or renal toxicity; PD ineffective in removing drug—one case reported	7-10,124
Acetazolamide	MD			Data from single case study	6
Allopurinol				No data available	
Amantadine	SD	SD			17,18
Amikacin	D	MD		Dialyzable to the same extent as other aminoglycosides; 50-70% of the loading dose may be given post-dialysis; plasma concentrations should be used as a guide to dosing	19-21
Amoxicillin	MD			Supplemental post-dialysis dose may be warranted—see reference 16	15,16
Amphotericin B	ND				11,12
Ampicillin	MD	ND		Supplemental post-dialysis dose may be warranted—see reference 13	9,13,14,22
Aspirin	D	D	D	Charcoal may be more effective than resin for hemoperfusion	5,23,24
Barbiturates:					
Pentobarbital	SD		SD-MD	Long-acting barbiturates are removed more than short-acting barbiturates; PD is considered much less effective in removing barbiturates than HD	5,23,25-29
Phenobarbital	MD-D	SD	D		
Carbamazepine				No data on the dialyzability of carbamazepine or its epoxide metabolite	29

Continued

Dialysis of Drugs

DRUG	HEMO-DIALYSIS	PERITONEAL DIALYSIS	HEMO-PERFUSION	COMMENTS	REFERENCES
Carbenicillin	MD				30-34
Cefaclor	MD			See Cefazolin	41,42
Cefamandole	MD			See Cefazolin	47-49
Cefazolin	MD	MD		Maintenance dose after dialysis may be necessary	35-40
Cephalothin	MD			See Cefazolin	46
Chloral Hydrate	D			Data are for the trichloroethanol active metabolite	50,51
Chloramphenicol	SD				52
Chlordiazepoxide	ND-SD			Active metabolites	23,29,53
Chlorpropamide		ND		Single case of PD did not decrease plasma chlorpropamide levels; high protein binding limits its dialyzability	54
Cimetidine	SD	SD		Supplemental doses after dialysis appear unnecessary; coincide doses around dialysis; PD studied in only 2 patients	55-62,129
Clindamycin	ND	ND			64-66
Clonidine	ND				63
Cloxacillin	ND				30
Colchicine	ND			Insufficient data	67
Diazepam	ND				29,68
Dicloxacillin	ND				29,69,70
Digoxin	ND	ND	ND		5,71,72

Continued

Dialysis of Drugs

DRUG	HEMO-DIALYSIS	PERITONEAL DIALYSIS	HEMO-PERFUSION	COMMENTS	REFERENCES
Diphenhydramine			ND	Hemoperfusion was not clinically effective in a case report of a diphenhydramine overdose	29,73
Doxycycline	ND				73
Erythromycin	SD				74
Ethambutol	SD				2
Ethchlorvynol	ND-SD	ND	SD-MD	Concentration-dependent kinetics	5,75,76, 122,123
Ethosuximide	MD-D			Hemodialysis potentially useful for overdosage	130
Flurazepam	ND				29,79
Furosemide				Insufficient data	
Gentamicin	D	MD		See Amikacin	78-81
Glutethimide	ND-SD		SD-MD	Insufficient information	5,82-85
Haloperidol				No data available; probably insignificant removal by dialysis	29
Heparin	ND	ND		No data available	121
Insulin	?				121
Kanamycin	D	MD		See Amikacin	19-21
Lidocaine	ND			Active metabolites with unknown dialysis characteristics	86,87
Lithium	D	D			88,89
Lorazepam	ND			See Diazepam	29,68
Meprobamate	MD	SD	SD	Insufficient information; few case reports with PD and hemoperfusion	90-92,125

Continued

Dialysis of Drugs

DRUG	HEMO-DIALYSIS	PERITONEAL DIALYSIS	HEMO-PERFUSION	COMMENTS	REFERENCES
Methaqualone	SD	SD	SD	Insufficient information	3,5,92
Methicillin	ND				30
Methyldopa	SD	SD		HD reported for 4 patients; PD reported for only 2 patients	93
Minoxidil				Insufficient data; probably not dialyzable	94
Moxalactam	D	SD		Give additional dose after HD	131-133
Nadolol	SD-MD				95
Nafcillin	ND				30,96
Oxacillin	ND				30
Oxazepam	ND			See Diazepam	29,68
Penicillin G	SD-MD			Insufficient data	30,97
Phenytoin	ND	ND	SD-MD		5,98-101
Prazosin	ND			Insufficient data; probably insignificantly dialyzed	102,103
Procainamide	MD				104-106
N-Acetylprocainamide (active metabolite of procainamide)	MD				104-106
Propoxyphene	ND	ND			107-110
Propranolol	ND				111,112
Quinidine	SD	SD			113,114
Reserpine				Insufficient information; probably not dialyzable	115

Continued

Dialysis of Drugs

DRUG	HEMO-DIALYSIS	PERITONEAL DIALYSIS	HEMO-PERFUSION	COMMENTS	REFERENCES
Sulfamethoxazole	SD-MD				29
Theophylline			D	Efficiently removed by hemoperfusion	5,126-128
Ticarcillin	MD			See Carbenicillin	30-34
Tobramycin	D	MD		See Amikacin	78-81
Tolbutamide	ND				121
Tricyclic Antidepressants				Insufficient data; probably not removed by hemoperfusion	5
Trimethoprim-Sulfamethoxazole	SD-MD				116
Vancomycin	ND	ND			117-119

References

1. Anderson RJ, Melikian DM, Gambertoglio JG et al. Current patterns of medication usage in the chronic dialysis unit. Kid Int (submitted 1982).

2. Lee CS, Marbury TC, Benet LZ. Clearance calculations in hemodialysis: application to blood, plasma, and dialysate measurements for ethambutol. J Pharmacokinet Biopharm 1980;8:69-81.

3. Takki S, Gambertoglio JG, Honda DH et al. Pharmacokinetic evaluation of hemodialysis in acute drug overdose. J Pharmacokinet Biopharm 1978;6:427-42.

4. Gibson TP, Nelson HA. Drug kinetics and artificial kidneys. Clin Pharmacokinet 1977;2:403-26.

5. Pond S, Rosenberg J, Benowitz NL et al. Pharmacokinetics of haemoperfusion for drug overdose. Clin Pharmacokinet 1979;4:329-54.

6. Vaziri ND, Saiki J, Barton CH et al. Hemodialyzability of acetazolamide. South Med J 1980;73:422-3.

7. Maclean D, Peters TJ, Brown RAG et al. Treatment of acute paracetamol poisoning. Lancet 1968;2:849-52.

8. Watanabe AS. Pharmacokinetic aspects of the dialysis of drugs. Drug Intell Clin Pharm 1977;11:407-16.

9. Winchester JF, Gelfand MC, Knepshield JH et al. Dialysis and hemoperfusion of poisons and drugs — update. Trans Am Soc Artif Intern Organs 1977;23:762-807.

10. Oie S. Lowenthal DT, Briggs WA et al. Effect of hemodialysis on kinetics of acetaminophen elimination by anephric patients. Clin Pharmacol Ther 1975;18:680-6.

11. Block ER, Bennett JE, Livoti LG et al. Flucytosine and amphotericin B: hemodialysis effects on the plasma concentration and clearance. Ann Intern Med 1974;80:613-7.

12. Bindschadler DD, Bennett JE. A pharmacologic guide to the clinical use of amphotericin B. J Infect Dis 1969;120:427-36.

13. Jusko WJ, Lewis GP, Schmitt GW. Ampicillin and hetacillin pharmacokinetics in normal and anephric subjects. Clin Pharmacol Ther 1972;14:90-9.

14. Kunin CM, Finkelberg Z. Oral cephalexin and ampicillin: antimicrobial activity, recovery in urine, and persistence in blood of uremic patients. Ann Intern Med 1970;72:349-56.

15. Oe PL, Simonian S, Verhoef J. Pharmacokinetics of the new penicillins. Chemotherapy 1973;19:279-88.

16. Francke EL, Appel GB, Neu HC. Kinetics of intravenous amoxicillin in patients on long-term dialysis. Clin Pharmacol Ther 1979;26:31-5.

17. Soung L-S, Ing TS, Daugirdas JT et al. Amantadine hydrochloride pharmacokinetics in hemodialysis patients. Ann Intern Med 1980;93 (part 1):46-9.

18. Ing TS, Mahurkar SD, Dunea G et al. Removal of amantadine hydrochloride by dialysis in patients with renal insufficiency. Can Med Assoc J 1976;115:515.

19. Madhavan T, Yaremchuk K, Levin N. Effect of renal failure and dialysis on the serum concentration of the aminoglycoside amikacin. Antimicrob Agents Chemother 1976;10:464-6.

20. Sarubbi FA, Hull JH. Amikacin serum concentrations: prediction of levels and dosage guidelines. Ann Intern Med 1978;89:612-8.

21. Regeur L, Colding H, Jensen H et al. Pharmacokinetics of amikacin during hemodialysis and peritoneal dialysis. Antimicrob Agents Chemother 1977;11:214-8.

22. Ruedy J. The effects of peritoneal dialysis on the physiological disposition of oxacillin, ampicillin and tetracycline in patients with renal disease. Can Med Assoc J 1966;94:257-61.

23. Schreiner GE, Teehan BP. Dialysis of poisons and drugs — annual review. Trans Am Soc Artif Intern Organs 1972;18:563.

24. Kallen RJ, Zaltzman S, Coe FL et al. Hemodialysis in children: technique, kinetic aspects related to varying body size, and application to salicylate intoxication, acute renal failure and some other disorders. Medicine 1966;45:1-45.

25. Bloomer HA, Maddock RK. An assessment of diuresis and dialysis for treating acute barbiturate poisoning. In: Matthew H, ed. Acute barbiturate poisoning. Amsterdam: Excerpta Medica, 1971:233-53.

26. Henderson LW, Merrill JP. Treatment of barbiturate intoxication. Ann Intern Med 1966;64:876-91.

27. Frank JT. Barbiturate intoxication. Drug Intell Clin Pharm 1973;7:309-16.

28. Hadden J, Johnson K, Smith S et al. Acute barbiturate intoxication. JAMA 1969;209:893-900.

29. Anderson RJ, Gambertoglio JG, Schrier RW, eds. Clinical use of drugs in renal failure. Springfield, IL: Charles C Thomas, 1976.

30. Barza M, Weinstein L. Pharmacokinetics of the penicillins in man. Clin Pharmacokinet 1976;1:297-308.

31. Hoffman TA, Cestero R, Bullock WE. Pharmacodynamics of carbenicillin in hepatic and renal failure. Ann Intern Med 1970;73:173-8.

32. Eastwood JB, Curtis JR. Carbenicillin administration in patients with severe renal failure. Br Med J 1968;1:486-7.

33. Hoffman TA, Cestero R, Bullock WE. Pharmacokinetics of carbenicillin in patients with hepatic and renal failure. J Infect Dis 1970;122 (Suppl):S75-7.

34. Latos DL, Bryan CS, Stone WJ. Carbenicillin therapy in patients with normal and impaired renal function. Clin Pharmacol Ther 1975;17:692-700.

35. Brogard JM, Pinget M, Brandt C et al. Pharmacokinetics of cefazolin in patients with renal failure; special reference to hemodialysis. J Clin Pharmacol 1977;17:225-30.

36. Craig CP, Rifkin SI. Pharmacokinetics and hemodialyzability of cefazolin in uremic patients. Clin Pharmacol Ther 1976;19:825-9.

37. McCloskey RV, Forland MF, Sweeney MJ et al. Hemodialysis of cefazolin. J Infect Dis 1973;128 (Suppl):S358-60.

38. Linquist JA, Siddiqui JY, Smith IM. Cephalexin in patients with renal disease. N Engl J Med 1970;283:720-3.

39. Kaye D, Younger N, Agarwal B. Pharmacology of intraperitoneal cefazolin in patients undergoing peritoneal dialysis. Antimicrob Agents Chemother 1978;14:318-21.

40. Levison ME, Levison SP, Ries K et al. Pharmacology of cefazolin in patients with normal and abnormal renal function. J Infect Dis 1973;128 (Suppl):S354-7.

41. Gartenberg G, Meyers BR, Hirschman SZ et al. Pharmacokinetics of cefaclor in patients with stable renal im-

pairment, and patients undergoing haemodialysis. J Antimicrob Chemother 1979;5:465-70.

42. Berman SJ, Boughton WH, Sugihara JG et al. Pharmacokinetics of cefaclor in patients with end stage renal disease and during hemodialysis. Antimicrob Agents Chemother 1978;14:281-3.

43. Kabins SA, Kelner B, Walton E et al. Cephalexin therapy as related to renal function. Am J Med Sci 1970;259:133-42.

44. Bailey RR, Gower PE, Dash CH. The effect of impairment of renal function and haemodialysis on serum and urine levels of cephalexin. Postgrad Med J 1970;46 (Suppl):60-4.

45. Reisberg BE, Mandelbaum JM. Cephalexin: absorption and excretion as related to renal function and hemodialysis. Infect Immun 1971;3:540-3

46. Venuto RC, Plaut ME. Cephalothin handling in patients undergoing hemodialysis. Antimicrob Agents Chemother 1970;10:50-2.

47. Gambertoglio JG, Aziz NS, Lin ET et al. Cefamandole kinetics in uremic patients undergoing hemodialysis. Clin Pharmacol Ther 1979;26:592-9.

48. Appel GB, Neu HC, Parry MF et al. Pharmacokinetics of cefamandole in the presence of renal failure and in patients undergoing hemodialysis. Antimicrob Agents Chemother 1976;10:623-5.

49. Campillo JA, Lanao JM, Dominguez-Gil A et al. Pharmacokinetics of cefamandole in patients undergoing hemodialysis. Int J Clin Pharmacol Biopharm 1979;17:416-20.

50. Stalker NE, Gambertoglio JG, Fukumitsu CJ et al. Acute massive chloral hydrate intoxication treated with hemodialysis: a clinical pharmacokinetic analysis. J Clin Pharmacol 1978;18:136-42.

51. Vaziri ND, Kumar KP, Mirahmadi K et al. Hemodialysis in treatment of acute chloral hydrate poisoning. South Med J 1977;70:377-8.

52. Slaughter RL, Cerra FB, Koup JR. Effect of hemodialysis on total body clearance of chloramphenicol. Am J Hosp Pharm 1980;37:1083-6.

53. Cruz IA, Cramer NC, Parrish AE. Hemodialysis in chlordiazepoxide toxicity. JAMA 1967;202:438-40.

54. Graw RG, Clarke PR. Chlorpropamide intoxication-treatment with peritoneal dialysis. Pediatrics 1970;45:106-9.

55. Vaziri ND, Ness RL, Barton CH. Peritoneal dialysis clearance of cimetidine. Am J Gastroenterol 1979;71:572-6.

56. Doherty CC, O'Connor FA, Buchanan KD et al. Cimetidine for duodenal ulceration in patients undergoing haemodialysis. Br Med J 1977;2:1506-8.

57. Jones RH, Lewin MR, Parsons V. Therapeutic effect of cimetidine in patients undergoing haemodialysis. Br Med J 1979;1:650-2.

58. Cutler RE, Blair AD. Abstract. In: Mackey BB, ed. 12th Annual Contractors' Conference of the Artificial Kidney Program, Bethesda, MD: National Institutes of Health, 1981. (NIH publication no. 81-1979):235.

59. Moran DM, Cersosimo RJ, Ziemniak J et al. Effect of hemodialysis on cimetidine pharmacokinetics. 2nd annual American College of Clinical Pharmacy Meeting 1981. Abstract.

60. Bjaeidager PAL, Jensen JB, Larsen N-E et al. Elimination of oral cimetidine in chronic renal failure and during haemodialysis. Br J Clin Pharmacol 1980;9:585-92.

61. Vaziri ND, Ness RL, Barton CH. Hemodialysis clearance of cimetidine. Arch Intern Med 1978;138:1685-6.

62. Personal Communication. Smith, Kline, and French Laboratories, March 27, 1979.

63. Hulter HN, Licht JH, Ilimicki LP et al. Clinical efficacy and pharmacokinetics of clonidine in hemodialysis and renal insufficiency. J Lab Clin Med 1979;94:223-31.

64. Eastwood JB, Gower PE. A study of the pharmacokinetics of clindamycin in normal subjects and patients with chronic renal failure. Postgrad Med J 1974;50:710-2.

65. Peddie BA, Dann E, Bailey RR. The effect of impairment of renal function and dialysis on the serum and urine levels of clindamycin. Austral NZ J Med 1975;5:198-202.

66. Malacoff RF, Finkelstein FO, Andriole VT. Effect of peritoneal dialysis on serum levels of tobramycin and clindamycin. Antimicrob Agents Chemother 1975;8:574-80.

67. Ellwood MG, Robb GH. Self-poisoning with colchicine. Postgrad Med J 1971;47:129-38.

68. Schreiner GE. Dialysis of poisons and drugs — annual review. Trans Am Soc Artif Intern Organs 1970;16:544.

69. Williams TW, Lawson SA, Brook MI et al. Effect of hemodialysis on dicloxacillin concentrations in plasma. Antimicrob Agents Chemother 1967;7:767-9.

70. McCloskey RV, Hayes CP. Plasma levels of dicloxacillin in oliguric patients and the effect of hemodialysis. Antimicrob Agents Chemother 1967;7:770-2.

71. Ackerman GL, Doherty JE, Flanigan WJ. Peritoneal dialysis and hemodialysis of tritiated digoxin. Ann Intern Med 1967;67:718-23.

72. Koup JR. Jusko WJ, Elwood CM et al. Digoxin pharmacokinetics: role of renal failure in dosage regimen design. Clin Pharmacol Ther 1975;18:9-21.

73. Whelton A, von Whittenau MS, Twomey TM et al. Doxycycline pharmacokinetics in the absence of renal function. Kidney Int 1974;5:365-71.

74. Vaziri ND, Cesario TC, Valenti J et al. Hemodialysis of erythromycin (letter). Drug Intell Clin Pharm 1980;14:549-51.

75. Tozer TN, Witt LD, Gee L et al. Evaluation of hemodialysis for ethchlorvynol overdose. Am J Hosp Pharm 1974;31:986-9.

76. Hedley-Whyte J, Laasberg LH. Ethchlorvynol poisoning: gas liquid chromatography in management. Anesthesia 1969;30:107-11.

77. Taclob L, Needle M. Drug-induced encephalopathy in patients on maintenance haemodialysis. Lancet 1976;2:704-5.

78. Christopher TG, Korn D, Blair AD et al. Gentamicin pharmacokinetics during hemodialysis. Kidney Int 1974;6:38-44.

79. Halpren BA, Axline SG, Coplon NS et al. Clearance of gentamicin during hemodialysis: comparison of four artificial kidneys. J Infect Dis 1976;133:627-36.

80. Jusko WJ, Baliah T, Kim KH et al. Pharmacokinetics of gentamicin during peritoneal dialysis in children. Kidney Int 1976;9:430-8.

81. Danish M, Schultz R, Jusko WJ. Pharmacokinetics of gentamicin and kanamycin during hemodialysis. Antimicrob Agents Chemother 1974;6:841-7.

82. Ozdemir AI, Tannenberg AM. Peritoneal and Hemodialysis for acute glutethimide overdosage. NY State J Med 1972;72:2076-9.

83. Chazan JA, Cohen JJ. Clinical spectrum of glutethimide intoxication: hemodialysis reevaluated. JAMA 1969;208:837-9.

84. King LRH, Decherd JF, Newton JL et al. A clinically efficient and economical lipid dialyzer. JAMA 1970;211:652-3.

85. Maher JF. Determinants of serum half-life of glutethimide in intoxicated patients. J Pharmacol Exp Ther 1970;174:450-5.

86. Collinsworth KA, Strong JM, Atkinson AJ et al. Pharmacokinetics and metabolism of lidocaine in patients with renal failure. Clin Pharmacol Ther 1975;18:59-64.

87. Thomson PD, Melmon KL, Richardson JA et al. Lidocaine pharmacokinetics in advanced heart failure, liver disease, and renal failure in humans. Ann Intern Med 1973;78:499-508.

88. Wilson HP, Donker AJM, Van Der Hem K et al. Peritoneal dialysis for lithium poisoning. Br Med J 1971;2:749-50.

89. Schou M, Amdisen A, Trap-Jensen J. Lithium poisoning. Am J Psychiatry 1968;4:520-6.

90. Maddock RK, Bloomer HA. Meprobamate overdosage: evaluation of its severity and methods of treatment. JAMA 1967;201:999-1003.

91. Castell DO, Sode J. Meprobamate intoxication treated with peritoneal dialysis. Illinois Med J 1976;131:298-9.

92. Proudfoot AT, Noble J, Nimmo J et al. Peritoneal dialysis and haemodialysis in methaqualone (Mandrax) poisoning. Scott Med J 1968;13:232-6.

93. Yeh BK, Dayton PG, Waters WC. Removal of alpha-methyldopa (Aldomet) in man by dialysis. Proc Soc Exp Biol Med 1970;135:840-3.

94. Limas CJ, Freis ED. Minoxidil in severe hypertension with renal failure. Am J Cardiol 1973;31:355-61.

95. Herrera J, Vukovich RA, Griffith DL. Elimination of nadolol by patients with renal impairment. Br J Clin Pharmacol 1979;7:2275-2315.

96. Rudnick M, Morrison G, Walker B et al. Renal failure, hemodialysis, and nafcillin kinetics. Clin Pharmacol Ther 1976;20:413-23.

97. Bryan CS, Stone WJ. "Comparably massive" penicillin G therapy in renal failure. Ann Intern Med 1975;82:189-95.

98. Adler DS, Martin E, Gambertoglio JG et al. Hemodialysis of phenytoin in a uremic patient. Clin Pharmacol Ther 1975;18:65-9.

99. Tenckhoff H, Sherrard DJ, Hickman RO et al. Acute diphenylhydantoin intoxication. Am J Dis Child 1968;116:422-5.

100. Martin E, Gambertoglio JG, Adler DS et al. Removal of phenytoin by hemodialysis in uremic patients. JAMA 1977;238:1750-3.

101. Rubinger D, Levy M, Roll D et al. Inefficiency of haemodialysis in acute phenytoin intoxication. Br J Clin Pharmacol 1979;7:405-7.

102. Hobbs DC, Twomey TM, Palmer RF. Pharmacokinetics of prazocin in man. J Clin Pharmacol 1978;18:402-6.

103. Curtis JR. Bateman FJA. Use of Prazocin in management of hypertension in patients with chronic renal failure and in renal transplant recipients. Br Med J 1975;4:432-4.

104. Atkinson AJ, Krumlovsky FA, Huang CM et al. Hemodialysis for severe procainamide toxicity: clinical and pharmacokinetic observations. Clin Pharmacol Ther 1976;20:585-92.

105. Gibson TP, Lowenthal DT, Nelson HA et al. Elimination of procainamide in end stage renal failure. Clin Pharmacol Ther 1975;17:321-9.

106. Gibson TP, Atkinson AJ, Matusik E et al. Kinetics of procainamide and N-acetyl procainamide in renal failure. Kidney Int 1977;12:422-9.

107. Gary NE, Maher JF, De Myttenaere MH et al. Acute propoxyphene hydrochloride intoxication. Arch Intern Med 1968;121:453-7.

108. Mauer SM, Paxson CL, von Hartizsch B et al. Hemodialysis in an infant with propoxyphene intoxication. Clin Pharmacol Ther 1974;17:88-92.

109. McCarthy WH, Keenan RL. Propoxyphene hydrochloride poisoning. JAMA 1964;187:164-5.

110. Karliner JS. Propoxyphene hydrochloride poisoning. JAMA 1967;199:152-5.

111. Lowenthal DT, Briggs WA, Gibson TP et al. Pharmacokinetics of oral propranolol in chronic renal disease. Clin Pharmacol Ther 1974;16:761-9.

112. Bianchetti G, Graziani G, Brancaccio D et al. Pharmacokinetics and effects of propranolol in terminal uraemic patients and in patients undergoing regular dialysis treatment. Clin Pharmacokinet 1976;1:373-84.

113. Woie L. Oyri A. Quinidine intoxication treated with hemodialysis. Acta Med Scand 1974;195:237-9.

114. Ueda CT, Hirschfeld DS, Scheinman MM et al. Disposition kinetics of quinidine. Clin Pharmacol Ther 1975;19:30-6.

115. Zsoter TT, Johnson GE, De Veber GA et al. Excretion and metabolism of reserpine in renal failure. Clin Pharmacol Ther 1973;14:325-30.

116. Craig WA, Kunin CM. Trimethoprim-Sulfamethoxazole: pharmacodynamic effects of urinary pH and impaired renal function. Ann Intern Med 1973;78:491-7.

117. Ayus JC, Eneas JF, Tong TG et al. Peritoneal clearance and total body elimination of vancomycin during chronic intermittent peritoneal dialysis. Clin Nephrol 1979;11:129-32.

118. Alexander MR. A review of vancomycin after 15 years of use. Drug Intell Clin Pharm 1974;8:520-4.

119. Lindholm DD, Murray JS. Persistence of vancomycin in the blood during renal failure and its treatment by hemodialysis. N Engl J Med 1966;274:1047-51.

120. Bennet WM, Muther RS, Parker RA et al. Drug therapy in renal failure: dosing guidelines for adults, part 1. Ann Intern Med 1980;93 (part 1):62-89.

121. Bennet WM, Muther RS, Parker RA et al. Drug therapy in renal failure: dosing guidelines for adults, part 11. Ann Intern Med 1980;93:286-325.

122. Benowitz N, Abolin C, Tozer T et al. Resin hemoperfusion in ethchlorvynol overdose. Clin Pharmacol Ther 1980;27:236-42.

123. Lynn RI, Honig CL, Jatlow PI et al. Resin hemoperfusion for treatment of ethchlorvynol overdose. Ann Intern Med 1979;91:549-53.

124. Rigby RJ, Thomson NM, Parkin GW et al. The treatment of paracetamol overdose with charcoal haemoperfusion and cysteamine. Med J Aust 1978;1:386-99.

125. Hoy WE, Rivero A, Marin MG et al. Resin hemoperfusion for treatment of a massive meprobamate overdose. Ann Intern Med 1980;93:455-6.

126. Russo ME. Management of theophylline intoxication with charcoal-column hemoperfusion. N Engl J Med 1979;300:24-6.

127. Ehlers SM, Zaske DE, Sawchuck RJ. Massive theophylline overdose: rapid elimination by charcoal hemoperfusion. JAMA 1978;240:474-5.

128. Lawyer C, Aitchison J, Sutton J et al. Treatment of theophylline neurotoxicity with resin hemoperfusion. Ann Intern Med 1978;88:516-7.

129. Hyneck ML, Murphy JF, Lipshultz DE. Cimetidine clearance during intermittent and chronic peritoneal dialysis. Am J Hosp Pharm 1981;38:1760-2.

130. Marbury TC, Lee C-s C,Perchalski RJ et al. Hemodialysis clearance of ethosuximide in patients with chronic renal disease. Am J Hosp Pharm 1981;38:1757-60.

131. Srinivasan S, Neu HC. Pharmacokinetics of moxalactam in patients with renal failure and during hemodialysis. Antimicrob Agents Chemother 1981;20:398-400.

132. Jacobson EJ, Zahrowski JJ, Nissenson AR. Moxalactam kinetics in hemodialysis. Clin Pharmacol Ther 1981;30:487-90.

133. Singlas E, Boutron HF, Merdjan H et al. Moxalactam kinetics during chronic ambulatory peritoneal dialysis. Clin Pharmacol Ther 1983;34:403-7.

3 BODY MEASUREMENTS

Creatinine Clearance Nomogram

Nomogram for Evaluation of the Endogenous Creatinine Clearance in Patients with Stable Renal Function.[a,b]

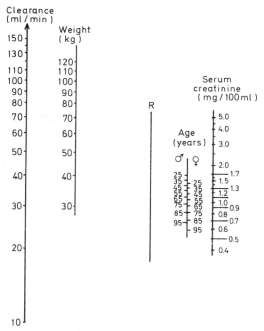

Use of the nomogram. Connect with a ruler the patient's weight on the second line from the left with the patient's age on the fourth line. Note the point of intersection on *R* and keep the ruler there. Turn the right part of the ruler to the appropriate serum creatinine value and the left side will indicate the clearance in ml/min.

a. From Kampmann J, Siersbaek-Nielsen K, Kristensen M et al. Rapid evaluation of creatinine clearance. Acta Med Scand 1974;196:517-20, reproduced with permission.
b. It has been found that the estimated creatinine clearance (by nomogram) more closely reflects the measured creatinine clearance in obese patients if these patients' weights are adjusted to the "lean body weight" before using the nomogram; see the formulas which follow.

Ideal Body Weight

Ideal Body Weight for Height

MALES

Height (cm)	Weight (kg)	Height (cm)	Weight (kg)	Height (cm)	Weight (kg)
145	51.9	159	59.9	173	68.7
146	52.4	160	60.5	174	69.4
147	52.9	161	61.1	175	70.1
148	53.5	162	61.7	176	70.8
149	54.0	163	62.3	177	71.6
150	54.5	164	62.9	178	72.4
151	55.0	165	63.5	179	73.3
152	55.6	166	64.0	180	74.2
153	56.1	167	64.6	181	75.0
154	56.6	168	65.2	182	75.8
155	57.2	169	65.9	183	76.5
156	57.9	170	66.6	184	77.3
157	58.6	171	67.3	185	78.1
158	59.3	172	68.0	186	78.9

FEMALES

Height (cm)	Weight (kg)	Height (cm)	Weight (kg)	Height (cm)	Weight (kg)
140	44.9	150	50.4	160	56.2
141	45.4	151	51.0	161	56.9
142	45.9	152	51.5	162	57.6
143	46.4	153	52.0	163	58.3
144	47.0	154	52.5	164	58.9
145	47.5	155	53.1	165	59.5
146	48.0	156	53.7	166	60.1
147	48.6	157	54.3	167	60.7
148	49.2	158	54.9	168	61.4
149	49.8	159	55.5	169	62.1

This table corrects the 1959 Metropolitan Standards to nude weight without shoe heels.Adapted from Jelliffe DB, The Assessment of the Nutritional Status of the Community, WHO, Geneva, 1966.

Lean Body Weight

Lean body weight (mass) is equal to total body weight minus the weight of body fat. The formulas below give the best estimate of lean body weight for drug dosing purposes.[1,2]

$$LBW \text{ (males)} = 1.10 \times weight - 128 \times (weight^2/height^2)$$
$$LBW \text{ (females)} = 1.07 \times weight - 148 \times (weight^2/height^2)$$

LBW = Lean body weight in kg
Weight = Total body weight in kg
Height = Height in cm

References

1. Hallynck TH, Soep HH, Thomis JA et al. Should clearance be normalised to body surface area or to lean body mass? Br J Clin Pharmacol 1981;11:523-6.
2. Hallynck TH, Soep HH, Thomis JA et al. Lean body mass and amikacin dosage. J Antimicrob Chemother 1980;6:286-8.

Surface Area Nomograms

Body Surface Area of Adults[a]

Nomogram for Determination of Body Surface Area from Height and Weight (Adults)

Height	Body surface area	Weight
cm 200 — 79 in	2.80 m²	kg 150 — 330 lb

A straight edge is placed from the patient's height in the left column to his weight in the right column and this intersect on the body surface area column indicates his body surface area.

a. From the formula of Du Bois and Du Bois, *Arch. intern. Med.*, **17,** 863 (1916):
$S = W^{0.425} \times H^{0.725} \times 71.84$, or $\log S = \log W \times 0.425 + \log H \times 0.725 + 1.8564$
(S = body surface in cm², W = weight in kg, H = height in cm)
Diem K, Lentner C, eds. Documenta Geigy scientific tables. 7th ed. Basle, Switzerland: Ciba-Geigy Ltd, 1970, reproduced with permission.

Body Surface Area of Children[a]

Nomogram for Determination of Body Surface Area from Height and Weight (Children)

Height	Body surface area	Weight

A straight edge is placed from the patient's height in the left column to his weight in the right column and this intersect on the body surface area column indicates his body surface area.

a. From the formula of Du Bois and Du Bois, *Arch. intern. Med.*, **17**, 863 (1916): $S = W^{0.425} \times H^{0.725} \times 71.84$, or $\log S = \log W \times 0.425 + \log H \times 0.725 + 1.8564$ ($S =$ body surface in cm^2, $W =$ weight in kg, $H =$ height in cm)

Diem K, Lentner C, eds. Documenta Geigy scientific tables. 7th ed. Basle, Switzerland: Ciba-Geigy Ltd, 1970, reproduced with permission.

4 *DIETARY CONSIDERATIONS*

**Potassium Content of Diet Supplements
Recommended Daily Dietary Allowances
Sodium Content of Selected Drugs
Sugar-Free Liquid Pharmaceuticals
Tyramine in Food and Beverages**

Potassium Content of Selected Foods and
Salt Substitutes[a,b]

BEVERAGES [8 fl ʒ]	MG	MEQ
Apple juice, canned	249	6.4
Apricot juice, nectar	372	9.5
Grape juice, canned	285	7.3
Grapefruit juice, canned	360	9.2
Milk, whole (high in sodium)	352	9.0
Milk, nonfat (high in sodium)	408	10.4
Orange juice, fresh or canned	496	12.7
Pineapple juice, canned	379	9.7
Prune juice, canned	563	14.4
Tangerine juice, canned	445	11.4
Tomato juice, canned (high in sodium)	544	13.9

FRUITS	MG	MEQ
Apricots, raw, 2-3 medium	281	7.2
Banana, raw, 1 medium	550	14.1
Cantaloupe, raw, ¼, 5-inch diameter	251	6.4
Dates, 10 medium	648	16.6
Figs, dried, 5 medium	640	16.4
Fruit cocktail, canned, 1 cup	330	8.4
Orange, raw, 1 medium	271	6.9
Peach, raw, 1 medium	202	5.2
Pear, raw, 1 medium	260	6.6
Prunes, dried, 5 large, raw	347	8.9
Raisins, dried, 2 tablespoonfuls	152	3.9
Strawberries, raw, 1 cup	246	6.3
Watermelon, 1 slice, 1½ X 6-inch diameter	600	15.3

VEGETABLES	MG	MEQ
Avocado, raw, ½ (California)	574	14.7
Avocado, raw, ½ (Florida)	924	23.6
Beans, green lima, cooked, ½ cup	338	8.6
Beans, red kidney, cooked, ½ cup	425	10.9
Broccoli, cooked, ⅔ cup	267	6.8

Continued

Potassium Content of Selected Foods and Salt Substitutes[a,b]

VEGETABLES	MG	MEQ
Brussels sprouts, cooked, ⅔ cup	273	7.0
Carrots, raw, 2 small	341	8.7
Mushrooms, raw, 4 large	414	10.6
Potato, baked, w/o skin, 2½-inch diam.	503	12.9
Spinach, cooked, ½ cup	291	7.4
Squash, winter, baked, ½ cup	461	11.8
Tomato, raw, 1 medium	366	9.4

SALT SUBSTITUTES	MG	MEQ
Adolph's, 1 packet	430	11.0
Co-Salt, 1 g	450	11.5
Diasal, 1 g	442	11.3
Lite-Salt, 1 g (high in sodium)	260	6.6
Neocurtasal, 1 g	470	12.1
Nu-Salt, 1 g	404	10.4
Salfree, 1 g	548	14.1

a. Food values adapted from Pennington JAT, Church HN. Food values of portions commonly used. 13th ed. Philadelphia: JB Lippincott, 1980, reproduced with permission.

b. Salt substitute values from Pearson RE, Fish KH. Potassium content of selected medicines, foods and salt substitutes. Hosp Pharm 1971;6:6-9, reproduced with permission. Product formulations are subject to change by manufacturer.

Recommended Daily Dietary Allowances,[a] Revised 1980[i]

| | Age | Weight | | Height | | Protein | MINERALS | | | | | |
	(years)	(kg)	(lb)	(cm)	(in)	(g)	Calcium (mg)	Phosphorus (mg)	Magnesium (mg)	Iron (mg)	Zinc (mg)	Iodine (mcg)
Infants	0.0–0.5	6	13	60	24	kg × 2.2	360	240	50	10	3	40
	0.5–1.0	9	20	71	28	kg × 2.0	540	360	70	15	5	50
Children	1–3	13	29	90	35	23	800	800	150	15	10	70
	4–6	20	44	112	44	30	800	800	200	10	10	90
	7–10	28	62	132	52	34	800	800	250	10	10	120
Males	11–14	45	99	157	62	45	1200	1200	350	18	15	150
	15–18	66	145	176	69	56	1200	1200	400	18	15	150
	19–22	70	154	177	70	56	800	800	350	10	15	150
	23–50	70	154	178	70	56	800	800	350	10	15	150
	51+	70	154	178	70	56	800	800	350	10	15	150
Females	11–14	46	101	157	62	46	1200	1200	300	18	15	150
	15–18	55	120	163	64	46	1200	1200	300	18	15	150
	19–22	55	120	163	64	44	800	800	300	18	15	150
	23–50	55	120	163	64	44	800	800	300	18	15	150
	51+	55	120	163	64	44	800	800	300	10	15	150
Pregnant						+30	+400	+400	+150	h	+5	+25
Lactating						+20	+400	+400	+150	h	+10	+50

Continued

Recommended Daily Dietary Allowances,[a] Revised 1980[i]

	Age (years)	FAT-SOLUBLE VITAMINS			WATER-SOLUBLE VITAMINS						
		Vitamin A (mcg RE)[b]	Vitamin D (mcg)[c]	Vitamin E (mg α-TE)[d]	Vitamin C (mg)	Thiamin (mg)	Riboflavin (mg)	Niacin (mg NE)[e]	Vitamin B-6 (mg)	Folacin[f] (mcg)	Vitamin B-12 (mcg)
Infants	0.0–0.5	420	10	3	35	0.3	0.4	6	0.3	30	0.5[g]
	0.5–1.0	400	10	4	35	0.5	0.6	8	0.6	45	1.5
Children	1–3	400	10	5	45	0.7	0.8	9	0.9	100	2.0
	4–6	500	10	6	45	0.9	1.0	11	1.3	200	2.5
	7–10	700	10	7	45	1.2	1.4	16	1.6	300	3.0
Males	11–14	1000	10	8	50	1.4	1.6	18	1.8	400	3.0
	15–18	1000	10	10	60	1.4	1.7	18	2.0	400	3.0
	19–22	1000	7.5	10	60	1.5	1.7	19	2.2	400	3.0
	23–50	1000	5	10	60	1.4	1.6	18	2.2	400	3.0
	51+	1000	5	10	60	1.2	1.4	16	2.2	400	3.0
Females	11–14	800	10	8	50	1.1	1.3	15	1.8	400	3.0
	15–18	800	10	8	60	1.1	1.3	14	2.0	400	3.0
	19–22	800	7.5	8	60	1.1	1.3	14	2.0	400	3.0
	23–50	800	5	8	60	1.0	1.2	13	2.0	400	3.0
	51+	800	5	8	60	1.0	1.2	13	2.0	400	3.0
Pregnant		+ 200	+ 5	+ 2	+ 20	+ 0.4	+ 0.3	+ 2	+ 0.6	+ 400	+ 1.0
Lactating		+ 400	+ 5	+ 3	+ 40	+ 0.5	+ 0.5	+ 5	+ 0.5	+ 100	+ 1.0

Continued

Footnotes to Recommended Daily Dietary Allowances,[a]
Revised 1980[i]

a. The allowances are intended to provide for individual variations among most normal persons as they live in the United States under usual environmental stresses. Diets should be based on a variety of common foods in order to provide other nutrients for which human requirements have been less well defined. See text for detailed discussion of allowances and of nutrients not tabulated. See Table 1 (p. 20) for weights and heights by individual year of age. See Table 3 (p. 23) for suggested average energy intakes. For the text and Tables referred to in these footnotes, see the text listed in footnote i.

b. Retinol equivalents. 1 retinol equivalent = 1 mcg retinol or 6 mcg β carotene. See text for calculation of vitamin A activity of diets as retinol equivalents.

c. As cholecalciferol. 10 mcg cholecalciferol = 400 IU of vitamin D.

d. α-tocopherol equivalents. 1 mg d-α tocopherol = 1 α-TE. See text for variation in allowances and calculation of vitamin E activity of the diet as α-tocopherol equivalents.

e. 1 NE (niacin equivalent) is equal to 1 mg of niacin or 60 mg of dietary tryptophan.

f. The folacin allowances refer to dietary sources as determined by *Lactobacillus casei* assay after treatment with enzymes (conjugases) to make polyglutamyl forms of the vitamin available to the test organism.

g. The recommended dietary allowance for vitamin B-12 in infants is based on average concentration of the vitamin in human milk. The allowances after weaning are based on energy intake (as recommended by the American Academy of Pediatrics) and consideration of other factors, such as intestinal absorption; see text.

h. The increased requirement during pregnancy cannot be met by the iron content of habitual American diets nor by the existing iron stores of many women; therefore the use of 30–60 mg of supplemental iron is recommended. Iron needs during lactation are not substantially different from those of nonpregnant women, but continued supplementation of the mother for 2–3 months after parturition is advisable in order to replenish stores depleted by pregnancy.

i. Food and Nutrition Board. Recommended dietary allowances. 9th ed. Washington, D.C.: National Academy of Sciences-National Research Council, 1980, reproduced with permission.

Sodium Content of Selected Drugs[a]

DRUGS (INJECTABLE FORMS UNLESS NOTED OTHERWISE)	MG	MEQ
Aminosalicylate Sodium, 1 g	108.7	4.7
Ampicillin Sodium, 1 g	66.7	2.9
Carbenicillin Disodium, 1 g	108.1 – 121.9[b]	4.7 – 5.3[b]
Cefazolin Sodium, 1 g	46.0 – 48.3	2.0 – 2.1
Cefotaxime Sodium, 1 g	50.5	2.2
Cephalothin Sodium, 1 g	63.2	2.8
Chloramphenicol Sodium Succinate, 1 g	51.8	2.3
Methicillin Sodium, 1 g	66.7	2.9
Mezlocillin Sodium, 1 g	42.6	1.85
Moxalactam Sodium, 1 g	88.0	3.8
Nafcillin Sodium, 1 g	66.7	2.9
Oxacillin Sodium, 1 g	64.4	2.8
Penicillin G Potassium, 1 million units	7.6	0.3
Penicillin G Sodium, 1 million units	46.0	2.0
Phenytoin Sodium, 1 g	88.0	3.8
Piperacillin Sodium, 1 g	42.6	1.85
Sodium Bicarbonate, 50 ml of 7.5%, 8.4%	1025.8, 1150.0	44.6, 50.0
Sodium Iodide, 1 g	156.0	6.8
Sodium Polystyrene Sulfonate, 1 g, oral	94.3[c]	4.1[c]
Thiopental Sodium, 1 g	86.8	3.8
Ticarcillin Disodium, 1 g	119.6[b]	5.2[b]

a. Product formulations, and hence sodium content are subject to change by manufacturer.
b. Sodium content per gram of free acid; actual vial content can be as high as 6.5 mEq per gram.
c. Total sodium content; however, only about 33% is liberated in clinical use.

Sugar-Free Liquid Pharmaceuticals[a,b]

ANALEPTICS
Cenalene, *Central*
Coramine, *Ciba*

ANALGESICS
Acetaminophen Elixir, *Beecham Labs, Lannett*
Covangesic, *Wallace*
Conex Liquid, *O'Neal, Jones & Feldman*
Conex c/Codeine Liquid, *O'Neal, Jones & Feldman*
Dolanex Elixir, *Lannett*
Elixir Aminodyne, *Bowman*
Paregoric USP, *Abbott*
SK-APAP Elixir, *SKF Labs*
Tylaprin Elixir, *Cenci*
Tylenol Drops, *McNeil*

ANTACIDS AND COMBINATIONS
Alternagel, *Stuart*
Alumihab Suspension, *Bowman*
Camalox Susp, *Rorer*
Creamalin, *Winthrop*
Delcid, *Merrell Dow*
Digestamic, *Metro Med*
Di-Gel Liquid (mint, lemon & orange flavored), *Plough*
Estomul-M Liquid, *Riker*
Gaviscon Liquid, *Marion*
Gelusil Liquid-Flavor Pack, *Warner-Chilcott*
Gelusil Liquid, *Warner-Chilcott*
Gelusil M Liquid, *Warner-Chilcott*
Kolantyl Gel, *Merrell Dow*
Maalox Susp, *Rorer*
Maalox Plus Susp, *Rorer*
Maalox Therapeutic Conc, *Rorer*
Magnatril Susp, *Lannett*
Magnesia and Alumina Oral Susp USP, *Abbott, Philips Roxane*
Malcogel, *Upjohn*
Milk of Bismuth, *Parke-Davis*
Milk of Magnesia USP, *Bowman*
Mylanta Liquid, *Stuart*
Mylanta II Liquid, *Stuart*
Nutragel, *Cenci*
Nutrameg, *Cenci*
Pepto-Bismol, *Norwich-Eaton*
Riopan Plus, *Ayerst*
Riopan Susp, *Ayerst*
Silain Gel Liquid, *Robins*
Titralac Liquid, *Riker*
Trisogel, *Lilly*
WinGel, *Winthrop*

ANTIASTHMATICS
Alevaire, *Breon*
Alupent Syrup, *Boehringer Ingelheim*
Bronkometer, *Breon*
Bronkosol, *Breon*
Elixir Adolphyllin, *Bowman*
Elixophyllin Elixir, *Cooper*
Elixicon Susp, *Cooper*
Ephed Organidin Elixir, *Wallace*
Isuprel Mistometer, *Breon*
Isuprel Solutions, *Breon*
Lanophyllin Elixir, *Lannett*
Lixaminol AT Elixir, *Ferndale*
Lixaminol Elixir, *Ferndale*
Lufyllin Elixir, *Wallace*
Mucomyst-10%, *Mead Johnson*
Mucomyst-20%, *Mead Johnson*
Metaprel Syrup, *Dorsey*
Mini-Lix Elixir, *Ferndale*
Mudrane GG Elixir, *Poythress*
Neothylline Elixir, *Lemmon*
Neothylline G, *Lemmon*
Organidin Soln, *Wallace*
Organaphen Elixir, *Wallace*
Somophyllin Oral Liquid, *Fisons*
Tedral Elixir, *Warner-Chilcott*
Theolixir, *Panray*
Theo-Organadin Elixir, *Wallace*
Theophyl-225 Elixir, *Knoll*
Theophylline Elixir, *Philips Roxane*

ANTICONVULSANTS
Mysolin Susp, *Ayerst*
Paradoine Solution, *Abbott*

ANTIDEPRESSANTS
Sinequan Oral Concentrate, *Pfizer*

ANTI-DIARRHEA AGENTS
Bismuth & Salol Comp c/Opium, *Zemmer*
Colonil Liquid, *Wallace*
Corrective Mixture, *Beecham Labs*
Corrective Mixture c/Paregoric, *Beecham Labs*
C-M c/Paregoric, *Beecham Labs*
Infantol Pink, *First Texas*
Infantol White, *First Texas*
Kao-Con, *Upjohn*
Kaolin Mixture c/Pectin NF, *Abbott*
Kaolin-Pectin Susp, *Philips Roxane*
Kaopectate, *Upjohn*
Kaopectate Concentrate, *Upjohn*
Ka-Thal-Pec Susp, *O'Neal, Jones & Feldman*

Continued

Sugar-Free Liquid Pharmaceuticals[a,b]

Konsyl Powder, *Burton-Barsons*
Lomotil Liquid, *Searle*
Opecto Elixir, *Bowman*
Paregoric, *Parke-Davis*
Paregoric USP, *Lannett, Philips Roxane*
Parepectolin, *Rorer*
Pecto-Kalin, *Lemmon*
Pectokay Mixture, *Bowman*
Pectokay Mixture c/Belladonna Alkaloids, *Bowman*
Pektamalt, *Warren-Teed*
Pepto-Bismol, *Norwich-Eaton*
Quintess, *Lilly*

ANTIFLATULENTS
Di-Gel Liquid (mint, lemon & orange flavored), *Plough*
Mylicon Drops, *Stuart*
Riopan-Plus, *Ayerst*

ANTIHISTAMINE-DECONGESTANTS
Ciramine, *Zemmer*
Covanamine, *Wallace*
Covangesic Liquid, *Wallace*
Dimetapp Elixir, *Robins*
Euphenex, *O'Neal, Jones & Feldman*
Euphenex c/Codeine, *O'Neal, Jones & Feldman*
Histatapp Elixir, *Upsher-Smith*
Isoclor Liquid, *Arnar-Stone*
Nasal Decongestant Elixir, *Bowman*
Phenergan Syrup, *Wyeth*
Phenergan Fortis Syrup, *Wyeth*
Ryna Liquid, *Wallace*
SK-Diphenhydramine, *SKF Labs*
Veltap Elixir, *Lannett*

ANTI-INFECTIVE AGENTS
Declomycin Syrup, *Lederle*
Furadantin Oral Susp, *Norwich-Eaton*
Furadantin Sodium Sterile, *Norwich-Eaton*
Furoxone Liquid, *Norwich-Eaton*
Mandelamine Susp/Forte, *Warner-Chilcott*
Minocin Syrup, *Lederle*
Mycifradin Sulfate Oral Solution, *Upjohn*
NegGram Susp, *Winthrop*
Nydrazid Syrup, *Squibb*
Proklar Susp, *O'Neal, Jones & Feldman*
Robitet Syrup, *Robins*
Rondomycin Syrup, *Wallace*
Sulfaloid Susp, *O'Neal, Jones & Feldman*
Terramycin Syrup, *Pfizer*
Tetracyn Syrup, *Pfipharmecs*
Vectrin Syrup, *Parke-Davis*
Vibramycin Syrup, *Pfizer*

ANTIPARKINSON AGENTS
Artane Elixir, *Lederle*

ANTISPASMODICS
Antrocol Elixir, *Poythress*
Pamine PB Drops, *Upjohn*
Spasmophen Elixir, *Lannett*

COUGH PREPARATIONS
Brown Mixture, *Bowman*
Brown Mixture, N.F., *Lannett*
Cerose, *Ives Labs*
Cerose DM, *Ives Labs*
Cetro-Cerose, *Ives Labs*
Cidicol, *Upjohn*
Clistin Expect, *McNeil*
Codimal DM, *Central*
Colrex Syrup, *Rowell*
Colrex Comp Elixir, *Rowell*
Colrex Expect, *Rowell*
Conar Liquid, *Beecham Labs*
Conex Liquid, *O'Neal, Jones & Feldman*
Coryban D Cough Syrup, *Pfipharmecs*
Guaiatrate, *Bowman*
Hycomine Syrup, *Endo*
Lanatuss, *Lannett*
Neo-Codenyl-M, *O'Neal, Jones & Feldman*
Neotuss, *O'Neal, Jones & Feldman*
Neotuss c/Codeine, *O'Neal, Jones & Feldman*
Nevicof, *Nevin*
Omni-Tuss, *Pennwalt*
Ornacol Liquid, *SKF Labs*
Potassium Iodide Liquid, *Philips Roxane*
Promex, *Lemmon*
Prunicodeine, *Lilly*
Queltuss, *O'Neal, Jones & Feldman*
Quiecof, *Nevin*
Quiecof-RX, *Nevin*
Robitussin-CF Liquid, *Robins*
Ryna-C, *Wallace*
Ryna-CX Liquid, *Wallace*
S-T Expectorant SF & D-F, *Scot-Tussin*
S-T Forte, Sugar-Free, *Scot-Tussin*
Scot-Tussin Sugar-Free, *Scot-Tussin*
Sorbutuss, *Dalin*
Syrup Bowtussin, *Bowman*
Toclonol Expect, *Cenci*
Toclonol Expect c/Codeine, *Cenci*
Tolu-Sed, *First Texas*
Tolu-Sed DM, *First Texas*
Tussar SF, *Armour*
Tussionex, *Pennwalt*
Tussi-Organidin Elixir, *Wallace*
Tussirex Sugar-Free, *Scot-Tussin*

Continued

Sugar-Free Liquid Pharmaceuticals[a,b]

Tuss-Ornade, *SKF Labs*

DENTAL PREPARATIONS
Astring-o-Sol, *Winthrop*
Ceetolan Concentrate Mouthwash,
    Lannett
Cepacol Mouthwash, *Merrell Dow*
Cepastat Mouthwash/Gargle, *Merrell Dow*
Chloraseptic Mouthwash & Gargle,
    Norwich-Eaton
Fluorigard Mouthrinse, *Colgate-Palmolive*
Luride Drops, *Hoyt*
Phos-Flur Rinse-Supplement, *Hoyt*
Point-Two Mouthrinse, *Hoyt*
PreviDent Disclosing Drops, *Hoyt*
Thera-Flur Gel-Drops, *Hoyt*

DIAGNOSTIC AGENTS
Gastrografin, *Squibb*

DIETARY SUBSTITUTES
Co-Salt, *Norcliff Thayer*
Ril-Sweet Concentrate, *Plough*
Ril-Sweet Sugar Concentrate, *Plough*
Sweeta Liquid, *Squibb*

IRON PREPARATIONS
Chel-Iron Drops, *Kinney*
Chel-Iron Liquid, *Kinney*
Ferrolip Syrup, *Flint*
Iberet Liquid, *Abbott*
Iberet-500 Liquid, *Abbott*
Niferex, *Central*
Toleron Susp, *Wallace*
Vita-Plus H Sugar-Free, *Scot-Tussin*
Vita-Plus H Half Strength Sugar-Free,
    Scot-Tussin

LAXATIVES
Agoral, *Warner-Chilcott*
Aromatic Cascara Fluidextract USP,
    *Abbott, Lannett, Parke-Davis, Philips
    Roxane*
Castor Oil (flavored), *Philips Roxane*
Castor Oil USP, *Lannett, Philips Roxane*
Castor Oil, *Squibb*
Colace, Liquid 1%, *Mead Johnson*
Cologel, *Lilly*
Doxinate Solution 5%, *Hoechst-Roussel*
Evac-Q-Mag, Magnesium Citrate Soln NF,
    Warren-Teed
Haley's MO, *Winthrop*
Hypaque oral powder (radiopaque), *Winthrop*

Kondremul, *Fisons*
Kondremul c/Cascara, *Fisons*
Kondremul c/Phenolphthalein, *Fisons*
Milkinol Liquid, *Kremers-Urban*
Milk of Magnesia, *Lilly, Parke-Davis, Squibb*
Milk of Magnesia-Cascara Susp, *Philips
    Roxane*
Milk of Magnesia-Mineral Oil Emulsion,
    Philips Roxane
Milk of Magnesia-Mineral Oil Emulsion
    (flavored), *Philips Roxane*
Milk of Magnesia USP, *Lannett, Philips
    Roxane*
Mineral Oil, *Squibb*
Mineral Oil USP, *Abbott, Philips Roxane*
Mint-O-Mag, *Squibb*
Neoloid, *Lederle*
Nujol Mineral Oil, *Plough*
Phospho-Soda, *Fleet*
Sodium Phosphate & Biphosphate Oral
    Solution USP, *Philips Roxane*

POTASSIUM PRODUCTS
Elixir Potassium Gluconate, *Bowman*
K-10 Solution, *Cenci*
Kaochlor S-F 10% Liquid, *Warren-Teed*
Kaochlor-Eff, *Warren-Teed*
Kaon-Cl 20% Liquid, *Warren-Teed*
Kaon Elixir grape and lemon-lime flavor,
    Warren-Teed
Kay Ciel Elixir, *Cooper*
Kay Ciel Powder, *Cooper*
Kaylixir, *Lannett*
Klor-Con Liquid 20%, *Upsher-Smith*
Klor-10% Liquid, *Upsher-Smith*
Klor-Con Powder, *Upsher-Smith*
Kloride Elixir, *Federal*
Klorvess Effervescent Tabs, *Dorsey*
Klorvess Granules, *Dorsey*
Kolyum Liquid, *Pennwalt*
Liquid Potassium Triplex, *Lilly*
Pan-Kloride Elixir, *Panray*
PfiKlor 10% Liquid, *Pfizer*
Potasalen Elixir, *Lannett*
Potassium Chloride 10% and 20%, *Cenci,
    Lederle*
Potassium Chloride Liquid 10%, *Abbott*
Potassium Chloride, 10% Solution, *Bowman*
Potassium Chloride Oral Solution USP
    5%, 10%, 20%, *Philips Roxane*
Potassium Chloride Powder, *Philips
    Roxane*
Potassium Gluconate, *Lederle*
Potassium Gluconate Elixir NF, *Philips
    Roxane*
Potassium Triplex, *Lilly*   Continued

Sugar-Free Liquid Pharmaceuticals[a,b]

SEDATIVES AND HYPNOTICS, TRANQUILIZERS

Amytal Elixir, *Lilly*
Butabarbital Sodium Elixir, *Lannett*
Butazem Elixir, *Zemmer*
Butisol Sodium Elixir, *McNeil*
Haldol Concentrate, *McNeil*
Hyonatol-B Elixir, *Bowman*
Lithonate-S, *Rowell*
Loxitane Oral Conc, *Lederle*
Mellaril Concentrate, *Sandoz*
Serentil Concentrate, *Boehringer Ingelheim*
Thorazine Concentrate, *SKF Labs*
Triclos, *Merrell Dow*
Vesprin High Potency Susp, *Squibb*
Vistaril Oral Susp, *Pfizer*

VITAMINS-NUTRITIONALS

Ad-Cebrin c/Fluoride Drops, *Lilly*
Aquasol A Drops, *USV Pharm*
B & C Liquid, *Nature's Bounty*
Ce-Vi-Sol Drops, *Mead Johnson*
Cod Liver Oil, *Squibb*
Cod Liver Oil (mint-flavored), *Squibb*
Drisdol in Propylene Glycol, *Winthrop*
Fluorac Drops, *USV Pharm*
Hycal, *Beecham Labs*
Incremin with Iron Syrup Vitamins B-1,
   B-6, B-12
Lysine/Iron, *Lederle*

Iron, B Complex & Vitamin C Liquid,
   Abbott
Lanoplex Elixir, *Lannett*
Lipotriad, *Cooper*
Liqui-Cee, *Arnar-Stone*
Lycolan Elixir, *Lannett*
MVI, *USV Pharm*
Novacebrin Drops, *Lilly*
Novacebrin c/Fluoride Drops, *Lilly*
Pediaflor, *Ross*
Poly-Vi-Flor Drops, *Mead Johnson*
Poly-Vi-Flor/Iron Drops, *Mead Johnson*
Poly-Vi-Sol Drops, *Mead Johnson*
Poly-Vi-Sol/Iron Drops, *Mead Johnson*
Protolan Liquid, *Lannett*
Super D Cod Liver Oil, *Upjohn*
Theragran Liquid, *Squibb*
Thi-Co-Lix, *Bowman*
Tri-Vi-Flor Drops, *Mead Johnson*
Tri-Vi-Sol Drops, *Mead Johnson*
Tri-Vi-Sol/Iron Drops, *Mead Johnson*
Vi-Daylin Drops, *Ross*
Vi-Daylin ADC Drops, *Ross*
Vi-Daylin ADC/Fluoride Drops, *Ross*
Vi-Daylin ADC Plus Iron Drops, *Ross*
Vi-Daylin/Fluoride Drops, *Ross*
Vi-Daylin Plus Iron Drops, *Ross*
Vi-Mix Drops, *Lilly*
Vi-Penta Infant Drops, *Roche*
Vi-Penta F Infant Drops, *Roche*
Vi-Penta Multivitamin Drops, *Roche*
Vi-Penta F Multivitamin Drops, *Roche*

a. Anon. Sugar-free liquid preparations. Am Drug 1979;178:62-5, reproduced with permission. Product formulations are subject to change by manufacturer.
b. Some of these products may contain sorbitol, xylitol or other sweeteners which can be partially metabolized to provide calories.

Tyramine in Food and Beverages[a]

FOOD OR BEVERAGE	ESTIMATED LEVELS[b]
Cheese	
American, processed	Low
Blue	Moderate to high
Boursault	Very high
Brick, natural	Moderate to high
Brie	Moderate to high
Camembert	Very high
Cheddar	Very high
Cottage cheese	Little or none
Cream cheese	Little or none
Emmenthaler	Very high
Gruyere	Moderate to high
Mozzarella	Moderate to high
Parmesan	Moderate to high

Continued

Tyramine in Food and Beverages[a]

FOOD OR BEVERAGE	ESTIMATED LEVELS[b]
Romano	Moderate to high
Roquefort	Moderate to high
Stilton	Very high
Meat and Fish	
Beef liver, unrefrigerated, fermented	Moderate
Caviar	High
Chicken liver, unrefrigerated, fermented	Moderate
Fish, unrefrigerated, fermented	Moderate
Fish, dried	Moderate
Herring, dried salted	Moderate to high
Herring, pickled, if spoiled	Highest levels found
Sausages, fermented:	Very high
Bologna	
Pepperoni	
Salami	
Summer sausage	
Other unrefrigerated, fermented meats	Moderate
Alcoholic Beverages	
Beer and Ale[c]	Low
Chartreuse[d]	Unknown
Drambuie[d]	Unknown
Sherry[d]	Low
Wine, red[e]	Low
Wine, white[f]	Little or none
Vegetables	
Avocado, particularly if overripe	Low to moderate
Fava beans, particularly if overripe	Contain dopamine
Fruit	
Bananas	Low
Figs, canned, particularly if overripe	Low to moderate
Others	
Caffeine, very large amounts	A weak pressor agent
Chocolate, very large amounts	Contains phenylethylamine, a weak pressor agent
Yeast extracts such as Marmite[g]	Very high

a. Anon. Monoamine oxidase inhibitors for depression. Med Lett Drugs Ther 1980;22:58-60, reproduced with permission.

b. The tyramine content of most foods is not entirely predictable. These estimates are taken from isolated reports, some based on small samples. The amount of tyramine in food and beverages could vary with different conditions, different samples and different manufacturers.

c. Fermentation of beer does not ordinarily involve processes that produce tyramine. Some imported beers have caused reactions in patients taking MAO inhibitors.

d. Some patients have had reactions.

e. Fermentation of wine does not ordinarily produce tyramine. However, contamination with other than the usual fermenting organisms and production of appreciable amounts of tyramine has occurred in Chianti and could occur in any red wine.

f. White wine is free of tyramine because it is made without the grape pulp and seeds, which may be the source of amino acids in red wine.

g. But baked goods do not contain appreciable amounts of tyramine.

5 DRUG-INDUCED DISCOLORATION OF FECES AND URINE

THE DRUGS AND DRUG CLASSES in the following tables have been associated with the discoloration of feces or urine. Drugs are listed generically, with a corresponding proprietary name given in parentheses.

Drugs Which May Discolor Feces

DRUG	COLOR PRODUCED
Antacids, Aluminum Hydroxide Types	Whitish or speckling
Antibiotics, Oral	Greenish gray
Anticoagulants, All	Pink to red or black**
Bismuth Containing Preparations	Greenish black
Charcoal	Black
1, 8-Dihydroxyanthraquinone*	Brownish staining of rectal mucosa
Dithiazanine (Delvex®)	Blue
Ferrous Salts	Black
Heparin	Pink to red or black**
Indocyanine Green	Green
Indomethacin (Indocin®)	Green due to biliverdinemia
Nonsteroidal Anti-Inflammatory Agents	Pink to red or black**
Oxyphenbutazone (Oxalid®, Tandearil®)	Pink to red or black**
Phenazopyridine (Pyridium®)	Orange-red
Phenylbutazone (Azolid®, Butazolidin®)	Pink to red or black**
Pyrvinium (Povan®)	Red
Rifampin (Rifadin®, Rimactane®)	Red-orange
Salicylates, Especially **Aspirin**	Pink to red or black**
Senna	Yellow

*Present in many combination products containing docusate sodium.
**These colors may indicate intestinal bleeding.

Drugs Which May Discolor Urine

DRUG	COLOR PRODUCED
Acetanilid	Yellow to red
Aminopyrine	Red
Aminosalicylic Acid (Pamisyl®)	Discoloration; red in hypochlorite solution**
Amitriptyline (Elavil®)	Blue-green
Anthraquinone Laxatives	Reddish in alkaline urine
Antipyrine	Yellow to red
Azuresin (Diagnex Blue®)	Blue or green
Chloroquine (Aralen®)	Rust yellow to brown
Chlorzoxazone (Paraflex®)	Orange to purplish red
Daunorubicin (Cerubidine®)	Red
Deferoxamine (Desferal®)	Reddish
1, 8-Dihydroxyanthraquinone*	Pink to red or red-brown
Dimethylsulfoxide (DMSO)	Reddish, due to hemoglobinuria
Doxorubicin (Adriamycin®)	Red
Emodin	Pink to red or red-brown in alkaline urine
Ethoxazene (Serenium®)	Orange to orange-red
Ferrous Salts	Black
Furazolidone (Furoxone®)	Rust yellow to brown
Indandiones	Orange in alkaline urine
Indomethacin (Indocin®)	Green due to biliverdinemia
Iron Sorbitex (Jectofer®)	Black
Levodopa (Dopar®, Larodopa®)	Dark on standing, possibly due to hypochlorite solution**
Methocarbamol (Robaxin®)	Dark on standing
Methyldopa (Aldomet®)	Dark on standing, possibly due to hypochlorite solution**
Methylene Blue	Blue or green
Metronidazole (Flagyl®)	Dark
Nitrofurantoin (Furadantin®, Macrodantin®)	Rust yellow to brown
Pamaquine (Plasmochin®)	Rust yellow to brown
Phenacetin	Dark brown to black on standing
Phenazopyridine (Pyridium®)	Orange to orange-red
Phenol (IV)	Green

Continued

Drugs Which May Discolor Urine

DRUG	COLOR PRODUCED
Phenolphthalein	Pink to purplish red in alkaline urine
Phenolsulfonphthalein (PSP)	Pink to red in alkaline urine
Phenothiazines	Pink to red or red-brown
Phensuximide (Milontin®)	Pink to red or red-brown
Phenytoin (Dilantin®)	Pink to red or red-brown
Primaquine	Rust yellow to brown
Quinacrine (Atabrine®)	Yellow, possibly upon urine acidification
Quinine	Brown to black
Resorcinol	Dark green
Riboflavin	Yellow fluorescence
Rifampin (Rifadin®, Rimactane®)	Bright red-orange
Sulfasalazine (Azulfidine®)	Orange-yellow in alkaline urine
Sulfonamides, Antibacterial	Rust yellow to brown
Tolonium (Blutene®)	Blue-green
Triamterene (Dyrenium®)	Pale blue fluorescence
Warfarin (Coumadin®)	Orange

*Present in many combination products containing docusate sodium.
**Hypochlorite solution in toilet bowl from prior use of chlorine bleach cleanser.

References

1. Baran RB, Rowles, B. Factors affecting coloration of urine and feces. J Am Pharm Assoc 1973;NS13:139-42, 155.

2. Block LH, Lamy PP. These drugs discolor the feces or urine. Am Prof Pharm 1968;34:27-9.

3. Bowling P, Belliveau RR, Butler TJ, Intravenous medications and green urine. JAMA 1981;246:216.

4. Devereaux MW, Mancall EL. Brown urine, bleach, and L-dopa. N Engl J Med 1974;291:1142.

5. Hansten PD. Drug interactions. 4th ed. Philadelphia: Lea & Febiger, 1979:444-8.

6. Lamy PP. Drug interactions: a growing problem. Hosp Formul 1975;10:60-95 passim.

7. Mercy Hospital (Rockville Centre, New York). Drugs and foods which may cause discoloration of the urine/feces. Pharm News! for Nurses 1973;7(March):1-2.

8. Meyers FH, Jawetz E, Goldfien A. Review of medical pharmacology. 7th ed. Los Altos, CA: Lange Medical Publications, 1980:704-17.

9. Muther RS, Bennett WM. Effects of dimethyl sulfoxide on renal function in man. JAMA 1980;244:2081-3.

10. Shirkey HC. Drugs that discolor the urine and feces. In: Shirkey HC, comp. Pediatric therapy. 6th ed. St. Louis: C.V. Mosby, 1980:163-6.

11. Strauss S. Patient dosage instructions: a guide for pharmacists. 3rd ed. Ambler, PA: IMS America, Ltd, 1975:64.

12. Wallach J. Alteration of laboratory test values by drugs. In: Wallach J, comp. Interpretation of diagnostic tests. 3rd ed. Boston: Little, Brown & Co., 1978:537-9, 547-8.

6 DRUG-INDUCED DISEASES

Introduction. The tables in this chapter provide the user with a ready source of information on a selected group of drug-induced diseases. These tables do not include all drugs reported to be the cause of a drug-induced disease, but every effort has been made to include those agents of major significance.

Each table identifies those drugs which are thought to be most frequently implicated in causing the disorder in question and, in most cases, some statement of the clinical significance of the problem is provided. References are listed which will lead the reader to the primary literature discussions and case reports of each particular drug-induced disorder. Since the format of each table is designed to best display the data available on the subject, it is imperative that the user read the introductory statement preceding the table to become aware of any abbreviations, symbols or other signs used to identify the nature and significance of the drug-induced problems discussed.

When several members of a drug class are known to be similarly capable of producing a disorder, the class name (eg, sulfonamides, phenothiazines) is used to conserve space. Occasionally, the available literature reports that a drug is a possible cause of a disorder, but fails to adequately characterize the frequency and severity of the adverse reaction. In these cases, the phrase "scattered reports only" appears in the discussion section of the table.

Drug-Induced Blood Dyscrasias

THE AGENTS IN THE FOLLOWING TABLE have been regularly reported to cause blood dyscrasias in man. Five major types of blood dyscrasias have been selected for inclusion in this table. These do not represent a complete list of drug-induced hematologic problems and the drugs selected for inclusion are not necessarily the only ones capable of producing these dyscrasias. For a more detailed list, the reader should consult reference 1. Excluded from the table are the cancer chemotherapeutic agents which are well known for producing dose-related bone marrow suppression. Those drugs which are thought to be one of the most common causes of a particular blood dyscrasia have been designated with a plus (+) symbol after the abbreviation identifying the dyscrasia. The following abbreviations are used to indicate the specific blood dyscrasia:

AA—Aplastic Anemia   HA—Hemolytic Anemia
AGN—Agranulocytosis,   MA—Megaloblastic Anemia
    Granulocytopenia   Th—Thrombocytopenia
    or Neutropenia

Drug-Induced Blood Dyscrasias

DRUG	NATURE OF DYSCRASIA	DISCUSSION
Acetaminophen	HA	Scattered reports only; may be an immune reaction[3,11]
	Th	Scattered reports only; has been seen in overdose; may be an immune reaction[1,2,11]
Acetazolamide	AA	11 cases in older literature[1,2,8]
	Th	10 cases in older literature[1,2,5]
Allopurinol	AGN	Scattered reports only[4,12]
Aminopyrine	AGN +	Results from an immune reaction and does not appear to be dose-related. The onset is sudden and may be encountered even after long-term therapy. Beware of the presence of this drug in foreign products and "herbal" preparations[1,2,4]
	HA	In G6PD deficiency (but not in blacks). May also result from an immune reaction[1,3]
Amphotericin B	AGN	Scattered reports only[13]
	HA	Rare; may be more common in patients with impaired renal function[1]
	Th	Scattered reports only[9,13]
Antidepressants, Tricyclic	AGN	Idiosyncratic reaction, probably resulting from a direct toxic effect rather than allergy. Most commonly encountered between the 2nd and 8th weeks of therapy[1-3,10,14]
Antipyrine	AGN	Scattered reports only[4]
	HA	In G6PD deficiency (but not in blacks)[1]
Arsenicals, Organic	AA	Seen both during and after the completion of therapy[1,8]

Continued

Drug-Induced Blood Dyscrasias

DRUG	NATURE OF DYSCRASIA	DISCUSSION
	AGN	Seen both during and after the completion of therapy[1]
	Th	Scattered reports only[1]
Ascorbic Acid	HA	In G6PD deficiency[1,6]
Aspirin	AA	Prevalence is quite low when the extensive use of the drug is taken into consideration. Often seen after long-term high-dose therapy (several kg total dose)[1,2,8,15]
	AGN	Rare; reported patients were usually taking other drugs capable of producing this dyscrasia[1,2,4]
	HA	In G6PD deficiency; usually requires infection or other complicating factors[1,2,6]
	Th	May occur in addition to the drug's effects on platelet adhesiveness. Some evidence for an immune reaction[1,2,5]
Captopril	AGN	Early reports suggest a prevalence of 3/1000; the reaction is gradual in development and usually begins 3–12 weeks after the initiation of therapy[4,16,17]
Carbamazepine	AA	Scattered reports only; onset may be delayed until weeks or months after the initiation of therapy[1,2]
	Th	Scattered reports only[1]
Cephalosporins	AGN	Rare; possibly the result of an immune reaction[1,2,4]
	HA	Positive direct Coombs' tests are common (3–75%, depending on the report) and may persist for up to 2 months after the discontinuation of therapy. Hemolysis is rare[1-3,9]
	Th	Rare; possibly the result of an immune reaction[1,2,5,9]
Chloramphenicol	AA +	Prevalence estimated at 1/18,000 to 1/50,000. Most cases develop after the discontinuation of therapy and most occur with oral therapy, suggesting the

Continued

Drug-Induced Blood Dyscrasias

DRUG	NATURE OF DYSCRASIA	DISCUSSION
		development of a toxic metabolite. Aplastic anemia should not be confused with the dose-related anemia seen with chloramphenicol (note: one case report suggests that a patient's dose-related anemia may have progressed to aplastic anemia, but most sources separate the origins of the two dyscrasias [1,2,8,9,18]
	AGN	Rare when compared with the prevalence of aplastic anemia [1,4]
	HA	In G6PD deficiency; usually requires infection or other complicating factors [1,6,9]
	Th	Scattered reports only; chloramphenicol-induced thrombocytopenia is usually a feature of aplastic anemia, rather than occurring alone [1]
Chlordiazepoxide	AGN	Scattered reports only [1,4]
Chloroquine	AGN	Scattered reports only [1,2]
	HA	Only a handful of cases have been reported; mechanism unclear [1,6]
	Th	Scattered reports only [1]
Chlorpropamide	AGN	Scattered reports only [1,2,4]
	Th	Scattered reports only [1]
Chlorthalidone		See Thiazide Diuretics
Cimetidine	AA	Scattered reports only, but they include at least 1 fatality [19]
	AGN	Reports are far less common than with **metiamide.** Some patients who developed agranulocytosis on metiamide have been successfully treated with cimetidine without reaction [2,4,20]
Clofibrate	AGN	Rare; seen with long-term therapy [1]
Contraceptives, Oral	MA	Results from impaired absorption or utilization of folate; of consequence only if the patient's dietary folate intake is inadequate [1,7]

Continued

Drug-Induced Blood Dyscrasias

DRUG	NATURE OF DYSCRASIA	DISCUSSION
Co-Trimoxazole		See Sulfonamides and Trimethoprim
Dapsone		See Sulfones
Diazoxide	HA	In G6PD deficiency[6]
Digitoxin	Th	Scattered reports only; evidence of an immune mechanism[2,5]
Dimercaprol	HA	In G6PD deficiency[1,6]
Dipyrone	AGN	Not dose-dependent[1]
Ethanol	HA	Most commonly encountered in chronic alcoholism[1]
	MA +	Results from malnutrition, decreased folate absorption or decreased folate utilization; responds rapidly to folate therapy[1,7]
	Th	Transient in many drinkers; persistent thrombocytopenia may accompany advanced alcoholic liver disease[1]
Fat Emulsions	HA	Scattered reports only[2]
	Th	Scattered reports only[2]
Furosemide	Th	Scattered reports only[1,2]
Gold Salts	AA	Not dose-dependent; may not be seen until after the drug has been discontinued; numerous fatalities have been reported[1,8]
	Th	Not dose- or duration-dependent; prevalence estimated at 1–3%; onset is usually seen during the loading phase of gold therapy (first 1000 mg), but may be delayed until after the drug has been discontinued. Mechanism is unclear; may be either marrow hypofunction or increased peripheral destruction of platelets[1,2,21]
Heparin	Th	Mild reductions in platelet count are common, but significant reductions are rare; highest prevalence is seen with beef lung derived products. Intermittent, continuous infusion and "mini-dose" regimens have all been implicated. Onset is rapid, but so is recovery after

Continued

Drug-Induced Blood Dyscrasias

DRUG	NATURE OF DYSCRASIA	DISCUSSION
		the discontinuation of the drug[1,2,5,22-24]
Hydralazine	Th	Appears to be quite rare, but 3 cases reported in neonates whose mothers were treated with hydralazine are disturbing[25]
Hydrochlorothiazide		See Thiazide Diuretics
Ibuprofen	Th	Scattered reports only with ibuprofen; isolated cases reported with many of the other newer nonsteroidal anti-inflammatory drugs[2]
Idoxuridine	Th	Onset usually after the drug has been discontinued; keep the total dose below 20 g to minimize the adverse effect[1,2]
Indomethacin	AA	Scattered reports only[1,2]
	AGN	Scattered reports only[1,24]
	Th	Mild impairment of platelet function is common, but thrombocytopenia is rare[1,2]
Interferon	AGN	Scattered reports only[2]
	Th	Scattered reports only[2]
Isoniazid	AGN	Scattered reports only; some evidence for an immune mechanism[1,4]
	Th	Scattered reports only; some evidence for an immune mechanism[1,5]
Levamisole	AGN	May be the result of an autoimmune reaction with a prevalence of 4% in some series. The presence of HLA B27 in seropositive rheumatoid arthritis patients is apparently an important predisposing factor[2,26,27]
Levodopa	HA	Autoimmune reaction; positive direct and indirect Coombs' tests are common, but hemolysis is rare. **Levodopa-carbidopa** combinations have also produced hemolysis[1-3]
Mefenamic Acid	HA	Autoimmune[1-3]
Mephenytoin	AA	Onset usually after several months of therapy[1,2,8]

Continued

Drug-Induced Blood Dyscrasias

DRUG	NATURE OF DYSCRASIA	DISCUSSION
	AGN	Rare; most return to normal 1–2 weeks after discontinuation of the drug, but some fatalities have been reported[1,4]
Methimazole	AA	Scattered reports only[8]
	AGN	Most cases are encountered in the first 9 weeks of therapy; a high percentage of the reported cases are in females[1,4]
Methyldopa	HA +	Autoimmune reaction; positive direct Coombs' test seen in 5–25% of patients, depending on dose; hemolysis in less than 1% and its onset is gradual after 6 months or more of therapy. Recovery is rapid after discontinuation of the drug[1-3]
	Th	Rare; may be a manifestation of an immune reaction[1,2]
Methylene Blue	HA	In G6PD deficiency[1,6]
Nalidixic Acid	HA	In G6PD deficiency; other causes of hemolysis may also be possible[1,2,9]
Nitrofurantoin	HA	In G6PD deficiency; also has been encountered with enolase deficiency (mechanism unknown)[1,2,6,9]
Oxprenolol	Th	Scattered reports only; also seen with some of the other β-blockers[2,28,29]
Oxyphenbutazone		See Phenylbutazone
Penicillamine	AA	Slow developing; results from direct toxicity[8,30]
	AGN	Most cases encountered during the first month of therapy[1,2,4]
	HA	Scattered reports only; may be due to G6PD deficiency or fluctuations in copper levels during therapy of Wilson's disease[2]
	Th	Scattered reports only; may be the result of an immune reaction; recovery is usually seen within 1–2 weeks after discontinuation of the drug[1,2]
Penicillins	AA	Prevalence very low when the extensive use of these drugs is considered[1,2,9]

Continued

Drug-Induced Blood Dyscrasias

DRUG	NATURE OF DYSCRASIA	DISCUSSION
	AGN	Rare; seen with high doses; semi-synthetic penicillins mentioned frequently in the reported cases[1,2,4,9]
	HA	Hemolysis rare; positive direct Coombs' tests seen with large IV doses[1-3,9]
	Th	Prevalence very low when the extensive use of these drugs is considered[1,2,5,9]
Phenacetin	HA	In G6PD deficiency; usually requires infection or other complicating factors. Hemolysis may also result from an immune reaction or direct drug toxicity[1,3,6]
Phenazopyridine	HA	Mechanism unknown; renal insufficiency or overdose may be contributing factors[1,2,6]
Phenindione	AGN	Usually seen as part of a hypersensitivity reaction; reported number of cases is impressive when the limited use of the drug is considered[1,2,4]
Phenobarbital	MA +	Similar to phenytoin; usually responds to folate administration[1,2,7]
Phenothiazines	AA	Scattered reports only[1]
	AGN +	Most common during the first 6 weeks of therapy and in older patients (less than 15% are under 40 yr). Rapid onset and lack of dose-dependence suggests an idiosyncratic mechanism[1,2,4,10]
	Th	Scattered reports only[1,5]
Phenylbutazone	AA +	With the more limited use of chloramphenicol, phenylbutazone is the major cause of drug-induced aplastic anemia. Onset after weeks to decades of therapy; fatality rate of about 50%[1,2,8]
	AGN +	No dose-dependence; onset after days to years of therapy[1,4]
	Th	Usually seen during the first 4 weeks of therapy[1,2,5]
Phenytoin	AA	Less than 25 cases reported, but the association with phenytoin is strong[1,2,8]

Continued

Drug-Induced Blood Dyscrasias

DRUG	NATURE OF DYSCRASIA	DISCUSSION
	AGN	Scattered reports only; onset after days to years of therapy[1,4]
	MA +	Results from impaired absorption or utilization of folate and responds to folate therapy (although folate replacement may lower phenytoin levels). Mild macrocytosis is very common (25% or more); onset is unpredictable, but it usually requires 6 or more months to develop[1,2,7]
	Th	Scattered reports only[1,2,5]
Primaquine	HA	In G6PD deficiency[1,2,6]
Primidone	MA +	Similar to phenytoin, but the prevalence may be lower; onset unpredictable, may be delayed for several years[1,2,7]
Procainamide	AGN	Most cases are encountered in the first 3 months of therapy[1,2,4,31]
Propranolol	Th	Scattered reports only; also seen with some of the other β-blockers[1,28]
Propylthiouracil	AA	Scattered reports only, but the association with propylthiouracil is strong[8]
	AGN	Exact mechanism is unclear, may be an immune reaction; most reported patients were receiving other drugs[1,2,4]
	Th	Scattered reports only[1,2]
Quinacrine	AA	About half of the reported cases were preceded by a rash or lichenoid eruption[1,2,8]
	HA	In G6PD deficiency; usually requires infection or other complicating factors[1,6]
Quinidine	AGN	An immune mechanism has been described[4]
	HA	In G6PD deficiency (but not in blacks). An immune mechanism has also been described[1-3]
	Th +	Caused by quinidine-specific antibodies; little or no cross-reactivity with quinine. Accounts for a significant percentage of drug-induced thrombocytopenia[1,2,5,32]

Continued

Drug-Induced Blood Dyscrasias

DRUG	NATURE OF DYSCRASIA	DISCUSSION
Quinine	AGN	Scattered reports only[1,4]
	HA	In G6PD deficiency (but not in blacks)[1-3]
	Th	Caused by quinine-specific antibodies, little or no cross-reactivity with quinidine[1,2,5,33]
Rifampin	HA	Rare, but a significant number of patients will have positive Coombs' tests; onset in hours in some sensitized patients[1,2]
	Th	Appears to result from an immune reaction[1,2,5,34]
Stibophen	HA	Immune mechanism; high fatality rate[1,3,5]
Streptomycin	AA	Has not clearly been established as a cause, but has been implicated in numerous cases[1,9]
	AGN	Has not clearly been established as a cause, but has been implicated in numerous cases[1,4,9]
	Th	Scattered reports only[1]
Sulfinpyrazone	AGN	Scattered reports only; seen in prolonged therapy[2]
	Th	Scattered reports only[2]
Sulfonamides, Antibacterial	AA +	Historically, an important cause of aplastic anemia, but most cases were reported following the use of older sulfonamides; rarely encountered with the products currently in use[1,2,8,9]
	AGN	Seen mostly with older products; rarely encountered with the products currently in use. Rapid onset suggest an immune mechanism[1,2,4,9]
	HA	In G6PD deficiency; also seen in nondeficient patients. **Sulfasalazine** is the most commonly used oxidative sulfonamide and its hemolysis is most common in slow acetylators[1,2,3,9]

Continued

Drug-Induced Blood Dyscrasias

DRUG	NATURE OF DYSCRASIA	DISCUSSION
Sulfones	AGN	Many cases are the result of combination therapy, so it is difficult to discern the influence of the sulfones[1,4]
	HA	In G6PD deficiency; may have other mechanism(s)[1,2,6]
Tetracyclines	AA	Scattered reports only[1,2]
	AGN	Scattered reports only; **doxycycline** mentioned often[1,2,4]
	Th	Scattered reports only[1,2,9]
Thiazide Diuretics	AA	Scattered reports only[1,2,8]
	AGN	Scattered reports only[1,2,4]
	HA	Exact mechanism is unclear, may be an immune reaction[1]
	Th	Mild thrombocytopenia is common, but severe cases are rare. May result from an immune reaction[1,2,5]
Tolbutamide	AA	Scattered reports only[1,8]
	Th	Scattered reports only; may result from an immune reaction[1]
Triamterene	MA	Few cases, but it is a potential inhibitor of dihydrofolate reductase; greatest risk among those with low folate levels prior to triamterene therapy (eg, alcoholics).[1,2,7]
Trimethadione	AA	Scattered reports only; seen in the first year of therapy[1,2,8]
	AGN	Scattered reports only; often seen in combination therapy[1,4]
Trimethoprim	AA	Rare; seen in combination therapy with sulfonamides[2,9]
	AGN	Rare; seen both in single and in combination therapy with sulfonamides, with the latter numerically more common[1,4,9]
	MA	Most cases seen after 1–2 weeks of therapy; may have small antifolate action in humans which becomes important only in patients with already re-

Continued

Drug-Induced Blood Dyscrasias

DRUG	NATURE OF DYSCRASIA	DISCUSSION
		duced folate levels (eg, alcoholics)[1,2,7,9]
	Th	Mild thrombocytopenia is common, but rarely severe. Most commonly encountered in combination therapy with sulfonamides[1,2,5,9]
Valproic Acid	Th	Exact prevalence or significance is undetermined[2]
Vancomycin	AGN	Scattered reports only; possibly an immune reaction[2,35]
Vitamin K	Th	In G6PD deficiency; usually requires infection or other complicating factors. Hemolysis from high doses contributes to kernicterus in neonates; rarely toxic in older children or adults[1,2,6]

References

1. Swanson M, Cook R. Drugs, chemicals and blood dyscrasias. Hamilton, IL: Drug Intelligence Publications, Inc. 1977.

2. Dukes MNG, ed. Meyler's side effects of drugs, 9th ed. Amsterdam: Excerpta Medica, 1980.

3. Petz LD. Drug-induced immune haemolytic anaemia. Clin Haematol 1980;9:455-82.

4. Young GAR, Vincent PC. Drug-induced agranulocytosis. Clin Haematol 1980;9:483-504.

5. Miescher PA, Graf J. Drug-induced thrombocytopenia. Clin Haematol 1980;9:505-19.

6. Gordon-Smith EC. Drug-induced oxidative haemolysis. Clin Haematol 1980;9:557-86.

7. Scott JM, Weir DG. Drug-induced megaloblastic change. Clin Haematol 1980;9:587-606.

8. Heimpel H, Heit W. Drug-induced aplastic anaemia: clinical aspects. Clin Haematol 1980;9:641-62.

9. Kucers A, Bennett NMcK. The use of antibiotics. 3rd ed. Philadelphia: JB Lippincott, 1979.

10. Klein DF, Gittelman R, Quitkin F et al. Diagnosis and drug treatment of psychiatric disorders: adults and children. 2nd ed. Baltimore: Williams & Wilkins, 1980.

11. Kornberg A, Polliack A. Paracetamol-induced thrombocytopenia and haemolytic anaemia. Lancet 1978;2:1159.

12. Hawson GAT, Bain BJ. Allopurinol and agranulocytosis. Med J Aust 1980;1:283-4.

13. Wilson R, Feldman S. Toxicity of amphotericin B in children with cancer. Am J Dis Child 1979;133:731-4.

14. Albertini RS, Penders TM. Agranulocytosis associated with tricyclics. J Clin Psychiatry 1978;39:483-5.

15. Eldar M, Aderka D, Shoenfeld Y et al. Aspirin-induced aplastic anaemia. S Afr Med J 1979;55:318.

16. Staessen J, Fagard R, Lijnen P et al. Captopril and agranulocytosis. Lancet 1980;1:926-7.

17. Capoten® Monograph. ER Squibb & Sons, 1981:51.

18. Daum RS, Cohen DL, Smith AL. Fatal aplastic anemia following apparent "dose-related" chloramphenicol toxicity. J Pediatr 1979;94:403-6.

19. Chang HK, Morrison SL. Bone-marrow suppression associated with cimetidine. Ann Intern Med 1979;91:580.

20. Carloss HW, Tavassoli M, McMillan R. Cimetidine-induced granulocytopenia. Ann Intern Med 1980;93:57-8.

21. Harth M, Hickey JP, Coulter WK et al. Gold-induced thrombocytopenia. J Rheumatol 1978;5:165-72.

22. Rector TS, Cipolle RJ, Seifert RD et al. Characteristics of heparin-associated thrombocytopenia. Am J Hosp Pharm 1979;36:1561-5.

23. Bell WR, Royall RM. Heparin-associated thrombocytopenia: a comparison of three heparin preparations. N Engl J Med 1980;303:902-7.

24. Ayars GH, Tikoff G. Incidence of thrombocytopenia in medical patients on "mini-dose" heparin prophylaxis. Am Heart J 1980;99:816.

25. Widerlov E, Karlman I. Storsater J. Hydralazine-induced neonatal thrombocytopenia. N Engl J Med 1980;303:1235.

26. Mielants H, Veys EM. A study of the hematological side effects of levamisole in rheumatoid arthritis with recommendations. J Rheumatol 1978;5(Suppl 4):77-83.

27. Drew SI, Carter BM, Nathanson DS et al. Levamisole-associated neutropenia and autoimmune granulocytotoxins. Ann Rheum Dis 1980;39:59-63.

28. Petrie JC, Galloway DB, Jeffers TA et al. Adverse reactions to beta-blocking drugs: a review. Postgrad Med J 1976;52(Suppl 4):63-9.

29. Dodds WN, Davidson RJL. Thrombocytopenia due to slow-release oxprenolol. Lancet 1978;2:683.

30. Kay AGL. Myelotoxicity of D-penicillamine. Ann Rheum Dis 1979;38:232-6.

31. Riker J, Baker J, Swanson M. Bone marrow granulomas and neutropenia associated with procainamide. Arch Intern Med 1978;138:1731-2.

32. Alperin JB, deGroot WJ, Cimo PL. Quinidine-induced thrombocytopenia with pulmonary hemorrhage. Arch Intern Med 1980;140:266-7.

33. Murray JA, Abbott I, Anderson DA et al. Bitter lemon purpura. Br Med J 1979;2:1551-2.

34. Hadfield JW. Rifampicin-induced thrombocytopenia. Postgrad Med J 1980;56:59-60.

35. Borland CDR, Farrar WE, Reversible neutropenia from vancomycin. JAMA 1979;242:2392-3.

Drug-Induced Hepatotoxicity

THE AGENTS IN THE FOLLOWING TABLE have been associated with drug-induced hepatotoxicity in man. They are classified according to the nature of the hepatic injury they are thought to produce. "Cytotoxic" injury refers to degeneration or necrosis of the hepatic parenchyma, while "cholestatic" injury means arrested bile flow and jaundice, with minimal histologic evidence of parenchymal injury. Liver damage produced by "intrinsic hepatotoxins" is characterized by its occurrence in a significant number of those exposed, by dose-dependency and by its reproducibility in laboratory animals. Liver damage resulting from "idiosyncratic reactions" occurs rarely, with few identifiable predisposing factors, and is usually not dose-dependent. Allergic hypersensitivity reactions are in the "idiosyncratic" category. The available literature may not permit accurate classification of some drugs; in these cases more than one classification is used. The following abbreviations are used to indicate the nature of the hepatic injury:

1—Cytotoxic, Intrinsic Hepatotoxin

2—Cytotoxic, Idiosyncracy

3—Cholestatic, Intrinsic Hepatotoxin

4—Cholestatic, Idiosyncracy

The table begins on page 75.

Drug-Induced Hepatotoxicity

DRUG	NATURE OF INJURY	CLINICAL SIGNIFICANCE AND COMMENTS
Acetaminophen	1	Hepatic damage may follow overdose with as little as 7.5 g, although doses of 140 mg/kg or more are usually needed to produce evidence of hepatotoxicity. These large doses saturate the normal metabolic pathways and produce large quantities of a toxic metabolite. This metabolite is usually eliminated after combination with glutathione, but glutathione stores can be depleted in acetaminophen overdoses leaving the toxic metabolite free to attack hepatic tissues resulting in a centrizonal hepatic necrosis. Acetaminophen hepatotoxicity is enhanced by **alcohol, barbiturates** or other hepatic enzyme inducers. Prompt therapy with exogenous sulfhydryl donors (most notably **cysteamine, methionine** and especially **N-acetylcysteine**) may reduce the risk of severe hepatic damage. Therapy with sulfhydryl donors is recommended if the 4 hr postingestion acetaminophen level exceeds 200 mg/L. Less destructive, but still detectable, hepatitis has been reported in patients taking therapeutic doses for a prolonged period of time[1-8]
Acetohexamide	2	Scattered reports only.[1,4,9]
Alcohol	1	Fatty infiltration of the liver can be found in 70-100% of alcoholics. Fatty liver is generally without physical manifestation, but 30% of patients progress to develop alcoholic hepatitis and about 10% develop cirrhosis. Malnutrition may contribute significantly to alcoholic liver disease and alcohol may potentiate the hepatotoxicity of other drugs[1,3]
Allopurinol	2,4	The number of cases in the literature is too small to permit accurate characterization of allopurinol hepatotoxicity. Granulomas, necrosis, portal inflammation and cholestasis have all been seen[1,10,11]
Aminosalicylic Acid	2	0.3-5% of patients taking aminosalicylic acid may develop a generalized hypersensitivity reaction. 25% of these patients will demonstrate evidence of hepatic injury as part of their hypersensitivity reaction; the fatality rate among them has been estimated to be as high as 10%. Withdrawal of the drug results in recovery in 1-6 weeks[1,4]

Continued

Drug-Induced Hepatotoxicity

DRUG	NATURE OF INJURY	CLINICAL SIGNIFICANCE AND COMMENTS
Androgens		See Steroids, C-17-α-alkyl
Antidepressants, Tricyclic	4	0.5-1% estimated prevalence[1-3,12]
Antimony Compounds	1	Actual hepatitis is rare, but laboratory evidence of hepatotoxicity can be seen in up to 65% of patients[1,3]
Arsenicals	1,4	Hepatitis may result from large doses, while cholestasis appears to be the result of hypersensitivity[1,3,4]
Asparaginase	1	Reversible fatty infiltration of the liver is seen in 50-90% of patients receiving this drug, apparently as a result of asparagine depletion. Daily doses may be more toxic than weekly doses[1-3,13]
Aspirin		See Salicylates
Azathioprine	4	Scattered reports only[1,3,4,14]
BCG Vaccine	2	Granulomatous hepatitis has been encountered in both healthy and immunosuppressed patients[1,2,15,16]
Benzodiazepines	4	Most published reports indicate that these compounds are associated with a low prevalence of cholestatic jaundice, but some evidence does exist for a possible cytotoxic reaction as well[1-4,17]
Carbamazepine	2,4	Scattered reports only, but one possible fatality[1-3,18]

Continued

Drug-Induced Hepatotoxicity

DRUG	NATURE OF INJURY	CLINICAL SIGNIFICANCE AND COMMENTS
Carbenicillin	2	Anicteric hepatotoxicity in up to 6% of patients receiving the drug[1,2,19]
Chlorambucil	2	Scattered reports only[1,3]
Chlordiazepoxide		See Benzodiazepines
Chlorpromazine		See Phenothiazines
Chlorpropamide	3	A relatively high prevalence of cholestatic hepatic changes has been decreased through the use of lower doses[1-4]
Contraceptives, Oral	3	Several hundred cases of jaundice have been reported with the onset of symptoms usually in the first few months of therapy. Patients who demonstrate jaundice during pregnancy have a greater chance of reacting similarly to oral contraceptives. Withdrawal of the drug is usually followed by prompt resolution of the jaundice. Oral contraceptives are also associated with a marked increase in the prevalence of hepatic adenomas and related benign tumors. These tumors may require resection. The frequency of gall bladder disease is also apparently increased by oral contraceptives[1-4,20,21]
Dantrolene	1	At least 0.8% of patients taking dantrolene develop laboratory evidence of hepatic dysfunction, with symptomatic hepatitis seen in about 0.4%; the fatality rate among jaundiced patients is about 25%. Predisposing factors seem to include dose (greater than 300 mg/day), sex (females > males), age (> 30 yr) and duration of therapy (at least 2 months)[1,2,22,23]
Diazepam		See Benzodiazepines

Continued

Drug-Induced Hepatotoxicity

DRUG	NATURE OF INJURY	CLINICAL SIGNIFICANCE AND COMMENTS
Disulfiram	2	Disulfiram-induced hepatitis appears rare, but its actual prevalence is difficult to determine because of the high frequency of liver disease in alcoholics[1,2,24]
Enflurane	2	A limited number of cases have been reported with symptoms resembling mild halothane hepatitis. Cross-reactivity with halothane has not been demonstrated[1,2,25,26]
Erythromycin Estolate	4	Jaundice is evident in 2–4% of patients while laboratory evidence of cholestasis is present in many more. The cholestatic reaction is the result of hypersensitivity and appears after 10–14 days of initial therapy or after 1–2 days in patients with a history of a previous exposure to the drug. Rapid reversal of symptoms follows withdrawal of the drug. One case has been associated with **erythromycin ethylsuccinate**[1-4,19,27,28]
Ethionamide	1	Hepatitis may be seen in 3–5% of patients with serum enzyme elevations in 10–30%. Onset of hepatitis is seen after 1–8 months of therapy[1-4,29]
Ferrous Salts	1	Hepatic necrosis may appear within 1–3 days of an acute overdose. The fatality rate is high if the patient is not treated promptly[1-3]
Flurazepam		See Benzodiazepines
Gold Salts	4	Rare cholestasis, primarily with gold sodium thiomalate[1,2,30]
Halothane	2	Despite extensive publicity, the actual frequency of fatal halothane hepatitis is low, ranging from 1:40,000 to 7:10,000. Susceptibility is enhanced in adults, females, obese patients and especially in patients with prior exposure to halothane. The mechanism of halothane hepatitis is hypersensitivity. Fever precedes jaundice in most patients and the onset of jaundice is usually

Continued

Drug-Induced Hepatotoxicity

DRUG	NATURE OF INJURY	CLINICAL SIGNIFICANCE AND COMMENTS
		between 3–14 days after exposure, with the shorter latent periods associated with prior halothane exposure. Halothane may cross-react with **methoxyflurane** [1-4,31]
Iron Salts		See Ferrous Salts
Isoniazid	1	Subclinical hepatitis (increased SGOT) is common (10–20%); this usually resolves rapidly following withdrawal of the drug and frequently without discontinuation of therapy. Clinical hepatitis is age-related; it is seldom seen in children and ranges from 0.5% in 20–35 year-olds to 3% in those over 50. The onset of symptoms may occur anytime during the first year of therapy, but over half of the cases develop during the first 3 months. The fatality rate is about 10% with a poorer prognosis associated with an onset of symptoms after more than 2 months of therapy [1-4,32,33]
Ketoconazole	2	Elevations in hepatic enzymes have been reported in a few patients, often reversing with continued therapy. Cases of hepatitis have been reported, one having been confirmed by rechallenge. Injury appears to be similar to methyldopa-induced hepatitis. Hepatitis has been reversible with drug discontinuation, [61,62] but at least one death has occurred
Mercaptopurine	1	Jaundice has been reported in 6–40% of patients, usually appearing after 1–2 months of therapy. The highest prevalence is associated with doses of 2.5 mg/kg/day or more [1-4]
Methimazole	4	While the prevalence of cholestasis is low, it may take 3–5 months for it to clear after withdrawal of the drug [1,3,4]
Methotrexate	1	Hepatic damage is dependent on dose and duration of therapy and may progress to cirrhosis if the drug is not stopped. Intermittent high doses may pose less of a threat than low daily doses.

Continued

Drug-Induced Hepatotoxicity

DRUG	NATURE OF INJURY	CLINICAL SIGNIFICANCE AND COMMENTS
		Hepatic fibrosis is not reflected by standard liver function tests and is best detected by biopsy[1-4,34]
Methoxyflurane	2	Very similar to halothane hepatitis and may cross-react with **halothane**[1-4,35]
Methyldopa	1	Small changes in liver function tests have been reported in up to 35% of patients taking methyldopa, but the prevalence of clinical hepatitis is probably less than 1% with an onset after 1–20 weeks of therapy. Hepatitis is more common in females. Most patients show rapid recovery after withdrawal of the drug. Most cases occur during the first 3 months of therapy, but some cases have occurred up to 2 years after beginning methyldopa. The fatality rate is no more than 10% among patients who develop hepatitis. There is evidence to support a hypersensitivity mechanism in some patients[1-4,36]
Mithramycin	1	Biochemical evidence of hepatotoxicity has been reported in virtually all patients in some studies. Intermittent rather than continuous dosing may provide some protection[1,4,37]
Niacin	3	Hepatic dysfunction has been reported in as many as a third of patients taking the drug with jaundice in 5%. Sustained-release products seem to be particularly prone to producing liver damage[1-3,38]
Nitrofurantoin	4	Hepatic damage from nitrofurantoin is rare. Cholestasis is the major presentation, but as many as 20 cases of chronic active hepatitis have been reported[1-4,39]
Penicillins	2	A number of the penicillins (most notably **carbenicillin, oxacillin, ampicillin** and **amoxicillin**) have been implicated in causing mild reversible hepatic dysfunction[1,3,4,19,40,41]
Phenacemide	2	With a prevalence of about 2%, this drug has the highest rate of hepatic injury of the anticonvulsants. The mechanism appears to be hypersensitivity[1,3]

Continued

Drug-Induced Hepatotoxicity

DRUG	NATURE OF INJURY	CLINICAL SIGNIFICANCE AND COMMENTS
Phenazopyridine	2	Hepatic injury with this drug is very rare and is usually accompanied by other signs of hypersensitivity.[1,3,4,42]
Phenobarbital	2	Hepatic injury with this drug is very rare and is usually accompanied by other signs of hypersensitivity, particularly cutaneous manifestations[1-3,43]
Phenothiazines	4	Current estimates of the prevalence of hypersensitivity cholestasis are about 1%, with the disorder following a benign course. Most reported cases are with **chlorpromazine**, but this may reflect the extensive early use of this drug[1-4,44]
Phenylbutazone	2,4	Most cases of phenylbutazone hepatotoxicity develop within the first month of therapy and many are accompanied by other signs of hypersensitivity. The overall prevalence is probably below 0.5%. The cholestatic form is benign, but the cytotoxic form has produced fatalities[1-4,45]
Phenytoin	2	Rare, but often fatal, hepatic damage has been associated with phenytoin therapy. It is invariably accompanied by other signs of hypersensitivity, frequently as part of a diffuse syndrome of lymphadenopathy, exfoliative dermatitis, high fever and leukopenia[1-4]
Progestogens		See Steroids, C-17-α-alkyl
Propoxyphene	4	Only a few cases of propoxyphene-induced cholestasis have been reported, but comments in the literature suggest that more have been observed[1-3,46]
Propylthiouracil	2	As with methimazole, the prevalence of hepatic dysfunction is quite low but, unlike methimazole, the damage is hepatocellular rather than cholestatic[1-3,47]
Pyrazinamide	1	Pyrazinamide-induced hepatitis is dependent on dose and duration of therapy. Daily doses of

Continued

Drug-Induced Hepatotoxicity

DRUG	NATURE OF INJURY	CLINICAL SIGNIFICANCE AND COMMENTS
Quinidine	2	20-30 mg/kg or weekly doses of 90 mg/kg are associated with a lower prevalence of hepatitis than with 40-50 mg/kg/day[1-3,48] Rare and usually accompanied by other signs of hypersensitivity, particularly fever[1-3,48]
Rifampin	1	Subclinical hepatitis has been observed in 10-30% of patients receiving rifampin, particularly during the first weeks of therapy; however, it is difficult to attribute these cases specifically to rifampin, because nearly all patients receive **isoniazid** simultaneously. Only a few of these patients suffer enough damage to produce jaundice. Pre-existing liver disease, alcohol consumption and the use of other hepatotoxic drugs such as isoniazid may increase the risk of liver damage[1-4,19]
Salicylates	1	Salicylate-induced hepatitis is rare, usually mild, readily reversible and most often associated with high-dose salicylate therapy such as that encountered in the management of rheumatoid arthritis[1,2,4,49]
Steroids, C-17-α-alkyl	3	Cholestasis is seen with a minimal amount of hepatic inflammation. The onset of jaundice may or may not be preceded by other clinical signs. The prevalence appears to be dose-related. Examples include **methyltestosterone, norethandrolone, methylandrostenolone, fluoxymesterone, norethindrone, norethynodrel** and **oxymetholone**[1-4,50]
Sulfonamides, Antibacterial	2	The newer short-acting sulfonamides are apparently less hepatotoxic than their long-acting predecessors, with most reported cases appearing before 1947. This could, of course, also reflect less interest in reporting the problem. Most cases of sulfonamide hepatotoxicity develop during the first 2 weeks of therapy and many are accompanied by other signs of hypersensitivity. The case fatality rate may be 10% or more[1-4,19,51,52]
Sulfones	1,2	Little definitive information is available on the hepatotoxicity of sulfones with

Continued

Drug-Induced Hepatotoxicity

DRUG	NATURE OF INJURY	CLINICAL SIGNIFICANCE AND COMMENTS
		evidence for both intrinsic hepatotoxic and hypersensitivity mechanisms. The prevalence of hepatic injury has been estimated at 5%[1,2]
Tetracyclines	1	Fatty infiltration of the liver has been encountered in patients receiving large doses of tetracyclines IV, usually in excess of 1.5 g/day. Contributing factors include pregnancy, malnutrition and impaired renal function, but hepatotoxicity has been encountered in patients demonstrating none of these. The fatality rate is very high. Oral therapy may also produce signs of hepatotoxicity, although far less frequently[1-4,19,53,54]
Thiazide Diuretics	4	Scattered reports only[1-3]
Tolbutamide	4	Scattered reports only[1,3,55]
Troleandomycin	1,4	30–50% of patients receiving the drug show some laboratory evidence of abnormal liver function and 5% develop jaundice. In general, the reaction is similar to that seen with **erythromycin estolate**, except that there is some evidence of intrinsic hepatotoxicity associated with troleandomycin or one of its metabolites[1-4,19,56]
Tromethamine	1	About one-third of neonates receiving tromethamine through the umbilical vein develop hemorrhagic liver necrosis. Liver damage is not seen when the drug is given through the umbilical artery[1,3,57]
Valproic Acid	2	Cases of fatal hepatitis resulting from valproic acid therapy are beginning to accumulate in the literature. The prevalence of nonfatal hepatic dysfunction has been reported to be as high as 44% in one series; hepatic damage does not appear to be dose-related. Serial liver function tests in asymptomatic patients probably do little to prevent the problem. Liver function tests may be of some value during the first 6 months of therapy in those at greatest risk (children with severe epilepsy associated with structural brain damage and mental retardation)[2,58-60]

References

1. Zimmerman HJ. Hepatotoxicity: the adverse effects of drugs and chemicals on the liver. New York: Appleton-Century-Crofts, 1978.

2. Dukes MNG, ed. Meyler's side effects of drugs. 9th ed. Amsterdam: Excerpta Medica, 1980.

3. Klatskin G. Toxic and drug-induced hepatitis. In: Schiff L, ed. Diseases of the liver. 4th ed. Philadelphia: JB Lippincott, 1975:604-710.

4. Sherlock S. Diseases of the liver and biliary system. 6th ed. Oxford: Blackwell, 1981:295-322.

5. Peterson RG, Rumack BH. Toxicity of acetaminophen overdose JACEP 1978;7:202-5.

6. McClain CJ, Kromhout JP, Peterson FJ, et al. Potentiation of acetaminophen hepatotoxicity by alcohol. JAMA 1980;244:251-3.

7. Barker JD, de Carle DJ, Anuras S. Chronic excessive acetaminophen use and liver damage. Ann Intern Med 1977;87:299-301.

8. Bonkowsky HL, Mudge GH, McMurtry RJ. Chronic hepatic inflammation and fibrosis due to low doses of paracetamol. Lancet 1978;1:1016-8.

9. Goldstein MJ, Rothenberg AJ. Jaundice in a patient receiving acetohexamide. N Engl J Med 1966;275:97-9.

10. Chawla SK, Patel HD, Parrino GR et al. Allopurinol hepatotoxicity: case report and literature review. Arthritis Rheum 1977;20:1546-9.

11. Swank LA, Chejfec G, Nemchausky BA. Allopurinol-induced granulomatous hepatitis with cholangitis and a sarcoid-like reaction. Arch Intern Med 1978;138:997-8.

12. Anderson BN, Henrikson IR. Jaundice and eosinophilia associated with amitriptyline. J Clin Psychiatry 1978;39:730-1.

13. Pratt CB, Simone JV, Zee P et al. Comparison of daily versus weekly L-asparaginase for the treatment of childhood acute leukemia. J Pediatr 1970;77:474-83.

14. Davis M, Eddleston ALWF, Williams R. Hypersensitivity and jaundice due to azathioprine. Postgrad Med J 1980;56:274-5.

15. d'Alessandri RM, Khakoo RA. Granulomatous hepatitis in a healthy adult following BCG injection into a plantar wart. Am J Gastroenterol 1977;68:392-5.

16. Aungst CW, Sokal JE, Jager BV. Complications of BCG vaccination in neoplastic disease. Ann Intern Med 1975;82:666-9.

17. Fang MH, Ginsberg AL, Dobbins WO. Cholestatic jaundice associated with flurazepam hydrochloride. Ann Intern Med 1978;89:363-4.

18. Zucker P, Daum F, Cohen MI. Fatal carbamazepine hepatitis. J Pediatr 1977;91:667-8.

19. Kucers A, Bennett NMcK. The use of antibiotics. Philadelphia: JB Lippincott, 1979.

20. Bennion LJ, Ginsberg RL, Garnick MB et al. Effects of oral contraceptives on the gallbladder bile of normal women. N Engl J Med 1976;294:189-92.

21. Edmondson HA, Henderson B, Benton B. Liver-cell adenomas associated with use of oral contraceptives. N Engl J Med 1976;294:470-2.

22. Utili R, Boitnott JK, Zimmerman HJ. Dantrolene-associated hepatic injury: incidence and character. Gastroenterology 1977;72:610-6.

23. Wilkinson SP, Portmann B, Williams R. Hepatitis from dantrolene sodium. Gut 1979;20:33-6.

24. Morris SJ, Kanner R, Chiprut RO et al. Disulfiram hepatitis. Gastroenterology 1978;75:100-2.

25. Ona FV, Patanella H, Ayub A. Hepatitis associated with enflurane anesthesia. Anesth Analg 1980;59:146-9.

26. Kline MM. Enflurane-associated hepatitis. Gastroenterology 1980;79:126-7.

27. Cacace LG, Schweigert BF, Gildon AM. Erythromycin estolate induced hepatotoxicity: report of a case and review of the literature. Drug Intell Clin Pharm 1977;11:22-5.

28. Sullivan D, Csuka ME, Blanchard B. Erythromycin ethylsuccinate hepatotoxicity. JAMA 1980;243:1074.

29. Conn HO, Binder HJ, Orr HD. Ethionamide-induced hepatitis: a review with a report of an additional case. Am Rev Resp Dis 1964;90:542-52.

30. Favreau M, Tannenbaum H, Lough J. Hepatic toxicity associated with gold therapy. Ann Intern Med 1977;87:717-9.

31. Inman WHW, Mushin WW. Jaundice after repeated exposure to halothane: a further analysis of reports to the Committee on Safety of Medicine. Br Med J 1978;2:1455-6.

32. Mitchell JR, Zimmerman HJ, Ishak KG et al. Isoniazid liver injury: clinical spectrum, pathology, and probable pathogenesis. Ann Intern Med 1976;84:181-92.

33. Black M, Mitchell JR, Zimmerman HJ. Isoniazid-associated hepatitis in 114 patients. Gastroenterology 1975;69:289-302.

34. McIntosh S, Davidson DL, O'Brien RT et al. Methotrexate hepatotoxicity in children with leukemia. J Pediatr 1977;90:1019-21.

35. Joshi PH, Conn HO. The syndrome of methoxyflurane-associated hepatitis. Ann Intern Med 1974;80:395-401.

36. Thomas E, Rosenthal WS, Zapiach L et al. Spectrum of methyldopa liver injury. Am J Gastroenterol 1977;68:125-33.

37. Kennedy BJ. Mithramycin therapy in advanced testicular neoplasms. Cancer 1970;26:755-66.

38. Einstein N, Baker A, Galper J et al. Jaundice due to nicotinic acid therapy. Am J Digest Dis 1975;20:282-6.

39. Hatoff DE, Cohen M, Schweigert BF et al. Nitrofurantoin: another cause of drug-induced chronic active hepatitis? Am J Med 1979;67:117-21.

40. Wilson FM, Belamaric J, Lauter CB et al. Anicteric carbenicillin hepatitis: eight episodes in four patients. JAMA 1975;232:818-21.

41. Bruckstein AH, Attia AA. Oxacillin hepatitis: two patients with liver biopsy, and review of the literature. Am J Med 1978;64:519-22.

42. Goldfinger SE, Marx S. Hypersensitivity hepatitis due to phenazopyridine hydrochloride. N Engl J Med 1972;286:1090-1.

43. Evans WE, Self TH, Weisburst MR. Phenobarbital-induced hepatic dysfunction. Drug Intell Clin Pharm 1976;10:439-43

44. Klein DF, Gittelman R, Quitkin F et al. Diagnosis and drug treatment of psychiatric disorders: adults and children. 2nd ed. Baltimore: Williams & Wilkins, 1980:195-7.

45. Fowler PD, Woolf D, Alexander S. Phenylbutazone and hepatitis. Rheumatol Rehabil 1975;14:71-5.

46. Ford MJ, Kellett RJ, Busuttil A et al. Dextropropoxyphene and jaundice. Br Med J 1977;2:674.

47. Weiss M, Hassin D, Bank H. Propylthiouracil-induced hepatic damage. Arch Intern Med 1980;140:1184-5.

48. Bramlet DA, Posalaky Z, Olson R. Granulomatous hepatitis as a manifestation of quinidine hypersensitivity. Arch Intern Med 1980;140:395-7.

49. Kanada SA, Kolling WM, Hindin BI. Aspirin hepatotoxicity. Am J Hosp Pharm 1978;35:330-6.

50. Murray-Lyon IM, Westaby D, Paradinas F. Hepatic complications of androgen therapy. Gastroenterology 1977;73:1461.

51. Dujovne CA, Chan CH, Zimmerman HJ. Sulfonamide hepatic injury: review of the literature and report of a case due to sulfamethoxazole. N Engl J Med 1967;277:785-8.

52. Stevenson DK, Christie DL, Haas JE. Hepatic injury in a child caused by trimethoprim-sulfamethoxazole. Pediatrics 1978;61:864-6.

53. Dowling HF, Lepper MH. Hepatic reactions to tetracycline. JAMA 1964;188:307-9.

54. Peters RL, Edmondson HA, Mikkelsen WP et al. Tetracycline-induced fatty liver in nonpregnant patients; a report of six cases. Am J Surg 1967;113:622-32.

55. Gregory DH, Zaki GF, Sarcosi GA et al. Chronic cholestasis following prolonged tolbutamide administration. Arch Path 1967;84:194-201.

56. Ticktin HE, Zimmerman HJ. Hepatic dysfunction and jaundice in patients receiving triacetyloleandomycin. N Engl J Med 1962;267:964-8.

57. Goldenberg VE, Wiegenstein L, Hopkins GB. Hepatic injury associated with tromethamine. JAMA 1968;205:81-4.

58. Anon. Sodium valproate and the liver. Lancet 1980;2:1119-20.

59. Ware S, Millward-Sadier GH. Acute liver disease associated with sodium valproate. Lancet 1980;2:1110-3.

60. Jeavons PM. Sodium valproate and acute hepatic failure. Develop Med Child Neurol 1980;22:547-8.

61. Petersen EA, Alling DW, Kirkpatrick CH. Treatment of chronic mucocutaneous candidiasis with ketoconazole. Ann Intern Med 1980;93:791-5.

62. Heiberg JK, Svejgaard E. Toxic hepatitis during ketoconazole treatment. Brit Med J 1981;283:825-6.

Drug-Induced Nephrotoxicity

THE AGENTS IN THE FOLLOWING TABLE have been associated with drug-induced nephrotoxicity. Each is accompanied by a brief description of the nature of its nephrotoxicity and references which will be of assistance to the reader who wants additional information. Not included in this table are drugs which produce nephrotoxicity as a result of damage to organs other than the kidney.

The table begins on page 86.

Drug-Induced Nephrotoxicity

DRUG	NATURE OF NEPHROTOXICITY
Acetaminophen	Proximal tubular necrosis has been reported, most frequently in association with hepatotoxicity seen in acute overdose. Whether the nephrotoxicity is a direct effect of acetaminophen or the result of the liver damage is the subject of some controversy, because it has been reported in cases where the only evidence of hepatotoxicity is mild elevation of serum enzymes. Acetaminophen has also been implicated in some cases of analgesic nephropathy (see Analgesics) and interstitial nephritis[1-3,8,9]
Allopurinol	Tubular necrosis with fibrinoid deposits has been seen in patients experiencing generalized hypersensitivity reactions to allopurinol. A few cases of interstitial nephritis have also been reported[1-3]
Aminoglycoside Antibiotics	Proximal tubular necrosis is a feature of all members of this antibiotic group. These drugs accumulate in renal tissues, but there does not appear to be a good correlation between renal tissue concentrations of individual aminoglycosides and their nephrotoxic potential. The reported frequency of nephrotoxicity varies widely, but has been as high as 20–30% in some series. The nephrotoxicity of aminoglycosides is shown below:

Nephrotoxic Potential

DRUG		DRUG	
Amikacin	+ +	Netilmicin	+ / + +
Gentamicin	+ +	Sisomicin	+ / + +
Kanamycin	+ +	Streptomycin	+
Neomycin	+ + +	Tobramycin	+

Aminoglycoside-induced acute renal failure is usually nonoliguric, which may delay its recognition. Monitoring of aminoglycoside plasma levels and renal function tests may be of value in recognizing nephrotoxicity. Aminoglycoside nephrotoxicity seems to correlate best with plasma trough concentrations of the antibiotics.

Continued

Drug-Induced Nephrotoxicity

DRUG	NATURE OF NEPHROTOXICITY
	Very early evidence of renal damage includes an increased number of casts in the urine and elevated urine levels of β_2-microglobulins and enzymes such as leucine aminopeptidase[1,2,4,6,10-13]
Amphotericin B	Some degree of nephrotoxicity is observed in almost all patients treated with amphotericin B. The drug causes renal vasoconstriction as well as glomerular and tubular damage. Distal tubular damage may lead to loss of concentrating ability, renal tubular acidosis and electrolyte disturbances, especially hypokalemia. These effects appear to be dose-related and many patients respond favorably to temporary drug discontinuation or a reduction in dose[1,2,4,7]
Ampicillin	See Penicillins
Analgesics	Analgesic nephropathy is a syndrome of papillary necrosis and progressive renal medullary impairment seen in persons who have chronically consumed large quantities of oral analgesic products. The syndrome is characterized by proteinuria, reduced urine concentrating ability and the presence of WBCs in the urine. Analgesic nephropathy is usually attributed to **phenacetin**, but the possible contribution of other analgesics, especially **salicylates**, cannot be ignored. Historically, this syndrome has been responsible for a significant percentage of chronic renal failure cases in some series. The withdrawal of phenacetin from nonprescription analgesics appears responsible for the recent decline in the number of reported cases of analgesic nephropathy. Mild cases are reversible, but severe cases may continue to deteriorate after the withdrawal of the offending drug[1,2,8]
Asparaginase	As many as 25% of patients treated with this drug show some evidence of nephrotoxicity (eg, casts, hematuria, albuminuria)[1]
Captopril	Proteinuria accompanies membranous glomerulonephritis in 3+ % of patients treated with captopril. The onset of proteinuria is often delayed until about the fourth month of therapy. The significance of the proteinuria is unknown since most patients improve despite continued therapy[14,15]
Carmustine	See Nitrosoureas

Continued

Drug-Induced Nephrotoxicity

DRUG	NATURE OF NEPHROTOXICITY
Cephalosporins	The cephalosporin (and cephamycin) antibiotics are capable of rarely producing interstitial nephritis similar to penicillins, although this has not yet been reported with some of the newly introduced members of the class. Cephaloridine is the most nephrotoxic of the cephalosporins, causing a dose-related acute tubular necrosis which may be the result of greater tubular cell uptake of the drug[1-5,16]
Cisplatin	Acute tubular necrosis is a major limiting factor in cisplatin therapy and appears more likely when the drug is administered repetitively at close time intervals. Forced hydration and diuretics may reduce renal toxicity. Urinary levels of N-acetyl-β-glucosaminidase, leucine aminopeptidase and β_2-microglobulins are sensitive, but nonspecific, indicators of nephrotoxicity. Most patients will recover in 3–4 weeks after discontinuation of the drug, but permanent damage has been reported[1,2,17,18]
Contrast Media	A variety of renal lesions have been associated with the use of radiocontrast media including osmotic nephrosis, medullary necrosis, proximal tubular vacuolation and necrosis as well as the deposition of oxalate crystals. The most common pattern is acute oliguric renal failure developing within 24 hr after the administration of the media and lasting 2–4 days. Most patients recover fully. The cholecystographic dyes appear to be more nephrotoxic than those used for urinary visualization. Vigorous hydration of the patient and limiting the total dose of iodine in the administered contrast media to 80 g or less may reduce the risk of nephrotoxicity[1,2,19-21]
Demeclocycline	This drug is capable of producing nephrogenic diabetes insipidus which is usually, but not always, dose-related. It has been used in the management of the syndrome of inappropriate antidiuretic hormone secretion. See also Tetracyclines[1,2,4,6]
Dextrans	Glomerulonephritis resulting from a hypersensitivity reaction has been reported (particularly with high molecular weight dextran), but the most common lesion is osmotic nephrosis and physical plugging of renal tubules with high viscosity urine. Adequate hydration of the patient minimizes this problem[1,2,22]
Fenoprofen	See Ibuprofen

Continued

Drug-Induced Nephrotoxicity

DRUG	NATURE OF NEPHROTOXICITY
Gold Salts	A lesion resembling membranous glomerulonephritis with proteinuria may be encountered in as many as 10% of patients receiving gold salts. Nephrotic syndrome is less common (0.3%). Occasional cases of acute tubular necrosis have also been reported. There is evidence for both immune and direct toxic mechanisms for gold nephrotoxicity[1,2,6,23,24]
Ibuprofen	All of the arylcarboxylic acid derived nonsteroidal anti-inflammatory agents can reduce creatinine clearance and produce a nonoliguric renal failure, probably as a result of renal circulatory changes brought about by the inhibition of prostaglandin synthesis. This effect tends to be relatively minor and is usually associated with long-term therapy. **Fenoprofen** and **naproxen** have been associated with the development of tubulo-interstitial nephritis and nephrotic syndrome. Withdrawal of the drug usually results in a reversal of symptoms[1-3,25-27]
Indomethacin	This drug has effects on creatinine clearance similar to other nonsteroidal anti-inflammatory agents (see Ibuprofen). This nonoliguric renal failure is of greatest concern in patients who are volume depleted or have other renal circulatory deficiencies[1,28,29]
Lithium	This drug can produce a nephrogenic diabetes insipidus which is, at least in part, dose-related. This effect is usually reversible with withdrawal of the drug, but some prolonged cases have been reported. Interstitial nephritis, renal fibrosis and glomerular atrophy have also been reported[1-3,30-33]
Lomustine	See Nitrosoureas
Methicillin	See Penicillins
Methotrexate	This drug is directly toxic to the kidney in large doses, producing acute tubular necrosis. Because methotrexate is significantly eliminated through the kidney, its nephrotoxicity compounds itself by causing the plasma levels of drug to rise. Close monitoring of methotrexate plasma levels may help to minimize nephrotoxicity[1,2,34,35]

Continued

Drug-Induced Nephrotoxicity

DRUG	NATURE OF NEPHROTOXICITY
Methoxyflurane	Nephrogenic diabetes insipidus has been reported with this drug. Proximal tubular damage and interstitial nephritis are also reported. The nephrotoxicity of methoxyflurane appears to be dose-related and may be due to increases in circulating fluoride ion concentrations. Urinary oxalate crystallization has also been reported following methoxyflurane anesthesia[1,2,36-38]
Naproxen	See Ibuprofen
Nitrosoureas	The nitrosoureas produce some degree of interstitial nephritis (resembling radiation nephritis) in almost all patients on long-term therapy[2,39,40]
Penicillamine	Slight to moderate proteinuria occurs in about 15% of patients on long-term therapy with penicillamine. The lesions appear to be perimembranous glomerulonephritis resulting from the deposition of antigen-antibody complexes on the renal basement membrane. Some patients may progress to nephrotic syndrome. Deaths have been reported in cases of glomerular damage without evidence of immune complex involvement[1,2,41]
Penicillins	Interstitial nephritis has been reported with a number of penicillins including **amoxicillin, ampicillin, carbenicillin, methicillin, nafcillin, oxacillin** and **penicillin G.** Methicillin is by far the most frequently implicated penicillin. The reason for its dominance is not known. Penicillin interstitial nephritis is an immune reaction which is most commonly encountered during a long course of drug therapy. The reaction is usually accompanied by other signs of hypersensitivity such as fever, rash and eosinophilia. Hematuria may also be encountered. The reduction in renal function may or may not be oliguric, so urine volume is not a good parameter to monitor[1-4,42]
Phenacetin	See Analgesics
Phenazopyridine	This drug may deposit in renal tubules (phenazopyridine stones) and interstitial tissues. Oliguria, casts, rising BUN and declining creatinine clearance are characteristic of phenazopyridine nephrotoxicity[1,2]

Continued

Drug-Induced Nephrotoxicity

DRUG	NATURE OF NEPHROTOXICITY
Phenylbutazone	Acute renal failure, papillary necrosis and interstitial nephritis have been seen in patients taking phenylbutazone with other anti-inflammatory drugs or with high doses of phenylbutazone alone[1-3]
Phenytoin	Interstitial nephritis and reversible acute renal failure can occur as part of a generalized hypersensitivity reaction to phenytoin, but this reaction is rare[1,43]
Polymyxins	Adverse reactions involving the kidney occur in about 20% of patients receiving polymyxins. Tubular necrosis is the most commonly described lesion, but interstitial nephritis has also been reported. High doses, long durations of therapy and renal impairment are predisposing factors. Polymyxin-induced renal damage is usually reversible, but some patients continue to deteriorate after the drug has been withdrawn[1,2,4,6]
Rifampin	There are scattered reports of rifampin-induced acute renal failure resulting from tubulo-interstitial nephritis. This appears to be a hypersensitivity reaction and is most frequently seen in intermittent dosage regimens[1-4,7,44]
Salicylates	See Analgesics
Semustine	See Nitrosoureas
Sulfonamides, Antibacterial	Early sulfonamides were poorly soluble and urinary crystallization was a common problem. Today, the prevalence of crystallization is less than 0.3% with the use of the more soluble sulfonamides and adequate hydration. Interstitial nephritis, glomerulonephritis and tubular necrosis have also been reported, although rarely. These reactions are probably allergic in origin[1-4,7,45]
Sulfones	Nephrotic syndrome is an occasional complication of sulfone therapy[2,46]
Tetracyclines	Fanconi syndrome, characterized by tubular damage with proteinuria, glycosuria, amino-aciduria and elec- Continued

Drug-Induced Nephrotoxicity

DRUG	NATURE OF NEPHROTOXICITY
	trolyte disturbances, was associated with the use of outdated early tetracycline products. This syndrome is no longer likely to occur, because of changes in the manufacturing process. The anti-anabolic effects of tetracyclines can contribute to azotemia in patients with pre-existing renal impairment[1,2,4,6]
Thiazide Diuretics	Occasional cases of interstitial nephritis have been reported. These cases may be the result of hypersensitivity reactions[3,47]
Triamterene	About 0.4% of renal calculi contain triamterene, some of which consist almost entirely of triamterene. One report has suggested that one in 1,500 users of the drug will develop triamterene-associated calculi during the course of a year. As a precaution, the drug probably should not be used in patients with a history of renal calculi[1,2,48]
Trimethadione	Nephrotic syndrome with significant proteinuria has been associated with trimethadione therapy. Early discontinuation of the drug usually results in complete recovery, but some deaths have been reported. The onset of the nephrotic syndrome may be delayed until after months or years of therapy[1,2,49]
Vancomycin	There were some reports of nephrotoxicity associated with early formulations of vancomycin. These reactions may have been due to impurities and nephrotoxicity is only rarely encountered with vancomycin now[1,4,6]

References

1. Dukes MNG, ed. Meyler's side effects of drugs. 9th ed. Amsterdam: Excerpta Medica, 1980.

2. Roxe DM. Toxic nephropathy from diagnostic and therapeutic agents: review and commentary. Am J Med 1980;69:759-66.

3. Linton AL, Clark WF, Driedger AA et al. Acute interstitial nephritis due to drugs: review of the literature with a report of nine cases. Ann Intern Med 1980;93:735-41.

4. Kucers A, Bennett NMcK. The use of antibiotics. 3rd ed. Philadelphia: JB Lippincott, 1979.

5. Appel GB, Neu HC. The nephrotoxicity of antimicrobial agents (first of three parts). N Engl J Med 1977;296:663-70.

6. Appel GB, Neu HC. The nephrotoxicity of antimicrobial agents (second of three parts). N Engl J Med 1977;296:722-8.

7. Appel GB, Neu HC. The nephrotoxicity of antimicrobial agents (third of three parts). N Engl J Med 1977;296:784-7.

8. Duggin GG. Mechanisms in the development of analgesic nephropathy. Kidney Int 1980;18:553-61.

9. Kleinman JG, Breitenfield RV, Roth DA. Acute renal failure associated with acetaminophen ingestion: report of a case and review of the literature. Clin Nephrol 1980;14:201-5.

10. Kaloyanides GJ, Pastoriza-Munoz E. Aminoglycoside nephrotoxicity. Kidney Int 1980;18:571-82.

11. DiPiro JT, Rush DS, Record KE et al. Gentamicin nephrotoxicity during dosing controlled by gentamicin serum levels. Drug Intell Clin Pharm 1980;14:53-5.

12. Schentag JJ, Gengo FM, Plaut ME et al. Urinary casts as an indicator of renal tubular damage in patients receiving aminoglycosides. Antimicrob Agents Chemother 1979;16:468-74.

13. Schentag JJ, Plaut ME. Patterns of urinary β_2-microglobulin excretion by patients treated with aminoglycosides. Kidney Int 1980;17:654-61.

14. Case DB, Atlas SA, Mouradian JA et al. Proteinuria during long-term captopril therapy. JAMA 1980;244:346-9.

15. Capoten® Monograph. ER Squibb & Sons, 1981:51.

16. Barza M. The nephrotoxicity of cephalosporins: an overview. J Infect Dis 1978;137(Suppl):S60-73.

17. Madias NE, Harrington JT. Platinum nephrotoxicity. Am J Med 1978;65:307-14.

18. Jones BR, Bhalla RB, Mladek J et al. Comparison of methods of evaluating nephrotoxicity of cis-platinum. Clin Pharmacol Ther 1980;27:557-62.

19. Mudge GH. Nephrotoxicity of urographic radiocontrast drugs. Kidney Int 1980;18:540-52.

20. Lang EK, Foreman J, Schlegel JU et al. The incidence of contrast medium induced acute tubular necrosis following arteriography. Radiology 1981;138:203-6.

21. Byrd L, Sherman RL. Radiocontrast-induced acute renal failure: a clinical and pathophysiologic review. Medicine 1979;58:270-9.

22. Van DenBerg CJ, Pineda AA. Plasma exchange in the treatment of acute renal failure due to low molecular-weight dextran. Mayo Clin Proc 1980;55:387-9.

23. Watanabe I, Whittier FC, Moore J et al. Gold nephropathy: ultrastructural, fluorescence, and microanalytic studies of two patients. Arch Pathol Lab Med 1976;100:632-5.

24. Robbins G, McIllmurray MB. Acute renal failure due to gold. Postgrad Med J 1980;56:366-7.

25. Kimberly RP, Bowden RE, Keiser HR et al. Reduction of renal function by newer nonsteroidal anti-inflammatory drugs. Am J Med 1978;64:804-7.

26. Handa SP. Renal effects of fenoprofen. Ann Intern Med 1980;93:508.

27. Wendland ML, Wagoner RD, Holley KE. Renal failure associated with fenoprofen. Mayo Clin Proc 1980;55:103-7.

28. Dunn MJ, Zambraski EJ. Renal effects of drugs that inhibit prostaglandin synthesis. Kidney Int 1980;18:609-22.

29. O'Meara ME, Eknoyan G. Acute renal failure associated with indomethacin administration. South Med J 1980;73:587-9.

30. Myers JB, Morgan TO, Carney SL et al. Effects of lithium on the kidney. Kidney Int 1980;18:601-8.

31. Hwang S, Tuason VB. Long-term maintenance lithium therapy and possible irreversible renal damage. J Clin Psychiatry 1980;41:11-9.

32. Vestergaard P, Amdisen A, Hansen HE et al. Lithium treatment and kidney function: a survey of 237 patients in long-term treatment. Acta Psychiatr Scand 1979;60:504-20.

33. Donker AJM, Prins E, Meijer S et al. A renal function study in 30 patients on long-term lithium therapy. Clin Nephrol 1979;12:254-62.

34. Condit PT, Chanes RE, Joel W. Renal toxicity of methotrexate. Cancer 1969;23:126-31.

35. Stoller RG, Hande KR, Jacobs SA et al. Use of plasma pharmacokinetics to predict and prevent methotrexate toxicity. N Engl J Med 1977;297:630-4.

36. Desmond JW. Methoxyflurane nephrotoxicity. Can Anaesth Soc J 1974;21:294-307.

37. Cousins MJ, Mazze RI. Methoxyflurane nephrotoxicity: a study of dose response in man. JAMA 1973;225:1611-6.

38. Mazze RI, Shue GL, Jackson SH. Renal dysfunction associated with methoxyflurane anesthesia: a randomized, prospective clinical evaluation. JAMA 1971;216:278-88.

39. Harmon WE, Cohen HJ, Schneeberger EE et al. Chronic renal failure in children treated with methyl CCNU. N Engl J Med 1979;300:1200-3.

40. Schacht RG, Baldwin DS. Chronic interstitial nephritis and renal failure due to nitrosourea (NU) therapy (abstract). Kidney Int 1978;14:661.

41. Falck HM, Tornroth T, Kock B et al. Fatal renal vasculitis and minimal change glomerulonephritis complicating treatment with penicillamine. Acta Med Scand 1979;205:133-8.

42. Appel GB. A decade of penicillin related acute interstitial nephritis—more questions than answers. Clin Nephrol 1980;13:151-4.

43. Michael JR, Mitch WE. Reversible renal failure and myositis caused by phenytoin hypersensitivity. JAMA

1976;236:2773-5.

44. Qunibi WY, Godwin J, Eknoyan G. Toxic nephropathy during continuous rifampin therapy. South Med J 1980;73:791-2.

45. Smith EJ, Light JA, Filo RS et al. Interstitial nephritis caused by trimethoprim-sulfamethoxazole in renal transplant recipients. JAMA 1980;244:360-1.

46. Belmont A. Dapsone-induced nephrotic syndrome. JAMA 1967;200:262-3.

47. Magil AB, Ballon HS, Cameron EC et al. Acute interstitial nephritis associated with thiazide diuretics: clinical and pathologic observations in three cases. Am J Med 1980;69:939-43.

48. Ettinger B, Oldroyd NO, Sorgel F. Triamterene nephrolithiasis. JAMA 1980;244:2443-5.

49. Heymann W. Nephrotic syndrome after use of trimethadione and paramethadione in petit mal. JAMA 1967;202:893-4.

Drug-Induced Oculotoxicity

THE AGENTS IN THE FOLLOWING TABLE have been associated with drug-induced ocular toxicity when administered *systemically*. Occasionally, nonspecific blurred vision occurs with almost all drugs; the drugs in this table are those having a definite association with a specific pattern of oculotoxicity. The oculotoxicity of each drug is briefly described and the discussions are accompanied by a list of references for the reader who wants additional information.

The table begins on page 95.

Drug-Induced Oculotoxicity

DRUG	NATURE OF OCULOTOXICITY
Anticholinergics	These drugs dilate the pupil (mydriasis) and may precipitate narrow angle glaucoma. With systemic administration, large doses are usually required to produce this effect and it is most commonly associated with potent anticholinergics such as **atropine**, **scopolamine** or **benztropine**. Patients who are being treated for narrow angle glaucoma should be able to tolerate systemic anticholinergic therapy, but should nevertheless avoid these drugs unless absolutely necessary. Patients with open angle glaucoma, particularly if treated, can receive anticholinergic medications without significant hazard. Blurring of vision can result from paralysis of accommodation (cycloplegia); photophobia is possible as a result of mydriasis. All of the ocular effects of anticholinergics are dose-related and reversible [1,2,4,5]
Antidepressants, Tricyclic	These drugs all possess anticholinergic properties and are capable of precipitating narrow angle glaucoma (see Anticholinergics). The frequency of blurred vision resulting from cycloplegia ranges from 10–20%. This effect is rarely troublesome and is reversible upon withdrawal of the drug. Gaze paralysis (ophthalmoplegia) has been occasionally encountered with tricyclic antidepressant overdosage. Ophthalmoplegia responds to IV **physostigmine** [1,2,4,6,7]
Antihistamines (H$_1$-blockers)	These drugs all possess some degree of anticholinergic activity and are capable of precipitating narrow angle glaucoma and cycloplegia (see Anticholinergics). These effects tend to be minor and are reversible upon withdrawal of the drug. Antihistamines may significantly reduce night vision [1,9,10]
Bromocriptine	Myopia appears to be a fairly common, but often unrecognized complication of bromocriptine therapy. It may be the result of lens swelling, but this has not been fully determined. This effect is reversible within 1–2 weeks after withdrawal of the drug [1,9,10]
Chloramphenicol	Optic neuritis has been reported in at least 23 patients receiving chloramphenicol. This effect has been encountered after as few as 17 days or as long as 2 years of therapy. Most of the cases have been reported in children with cystic fibrosis, but the association with this disorder is unclear. Both permanent visual impairment and recovery after withdrawal have been reported. It has been suggested that large doses of B vitamins may have a beneficial effect, but no definitive data have been presented [11-15]

Continued

Drug-Induced Oculotoxicity

DRUG	NATURE OF OCULOTOXICITY
Chloroquine	The oculotoxicity of chloroquine limits its usefulness. Two general types of ocular changes are associated with chloroquine use: corneal deposits and retinopathy. About 50% of the patients treated with chloroquine demonstrate corneal deposits and less than one-half of these have visual impairment resulting from the deposits. Opacities present as punctate or whirling patterns and are usually reversible when chloroquine is withdrawn. Early changes in the retina (deposition of pigment in the macula) are usually asymptomatic and reversible. More advanced damage includes hyperpigmentation of the macula with one or more concentric rings of alternating hypo- and hyperpigmentation ("bull's eye" retinopathy). Patients complain of reading difficulty, blurred vision, visual field defects (scotomas) and photophobia; some may also report defective color vision and light flashes. Chloroquine retinopathy is dose-related, with the majority of patients having taken more than 250 mg/day for longer than 2 years. The prevalence of chloroquine retinopathy increases with age. Prognosis is uncertain; the vision of many patients may continue to deteriorate after withdrawal of the drug[1-3,16-19]
Clomiphene	Approximately 2–10% of patients taking clomiphene complain of visual disturbances, most commonly blurred vision; these will disappear after the drug is withdrawn[2,22,23]
Contraceptives, Oral	A variety of retinal vascular disorders have been attributed to oral contraceptives. The association between contraceptive use and these vascular changes remains to be fully determined. Some oral contraceptive users cannot tolerate contact lenses, possibly due to ocular edema[2,20,21]
Corticosteroids	These drugs are capable of producing a variety of ocular disorders, most notably glaucoma and cataracts. Steroid-induced increases in intra-ocular pressure appear to be dose-related and may persist for several months after withdrawal of the drug. The exact mechanism is unknown, but some have proposed that the accumulation of mucopolysaccharides may play a role. Steroid-induced cataracts (usually posterior subcapsular) are found in 10–20% of patients on long-term corticosteroid therapy. Cataract formation is not dose-dependent and some patients may improve despite continued therapy[1-3,24,25]
Cyclophosphamide	One report shows a high prevalence (17%) of transient reversible blurred vision during cyclophosphamide therapy. Recovery took from 1 hour to 14 days[25] Continued

Drug-Induced Oculotoxicity

DRUG	NATURE OF OCULOTOXICITY
Digitalis Glycosides	The most unique feature of the ocular effects of these drugs is the frosted or snowy appearance of objects or the presence of colored halos around them. These effects are most noticeable in bright light. Color vision may be affected so that objects appear yellow or green (other colors have been reported, but far less frequently). Digitalis glycosides have also been reported to produce photophobia, blurred vision, scotoma and flickering or light flashes before the eyes. Ocular side effects are seen in as many as 25% of digitalis intoxication patients. These effects are usually reversible upon withdrawal of the drug[1-3,27]
Disulfiram	A small number of cases of retrobulbar neuritis, with a dramatic decline in visual acuity and impairment of color vision, have occurred. In most cases, vision returned to normal after the drug was discontinued[1,2]
Ethambutol	Retrobulbar neuritis is the primary ocular complication of ethambutol therapy. Symptoms include blurred vision, scotoma and reduction of the visual field. Color vision defects are also encountered, usually presenting as a reduction in green perception. These effects are dose-related, occurring most frequently with doses of 25 mg/kg/day or more, and are slowly reversible after drug withdrawal. Doses of 10-15 mg/kg/day appear relatively free of ocular side effects[1-3,11,12]
Fluorouracil	Excessive lacrimation can be expected in about 50% of patients treated with systemic fluorouracil; this effect is reversible. Some patients develop potentially irreversible fibrosis of the tear duct (dacryostenosis), if the drug is not withdrawn[28-30]
Gold Salts	These drugs can produce microscopic crystalline deposits in the cornea, most commonly in the superficial layers. This effect is dose-related and rarely encountered until the total dose of gold exceeds 1 g. The deposits slowly resolve after withdrawal of gold therapy. The accumulation of gold in the cornea does not appear to affect vision and is not a reason to stop gold therapy[1,2,31]
Hydroxychloroquine	This drug can produce the same spectrum of ocular toxicity as chloroquine (see Chloroquine), but the prevalence appears to be less[2,3,32]

Continued

Drug-Induced Oculotoxicity

DRUG	NATURE OF OCULOTOXICITY
Indomethacin	A number of ocular effects, including blurred vision, corneal deposits and a variety of retinopathies, have been attributed to indomethacin. The recent literature, however, is devoid of any reports of indomethacin-induced oculotoxicity, and the latest published data fail to support the earlier reports of these effects [1-3, 33, 34]
Isoniazid	Optic neuritis is one of the possible neuropathies resulting from isoniazid. It occurs infrequently and most often in malnourished or alcoholic patients. It responds to **pyridoxine therapy** [1-3]
Metoprolol	Eye discomfort has been reported in 20% of patients in one study. Typical symptoms include ocular pain and conjunctival dryness. In view of the reports of ocular toxicity with other beta-adrenergic blockers (see Practolol and Propranolol), patients on metoprolol should be closely monitored for ocular effects [35, 36]
Oxygen	Retrolental fibroplasia is a significant complication of oxygen therapy in neonates, particularly premature or other low birth weight neonates. The risk of retrolental fibroplasia in these patients increases whenever the inspired air oxygen concentration exceeds normal [1, 2, 37, 38]
Phenothiazines	Lesions of the lens, cornea and retina are the most important features of phenothiazine-induced ocular toxicity. White to yellow-brown deposits in the lens are most frequently seen with long-term, high-dose (>1 kg total) **chlorpromazine therapy**. Similar deposits can also be found in the corneas of chlorpromazine-treated patients. Epithelial keratopathy, possibly resulting from a photosensitivity reaction, can occur after only a few months of high-dose therapy. It is characterized by a diffuse opacification of the corneal epithelium. Lens and corneal deposits usually do not interfere with vision, and all of these effects may be slowly reversible. **Thioridazine** is also capable of producing lens and corneal deposits, but it is most noted for pigmentary retinopathy. As with most phenothiazine-induced ocular effects, pigmentary retinopathy is dose-related. Patients may complain of blurred vision, decreased night vision, brown discoloration of vision and scotoma. Vision may improve if the drug is withdrawn soon enough; however, some cases have continued to deteriorate despite drug withdrawal. Phenothiazines possess mild anticholinergic effects and may precipitate narrow angle glaucoma [1-4, 6, 39]

Continued

Drug-Induced Oculotoxicity

DRUG	NATURE OF OCULOTOXICITY
Practolol	This beta-adrenergic blocker has been reported to produce a reduction in tear production, subconjunctival fibrosis and occasionally corneal ulcerations. This effect is related to an increased level of circulating anti-nuclear antibodies which may have an affinity for squamous epithelium[40,41]
Propranolol	A reduction in tear production can result in a hot, dry and gritty sensation in the eye during propranolol therapy. This effect is rapidly reversible upon withdrawal of the drug[2,42,43]
Quinidine	Amblyopia, scotoma, double or blurred vision, impaired color vision and, very rarely, blindness have been associated with quinidine overdose. Most quinidine-induced ocular changes are transient[2,3,44]
Quinine	Loss of visual acuity and reduction of the visual field to the point of blindness can be encountered with quinine therapy or overdosage. These effects are usually reversible and may be the result of changes in the retinal vasculature[1,2,45]
Rifampin	Exudative conjunctivitis, ocular pain and orange staining of tears and contact lenses have been reported with rifampin. These rare effects are rapidly reversible[1,2,46,47]
Sympathomimetics	These drugs are capable of dilating the pupil and precipitating narrow angle glaucoma. The risk of this reaction is slight unless large doses are administered[2,4]
Tamoxifen	Fine, white, refractile retinal opacities have been reported in patients taking tamoxifen; some corneal opacities have also been reported. These lesions have been associated with reduced visual acuity[48,49]

References

1. Dukes MNG, ed. Meyler's side effects of drugs. 9th ed. Amsterdam: Excerpta Medica, 1980.

2. Fraunfelder FT. Drug-induced ocular side effects and drug interactions. Philadelphia: Lea & Febiger, 1976.

3. Applebaum M. Drug toxicity and visual fields. J Am Optom Assoc 1980;51:859-62.

4. Durkee DP, Bryant BG. Drug therapy reviews: drug therapy of glaucoma. Am J Hosp Pharm 1978;35:682-90.

5. Hiatt RL, Fuller IB, Smith L et al. Systemically administered anticholinergic drugs and intraocular pressure. Arch Ophthalmol 1970;84:735-40.

6. Klein DF, Gittelman R, Quitkin F et al. Diagnosis and drug treatment of psychiatric disorders: adults and children. 2nd ed. Baltimore: Williams & Wilkins, 1980.

7. Smith MS. Amitriptyline ophthalmoplegia. Ann Intern Med 1979;91:793.

8. Luria SM, Kinney JAS, McKay CL et al. Effects of aspirin and dimenhydrinate (Dramamine) on visual processes. Br J Clin Pharmacol 1979;7:585-93.

9. Calne DB, Plotkin C, Williams AC et al. Long-term treatment of parkinsonism with bromocriptine. Lancet 1978;1:735-8.

10. Manor RS, Dickerman Z, Llaron Z. Myopia during bromocriptine treatment. Lancet 1981;1:102.

11. Dukes MNG, ed. Side effects of drugs, annual 4. Amsterdam: Excerpta Medica, 1980.

12. Kucers A, Bennett NMcK. The use of antibiotics. 3rd ed. Philadelphia: JB Lippincott, 1979.

13. Cocke JG. Chloramphenicol optic neuritis: apparent protective effects of very high daily doses of pyridoxine and cyanocobalamin. Am J Dis Child 1967;114:424-6.

14. Cocke JG, Brown RE, Geppert LJ. Optic neuritis with prolonged use of chloramphenicol. J Pediatr 1966;68:27-31.

15. Huang NN, Harley RD, Promadhattavedi V et al. Visual disturbances in cystic fibrosis following chloramphenicol administration. J Pediatr 1966;68:32-44.

16. Ogawa S, Kurumatani N, Shibaike N et al. Progression of retinopathy long after cessation of chloroquine therapy. Lancet 1979;1:1408.

17. Marks JS, Power BJ. Is chloroquine obsolete in the treatment of rheumatic disease? Lancet 1979;1:371-3.

18. Elman A, Gullberg R, Nilsson E et al. Chloroquine retinopathy in patients with rheumatoid arthritis. Scand J Rheumatol 1976;5:161-6.

19. Bernstein HN. Chloroquine ocular toxicity. Surv Ophthalmol 1967;12:415-47.

20. Svarc ED, Werner D. Isolated retinal hemorrhages associated with oral contraceptives. Am J Ophthalmol 1977;84:50-5.

21. Perry HD, Mallen FJ. Cilioretinal artery occlusion associated with oral contraceptives. Am J Ophthalmol 1977;84:56-8.

22. MacGregor AH, Johnson JE, Bunde CA. Further clinical experience with clomiphene citrate. Fertil Steril 1968;19:616-22.

23. Roch LM, Gordon DL, Barr AB et al. Visual changes associated with clomiphene citrate therapy. Arch Ophthalmol 1967;77:14-7.

24. Skalka HW, Prchal JT. Effect of corticosteroids on cataract formation. Arch Ophthalmol 1980;98:1773-7.

25. Forman AR, Loreto JA, Tina LU. Reversibility of corticosteroid-associated cataracts in children with the nephrotic syndrome. Am J Ophthalmol 1977;84:75-8.

26. Kende G, Sirkin SR, Thomas PRM et al. Blurring of vision: a previously undescribed complication of cyclophosphamide therapy. Cancer 1979;44:69-71.

27. Robertson DM, Hollenhorst RW, Callahan JA. Ocular manifestations of digitalis toxicity. Arch Ophthalmol 1966;76:640-5.

28. Christophidis N, Vajda FJE, Lucas I et al. Ocular side effects with 5-fluorouracil. Aust NZ J Med 1979;9:143-4.

29. Christophidis N, Lucas I, Vajda FJE et al. Lacrimation and 5-fluorouracil. Ann Intern Med 1978;89:574.

30. Haidak DJ, Hurwitz BS, Yeung KY. Tear-duct fibrosis (dacryostenosis) due to 5-fluorouracil. Ann Intern Med 1978;88:657.

31. Bron AJ, McLendon BF, Camp AV. Epithelial deposition of gold in the cornea in patients receiving systemic therapy. Am J Ophthalmol 1979;88:354-60.

32. Rynes RI, Krohel G, Falbo A et al. Ophthalmologic safety of long-term hydroxychloroquine treatment. Arthritis Rheum 1979;22:832-6.

33. Carr RE, Siegel IM. Retinal function in patients treated with indomethacin. Am J Ophthalmol 1973;75:302-6.

34. Burns CA. Indomethacin, reduced retinal sensitivity, and corneal deposits. Am J Ophthalmol 1968;66:825-35.

35. McNeil JJ, Louis WJ, Doyle AE et al. Comparison of metoprolol and pindolol in the treatment of mild to moderate hypertension: a double-blind crossover study. Med J Aust 1979;1:431-3,61.

36. Scott D. Another beta-blocker causing eye symptoms? Br Med J 1977;2:1221.

37. Betts EK, Downes JJ, Schaffer DB et al. Retrolental fibroplasia and oxygen administration during general anesthesia. Anesthesiology 1977;47:518-20.

38. Committee on Fetus and Newborn, American Academy of Pediatrics. History of oxygen therapy and retrolental fibroplasia. Pediatrics 1976;57(suppl):591-642.

39. Bond WS, Yee GC. Ocular and cutaneous effects of chronic phenothiazine therapy. Am J Hosp Pharm 1980;37:74-8.

40. Garner A. Rahi AHS. Practolol and ocular toxicity: antibodies in serum and tears. Br J Ophthalmol 1976;60:684-5.

41. Rahi AHS, Chapman CM, Garner A et al. Pathology of practolol-induced ocular toxicity. Br J Ophthalmol 1976;60:312-23.

42. Halloran TJ. Propranolol and eye symptoms. JAMA 1979;241:2784-5.

43. Cubey RB, Taylor SH. Ocular reaction to propranolol and resolution on continued treatment with a different beta-blocking drug. Br Med J 1975;4:327-8.

44. Abrams J. Quinidine toxicity: a review. Rocky Mt Med J 1973;70(May):31-4.
45. Valman HB, White DC. Stellate block for quinine blindness in a child. Br Med J 1977;1:1065.
46. Lyons RW. Orange contact lenses from rifampin. N Engl J Med 1979;300:372-3.
47. Cayley FE, Majumdar SK. Ocular toxicity due to rifampicin. Br Med J 1976;1:199-200.
48. McKeown CA, Swartz M, Blom J et al. Tamoxifen retinopathy. Br J Ophthalmol 1981;65:177-9.
49. Kaiser-Kupfer MI, Lippman ME. Tamoxifen retinopathy. Cancer Treat Rep 1978;62:315-20.

Drug-Induced Ototoxicity

THE AGENTS IN THE FOLLOWING TABLE have been reported to cause ototoxicity in man. Ototoxicity can affect hearing (auditory or cochlear function), balance (vestibular function) or both, depending upon the drug. The most common form of ototoxicity is tinnitus, characterized by the perception of a ringing or buzzing sound in the ears. Drugs of almost every class have been reported to produce tinnitus, as have placebos. The only drugs represented in this table are those which have demonstrated a clear capability of producing a measurable hearing or vestibular defect.

The table begins on page 102.

Drug-Induced Ototoxicity

DRUG	NATURE OF OTOTOXICITY
Aminoglycoside Antibiotics	Ototoxicity takes two forms, cochlear and vestibular. Cochlear presents as a progressive hearing loss starting with the highest tones and progressing toward lower tones. Thus, significant damage may have been done before the patient is cognizant of it. Vestibular damage presents as dizziness, vertigo or ataxia. Both forms of ototoxicity are usually bilateral and potentially reversible, but permanent damage is common and damage may progress after the discontinuation of aminoglycoside therapy. Most aminoglycoside-induced ototoxicity is associated with parenteral therapy, but it has followed topical, oral and irrigation use of these drugs, particularly with **neomycin.** In general, a patient should receive no more drug by these routes than by injection. Predisposing factors for ototoxicity include: reduced renal function; prolonged therapy (>2–3 weeks); plasma levels exceeding the therapeutic range; previous aminoglycoside use; use of other ototoxic drugs; dehydration and old age. Serial audiometry may be useful in early detection of ototoxicity. Each aminoglycoside antibiotic has a slightly different spectrum of ototoxicity; the table below will serve as a general guide:[1-9]

Ototoxic Potential

DRUG	COCHLEAR	VESTIBULAR
Amikacin	+ +	+
Gentamicin	+	+ +
Kanamycin	+ +	+
Neomycin	+ + + +	+
Netilmicin	+	+ +
Sisomicin	+	+ +
Streptomycin	+	+ + +
Tobramycin	+	+ / + +

Continued

Drug-Induced Ototoxicity

DRUG	NATURE OF OTOTOXICITY
Chloroquine	Nerve deafness is a rare, but consistent feature of chloroquine therapy. Its onset is often delayed and it has usually been thought of as irreversible and only accompanying long-term therapy. A partially reversible case and a case resulting from only 1 g of chloroquine have been reported[1-4,10,11]
Cisplatin	Hearing loss has been reported in an estimated 6% of patients receiving cisplatin, with tinnitus and audiogram abnormalities being reported in a much larger percentage of patients. Audiogram changes usually appear within 4 days after drug administration and high frequencies are lost first. The effects are dose-related and may be permanent[1,2,12,13]
Erythromycin	Reversible hearing loss has occasionally followed high-dose parenteral and oral therapy. The hearing loss does not seem to be due to any particular salt form. Impaired hepatic and renal function may contribute to the hearing loss[1-4,14-17]
Ethacrynic Acid and Furosemide	Rapid-onset hearing loss is a frequent feature of high-dose, rapid IV administration of these drugs. Renal failure is usually listed as a predisposing cause, but renal failure patients are the only ones likely to receive large IV doses. The hearing loss is usually transient, but permanent hearing loss has been reported, more often with ethacrynic acid than with furosemide. Administration of other ototoxic drugs such as **aminoglycoside** antibiotics may contribute to the hearing loss. Vestibular toxicity and hearing loss after oral administration have been encountered[1-4,18-22]
Minocycline	Reversible vestibular toxicity, manifested primarily by dizziness, loss of balance and lightheadedness, has been associated with minocycline therapy. This effect has been noted in as many as two-thirds of women patients in one study and appears to be dose-related. Women are significantly more susceptible than men[1-4,23-25]
Quinidine	Tinnitus and reversible hearing loss are well-known complications of quinidine therapy. Permanent hearing loss has been reported, but is uncommon[1-4]

Continued

Drug-Induced Ototoxicity

DRUG	NATURE OF OTOTOXICITY
Salicylates	Tinnitus, high frequency hearing loss and occasional vertigo are common features of salicylate intoxication. Hearing loss appears to be related to the salicylate plasma level, although there is a significant interpatient variability in the threshold plasma level at which it is first detected. Most patients demonstrating ototoxicity from salicylates are chronically receiving large doses, such as those used in rheumatoid arthritis. Salicylate ototoxicity, even if severe, is usually reversible, but permanent hearing loss has been reported[1-4,26,27]
Vancomycin	Transient and permanent hearing loss, often preceded by tinnitus, have been encountered. It is suggested that these effects are associated with high plasma levels of vancomycin; however, evidence for this is inconclusive. In the majority of cases reported, vancomycin was used either following or in combination with other potentially ototoxic drugs. The use of other ototoxic antibiotics may increase the risk of vancomycin ototoxicity[1,2,4,28]

References

1. Dukes MNG, ed. Meyler's side effects of drugs. 9th ed. Amsterdam: Excerpta Medica, 1980.
2. Brummett RE. Drug-induced ototoxicity. Drugs 1980;19:412-28.
3. Hybels RL. Drug toxicity of the inner ear. Med Clin North Am 1979;63:309-19.
4. Marlowe FI. Ototoxic agents. Otolaryngol Clin North Am 1978;11:791-800.
5. Black RE, Lau WK, Weinstein RJ et al. Ototoxicity of amikacin. Antimicrob Agents Chemother 1976;9:956-61.
6. Kalbian VV. Deafness following oral use of neomycin. South Med J 1972;65:499-501.
7. Masur H, Whelton PK, Whelton A. Neomycin toxicity revisited. Arch Surg 1976;111:822-5.
8. Bamford MFM, Jones LF. Deafness and biochemical imbalance after burns treatment with topical antibiotics in young children. Arch Dis Child 1978;53:326-9.
9. Smith CR, Lipsky JJ, Lietman PS. Relationship between aminoglycoside-induced nephrotoxicity and auditory toxicity. Antimicrob Agents Chemother 1979;15:780-2.
10. Dwivedi GS, Mehra YN. Ototoxicity of chloroquine phosphate. J Laryngol Otol 1978;92:701-3.
11. Mukherjee DK. Chloroquine ototoxicity—a reversible phenomenon? J Laryngol Otol 1979;93:809-15.
12. Helson L, Okonkwo E, Anton L et al. Cis-platinum ototoxicity. Clin Toxicol 1978;13:469-78.
13. Von Hoff DD, Schilsky R, Reichert CM et al. Toxic effects of cis-dichlorodiammineplatinum (II) in man. Cancer Treat Rep 1979;63:1527-31.
14. Eckman MR, Johnson T, Riess R. Partial deafness after erythromycin. N Engl J Med 1975;292:649.
15. Quinnan GV, McCabe WR. Ototoxicity of erythromycin. Lancet 1978;1:1160-1.
16. Mery J-P, Kanfer A. Ototoxicity of erythromycin in patients with renal insufficiency. N Engl J Med 1979;301:944.
17. Thompson P, Wood RP, Bergstrom L. Erythromycin ototoxicity. J Otolaryngol 1980;9:60-2.
18. Schneider WJ, Becker EL. Acute transient hearing loss after ethacrynic acid therapy. Arch Intern Med 1966;117:715-7.
19. Matz GJ. The ototoxic effects of ethacrynic acid in man and animals. Laryngoscope 1976;86:1065-86.
20. Mathog RH. Vestibulotoxicity of ethacrynic acid. Laryngoscope 1977;87:1791-808.
21. Keefe PE. Ototoxicity from oral furosemide. Drug Intell Clin Pharm 1978;12:428.
22. Gallagher KL, Jones JK. Furosemide-induced ototoxicity. Ann Intern Med 1979;91:744-5.
23. Schofield CBS, Masterton G. Vestibular reactions to minocycline. Morbid Mortal Wkly Rep 1976;25:31.
24. Gump DW, Ashikaga T, Fink TJ et al. Side effects of minocycline: different dosage regimens. Antimicrob Agents Chemother 1977;12:642-6.
25. Greco TP, Bonadio M, Lee RV et al. Minocycline toxicity: experience with an altered dosage regimen. Curr Ther Res 1979;25:193-201.
26. Miller RR. Deafness due to plain and long-acting aspirin tablets. J Clin Pharmacol 1978;18:468-71.
27. Jardini L, Findlay R, Burgi E et al. Auditory changes associated with moderate blood salicylate levels. Rheumatol Rehabil 1978;17:233-6.
28. Geraci JE, Heilman FR, Nichols DR et al. Antibiotic therapy of bacterial endocarditis VII. Vancomycin for acute micrococcal endocarditis. Proc Staff Meetings Mayo Clin 1958;33:172-81.

Drug-Induced Skin Disorders

THE AGENTS IN THE FOLLOWING TABLE have been reported to cause a variety of skin disorders. The most serious skin disorders are exfoliative dermatitis, lupus erythematosus-like reactions, Stevens-Johnson syndrome and toxic epidermal necrolysis, all of which may be life-threatening; the other reported skin disorders are less severe, but still serious. Drugs believed to be among the most common causes of a particular skin disorder are designated by "XX" in the table.

Only skin disorders resulting from systemic administration of drugs are represented in this table. For skin disorders caused by topical administration of drugs see: Cronin E. Contact dermatitis. Edinburgh: Churchill Livingstone, 1980. The following abbreviations are used to indicate specific skin disorders:

> AE—Acneiform Eruptions
> AI —Alopecia
> ED—Exfoliative Dermatitis
> EM—Erythema Multiforme
> FE —Fixed Eruptions
> LE —Lupus Erythematosus-Like Reactions

Continued

Ph —Photosensitivity Reactions
SJ —Stevens-Johnson Syndrome
TN—Toxic Epidermal Necrolysis

Drug-Induced Skin Disorders

DRUG	AE	AI	ED	EM	FE	LE	Ph	SJ	TN	REFERENCES
Acetazolamide				X						1
Allopurinol		X	X						X	1,3–6
Aminopyrine			XX		X			XX	XX	2
Aminosalicylic Acid			XX		X	X				1–5
Amphetamines		X								6
Androgens	XX									2
Antipyrine			XX	X	X			XX	XX	1–3,5
Arsenicals, Organic		X	X				X			1,3,5
Aspirin				X	X			X	X	1,3–5
Barbiturates	X		X	X	XX		X	XX	X	1–5
Bleomycin		X								4,5
Boric Acid		X								1,2,6
Bromides	XX									1–3,5
Busulfan		X								4,5
Carbamazepine			XX					XX		2
Chloramphenicol									X	2
Chlordiazepoxide					X		X			2,3
Chloroquine			X				X			1–3
Chlorpropamide			X	X		X	X	XX	XX	2–5
Clofibrate		X								1,5,6
Colchicine		X								1,3,6
Contraceptives, Oral	X	X			X		X			1,4–6
Corticosteroids	XX									1–5
Corticotropin	XX									2–5
Cyclophosphamide		X								3–5
Cytarabine		X								4,5
Dacarbazine		X								4,5
Dactinomycin	X									4
Dapsone					X					2,3
Daunorubicin		X								4,5
Dextran		X								2
Diphenhydramine							X			3,5
Doxorubicin		X								1,4,5

Continued

Drug-Induced Skin Disorders

DRUG	AE	AI	ED	EM	FE	LE	Ph	SJ	TN	REFERENCES
Ethosuximide						X				1,3
Fluorouracil		X								4,5
Gold Salts			X		X		X		X	1–3,5
Griseofulvin				X	X	X	X			1–5
Heparin		X								1–6
Hydralazine						XX				1–5
Hydroxyurea		X								4,5
Iodides	XX									1–5
Isoniazid	X		X			XX	X			2–5
Lithium	X									1,4
Meprobamate					X					4
Mercurials			X							2,3,5
Methotrexate		X								3–5
Methyldopa						X				5
Morphine					X					2
Nalidixic Acid		X					X			1–4
Nitrofurantoin			X			X		X	X	1,2
Oxyphenbutazone			XX	X	XX			XX	XX	1–4
Penicillamine						X				3
Penicillins				X		X		X	X	2–5
Pentazocine			X		X					2,5
Phenacetin					XX					2,4,5
Phenindione		X	XX	X						1,2
Phenolphthalein				X	XX				X	1,2,4,5
Phenothiazines			X	X		X	XX			2–5
Phenylbutazone			XX	X	XX	X		XX	XX	1–5
Phenytoin	XX		XX	X		XX	X	XX	XX	1–5
Practolol			X			X				2,3
Primidone						X			X	1
Procainamide						XX				1–5
Progestogens	X				X	X				2
Propranolol		X								6
Propylthiouracil		X				X				2–6
Psoralens	X						XX			1–5
Quinacrine		X	X							1,2,5
Quinidine			X		X			X		1,2,5
Quinine			X		X			X		2,5

Continued

Drug-Induced Skin Disorders

DRUG	AE	AI	ED	EM	FE	LE	Ph	SJ	TN	REFERENCES
Reserpine						X				2,3
Streptomycin			X			X				2,3,5
Sulfonamides			X	X	X	X	XX	XX	XX	1-5
Tetracyclines					X	X	XX		X	1-5
Thiazides				X			XX			1-5
Tolbutamide			X				X			1-5
Trimethadione	X	X	X	X		X	X	X		1-6
Vitamin A		X								3,5,6
Vinblastine		X								4
Vincristine		X								4
Warfarin		X								2-6

References

1. Dukes MNG, ed. Meyler's side effects of drugs. 9th ed. Amsterdam: Excerpta Medica, 1980.

2. Drug reactions. In: Stewart WD, Danto JS, Maddin S. Dermatology. 4th ed. St. Louis: CV Mosby, 1978:183-211.

3. Baker H. Drug reactions. In: Rook A, Wilkinson DS, Ebling FJG, eds. Textbook of dermatology. Oxford: Blackwell Scientific Publications, 1979:1111-49.

4. Wintroub BU, Shiffman NJ, Arndt KA. Adverse cutaneous reactions to drugs. In: Fitzpatrick TB, Eisen AZ, Wolff K et al, eds. Dermatology in general medicine. 2nd ed. New York: McGraw-Hill, 1979:555-67.

5. Beerman H, Kirshbaum BA. Drug eruptions (dermatitis medicamentosa). In: Moschella SL, Pillsbury DM, Hurley HJ, eds. Dermatology. Philadelphia: WB Saunders, 1975:350-84.

6. Reeves JRT, Maibach HI. Drug and chemical induced hair loss. In: Marzulli FN, Maibach HI, eds. Dermatotoxicology and pharmacology. New York: John Wiley & Sons, 1977:487-500.

7 *DRUG INTERACTIONS*

THE FOLLOWING IS A LIST OF THOSE DRUG INTERACTIONS which are most likely to be important in clinical practice. Minor or poorly documented interactions have been omitted, as have obvious interactions such as drugs with pharmacological actions which are clearly similar (barbiturates-glutethimide) or opposite (isoproterenol-propranolol). For a more comprehensive review, the reader is directed to references 1 and 2 at the end of the chapter. It is important to remember that the presence of a drug interaction in this list does not imply that the two drugs should not be used together. In the vast majority of cases, the drugs may be used concomitantly as long as appropriate measures are taken.

In preparing this chapter, collective drug group or drug class names have been used whenever possible; drugs which are a member of one of these groups are not listed individually. The following drug group names are used:

Aminoglycoside Antibiotics	Methenamine Compounds
Amphetamines	Monoamine Oxidase Inhibitors
Anabolic Steroids	Narcotic Analgesics
Antacids, Oral	Penicillins
Anticholinergics	Phenothiazines
Anticoagulants, Oral	Polymyxin Antibiotics
Antidepressants, Tricyclic	Potassium Salts
Antidiabetic Agents	Salicylates
Barbiturates	Skeletal Muscle Relaxants
Benzodiazepines	(Surgical)
Beta-Adrenergic Blockers	Sulfonamides, Antibacterial
Cephalosporins	Sympathomimetics
Contraceptives, Oral	Tetracyclines
Corticosteroids	Thiazide Diuretics
Digitalis Glycosides	Thyroid Hormones
Iron Preparations	

The table begins on page 110.

Drug Interactions

DRUG	INTERACTION AND COMMENTS

Acetazolamide—*quinidine:* alkalinization of the urine may decrease quinidine elimination, increasing the risk of quinidine toxicity[1]

—see also Methenamine Compounds; Salicylates; Sympathomimetics

Alcohol—*chloral hydrate:* may inhibit each other's metabolism and prolong CNS depression; may also produce vasodilation and hypotension[1,2]

—*disulfiram:* ingestion of even small amounts of alcohol may produce the disulfiram reaction, consisting of vasodilation, hypotension, nausea, vomiting, chest pain, weakness and confusion; patients should also be warned about contact with products whose alcohol content may not be obvious (eg, pharmaceuticals, topical preparations)[1]

—*guanethidine:* alcohol-induced vasodilation may accentuate guanethidine's orthostatic hypotension[1,2]

—*methotrexate:* chronic co-administration may increase the risk of methotrexate-induced liver damage; patients receiving methotrexate should minimize their consumption of alcohol[1]

—*metronidazole:* disulfiram-like reactions have been reported, but are not a consistent problem; although these reactions are not common, patients should be warned about the possibility of their existence[1,2]

—*nitroglycerin:* the vasodilation produced by both drugs may combine to produce significant hypotension[1]

—*phenytoin:* chronic use of large quantities of alcohol may stimulate the metabolism of phenytoin; monitor phenytoin levels in alcoholics[1,2]

—see also Anticoagulants, Oral; Antidiabetic Agents; Salicylates

Allopurinol—*azathioprine:* allopurinol inhibits the metabolism of mercaptopurine (active metabolite of azathioprine) to inactive products, resulting in increased mercaptopurine toxicity; when co-administration cannot be avoided, the azathioprine dose should be reduced[1,2]

—*cyclophosphamide:* cyclophosphamide-induced bone marrow suppression may be enhanced by allopurinol administration; mechanism is unknown[1,2]

—*mercaptopurine:* see Allopurinol—azathioprine

—see also Anticoagulants, Oral

Amantadine: see Anticholinergics

Amiloride: see Potassium Salts—spironolactone

Aminoglycoside Antibiotics—*amphotericin B:* possible additive nephrotoxicity; monitor renal function[1]

Continued

Drug Interactions

DRUG	INTERACTION AND COMMENTS

—*cephalosporins:* additive nephrotoxicity is a possibility; prolonged therapy merits repeated renal function tests[1]

—*digitalis glycosides:* oral neomycin may impair digoxin absorption; monitor digoxin levels if chronic oral neomycin therapy is begun[1]

—*ethacrynic acid:* additive ototoxicity has been reported—impaired renal function is an important predisposing factor[1,2]

—*methoxyflurane:* additive nephrotoxicity is a possibility; less nephrotoxic antibiotics should be used whenever possible[1]

—*penicillins:* the absorption of oral penicillin V is impaired by as much as 50% by oral neomycin; use parenteral penicillin until neomycin therapy is completed; also, carbenicillin appears to inactivate gentamicin when mixed in vitro, and possibly also in patients with severe renal impairment[1]

—*skeletal muscle relaxants (surgical):* aminoglycoside antibiotics are capable of producing neuromuscular blockade which can enhance that of the muscle relaxant by prolonging recovery time and sometimes causing respiratory paralysis; avoid co-administration when ventilatory assistance equipment is not available[1,2]

Aminophylline: see Theophylline

Aminosalicylic Acid (PAS)—_probenecid:_ renal elimination of PAS may be greatly impaired by probenecid, requiring reduction of PAS dose to avoid toxicity[1,2]

Ammonium Chloride—_spironolactone:_ large doses of ammonium chloride (eg, for acidification of the urine) may result in systemic acidosis in the presence of spironolactone[1]

Amphetamines: see Sympathomimetics

Amphotericin B: see Aminoglycoside Antibiotics; Corticosteroids; Digitalis Glycosides

Anabolic Steroids—_anticoagulants, oral:_ although mechanism is unknown, increase in anticoagulant activity is commonly encountered; monitor prothrombin time carefully[1,2]

—*antidiabetic agents:* enhanced hypoglycemic effect; antidiabetic agent dosage adjustments may be required[1]

Antacids, Oral—_digitalis:_ antacids may reduce the extent of digoxin absorption; give digoxin 2 hr before antacids[1]

—*iron preparations:* magnesium trisilicate and carbonate-containing products have been shown to interfere with iron absorption; separate doses by 2 hr[1,2]

—*isoniazid:* aluminum-containing antacids may interfere with isoniazid absorption; separate doses by 2 hr or select another antacid[1,2]

Continued

Drug Interactions

DRUG	INTERACTION AND COMMENTS

—*quinidine:* antacid-induced increases in urinary pH can decrease the amount of quinidine excreted by the kidney; watch for evidence of increased quinidine effect[1,2]

—*salicylates:* significantly reduced salicylate levels, due to enhanced renal elimination of salicylate; plasma salicylate levels should be monitored in patients requiring long-term salicylate therapy[27]

—*sodium polystyrene sulfonate resin:* the resin can bind magnesium and calcium ions from the antacid in the gut, resulting in systemic alkalosis; rectal use of the resin may avoid this problem[1]

—*tetracyclines:* antacids containing di- or trivalent ions interfere with the absorption of orally administered tetracyclines; separate doses by 2 hr[1,2]

—*thiazide diuretics:* large doses of calcium antacids may produce hypercalcemia in presence of thiazides; mechanism is thiazide-induced reduction in urinary calcium excretion[4]

Anticholinergics—*amantadine:* amantadine potentiates the effects of high doses of anticholinergics, especially the CNS activity[1]

Anticoagulants, Oral—*alcohol:* increases in anticoagulant activity have been noted with large doses of alcohol, but the mechanism has not been clearly defined; 1 or 2 drinks not likely to have any effect[1,2]

—*allopurinol:* increase in anticoagulant activity in some patients; monitor prothrombin time[1,2]

—*antidiabetic agents:* dicumarol may inhibit sulfonylurea metabolism while sulfonylureas may displace dicumarol from plasma protein binding sites, increasing anticoagulant effect; the use of warfarin may reduce the significance of this interaction[1,2]

—*barbiturates:* decreased anticoagulant effect, mostly due to stimulation of hepatic metabolism of the anticoagulant; monitor prothrombin time carefully if the barbiturate is being used as an anticonvulsant; benzodiazepines are more suitable if only sedative or hypnotic effects are desired[1,2]

—*carbamazepine:* decreased anticoagulant effect, most likely due to stimulation of hepatic metabolism of anticoagulant; monitor prothrombin time[1,2]

—*chloral hydrate:* chloral hydrate temporarily increases hypoprothrombinemic effect of warfarin, due to plasma protein binding displacement; chronic therapy with both drugs unlikely to cause problems[1]

—*chloramphenicol:* marked increase in dicumarol activity is well documented; while less evidence is available for warfarin, caution is nevertheless advised[1,2]

—*cholestyramine:* decreased absorption of warfarin; separate ad-

Continued

Drug Interactions

DRUG	INTERACTION AND COMMENTS

ministration by 6 hr; some interaction occurs even if doses are separated, due to enterohepatic circulation of anticoagulant[1,2]

—*cimetidine:* enhanced hypoprothrombinemic response to warfarin probably due to inhibition of warfarin metabolism; may necessitate reduction in warfarin dose[1]

—*clofibrate:* well documented increase in anticoagulant activity; monitor prothrombin time carefully[1,2]

—*dextrothyroxine:* well documented increase in anticoagulant effect; monitor prothrombin time[1,2]

—*diazoxide:* may displace coumarin anticoagulants from plasma protein binding sites; anticoagulant dose may need to be altered if use of diazoxide is planned[1,2]

—*disulfiram:* increased anticoagulant acitivity due to inhibition of metabolism; monitor prothrombin time carefully[1,2]

—*ethacrynic acid:* may displace coumarin anticoagulants from plasma protein binding sites; furosemide apparently does not have this effect and is the preferred loop diuretic[1,2]

—*glucagon:* enhanced anticoagulant activity, mechanism unknown; monitor prothrombin time[1,2]

—*glutethimide:* decreased anticoagulant effect, probably due to stimulation of hepatic metabolism of anticoagulant; benzodiazepine sedative-hypnotics are preferred in patients taking oral anticoagulants[1,2]

—*griseofulvin:* decreased anticoagulant effect has been reported; monitor prothrombin time[1,2]

—*indomethacin:* does not affect hypoprothrombinemic response to oral anticoagulants in most patients; use caution, due to possible GI bleeding and antiplatelet effect of indomethacin[1]

—*metronidazole:* enhanced hypoprothrombinemic response to warfarin due to inhibition of metabolism; monitor prothrombin time[1]

—*oxyphenbutazone:* marked increase in anticoagulant effect due to inhibition of metabolism and displacement of anticoagulant from plasma protein binding sites; monitor prothrombin time carefully[1,2]

—*phenylbutazone:* response same as oxyphenbutazone

—*phenytoin:* dicumarol may inhibit phenytoin metabolism, while phenytoin may stimulate dicumarol metabolism; the use of warfarin may reduce the significance of this interaction; but, watch for evidence of reduced warfarin effect due to phenytoin-induced enzyme stimulation[1,2]

Continued

Drug Interactions

DRUG	INTERACTION AND COMMENTS

—*quinidine:* enhanced hypoprothrombinemic response to warfarin in an occasional patient; monitor prothrombin time[1]

—*rifampin:* may decrease anticoagulant activity by stimulating warfarin metabolism; monitor prothrombin time[1,2]

—*salicylates:* large doses of salicylates increase anticoagulant effect; monitor prothrombin time; smaller doses may cause problems due to possible GI bleeding and antiplatelet effect[1,2]

—*sulfonamides:* some sulfonamides may enhance hypoprothrombinemic response to oral anticoagulants; monitor prothrombin time[1]

—*thyroid hormones:* increased anticoagulant effect, probably due to increased catabolism of clotting factors; monitor prothrombin time carefully[1,2]

—*trimethoprim/sulfamethoxazole:* well documented increase in hypoprothrombinemic response to warfarin; does not occur in all patients; probably due to sulfamethoxazole; monitor prothrombin time[1]

—see also Anabolic Steroids

Antidepressants, Tricyclic—*barbiturates:* may stimulate antidepressant metabolism; watch for evidence of reduced antidepressant effect[1,2]

—*bethanidine:* antidepressants inhibit the uptake (and therefore action) of bethanidine by the adrenergic neurons; use another antihypertensive agent (but not guanethidine or clonidine)[1,2]

—*clonidine:* reduced antihypertensive response to clonidine; use another antihypertensive (but not bethanidine or guanethidine)[1]

—*guanethidine:* antidepressants inhibit the uptake (and therefore action) of guanethidine by the adrenergic neurons; effects noted after 2 days of antidepressant therapy; use another antihypertensive agent (but not bethanidine or clonidine)[1,2]

—*monoamine oxidase inhibitors:* symptoms of CNS stimulation with convulsions and death have been reported; combination can be used if large doses are avoided and patient closely monitored[1,2]

—*sympathomimetics:* tricyclic antidepressant therapy may increase pressor response to parenteral epinephrine, norepinephrine, phenylephrine and possibly other sympathomimetics; effect of oral or nasal sympathomimetics not established, but caution is warranted; monitor blood pressure when sympathomimetics are given to patients receiving tricyclic antidepressants[1]

Antidiabetic Agents—*alcohol:* alcohol may enhance the risk of lactic acidosis in patients receiving phenformin; disulfiram-like reactions have occurred with sulfonylureas and patients should be warned of the possibility of their occurrence[1,2]

Continued

Drug Interactions

DRUG	INTERACTION AND COMMENTS

—*beta-adrenergic blockers:* prolongation of hypoglycemic episodes; inhibition of tachycardia and tremors as signs of hypoglycemia (sweating is not inhibited); hypertension during hypoglycemia; selective β-blockers (eg, metoprolol) less likely to cause problems with antidiabetics than nonselective types (eg, nadolol, propranolol)[30]

—*chloramphenicol:* prolonged half-lives have been reported for tolbutamide and chlorpropamide, probably resulting from inhibition of metabolism; reduction of sulfonylurea dosage may be necessary if prolonged use of chloramphenicol is planned[1,2]

—*clofibrate:* enhanced hypoglycemic effect of sulfonylureas may occur; may require adjustment of sulfonylurea dose[1]

—*corticosteroids:* corticosteroids may increase circulating glucose levels and adjustment of antidiabetic drug dose may be required[1,2]

—*methyldopa:* reduced tolbutamide metabolism; possible enhanced tolbutamide hypoglycemia; effect on other sulfonylureas not known[20]

—*monoamine oxidase inhibitors:* MAO inhibitors may interfere with the normal adrenergic response to hypoglycemia, prolonging the action of antidiabetic agents; the MAO inhibitors should be avoided in diabetics[1,2]

—*phenylbutazone:* prolongs the action of the active metabolite of acetohexamide and may enhance the activity of tolbutamide by inhibiting its metabolism or displacing it from plasma protein binding sites; chlorpropamide may also be enhanced; use alternative to phenylbutazone[1,2]

—*rifampin:* stimulates metabolism of tolbutamide and possibly other sulfonylureas; may require increased sulfonylurea dose[1]

—*salicylates:* enhanced response to sulfonylureas is possible; several possible mechanisms; reduction of antidiabetic agent dosage may be necessary if prolonged high-dose use of salicylates is planned; chlorpropamide most likely to be affected[1,2]

—*sulfonamides, antibacterial:* several sulfonamides have been reported to increase the activity of sulfonylureas by inhibition of metabolism or displacement from plasma protein binding sites; use another antibiotic whenever possible[1,2]

—*thiazide diuretics:* thiazides may aggravate diabetes; increased doses of antidiabetic agents may be needed to maintain control; patients stabilized on both drugs are not likely to have problems[1,2]

—*thyroid hormones:* may increase antidiabetic drug requirements; mechanism unknown[1]

—see also Anabolic Steroids; Anticoagulants, Oral

Continued

Drug Interactions

DRUG	INTERACTION AND COMMENTS

Azathioprine: see Allopurinol

Barbiturates—*contraceptives, oral:* barbiturates may stimulate metabolism of contraceptive hormones; menstrual irregularities and unplanned pregnancies may occur; more likely with low-dose oral contraceptives[1,28]

—*corticosteroids:* phenobarbital has been shown to increase the metabolism of corticosteroids; patients may require increased doses of corticosteroids[1,2]

—*griseofulvin:* significant impairment of griseofulvin absorption; numerous small doses of griseofulvin may provide greater absorption than single large doses[1,2]

—*phenothiazines:* barbiturates may enhance phenothiazine metabolism; possible decrease in antipsychotic effect[1]

—*quinidine:* barbiturates may enhance quinidine metabolism; monitor for reduced quinidine effect[1]

—*tetracyclines:* barbiturates may enhance doxycycline metabolism; possible decrease in antimicrobial effect[1]

—*valproic acid:* valproic acid inhibits phenobarbital metabolism; reduced phenobarbital dosage may be necessary[31]

—see also Anticoagulants, Oral; Antidepressants, Tricyclic

Benzodiazepines—*cimetidine:* cimetidine may inhibit the elimination of chlordiazepoxide and diazepam, but not lorazepam or oxazepam; reduction in diazepam or chlordiazepoxide dose may be necessary[10,11]

—*disulfiram:* disulfiram may inhibit the elimination of chlordiazepoxide and diazepam, but not lorazepam or oxazepam; reduction in diazepam or chlordiazepoxide dose may be necessary[16,25]

Beta-Adrenergic Blockers—*cimetidine:* enhanced propranolol effect; may require reduced propranolol dose[32]

—*clonidine:* combined use of clonidine and propranolol may result in *hyper*tensive reactions, especially if clonidine is rapidly withdrawn[1]

—*digitalis glycosides:* β-blockers may worsen congestive heart failure or digitalis-induced bradycardia[1]

—*indomethacin:* antihypertensive effect of β-blockers may be inhibited; mechanism may be prostaglandin inhibition[1]

—*sympathomimetics:* epinephrine may produce hypertensive reactions in patients on propranolol (and probably other nonselective blockers such as nadolol); may also occur with other sym-

Continued

Drug Interactions

DRUG	INTERACTION AND COMMENTS

pathomimetics such as phenylephrine and phenylpropanolamine; avoid such combinations if possible; if used, monitor carefully for hypertensive response[1]

—*theophylline:* mutual inhibition may occur; β-blockers (especially nonselective) may worsen asthma[1]

—see also Antidiabetic Agents; Digitalis Glycosides

Bethanidine: see Antidepressants, Tricyclic

Bismuth Subsalicylate—*tetracycline:* bismuth subsalicylate (Pepto-Bismol®) may reduce GI absorption of tetracycline; separate doses by 2 hr, with tetracycline given first[2]

Calcium Salts: see Digitalis Glycosides

Carbamazepine: see Anticoagulants, Oral; Tetracyclines

Cephalosporins—*furosemide:* additive nephrotoxicity is a possibility; large doses of cephalosporins merit repeated renal function tests[1,2]

—*polymyxin antibiotics:* additive nephrotoxicity is a possibility; unavoidable co-administration merits repeated renal function tests[1,2]

—*probenecid:* renal elimination of cephalosporins is reduced[1,2]

—see also Aminoglycoside Antibiotics

Chloral Hydrate—*furosemide:* IV furosemide may produce flushing, sweating and blood pressure variations in patients on chloral hydrate[1]

—see also Alcohol; Anticoagulants, Oral

Chloramphenicol—*phenytoin:* concomitant therapy may result in enhanced phenytoin levels through inhibition of phenytoin metabolism; use another antibiotic whenever possible[1,2]

—see also Anticoagulants, Oral; Antidiabetic Agents

Chlorthalidone: see Digitalis Glycosides

Cholestyramine: see Anticoagulants, Oral; Digitalis Glycosides; Thyroid Hormones

Cimetidine—*theophylline:* cimetidine may reduce the elimination of theophylline; watch for evidence of theophylline toxicity; reduced theophylline dosage may be required[24]

—see also Anticoagulants, Oral; Benzodiazepines

Clofibrate—*furosemide:* clofibrate-induced myopathy (eg, muscle pain, stiffness) may be more likely in presence of furosemide; hypoalbuminemia is also a predisposing factor[1]

Continued

Drug Interactions

DRUG	INTERACTION AND COMMENTS

—see also Anticoagulants, Oral; Antidiabetic Agents

Clonidine—*levodopa:* antiparkinson effect of levodopa may be inhibited; avoid combined use or monitor closely for impaired levodopa effect[1]

—see also Antidepressants, Tricyclic; Beta-Adrenergic Blockers

Contraceptives, Oral—*penicillins:* ampicillin may interfere with enterohepatic circulation of contraceptive hormones; menstrual irregularities and unplanned pregnancies may occur; more likely with low-dose oral contraceptives; use alternative contraception instead of, or in addition to oral contraceptives while on ampicillin[1,28]

—*phenytoin:* oral contraceptive metabolism may be increased; menstrual irregularities and unplanned pregnancies may occur; more likely with low-dose oral contraceptives[28]

—*rifampin:* rifampin may interfere with the action of oral contraceptives, increasing the risk of unplanned pregnancy; other methods of birth control should be used[1,28]

—*tetracyclines:* possibly same effect as penicillins (above)

—see also Barbiturates

Corticosteroids—*amphotericin B:* enhancement of amphotericin B-induced potassium depletion; monitor serum potassium levels regularly and supplement with potassium salts, if necessary[1]

—*ethacrynic acid:* enhancement of potassium depletion; monitor serum potassium levels regularly and supplement with potassium chloride, if necessary[1]

—*furosemide:* enhancement of potassium depletion; monitor serum potassium levels regularly and supplement with potassium chloride, if necessary[1]

—*phenytoin:* increase in dexamethasone metabolism; other corticosteroids may be similarly affected[1,2]

—*rifampin:* increase in corticosteroid metabolism; may require increased corticosteroid dose[1]

—*salicylates:* decreased salicylate levels, possibly due to corticosteroid effects on salicylate elimination; salicylate intoxication possible if patient is on large doses of salicylate and corticosteroid is reduced[1,2]

—*thiazide diuretics:* enhancement of potassium depletion; monitor serum potassium levels regularly and supplement with potassium chloride, if necessary[1]

—see also Antidiabetic Agents; Barbiturates

Continued

Drug Interactions

DRUG	INTERACTION AND COMMENTS

Cyclophosphamide: see Allopurinol

Dapsone—*probenecid:* probenecid may reduce the renal elimination of dapsone; reduction of dapsone dosage may be required[1,2]

Dextrothyroxine: see Anticoagulants, Oral

Diazoxide: see Anticoagulants, Oral

Digitalis Glycosides—*amphotericin B:* amphotericin B-induced potassium loss may contribute to the digitalis toxicity; monitor serum potassium levels regularly and supplement with potassium salts, if necessary[1,2]

—*calcium salts:* both have similar myocardial actions; avoid parenteral calcium salts[1,2]

—*cholestyramine:* may bind digitoxin (and possibly digoxin) in the gut; separate doses and monitor for reduced digitalis effect[1,2]

—*chlorthalidone:* see Digitalis Glycosides—thiazide diuretics

—*ethacrynic acid:* see Digitalis Glycosides—thiazide diuretics

—*furosemide:* see Digitalis Glycosides—thiazide diuretics

—*kaolin-pectin:* reduced GI absorption of digoxin; give digoxin 2 or more hr before kaolin-pectin[1]

—*penicillamine:* reduced plasma digoxin levels may occur; assess need for increase in digoxin dose[15]

—*quinidine:* reduced renal clearance and tissue binding of digoxin resulting in average twofold increase in plasma digoxin; digitoxin may also be affected, probably by different mechanisms; monitor clinically for increased digitalis effect, plasma digoxin levels useful; may necessitate reduction in digitalis dose[1,29]

—*rifampin:* enhanced hepatic metabolism of digitoxin; monitor for reduced digitoxin effect; digoxin probably less likely to interact with rifampin[1]

—*spironolactone:* reduced elimination of digitoxin and digoxin reported, but spironolactone metabolites may also produce false increases in plasma levels of digitalis glycosides by some methods; watch especially for clinical evidence of excessive digitalis effect[1,17]

—*sulfasalazine:* reduced GI absorption of digoxin; spacing doses may not avoid interaction; monitor for reduced digoxin effect[1]

—*thiazide diuretics:* diuretic-induced potassium loss may contribute to digitalis intoxication; monitor serum potassium levels and supplement with potassium chloride or give a potassium-sparing diuretic[1,2]

—see also Aminoglycoside Antibiotics; Antacids, Oral

Continued

Drug Interactions

DRUG	INTERACTION AND COMMENTS

Disulfiram—*isoniazid:* mental changes may result from effects of both drugs on metabolism of adrenergic neurotransmitters; avoid the use of disulfiram in patients who must take isoniazid[1]

—*metronidazole:* confusion and psychotic episodes have been reported; avoid combination or monitor for psychiatric reactions[1]

—*phenytoin:* disulfiram inhibits the inactivation of phenytoin by the liver; dosage adjustments may be necessary[1,2]

—see also Alcohol; Anticoagulants, Oral; Benzodiazepines

Dopamine—*phenytoin:* IV phenytoin has produced hypotension in severely ill patients receiving IV dopamine; monitor blood pressure carefully if combination used[13]

Erythromycin—*theophylline:* erythromycin may reduce theophylline elimination in some patients; risk of theophylline toxicity is greatest in patients on relatively large doses of theophylline[12]

Estrogens: see Contraceptives, Oral

Ethacrynic Acid: see Aminoglycoside Antibiotics; Anticoagulants, Oral; Corticosteroids; Digitalis Glycosides

Furosemide—*indomethacin:* the hypotensive and natriuretic effects of furosemide may be inhibited by indomethacin; possible need for increased furosemide dosage[8]

—see also Cephalosporins; Chloral Hydrate; Clofibrate; Corticosteroids; Digitalis Glycosides

Glucagon: see Anticoagulants, Oral

Glutethimide: see Anticoagulants, Oral

Griseofulvin: see Anticoagulants, Oral; Barbiturates

Guanethidine: see Alcohol; Antidepressants, Tricyclic; Phenothiazines; Sympathomimetics

Haloperidol—*methyldopa:* combined use may result in dementia (eg, confusion, disorientation); avoid combination or monitor for adverse psychiatric effects[1]

Heparin: see Salicylates

Indomethacin—*lithium carbonate:* indomethacin may reduce renal clearance of lithium; reduction in lithium dosage may be necessary[9]

—see also Anticoagulants, Oral; Beta-Adrenergic Blockers; Furosemide; Sympathomimetics; Thiazide Diuretics

Iron Preparations—*tetracyclines:* decreased tetracycline absorption,

Continued

Drug Interactions

DRUG	INTERACTION AND COMMENTS

probably due to chelation in the gut; separate doses by at least 2 hr[1,2]

—*vitamin E:* large doses of vitamin E impair the utilization of iron in patients with iron deficiency anemia; avoid vitamin E use in such patients[1]

—see also Antacids, Oral

Isoniazid—*phenytoin:* isoniazid inhibits the hepatic metabolism of phenytoin, increasing the risk of toxicity, particularly in slow acetylators; reduction of phenytoin dose may be required[1,2]

—*rifampin:* metabolism of isoniazid to hepatotoxic metabolites may be enhanced by rifampin; avoid use or monitor carefully for hepatotoxicity[1]

—see also Antacids, Oral; Disulfiram

Kaolin-Pectin—*lincomycin:* marked decrease in absorption of lincomycin from the GI tract; avoid concurrent use (note that diarrhea may be a sign of impending pseudomembranous colitis)[1,2]

—see also Digitalis Glycosides

Levodopa—*papaverine:* antiparkinson effect of levodopa may be inhibited; avoid papaverine in such patients[1]

—*phenytoin:* antiparkinson effect of levodopa may be inhibited; if phenytoin must be used in a patient on levodopa, monitor for reduced levodopa response; theoretically, increasing levodopa dose might restore antiparkinson response[1]

—*pyridoxine:* pyridoxine increases levodopa metabolism, significantly decreasing its effectiveness; this interaction is not encountered if a peripheral decarboxylase inhibitor is used in conjunction with levodopa[1,2]

—see also Clonidine; Monoamine Oxidase Inhibitors; Phenothiazines

Lincomycin: see Cyclamates; Kaolin-Pectin

Lithium Carbonate—*methyldopa:* patients on lithium may develop signs of lithium intoxication in presence of methyldopa; plasma lithium not elevated; if interaction occurs, select another antihypertensive[19]

—*phenytoin:* signs of lithium toxicity may occur with combined use in absence of increased plasma lithium; monitor for clinical evidence of lithium toxicity if combined use cannot be avoided[23]

—*sodium chloride:* excess sodium increases lithium excretion, while sodium deficiency may promote lithium retention and increase the risk of toxicity; patients taking lithium should not be on low salt diets[1]

Continued

Drug Interactions

DRUG	INTERACTION AND COMMENTS

—see also Indomethacin; Thiazide Diuretics

Mefenamic Acid: see Anticoagulants, Oral

Mercaptopurine: see Allopurinol

Methenamine Compounds—*acetazolamide:* the alkaline urine resulting from acetazolamide therapy inhibits the conversion of methenamine to its active form, formaldehyde; select an alternative for one of the drugs[1,2]

—*sodium bicarbonate:* the alkaline urine resulting from bicarbonate therapy inhibits the conversion of methenamine to its active form, formaldehyde; select an alternative for one of the drugs[1]

Methotrexate—*para-aminobenzoic acid (PABA):* PABA may displace methotrexate from plasma protein binding sites; do not give PABA-containing products during methotrexate therapy[1,2]

—*phenylbutazone:* possible increase in methotrexate plasma levels; monitor for methotrexate toxicity[1]

—*probenecid:* reduced renal excretion of methotrexate; may necessitate decreases in methotrexate dose[1]

—see also Alcohol; Salicylates

Methoxyflurane: see Aminoglycoside Antibiotics; Tetracyclines

Methyldopa: see Antidiabetic Agents; Haloperidol; Lithium Carbonate; Sympathomimetics

Metronidazole: see Alcohol; Anticoagulants, Oral; Disulfiram

Monoamine Oxidase (MAO) Inhibitors—*levodopa:* co-administration may lead to increased levels of dopamine and norepinephrine, hypertensive reaction may occur; carbidopa seems to protect against this interaction[1,2]

—*narcotic analgesics:* use with meperidine has produced a variety of reactions, including hypertension, excitement, rigidity and occasionally, hypotension and coma; other narcotics are apparently safer[1,2]

—*sympathomimetics:* indirect-acting agents such as amphetamines, ephedrine, metaraminol, phenylpropanolamine, pseudoephedrine and possibly methylphenidate may produce a hypertensive crisis in patients on MAO inhibitors; of the direct-acting agents, phenylephrine may also produce hypertension in patients on MAO inhibitors, while the response to epinephrine and norepinephrine is minimally affected[1]

—see also Antidepressants, Tricyclic; Antidiabetic Agents

Narcotic Analgesics—*rifampin:* may stimulate metabolism of meth-

Continued

Drug Interactions

DRUG	INTERACTION AND COMMENTS

adone; withdrawal symptoms possible in patients on methadone maintenance[1]

—see also Monoamine Oxidase Inhibitors

Nitroglycerin: see Alcohol

Norepinephrine—*methyldopa:* possible increase in pressor response to norepinephrine; mechanism not established[1]

Oxyphenbutazone: see Anabolic Steroids; Anticoagulants, Oral

Papaverine: see Levodopa

Para-Aminobenzoic Acid: see Methotrexate; Sulfonamides, Antibacterial

Penicillamine: see Digitalis Glycosides

Penicillins—*probenecid:* renal elimination of penicillin is reduced; this may be used to therapeutic advantage when high levels of penicillin are desired[2]

  —*tetracyclines:* bacteriostatic agents, such as tetracyclines, inhibit bacterial growth, while penicillins require actively growing bacteria to exert their effect; co-administration could nullify the action of the penicillins (may also occur with other bacteriostatic agents); however, clinical problems are probably infrequent in patients receiving adequate doses of both drugs[1,2]

—see also Aminoglycoside Antibiotics; Contraceptives, Oral

Phenothiazines—*guanethidine:* phenothiazines may inhibit the uptake of guanethidine by the adrenergic neurons, thereby reducing its hypotensive effects; at the same time, phenothiazines possess hypotensive effects of their own, so use of both drugs requires close monitoring of blood pressure[1,2]

  —*levodopa:* levodopa does not block phenothiazine-induced extrapyramidal symptoms, while phenothiazines may inhibit the antiparkinson activity of levodopa[1,2]

—see also Barbiturates

Phenylbutazone—*phenytoin:* phenylbutazone appears to inhibit phenytoin metabolism; this may necessitate reduction in phenytoin dosage[1]

—see also Anticoagulants, Oral; Antidiabetic Agents; Methotrexate

Phenylephrine: see Sympathomimetics

Phenylpropanolamine: see Sympathomimetics

Phenytoin—*theophylline:* theophylline may reduce plasma phenytoin;

Continued

Drug Interactions

DRUG	INTERACTION AND COMMENTS

watch for altered phenytoin response if theophylline is started or stopped; plasma phenytoin determinations may be useful[5]

—*valproic acid:* valproic acid displaces phenytoin from plasma protein binding; total plasma phenytoin levels are reduced; free phenytoin increases only temporarily, so a change in phenytoin dose is usually not necessary[6,7]

—see also Alcohol; Anticoagulants, Oral; Chloramphenicol; Contraceptives, Oral; Corticosteroids; Disulfiram; Dopamine; Isoniazid; Levodopa; Lithium Carbonate; Phenylbutazone; Sulfonamides, Antibacterial; Tetracyclines

Polymyxin Antibiotics: see Cephalosporins

Potassium Salts—*spironolactone:* serious hyperkalemia may result if potassium salts and a potassium-sparing compound such as amiloride, spironolactone or triamterene are given to the same patient; monitor serum potassium levels very carefully[1,2]

—*amiloride, triamterene:* see Potassium Salts—spironolactone

Probenecid: see Aminosalicylic Acid; Cephalosporins; Dapsone; Indomethacin; Methotrexate; Penicillins; Salicylates

Pyridoxine: see Levodopa

Quinidine—*rifampin:* rifampin stimulates quinidine metabolism; quinidine dose may need to be increased if combination cannot be avoided[22]

—*sodium bicarbonate:* alkalinization of the urine may decrease quinidine elimination, thereby increasing the risk of quinidine toxicity[1]

—see also Acetazolamide; Antacids, Oral; Anticoagulants, Oral; Barbiturates; Digitalis Glycosides

Rifampin: see Anticoagulants, Oral; Antidiabetic Agents; Contraceptives, Oral; Corticosteroids; Digitalis Glycosides; Isoniazid; Narcotic Analgesics; Quinidine

Salicylates—*acetazolamide:* acetazolamide may enhance renal salicylate excretion and increase salicylate penetration into the brain; latter effect may produce CNS salicylate toxicity if patient is on large doses of salicylate[1,14]

—*alcohol:* enhanced risk of GI blood loss[1,2]

—*heparin:* aspirin effects on platelet adhesiveness might leave the heparin-treated patient more prone to hemorrhage[1,2]

—*methotrexate:* salicylates displace methotrexate from plasma protein binding sites and also inhibit its renal elimination, thus greatly increasing the risk of methotrexate toxicity; do not give salicylates

Continued

Drug Interactions

DRUG	INTERACTION AND COMMENTS

to patients taking methotrexate; warn patient about the use of OTC products which contain salicylates[1,2]

—*probenecid:* salicylates inhibit the uricosuric effects of probenecid, particularly with large doses of salicylate; occasional small doses present no problem[1]

—*sulfinpyrazone:* salicylates inhibit the uricosuric effects of sulfin-pyrazone; occasional small doses present no problem[1,2]

—see also Antacids, Oral; Anticoagulants, Oral; Antidiabetic Agents; Corticosteroids

Sodium Bicarbonate: see Methenamine Compounds; Quinidine; Sym-pathomimetics; Tetracyclines

Sodium Chloride: see Lithium Carbonate

Sodium Polystyrene Sulfonate Resin: see Antacids, Oral

Spironolactone: see Ammonium Chloride; Digitalis Glycosides; Potassium Salts

Sulfinpyrazone: see Salicylates

Sulfonamides, Antibacterial—*para-aminobenzoic acid:* PABA antagonizes the antibacterial effects of the sulfonamides which work by competing with PABA in bacteria[1]

—*phenytoin:* sulfonamides have been variously reported to inhibit the metabolism of phenytoin and to displace it from plasma protein bind-ing sites; monitor plasma phenytoin levels if more than a few days of sulfonamide therapy are planned[1,2]

—see also Anticoagulants, Oral; Antidiabetic Agents; Digitalis Glycosides

Sympathomimetics—*acetazolamide:* alkalinization of the urine decreases elimination of amphetamines, pseudoephedrine and possibly other sympathomimetics[1]

—*guanethidine:* sympathomimetics with indirect-activity, such as am-phetamines and ephedrine, may inhibit antihypertensive effect of guanethidine; direct-acting sympathomimetics, such as norepinephrine and phenylephrine, may produce an exaggerated response in patients on guanethidine; avoid sympathomimetics, if possible, in patients on guanethidine[1]

—*indomethacin:* indomethacin may predispose to phenylpropanolamine-induced hypertension; might also occur with other sympathomimetics[26]

—*methyldopa:* possible increase in pressor response to norepinephrine; mechanism not established[1]

Continued

Drug Interactions

DRUG	INTERACTION AND COMMENTS

—*sodium bicarbonate:* alkalinization of the urine decreases elimination of amphetamines, pseudoephedrine and possibly other sympathomimetics[1]

—see also Antidepressants, Tricyclic; Beta-Adrenergic Blockers; Monoamine Oxidase Inhibitors

Tetracyclines—*carbamazepine:* carbamazepine may stimulate doxycycline metabolism; possible decrease in antimicrobial effect[1]

—*methoxyflurane:* additive nephrotoxicity has been reported[1,2]

—*phenytoin:* phenytoin may stimulate doxycycline metabolism; possible decrease in antimicrobial effect[1]

—*zinc:* large doses of zinc (eg, 200 mg) may reduce tetracycline absorption; space doses by 2 hr or more and give tetracycline first[1]

—see also Antacids, Oral; Barbiturates; Bismuth Subsalicylate; Contraceptives, Oral; Iron Preparations; Penicillins

Theophylline—*troleandomycin:* elevated plasma theophylline levels may occur; mechanism is probably inhibition of theophylline metabolism; may need to reduce theophylline dose[1]

—*vaccination, influenza:* theophylline elimination may be reduced following influenza vaccination; watch for evidence of theophylline toxicity[18]

—see also Beta-Adrenergic Blockers; Cimetidine; Erythromycin; Phenytoin

Thiazide Diuretics—*indomethacin:* indomethacin may inhibit the natriuretic and antihypertensive effects of thiazides; dosage changes may be needed if combination cannot be avoided[8,21]

—*lithium carbonate:* chronic diuretic use may result in decreased lithium elimination; monitor plasma lithium levels until the patient is stabilized in the therapeutic range[1,2]

—see also Antidiabetic Agents; Corticosteroids; Digitalis Glycosides

Thyroid Hormones—*cholestyramine:* cholestyramine binds both T_3 and T_4 in the gut, preventing their absorption; separate doses by at least 4 hr[1,2]

—see also Anticoagulants, Oral; Antidiabetic Agents

Triamterene: see Potassium Salts

Trimethoprim/Sulfamethoxazole: see Anticoagulants, Oral

Troleandomycin: see Theophylline

Vaccination, Influenza: see Theophylline

Continued

Drug Interactions

DRUG	INTERACTION AND COMMENTS

Valproic Acid: see Barbiturates; Phenytoin

Vitamin E: see Iron Preparations

Zinc: see Tetracyclines

References

1. Hansten PD. Drug interactions. 4th ed. Philadelphia: Lea & Febiger, 1979.
2. American Pharmaceutical Association. Evaluations of drug interactions. 2nd ed. Washington, 1976 (Suppl. 1978).
3. Albert KS, Welch RD, DeSante KA et al. Decreased tetracycline bioavailability caused by a bismuth subsalicylate antidiarrheal mixture. J Pharm Sci 1979;68:586-8.
4. Hakim R, Tolis G, Goltzman D et al. Severe hypercalcemia associated with hydrochlorothiazide and calcium carbonate therapy. Can Med Assoc J 1979;121:591-4.
5. Taylor JW, Hendeles L, Weinberger M et al. The interaction of phenytoin and theophylline (abstract). Drug Intell Clin Pharm 1980;14:638.
6. Bruni J, Wilder BJ, Willmore LJ et al. Valproic acid and plasma levels of phenytoin. Neurology 1979;29:904-5.
7. Monks A, Richens A. Effect of single doses of sodium valproate on serum phenytoin levels and protein binding in epileptic patients. Clin Pharmacol Ther 1980;27:89-95.
8. Hansten PD. Furosemide and indomethacin. Drug Interactions Newsletter 1981;1:1-3.
9. Frolich JC, Leftwich R, Ragheb M et al. Indomethacin increases plasma lithium. Br Med J 1979;1:1115-6.
10. Klotz U, Reimann I. Delayed clearance of diazepam due to cimetidine. N Engl J Med 1980;302:1012-4.
11. Patwardhan RV, Yarborough GW, Desmond PV et al. Cimetidine spares the glucuronidation of lorazepam and oxazepam. Gastroenterology 1980;79:912-6.
12. Hansten PD. Erythromycin and theophylline. Drug Interactions Newsletter 1981;1:5-6.
13. Bivins BA, Rapp RP, Griffen WO et al. Dopamine-phenytoin interaction. Arch Surg 1978;113:245-9.
14. Anderson CJ, Kaufman PL, Sturm RJ. Toxicity of combined therapy with carbonic anhydrase inhibitors and aspirin. Am J Ophthalmol 1978;86:516-9.
15. Moezzi B, Fatourechi V, Khozain R et al. The effect of penicillamine on serum digoxin levels. Jap Heart J 1978;19:366-70.
16. MacLeod SM, Sellers EM, Giles HG et al. Interaction of disulfiram with benzodiazepines. Clin Pharmacol Ther 1978;24:583-9.
17. Carruthers SG, Dujovne CA. Cholestyramine and spironolactone and their combination in digitoxin elimination. Clin Pharmacol Ther 1980;27:184-7.
18. Renton KW, Gray JD, Hall RI. Decreased elimination of theophylline after influenza vaccination. Can Med Assoc J 1980;123:288-90.
19. Hansten PD. Lithium and methyldopa. Drug Interactions Newsletter 1981;1:11.
20. Gachalyi B, Tornyossy M, Vas A et al. Effect of alphamethyldopa on the half-lives of antipyrine, tolbutamide and D-glucaric acid excretion in man. Int J Clin Pharmacol Ther Toxicol 1980;18:133-5.
21. Watkins J, Abbott EC, Hensby CN et al. Attenuation of hypotensive effect of propranolol and thiazide diuretics by indomethacin. Br Med J 1980;281:702-5.
22. Twum-Barima Y, Carruthers SG. Evaluation of rifampin-quinidine interaction (abstract). Clin Pharmacol Ther 1980;27:290.
23. MacCallum WAG. Interaction of lithium and phenytoin. Br Med J 1980;1:610.
24. Jackson JE, Powell JR, Wandell M et al. Cimetidine-theophylline interaction (abstract). Pharmacologist 1980;22:231.
25. Sellers EM, Giles HG, Greenblatt DJ et al. Differential effects on benzodiazepine disposition by disulfiram and ethanol. Arzneim Forsch 1980;30:882-6.
26. Lee KY, Beilin LJ, Vandongen R. Severe hypertension after ingestion of an appetite suppressant (phenylpropanolamine) with indomethacin. Lancet 1979;1:1110-1.
27. Hansten PD, Hayton WL. Effect of antacid and ascorbic acid on serum salicylate concentration. J Clin Pharmacol 1980;20:326-31.
28. Hansten PD. Drug interactions that inhibit oral contraceptive efficacy. Drug Interactions Newsletter 1981;1:9-11.
29. Hansten PD. Quinidine and digoxin. Drug Interactions Newsletter 1981;1:13-5.
30. Hansten PD. Beta-blocking agents and antidiabetic drugs. Drug Intell Clin Pharm 1980;14:46-50.
31. Patel IH, Levy RH, Cutler RE. Phenobarbital-valproic acid interaction. Clin Pharmacol Ther 1980;27:515-21.
32. Feely J, Wilkinson GR, Wood AJJ. Reduction of liver blood flow and propranolol metabolism by cimetidine. N Engl J Med 1981;304:692-5.

8 DRUGS AND BREAST FEEDING

WITH THE INCREASING POPULARITY OF BREAST FEEDING, the clinician often must weigh the benefits versus risks of drug therapy in the lactating woman. Unfortunately, reliable information on drug use during lactation is not readily available. Only recently have thorough, pharmacokinetically sound studies in humans been performed and many important drugs have yet to be adequately studied.[1] Recent publications have described the physicochemical and pharmacokinetic factors involved in drug transfer into milk as derived from animal and human data.[2-4] These factors are briefly discussed below.

Physicochemical Factors. Small water-soluble nonelectrolytes pass into milk by simple diffusion through pores in the lipoid membrane separating plasma from milk. Equilibration with plasma is usually rapid and milk levels approximate plasma levels. The lipid soluble, unionized forms of larger molecules pass through the lipoid membrane. Because the pH of milk is generally lower than plasma, milk can act as an "ion trap" for basic compounds. At equilibrium, these compounds attain high levels in milk relative to plasma. Conversely, acidic drugs tend to be inhibited from entering milk. The pKa of weak electrolytes is the primary determinant of their equilibrium concentration in milk, with the oil/water partition coefficient being of lesser importance.

Pharmacokinetic Factors. The oil/water partition coefficient is the major determinant of the *rate* of passage into milk. With drugs having a short half-life, the rate of passage into milk is very important in determining the concentration of drug in milk. Their concentration in plasma falls to low levels before high concentrations are attained in milk. Drugs having a long half-life reach concentrations in milk more closely resembling equilibrium conditions than those with short half-lives. Protein binding can also be a factor in the passage of drugs into milk. Binding of drugs is much more avid to plasma proteins than to milk proteins and highly protein-bound drugs do not attain high concentrations in milk.

Clinical Considerations

When it appears necessary to administer a drug to a breast feeding mother, several factors should be considered.

Maternal Factors. There are often several choices of drugs and routes of administration available to use in a given condition. Other times, drugs are prescribed which have only a slight or transient benefit to the patient. During breast feeding, consideration should be given to the use of alternative drugs, dosing regimens and routes of administration, as well as to the discontinuation of drug therapy, to minimize the risks of infant drug exposure.

Infant Factors. Acute, dose-related toxic effects in infants are rather uncommon; however, drug behavior is often not predictable because of immature excretory mechanisms. This is especially true in neonatal and preterm infants. Another type of dose-related phenomenon may occur in infants receiving low levels of antibiotics in milk. Although insignificant pharmacologically, levels may be sufficient to upset the GI flora and produce candidiasis, diarrhea or thrush. An additional possibility is sensitization of infants to drugs. Any allergenic drug can probably pass into milk in sufficient quantities to sensitize the infant or cause allergic reactions.

Idiosyncratic (nonallergic, non-dose-related) reactions can also be precipitated in susceptible infants. Hemolysis by oxidizing agents in milk has been reported in G6PD deficient infants. Neonates, and especially preterm infants, are also susceptible to hemolysis by oxidizing agents. Other apparently non-dose-related reactions such as blood dyscrasias and hepatotoxicity have not been reported, but should be considered before prescribing drugs capable of producing these reactions.

The long-term effects of most potent drugs and environmental chemicals on breast-fed infants are unknown. In addition to agents specifically listed in the table, several groups of drugs should be considered potentially hazardous when used continuously throughout lactation. These include anticonvulsants, antituberculars, corticosteroids, hypotensive agents, psychotherapeutic agents and sex hormones.

Use of the Table. In a previous review, data from the primary literature were compiled in a standardized format.[1] In this chapter, previous data and all new reports are summarized in narrative format. For specific numerical data, consult the references listed.

The table begins on page 130.

Drugs Excreted Into Breast Milk

DRUG	NATURE OF EFFECT
ALCOHOL	
Alcohol	Alcohol equilibrates rapidly between blood and milk; milk levels are about 90–95% of simultaneous blood levels. Low to moderate maternal intake appears to produce no effects in the infant; however, prolonged intake of large amounts, as in the alcoholic, may be detrimental. One case of drunkenness has been reported in an 8-day old infant whose mother drank 750 ml of port wine in a 24-hr period.[1] A case report of pseudo-Cushing's syndrome has been reported in an infant whose mother drank "at least 50 12-ounce cans of beer weekly plus generous amounts of more concentrated alcoholic beverages".[5] Doses of alcohol higher than 1 g/kg may inhibit the milk ejection reflex and doses higher than 2 g/kg probably completely block suckling-induced oxytocin release.[1] Alcohol should be used in moderation during lactation. There is no evidence that beer stimulates lactation other than through a tension-relieving effect on the mother
ANALGESICS AND ANTIPYRETICS	
Acetaminophen	Peak acetaminophen concentrations occur 1–2 hr after a dose; amounts ingested by infants are small and appear to be harmless.[6,7]
Aspirin	See Salicylate
Narcotics	Narcotics in analgesic doses are excreted in small amounts which seem insignificant. Those studied have been **butorphanol** 1–2 mg IM and 8 mg PO,[8] **codeine** 60 mg PO,[1,7] **meperidine** 50–100 mg IM[9,10] and **morphine** 16 mg parenterally[1]
	Heroin abuse can result in high enough milk levels to cause addiction or alleviate withdrawal symptoms in infants; however, breast feeding is not reliable enough to be used as a method of preventing withdrawal.[1,2]

Continued

Drugs Excreted Into Breast Milk

DRUG	NATURE OF EFFECT
	Although **methadone** maintenance is not a contraindication to breast feeding,[11,13] it is best to skip breast feeding 3-4 hr after the dose when peak milk levels occur.[1,13] One death has been reported in a malnourished 5-week old infant whose mother was on methadone maintenance. Methadone was detected in the infant on autopsy, but it is unclear what part the drug played in the infant's death[14]
Nonsteroidal Anti-Inflammatory Agents	Nonsteroidal anti-inflammatory agents have not been well studied in breast milk; however, small amounts of several agents have been detected. These include **indoprofen, mefenamic acid, naproxen, oxyphenbutazone** and **phenylbutazone**.[1,15-18] A one-week old infant, whose mother was taking **indomethacin**, had two generalized seizures, but drug levels were not measured in milk or in the infant.[19] All of these agents should be used with caution during breast feeding because of the lack of information about their use
Phenacetin	Phenacetin enters milk in small quantities which seem harmless[7]
Salicylate	Salicylate enters milk in low concentrations relative to plasma.[1,7,20-23] At high doses, salicylate has a long half-life in the mother and may accumulate in infants, particularly neonates; caution should be used when high doses are being given. Occasional **aspirin** in low doses should pose no hazards to the infant except for the potential antiplatelet effect. Avoiding breast feeding for an hr after a dose should obviate this effect
ANTICHOLINERGIC AGENTS	Excretion of anticholinergics into milk has not been studied. Theoretical hazards are anti-cholinergic effects such as drying of secretions, temperature elevations and CNS disturbances in the infant. Observe infants carefully if anticholinergics are used. Theoretically, anticholinergics can decrease milk flow by decreasing oxytocin secretion and release,[24] but this has not been documented

Continued

Drugs Excreted Into Breast Milk

DRUG	NATURE OF EFFECT
ANTICOAGULANTS	The two most commonly used anticoagulants, **heparin** and **warfarin**, are safe to use during breast feeding.[1,25] Heparin does not pass into milk; amounts of warfarin in milk are insignificant and cause no problems. Great caution should be used with other anticoagulants, particularly **indandiones**[1]
ANTICONVULSANTS	
Carbamazepine	Carbamazepine and its major metabolite are excreted in milk and can be detected in nursing infants; infant plasma concentrations are subtherapeutic and no effects have been seen in infants. Carbamazepine appears to be safe during lactation[1,26-28]
Ethosuximide	Ethosuximide milk levels approximate maternal plasma, but amounts ingested are not expected to cause harm to the infant[1,28,29]
Phenobarbital	Phenobarbital has a pKa near the pH of plasma; therefore, slight variations in milk pH cause marked changes in the amount transferred to milk. Although phenobarbital is generally safe, some infants may receive enough to cause drowsiness; enzyme induction may also occur[1,28]
Phenytoin	Phenytoin is excreted in small amounts; however, occasionally infants may experience idiosyncratic reactions or enzyme induction may occur. One case of cyanosis and methemoglobinemia may have been caused by phenytoin in milk[1,30]
Primidone	Primidone passes well into milk; its metabolites, especially **phenobarbital**, may reach significant levels. Drowsiness has occurred, but no serious reactions are expected[27,28,31,32]
Valproic Acid	Valproic acid passes poorly into milk, but is detectable. Caution should be used until more is known about this drug, particularly with respect to hepatic damage[31,33,34]

Continued

Drugs Excreted Into Breast Milk

DRUG	NATURE OF EFFECT
ANTIHISTAMINE DRUGS	Although it has been stated that antihistamines (through their anticholinergic effects) could decrease milk flow, this is not the case (see Anticholinergics). Excretion of antihistamines into milk has not been quantitated; however, most sources consider them safe during lactation (see also Sympathomimetics)
ANTI-INFECTIVE AGENTS	
Aminoglycosides	Aminoglycosides are very polar and pass poorly and irregularly into milk; milk concentrations do not fluctuate as widely or as rapidly as plasma levels.[1,35-38] Pharmacologic or toxic effects in infants are unlikely, due to the small amounts in milk; however, infants should be observed for disruption of the GI flora, such as thrush or diarrhea
Cephalosporins	Cephalosporins are not excreted in milk in sufficient quantities to treat infections in infants, but do appear in trace amounts which could lead to allergic sensitization or disruption of the GI flora. Breast feeding is not contraindicated, but infants should be observed for rashes, thrush or diarrhea[39-45]
Penicillins	Penicillins are not excreted in milk in sufficient quantities to treat infections in infants, but do appear in trace amounts which could lead to allergic sensitization or disruption of the GI flora. Breast feeding is not contraindicated, but infants should be observed for rashes, thrush or diarrhea.[1,44,45]
Plasmodicides	**Chloroquine** has not been detected in milk, although studies are not adequate. **Quinine** is excreted in insignificant amounts. **Pyrimethamine** may be excreted in sufficient quantities to treat or protect infants less than 6 months of age against malaria, but this is not a reliable method of drug administration[1,2]
Sulfonamides	Sulfonamides are not absolutely contraindicated, but do pass in sufficient quantities to have Continued

Drugs Excreted Into Breast Milk

DRUG	NATURE OF EFFECT
	caused hemolytic anemia in G6PD deficient infants. Cautious use and careful observation is mandatory, especially in neonates and premature infants. Avoid long-acting sulfas and those associated with G6PD deficiency.[1] **Sulfisoxazole** is excreted only in small amounts and appears to be safe in healthy infants; use caution in stressed or premature infants.[46] **Sulfasalazine's** metabolites, **sulfapyridine** and **5-aminosalicylate** are found in milk, but in quantities that seem to pose no hazard to infants with usual doses of sulfasalazine[47-49]
Tetracyclines	Tetracyclines could theoretically cause mottling of teeth if absorbed by the infant. Calcium in milk apparently inhibits absorption, so toxicity is unlikely; nevertheless, other less potentially toxic alternatives are available for most infections[1]
Urinary Germicides	**Methenamine** hippurate and mandelate pass into milk in very small quantities and seem safe to use.[1,50] **Nalidixic acid** has been associated with one case of hemolytic anemia in a breast-fed infant and should be used cautiously, if at all. **Nitrofurantoin** is excreted in pharmacologically insignificant amounts, but caution is advised in neonates, premature infants and those with G6PD deficiency[1]
Miscellaneous Anti-Infective Agents	**Amantadine** is contraindicated according to the manufacturer; it reportedly may cause vomiting, urinary retention and skin rashes in infants[1]
	Chloramphenicol levels are not sufficient to induce "grey baby" syndrome, but may be enough to harm bone marrow. Additionally, a number of adverse reactions in infants, including refusal of the breast, falling asleep during feeding and vomiting after feeding have occurred. Breast feeding is contraindicated during chloramphenicol treatment[1]
	Clindamycin is excreted in small amounts in milk.[1] It is not known what effects these levels may have on infants' GI flora (eg, induction of pseudomembranous colitis), so it is best avoided, if possible

Continued

Drugs Excreted Into Breast Milk

DRUG	NATURE OF EFFECT
	Cycloserine is excreted in small amounts, but no adverse reactions have been reported in infants[1]
	Erythromycin is excreted in small amounts and may disrupt the GI flora leading to thrush or candidiasis; however, the drug is generally safe, with few hazards to the infant[1,2]
	Isoniazid is excreted and should be used with caution during lactation. Hepatic damage might occur[51]
	Lincomycin is excreted, but no adverse effects have been reported.[1] See Clindamycin
	Metronidazole is detectable in plasma in small amounts in some infants. The dose in milk is too small to cause immediate reactions and no adverse systemic or GI effects have been reported. Because of possible carcinogenicity, it seems prudent to avoid the drug, or if essential to treat trichomoniasis, to give it as a single 2 g dose and use an alternative feeding method for 12-24 hr[52,53]
	Novobiocin carries the risk of causing hyperbilirubinemia and kernicterus in the infant. Although no infant toxicities have been reported, safer drugs should be used[1]
	Trimethoprim is excreted and infants absorb about 0.75-1 mg daily; this amount is probably not harmful[1]
ANTINEOPLASTIC AGENTS	Breast feeding is generally considered to be contraindicated in women receiving antineoplastic drugs
Busulfan	Busulfan was taken by one woman in a dose of 4 mg daily for 5 weeks while breast feeding with no adverse effects on her infant's leukocytes or hemoglobin. This study is by no means conclusive, however[54] Continued

Drugs Excreted Into Breast Milk

DRUG	NATURE OF EFFECT
Cyclophosphamide	Cyclophosphamide is detectable in milk, and two cases of bone marrow depression have been reported in infants of women receiving the drug[55,56]
Methotrexate	Methotrexate was measured in milk in one study. The authors concluded that breast feeding presents little hazard if bottle feeding is not possible; however, this study is not conclusive[1]
CARDIOVASCULAR DRUGS	
Alpha-Adrenergic Blocking Agents	**Phentolamine** can lower elevated serum prolactin levels[57]
Beta-Adrenergic Blocking Agents	Beta-adrenergic blocking agents are excreted in milk at levels often greater than the peak plasma level, because of their lipid solubility, pKa's and low protein binding. While all are excreted in relatively small amounts, caution should be used in premature or sick infants. **Propranolol** appears to provide the greatest margin of safety of the drugs studied (**atenolol, metoprolol, nadolol, propranolol** and **sotalol**).[1,58-61] Beta blockade does not lower prolactin levels in hyperprolactinemia[57]
Cardiac Drugs	**Digoxin** is excreted in milk in levels approaching maternal plasma. This constitutes an insignificant dose for the infant. Breast feeding is safe during digoxin therapy.[62-66] **Quinidine sulfate** excretion appears to be insignificant, but some authors warn against breast feeding because of potential accumulation and thrombocytopenia. Data are not conclusive, however[67]
Hypotensive Agents	**Captopril** is found in very small amounts and no adverse effects have occurred in infants.[68] **Methyldopa** appears to be excreted in insignificant amounts.[69] **Reserpine** may cause nasal stuffiness and increase tracheobronchial secretions. Because safer alternatives are available, reserpine should be avoided[1]

Continued

Drugs Excreted Into Breast Milk

DRUG	NATURE OF EFFECT
HORMONES AND SYNTHETIC SUBSTITUTES	
Corticosteroids	Corticosteroids have not been studied sufficiently to assess their potential for harm to the infant. Extremely small amounts of **prednisone** and **prednisolone** have been found in the human studies available, but very few subjects have been studied. One study found that an infant would receive only 47 mcg of prednisone daily with a maternal dose of 50 mg/day. The long-term effects of continual small doses of corticosteroids are unknown; many sources advise against breast feeding during corticosteroid intake. Low-dose, short-duration therapy probably poses no great hazard to the infant[1,70,71]
Sex Hormones	*Suppression of Lactation* **Estrogens, estrogen/progestogen** and **estrogen/androgen** combinations are used to suppress lactation; however, even in high doses, these agents are not always effective because of the numerous factors affecting lactation. The most important factor is cessation of breast feeding, which alone is quite effective. Because of concern with the possibility of thrombophlebitis and other adverse steroid effects, there is a trend toward the use of **bromocriptine** to suppress lactation[1,72,73] In the small doses used in **oral contraceptives**, sex steroids seem to have little effect on milk flow in the majority of women. With older, high-estrogen contraceptives, lactation could be suppressed sufficiently to cause discontinuation of breast feeding. When present-day, low-estrogen contraceptives are begun 3 weeks postpartum, when lactation is well established, this effect does not occur. **Progestogens** used singly in oral and depot forms for contraception affect milk flow adversely only at high doses (300 mg IM depot **medroxyprogesterone**), but not at lower doses (150 mg IM)[1,74,75] *Milk Composition* Some studies have shown a decrease in protein, fat and minerals in the milk of mothers using older, high-estrogen oral contraceptives. Newer, low-estrogen combination and progestogen-only types Continued

Drugs Excreted Into Breast Milk

DRUG	NATURE OF EFFECT
	decrease protein slightly, but levels remain within the normal range in well-nourished women. These changes in the milk of poorly nourished women (eg, in developing countries) may be of greater significance.[75] Large (600 mg) IM doses of depot medroxyprogesterone acetate (DMPA) used as a contraceptive significantly reduce the nutrient quality of milk, while the usual dose of 150 mg increases protein content[1,74,76]
	Transmission of Drugs Three cases of contraceptives possibly causing breast enlargement in infants and proliferation of the vaginal epithelium in female infants have been attributed to combination oral contraceptives; however, a cause-and-effect relationship has not been firmly established.[1,77] Assays of estrogens and progestogens in milk show that both are found in low levels.[78-83] Although amounts received by infants are small and are readily metabolized,[84] there is concern over the long-term effects of steroids, especially estrogens, in breast-fed infants. Follow-up of infants breast-fed during maternal use of DMPA, although not conclusive, has shown no adverse effects on growth and development. If hormonal contraception is essential, low-dose oral progestogen or IM DMPA are the safest methods[76,85,86]
Thyroid and Antithyroid	**Antithyroid.** In the past, it was felt that any antithyroid therapy was a contraindication to breast feeding. While use of I-131 remains a contraindication,[1] recent studies on the **thionamides** now in use indicate that **propylthiouracil** may be excreted in small enough amounts to be used during lactation.[87,88] This cannot necessarily be said for **methimazole**, however.[87,89] Careful monitoring of the infant is mandatory because of the limited knowledge of the safety of propylthiouracil
	Thyroid. With recent improvements in assay methods, thyroid hormones have been detected in breast milk, although there has been considerable quantitative variation among studies. Formula and cow's milk have negligible amounts of thyroid hormones, but levels in human milk are apparently sufficient to attenuate congenital hypothyroidism.[90-94] Breast feeding does not interfere with screening for hypothyroidism during the first week of life; however, screening after this time should include thyroxine and TSH measurements[95]

Continued

Drugs Excreted Into Breast Milk

DRUG	NATURE OF EFFECT
DIURETICS	
Diuretics	Diuretics can cause a decrease in production of milk and have been used to suppress postpartum lactation.[1,96] No adverse effects in infants have been reported due to diuretics in milk.[1,97,98] Long-acting agents such as **chlorthalidone** should be avoided because of the possibility of accumulation in the neonate. Theoretically, thrombocytopenia or other allergic reactions to **sulfonamide diuretics** could occur
GASTROINTESTINAL DRUGS	
Cathartics and Laxatives	Cathartics and laxatives that are nonabsorbable, such as bulk forming, osmotic and stool softening types cause no problems. Some **anthraquinone derivatives** such as **cascara** and **danthron** should probably be avoided and others, such as **aloe** and **senna**, may cause problems if high doses are used[1]
Cimetidine	Cimetidine should be used with caution because unexpectedly large amounts are found in milk and its effects in infants are unknown.[99] Because of its pKa, there may be large intersubject variation in its excretion. Cimetidine can also increase serum prolactin and induce galactorrhea[100]
Metoclopramide	Metoclopramide is excreted in small amounts that appear to be harmless in infants.[101] It seems to improve defective lactation by increasing prolactin[102,103] and may cause galactorrhea.[104] A related agent, **sulpiride**, also increases prolactin levels and milk yields. It is not detectable in milk[105,106]
PSYCHOTHERAPEUTIC AGENTS	
Antidepressants	Tricyclic antidepressants have not been well studied in breast feeding; however, only minute

Continued

Drugs Excreted Into Breast Milk

DRUG	NATURE OF EFFECT
	quantities have been found in milk. Amounts seem insufficient to affect the infant, but there is no consensus on the safety of breast feeding during tricyclic use. Therefore, close monitoring and caution is warranted during breast feeding[1,107-112]
Tranquilizers	
	Butyrophenones. Haloperidol has been studied in only 2 patients; small quantities have been found which did not affect the infants, but long-term effects are unknown[113,114]
	Phenothiazines pass into milk somewhat unpredictably, but usually in insignificant amounts.[1,107,115,116] Drowsiness with the more sedating agents, such as **chlorpromazine**, has occurred.[116] Other effects, such as extrapyramidal symptoms, seem possible, but have not been reported. Only scanty long-term follow-up has been reported with no adverse effects noted;[117] continuous observation is recommended during long-term use
Lithium	Lithium in milk can adversely affect the infant when lithium elimination in infants is impaired, as in dehydration or in neonates and premature infants (who may already have lithium in plasma acquired transplacentally).[118-121] The long-term effects of lithium in infants are not known, and some authors consider lithium therapy a contraindication to breast feeding.[107,121] Lithium should be used cautiously during lactation, and breast feeding discontinued if infant effects occur
SEDATIVES AND HYPNOTICS	Most sedative-hypnotics pass into breast milk in measurable and potentially significant amounts. Sedative-hypnotic intake should be minimized during lactation; and, agents with unique toxicities in the infant (eg, bromides, diazepam) should be avoided
Barbiturates	Barbiturates can stimulate metabolism of endogenous compounds in the infant if small amounts pass into milk. "Short-acting" agents appear to be preferable to "long-acting" agents, because smaller amounts are excreted in milk. High single doses may have more potential for causing infant drowsiness than do multiple small doses.[1] See also Anticonvulsants

Continued

Drugs Excreted Into Breast Milk

DRUG	NATURE OF EFFECT
Benzodiazepines	Benzodiazepines pass into milk in small amounts, but can accumulate in infants, especially neonates, because of their immature excretory mechanisms. Drugs with long-acting metabolites, such as **diazepam**, are particularly troublesome and have caused adverse effects in infants. It is not possible to avoid peak metabolite milk levels, because they occur up to 1–2 days after the dose. Benzodiazepines should be avoided during breast feeding[1,122-124]
Bromides	Bromides have caused drowsiness and rash and should be avoided during breast feeding[1]
Chloral Hydrate	Chloral hydrate and its metabolite, **trichloroethanol** reached 50–100% of maternal blood levels in most of 50 women given 1.3 g rectally. Drug and metabolites were detectable for up to 24 hr; the maximum dose that an infant could have received approximates a sedative dose. In another study, drowsiness was noted in 1 infant the morning after a bedtime hypnotic dose of a chloral hydrate derivative in the mother[1]
Ether	Ether milk levels are about equal to blood levels for 8–10 hr[1]
Glutethimide	Glutethimide has been detected in minute amounts 8–12 hr after a dose[1]
Halothane	Halothane milk levels equal or surpass levels in maternally inhaled air[125]
Meprobamate	Meprobamate concentrations peak in milk at 4 hr, 2 hr after peak plasma levels[1]
Phenobarbital	See Anticonvulsants
MISCELLANEOUS AGENTS	
Caffeine	Caffeine is excreted in relatively small amounts; most infants are not affected at usual levels of maternal intake.[126-128] However, one infant reportedly developed jitteriness with very high maternal intake (4–5 cups of coffee and 2–3 480 ml bottles of cola daily)[129]

Continued

Drugs Excreted Into Breast Milk

DRUG	NATURE OF EFFECT
Dihydrotachysterol	Dihydrotachysterol is considered contraindicated during breast feeding by some authors, because of renal calcifications that occurred in animal studies[1]
Ergot Alkaloids	**Bromocriptine** inhibits lactation by suppressing prolactin release;[1,73] and rebound galactorrhea has been reported following withdrawal of high-dose bromocriptine.[130] Related agents, **lisuride** and **metergoline**, also inhibit lactation[131-132]
	While **ergonovine** has been reported to lower prolactin levels slightly, **methylergonovine** does not, nor is it found in milk in significant quantities.[1,133] It appears that short-term, low-dose regimens of these two agents postpartum pose no hazard to the infant nor do they affect milk flow
	Older crude ergot preparations were found to produce toxic effects in infants, but they are no longer used.[1] The use and excretion of **ergotamine** during lactation has not been studied and its long-term use in migraine probably should be avoided during lactation until it has been studied
Gold	Gold is excreted in milk and can be detected in the blood and urine of nursing infants. The exact amounts of gold that infants receive has not been well quantified, but sufficient amounts may be ingested to cause adverse effects.[134-136] Gold therapy may be a reason for withholding breast feeding
Iodides	Iodides are probably contraindicated during breast feeding because of possible thyroid suppression and rashes.[1] **Iopanoic acid** contains free iodide which can be detected in milk. Although no adverse effects have been reported in infants, breast feeding should probably be withheld for 24–36 hr after a dose
Oxytocin	Oxytocin, as a nasal spray, brings about milk ejection, thus facilitating breast feeding and increasing milk volume in the mothers of premature infants[1,137]

Continued

Drugs Excreted Into Breast Milk

DRUG	NATURE OF EFFECT
Sympathomimetics	One anecdotal case exists of infant irritability, crying and disturbed sleep during maternal intake of a long-acting preparation containing **pseudoephedrine** and **dexbrompheniramine**.[138] In general, sympathomimetics are safe, but infants should be carefully observed with maternal use of high doses and long-acting products. Theoretically, sympathomimetics can decrease milk flow by central inhibition of secretion and release of oxytocin and by peripheral vasoconstriction which limits the access of oxytocin to myoepithelial cells in the breast.[24] However, this effect has not been documented
Theobromine	Theobromine from chocolate is excreted in amounts that are not pharmacologically significant in most infants, but could produce effects in sensitive infants or with high maternal intake[139]
Theophylline	Theophylline has been reported to cause irritability and fretful sleep in one infant.[1] Sustained-release products and continuous infusion (of **aminophylline**) should tend to maximize the dose received by infants, but amounts in infant plasma should remain below the therapeutic range in most cases.[1,140] There is no need to avoid theophylline products, but infant plasma levels should be measured if side effects occur
Tolbutamide	Tolbutamide is excreted in very small amounts which should cause no harm[1]
Vaccines	Much contradictory literature on **poliovirus** has been published about the possibility that antibodies in milk could prevent active immunization in infants. It has been recommended that breast feeding be withheld for 2–6 hr before and after immunization; however, if infants are immunized after 6 weeks of age, breast feeding has a negligible effect on antibody titers.[1] **Rubella** (Cadenhill strain) is apparently not transferred to infants via milk[1]

References

1. Anderson PO. Drugs and breast feeding: a review. Drug Intell Clin Pharm 1977;11:208-23. Revised and reprinted in Knoben JE, Anderson PO, Watanabe AS, eds. Handbook of clinical drug data. 4th ed. Hamilton, IL: Drug Intelligence Publications, 1978:89-118.

2. Anderson PO. Drugs and breast feeding. Semin Perinatol 1979;3:271-8.

3. Wilson JT, Brown RD, Cherek DR et al. Drug excretion in human milk: principles, pharmacokinetics and projected consequences. Clin Pharmacokinet 1980;5:1-65. Revised and reprinted as Wilson JT, ed. Drugs in breast milk. New York: ADIS Press, 1981.

4. Rasmussen F. Excretion of drugs by milk. In: Brodie BB, Gillette JR, eds. Concepts in biochemical pharmacology, part 1. New York: Springer-Verlag, 1971:390-402.

5. Binkiewicz A, Robinson MJ, Senior B. Pseudo-Cushing syndrome caused by alcohol in breast milk. J Pediatr 1978;93:965-7.

6. Berlin CM, Yaffe SJ, Ragni M. Disposition of acetaminophen in milk, saliva and plasma of lactating women. Pediatr Pharmacol 1980;1:135-41.

7. Findlay JWA, DeAngelis RL, Kearney MF et al. Analgesic drugs in breast milk. Clin Pharmacol Ther 1981;29:625-33.

7a. Bitzen P-O et al. Eur J Clin Pharmacol 1981;20:123-5.

8. Pittman KA, Smyth RD, Losada M et al. Human perinatal distribution of butorphanol. Am J Obstet Gynecol 1980;138:797-800.

9. Peiker G, Muller B, Inh W et al. Ausscheidung von pethidine durch die muttermilch. Zentralb Gynaekol 1980;102:537.

10. Freeborn SF, Calvert RT, Black P et al. Saliva and blood pethidine concentrations in the mother and the newborn baby. Br J Obstet Gynaecol 1980;87:966-9.

11. Kreek MJ, Schecter A, Gutjahr CL et al. Analysis of methadone and other drugs in maternal and neonatal body fluids: use in evaluation of symptoms in a neonate of mother maintained on methadone. Am J Drug Alcohol Abuse 1974;1:409-19.

12. Shaffer H. Methadone and pregnancy: perspectives and prescriptions. J Psychedelic Drugs 1979;11:191-202.

13. Anon. Methadone in breast milk. Med Lett Drugs Ther 1979;21:52.

14. Smialek JE, Monforte JR, Aranow R et al. Methadone deaths in children: a continuing problem. JAMA 1977;238:2516-7.

15. Lakings DB, Lizarraga C, Haggerty WJ et al. High-performance liquid chromatographic microdetermination of indoprofen in human milk. J Pharm Sci 1979;68:1113-6.

16. Strobel E, Herrmann B. Zur frage des ubergangs von oxyphenbutazon den fetalen kreislauf und die muttermilch. Arznemein Forsch 1962;12:302-5.

17. Leuxner E, Pulver R. Verabreichung von irgapyrin bei schwangeren und wochnerinnen. Schweigeisch Med Mchschr 1956;98:84-7.

18. Gensichen E, Klingmuller V. Verlauf der konzentrationen von phenylbutazon und isopyrin im serum, nabelschnurserum und frauenmilch. N-S Arch Exp Path Pharmakol 1963;246:52.

19. Eeg-Olofsson O, Elwin C-E, Steen B. Convulsions in a breast-fed infant after maternal indomethacin. Lancet 1978;2:215.

20. Berlin CM Jr, Pascuzzi MJ, Yaffe SJ. Excretion of salicylate in human milk (abstract). Clin Pharmacol Ther 1980;27:245-6.

21. Erickson SH, Oppenheim GL. Aspirin in breast milk. J Fam Pract 1979;8:189-90.

22. Levy G. Salicylate pharmacokinetics in the human neonate. In: Morselli PL, Sarattini S, Sereni F, eds. Basic and therapeutic aspects of perinatal pharmacology. New York: Raven Press, 1975:319-30.

23. Levy G. Clinical pharmacokinetics of aspirin. J Pediatr 1978;62(Suppl):867-72.

24. Tucker HA. Endocrinology of lactation. Semin Perinatol 1979;3:199-223.

25. Orme ML'E, Lewis PJ, DeSwiet et al. May mothers given warfarin breast-feed their infants? Br Med J 1977;1:1564-5.

26. Pynnonen S, Kanto J, Sillanpaa M et al. Carbamazepine: placental transport, tissue concentrations in foetus and newborn and level in milk. Arch Pharmacol Toxicol 1977;41:244-53.

27. Niebyl JR, Blake DA, Freeman JM et al. Carbamazepine levels in pregnancy and lactation. Obstet Gynecol 1979;53:139-40.

28. Kaneko S, Sato T, Suzuki K. The levels of anticonvulsants in breast milk. Br J Clin Pharmacol 1979;7:624-6.

29. Koup JR, Rose JQ, Cohen ME. Ethosuximide pharmacokinetics in a pregnant patient and her newborn. Epilepsia 1978;19:535-9.

30. Rane A, Garle M, Borga O et al. Plasma disappearance of transplacentally transferred diphenylhydantoin in the newborn studied by mass fragmentography. Clin Pharmacol Ther 1974;15:39-45.

31. Espir MLE, Benton P, Will E et al. Sodium valproate (Epilim)—some clinical and pharmacological aspects. In: Legg NJ, ed. The treatment of epilepsy. Turnbridge Wells, England: MCS Consultants, 1976:145-51.

32. Nau H, Rating D, Hausing I et al. Placental transfer and pharmacokinetics of primidone and its metabolites phenobarbital, PEMA and hydroxyphenobarbital in neonates and infants of epileptic mothers. Eur J Clin Pharmacol 1980;18:31-42.

33. Alexander FW. Sodium valproate and pregnancy. Arch Dis Child 1979;54:240-5.

34. Dickinson RG, Harland RC, Lynn RK et al. Transmission of valproic acid (Depakene) across the placenta: half-life of the drug in mother and baby. J Pediatr 1979;94:832-5.

35. Takase Z, Shirafuji M, Uchida M. Fundamental studies and clinical trials with sisomycin in obstetrics and gynecology. Chemotherapy (Tokyo) 1978:26:298-302.

36. Takase Z, Shirafuji H, Uchida M et al. Laboratory and clinical studies on tobramycin in the field of obstetrics and gynecology. Chemotherapy (Tokyo) 1975;23:1402-7.

37. Uwaydah M, Bibia S, Salam S. Therapeutic efficacy of tobramycin—a clinical and laboratory evaluation. J Antimicrob Chemother 1975;1:429-37.

38. Fujimori H, Imai S. Studies of dihydrostreptomycin administered to the pregnant and transferred to their fetuses. J Japanese Obstet Gynecol Soc 1957;4:133-49.

39. Yoshioka H, Cho K, Takimoto M et al. Transfer of cefazolin into human milk. J Pediatr 1979;94:151-2.

40. Kobyletzki D, Sas D, Dingeldein E et al. Pharmacokinetic investigations of cefazedone in gynecology and obstetrics. Arznzeim Forsch 1979;29:1763-8.

41. Santo GH, Huch A. Übergang von cefoxitin in muttermilch. Infection 1979;7(Suppl):590-1.

42. Geddes AM, Schnurr LP, Ball AP et al. Cefoxitin: a hospital study. Br Med J 1977;1:1126-8.

43. Matsuda S, Tanno M, Kashiwagura T et al. Basic and clinical studies on cefotiam (SCE-963) in the field of obstetrics and gynecology. Chemotherapy (Tokyo) 1979;27(S-3):655-60.

44. Mischler TW, Corson SL, Larranaga A et al. Cephradine and epicillin in body fluids of lactating and pregnant women. J Reprod Med 1978;21:130-6.

45. Kafetzis DA, Siafas CA, Georgakopoulos PA et al. Passage of cephalosporins and amoxicillin into the breast milk. Acta Paediatr Scand 1981;70:285-8.

46. Kauffman RE, O'Brien C, Gilford P. Sulfisoxazole secretion into human milk. J Pediatr 1980;97:839-41.

47. Jarnerot G, Into-Malmberg M-B. Sulfasalazine treatment during breast feeding. Scand J Gastroenterol 1979;147:869-71.

48. Kahn AKA, Truelove SC. Placental and mammary transfer of sulfasalazine. Br Med J 1979;2:1553.

49. Berlin CM Jr, Yaffe SJ. Disposition of salicylazosulfapyridine (Azulfidine) and metabolites in human breast milk. Develop Pharmacol Ther 1980;1:31-9.

50. Allgen LG, Holmberg G, Persson B et al. Biological fate of methenamine in man. Acta Obstet Gynecol Scand 1979;58:287-93.

51. Berlin CM, Lee C. Isoniazid and acetylisoniazid disposition in human milk, saliva and plasma (abstract). Fed Proc 1979;38(3) (part 1):426.

52. Moore B, Collier J. Drugs and breast feeding. Br Med J 1979;2:211.

53. Erickson SH, Oppenheim GL, Smith GH. Metronidazole in breast milk. Obstet Gynecol 1981;57:48-50.

54. Bounameaux Y, Durenne JM. Un cas de luecemie chez une femme allaite: effects du traitment par le busulfan sur le nourisson. Ann Soc Belge Med Trop 1964;44:381-4.

55. Amato D, Niblett JS. Neutropenia from cyclophosphamide in breast milk. Med J Aust 1977;1:383-4.

56. Durodola JI. Administration of cyclophosphamide during late pregnancy and early lactation: a case report. J Natl Med Assoc 1979;71:165-6.

57. Board JA, Fierro RJ, Wasserman HJ et al. Effects of α- and β- adrenergic blocking agents on serum prolactin levels in women with hyperprolactinemia and galactorrhea. Am J Obstet Gynecol 1977;127:285-7.

58. Sandstrom B, Regardh C-G. Metoprolol secretion into breast milk. Br J Clin Pharmacol 1980;9:518-9.

59. Heel RC, Brogden RN, Pakes GE et al. Nadolol: a review of its pharmacological properties and therapeutic efficacy in hypertension and angina pectoris. Drugs 1980;20:1-23.

60. Baver JH, Pape B, Zajicek J et al. Propranolol in human plasma and breast milk. Am J Cardiol 1979;43:860-2.

61. O'Hare MF, Murnaghan GA, Russell CJ et al. Sotalol as a hypotensive agent in pregnancy. Br J Obstet Gynaecol 1980;87:814-20.

61a. Liedholm H. Eur J Clin Pharmacol 1981;20:229.

61b. Devlin RG et al. Br J Clin Pharmacol 1981;12:393.

62. Levy M, Granit L, Laufer N. Excretion of drugs in milk. N Engl J Med 1977;297:789.

63. Loughnan PM. Digoxin excretion in human breast milk. J Pediatr 1978;92:1019-20.

64. Chan V, Tse TF, Wong V. Transfer of digoxin across the placenta and into breast milk. Br J Obstet Gynaecol 1978;85:605-9.

66. Finley JP, Waxman MB, Wong PY et al. Digoxin excretion in human milk. J Pediatr 1979;94:339-40.

67. Hill LM, Malkasin GD. The use of quinidine sulfate throughout pregnancy. Obstet Gynecol 1979;54:366-8.

68. Devlin RG, Fleiss PM. Captopril in human blood and breast milk. J Clin Pharmacol 1981;21:110-3.

69. Jones HMR, Cummings AJ. A study of the transfer of α-methyldopa to the human fetus and newborn infant. Br J Clin Pharmacol 1978;6:432-4.

70. Berlin CM, Kaiser DG, Demers L. Excretion of prednisone and prednisolone in human milk. Pharmacologist 1979;21:264.

71. Sagraves R, Kaiser D, Sharpe GL. Prednisone and prednisolone concentrations in the milk of a lactating mother (abstract). Drug Intell Clin Pharm 1981;15:484.

72. Rosa FW. Resolving the ''public health dilemma'' of steroid contraception and its effects on lactation. Am J Public Health 1976;66:791-2.

73. Harrison RG. Suppression of lactation. Semin Perinatol 1979;3:287-97.

74. Toddywalla VS, Joshi L, Virker K. Effect of contraceptive steroids on human lactation. Am J Obstet Gynecol 1977;127:245-9.

75. Lonnerdal B, Forsum E, Hambraeus L. Effect of oral contraceptives on composition and volume of breast milk. Am J Clin Nutr 1980;33:816-24.

76. IPPF International Medical Advisory Panel. Injectable contraception. IPPF Med Bull 1980;14(6):1-3.

77. Nilsson S, Nygren K-G, Johansson EDB. Ethinyl estradiol in human plasma after oral administration. Contraception 1978;17:131-9.

78. Saxena BN, Shrimanker K, Grudzinskas JG. Levels of contraceptive steroids in breast milk and plasma of lactating women. Contraception 1977;16:605-13.

79. Nilsson S, Nygren K-G, Johansson EDB. Megestrol acetate concentrations in plasma and milk during administration of an oral contraceptive containing 4 mg megestrol acetate to nursing women. Contraception 1977;16:615-24.

80. Thomas MJ, Danutra V, Read GF et al. The detection and measurement of d-norgestrel in human milk using sephadex LH 20 chromatography and radioimmunoassay. Steroids 1977;30:349-61.

81. Nilsson S, Nygren K-G, Johansson EDB. Transfer of estradiol to human milk. Am J Obstet Gynecol 1978;132:653-7.

82. Toddywalla VS, Mehta S, Virkar KD et al. Release of 19-nor-testosterone type of contraceptive steroids through different drug delivery systems into the serum and breast milk of lactating women. Contraception 1980;21:217-23.

83. Stoppelli I, Rainer E, Humpel M. Transfer of cyproterone to the milk of lactating women. Contraception 1980;22:485-93.

84. Nilsson S, Nygren K-G, Johansson EDB. d-Norgestrel concentrations in maternal plasma, milk and child plasma during administration of oral contraceptives to nursing women. Am J Obstet Gynecol 1977;129:178-84.

85. Nilsson S, Nygren K-G. Transfer of contraceptive steroids to human milk. Res Reprod 1979;11(1):1-2.

86. Kincl FA. Debate on the use of hormonal contraceptives during lactation. Res Reprod 1980;12(2):1.

87. Low LCK, Lang J, Alexander WD. Excretion of carbimazole and propylthiouracil in breast milk. Lancet 1979;2:1011.

88. Kampmann JP, Hansen JM, Johansen K et al. Propylthiouracil in human milk: revision of a dogma. Lancet 1980;1:736-8.

89. Tegler L, Lindstrom B. Antithyroid drugs in milk. Lancet 1980;2:591.

90. Sack J, Amado O, Lunefeld B. Thyroxine concentration in human milk. J Clin Endocrinol Metab 1977;45:171-3.

91. Bode HH, Vanjonack WJ, Crawford JD. Mitigation of cretinism by breast-feeding. Pediatrics 1978;62:13-6.

92. Varma SK, Collins M, Row A et al. Thyroxine, tri-iodothyronine and reverse tri-iodothyronine concentrations in human milk. J Pediatr 1978;93:803-6.

93. Man EB, Benotti J. Butanol-extractable iodine in human and bovine colostrum and milk. Clin Chem 1969;15:1141-6.

94. Strbak V, Macho R, Korvak R et al. Thyroxine (by competitive protein binding analysis) in human and cow milk and in infant formulas. Endocrinol Exp 1976;10:167-74.

95. Abbassi V, Steinout TA. Successful diagnosis of congenital hypothyroidism in four breast-fed infants. J Pediatr 1980;97:259-61.

96. Cominos DC, Van Der Walt A, Van Rooyen AJL. Suppression of postpartum lactation with furosemide. S Afr Med J 1976;50:251-2.

97. Phelps DC, Karim A. Spironolactone: relationship between concentration of dethioacetylated metabolite in human serum and milk. J Pharm Sci 1977;66:1203.

98. Mulley BA, Parr GD, Pau WK et al. Placental transfer of chlorthalidone and its metabolites in maternal milk. Eur J Clin Pharmacol 1978;13:129-31.

99. Somogi A, Gugler R. Cimetidine excretion into breast milk. Br J Clin Pharmacol 1979;7:627-9.

100. Bateson MC, Browning MCK, Maconnachie A. Galactorrhea with cimetidine. Lancet 1977;1:247-8.

101. Lewis PJ, Devenish C, Kahn C. Controlled trial of metoclopramide in the initiation of breast feeding. Br J Clin Pharmacol 1980;9:217-9.

102. Guzman V, Toscano G, Canales ES et al. Improvement of defective lactation by using oral metoclopramide. Acta Obstet Gynecol Scand 1979;58:53-5.

103. Kauppila A, Kivinen S, Ylikorkala A. A dose response relation between improved lactation and metoclopramide. Lancet 1981;1:1175-7.

104. Finnis WA, Bird CE, Wilson DL. Metoclopramide hydrochloride and galactorrhea. Can Med Assoc J 1976;115:845.

105. Badraoui MHH, Hefnawi F, Hegab M et al. The effect of a nonhormonal drug used as a contraceptive method and lactation stimulant after delivery. Fertil Steril 1978;30:742.

106. Aono T, Shioji T, Aki T et al. Augmentation of puerperal lactation by oral administration of sulpiride. J Clin Endocrinol Metab 1979;48:478-82.

107. Ananth J. Side effects in the neonate from psychotropic agents excreted through breast feeding. Am J Psychiatry 1978;135:801-5.

108. Gelenberg AJ. Amoxapine, a new antidepressant, appears in milk. J Nerv Ment Dis 1979;167:635-6.

109. Rees JA, Glass RC, Sporne GA. Serum and breast milk concentration of dothiepin. Practitioner 1976;217:686.

110. Sovner R, Orsulak PJ. Excretion of imipramine and desipramine in human breast milk. Am J Psychiatry 1979;136:451-2.

111. Erickson SJ, Smith GH, Heidrich F. Tricyclics and breast feeding. Am J Psychiatry 1979;136:1483.

112. Bader TF, Newman K. Amitriptyline in human breast milk and the nursing infant's serum. Am J Psychiatry 1980;137:855-6.

113. Stewart RB, Karas B, Springer PK. Haloperidol excretion in human milk. Am J Psychiatry 1980;137:849-50.

114. Whalley LJ, Blain PG, Prime JK. Haloperidol secreted in breast milk. Br Med J 1981;282:1746-7.

115. Citterio C. Riconoscimento e dosaggio di derivati fenotiazinici nella secrezione lattea. Neuropsichiatria 1964;20:141-6.

116. Wiles DH, Orr MW, Kolakowska T. Chlorpromazine levels in plasma and milk of nursing mothers. Br J Clin Pharmacol 1978;5:272-3.

117. Kris EB, Carmichael DM. Chlorpromazine maintenance therapy during pregnancy and confinement. Psychiatric Quarterly 1957;31:690-5.

118. Skavsig OB, Schou M. Diegivning under litiumbehandling. Ugeskr Laeg 1977;139:400-401.

119. Schou M, Weinstein MR. Problems of lithium maintenance treatment during pregnancy, delivery and lactation. Agressologie 1980;21(special issue A):7-9.

120. Rane A, Tomson G, Bjarke B. Effects of maternal lithium therapy in a newborn infant. J Pediatr 1978;93:296-7.

121. Tunnessen WW, Hertz CG. Toxic effects of lithium in newborn infants: a commentary. J Pediatr 1972;81:804-7.

122. Rey E, Giraux P, d'Athis P et al. Pharmacokinetics of the placental transfer and distribution of clorazepate and its metabolite nordiazepam in the fetoplacental unit and in the neonate. Eur J Clin Pharmacol 1979;15:181-5.

123. Kanto J, Aaltonen L, Kangas L et al. Placental transfer and breast milk levels of flunitrazepam. Curr Ther Res 1979;26:539-46.

124. Pacifici GM, Placidi GF. Rapid and sensitive electron-capture gas chromatographic method for the determination of pinazepam and its metabolites in human plasma, urine and milk. J Chromatogr 1977;135:133-9.

125. Cote CJ, Kenepp NB, Reed SB et al. Trace concentrations of halothane in human breast milk. Br J Anaesth 1976;48:541-3.

126. Tyrala EE, Dodson WE. Caffeine secretion into breast milk. Arch Dis Child 1979;54:787-800.

127. Hill R, Craig JP, Chaney MD et al. Utilization of over-the-counter drugs during pregnancy. Clin Obstet Gynecol 1977;20:381-4.

128. Brazier J-L, Renaur H, Ribon B et al. Plasma xanthine levels in low birthweight infants treated or not treated with theophyllline. Arch Dis Child 1979;54:194-9.

129. Rivera-Calimlin L. Drugs in breast milk. Drug Ther (Dec) 1977:59-63.

130. Pentland B, Sawers JSA. Galactorrhoea after withdrawal of bromocriptine. Br Med J 1980;281:716.

131. De Cecco L, Venturini PL, Ragni N et al. Effect of lisuride on inhibition of lactation and serum prolactin. Br J Obstet Gynaecol 1979;86:905-8.

132. Delitala G, Masala A, Alagna S et al. Metergoline in the inhibition of puerperal lactation. Br Med J 1977;1:744-6.

133. Erkkola R, Kanto J, Allonen H et al. Excretion of methylergometrine (methylergonovine) into the human breast milk. Int J Clin Pharmacol 1978;16:579-80.

134. Blau SP. Metabolism of gold during lactation. Arthritis Rheum 1973;16:777-8.

135. Gottlieb NL. Suggested errata. Arthritis Rheum 1974;17:1057.

136. Bell RAF, Dale IM. Gold secretion in maternal milk. Arthritis Rheum 1976;19:1374.

137. Ruis H, Rolland R, Doesburg W et al. Oxytocin enhances onset of lactation among mothers delivering prematurely. Br Med J 1981;283:340-2.

138. Mortimer EA. Drug toxicity from breast milk? Pediatrics 1977;60:781-2.

139. Resman BH, Blumenthal HP, Jusko WJ. Breast milk distribution of theobromine from chocolate. J Pediatr 1977;91:477-80.

140. Stec GP, Greenberger P, Ruo TI et al. Kinetics of theophylline transfer into breast milk. Clin Pharmacol Ther 1980;28:404-8.

9 DRUGS AND PREGNANCY

THE USE OF ANY THERAPEUTIC AGENT DURING PREGNANCY is associated with risks both to the woman and to her unborn child. The fetus is the inadvertent recipient of almost all medication taken by the pregnant woman. Generally, no fetal effect is intended, but many effects may be encountered during therapy of the pregnant woman. In addition, altered physiology associated with pregnancy may change accepted pharmacokinetic parameters and may make certain therapies more hazardous during this period. Therapy of the nonpregnant woman of reproductive age must also be undertaken with caution as many agents may affect the embryo before pregnancy is detectable.

Changes in maternal physiology are exemplified by the fact that the blood volume increases by approximately 20 to 30% throughout pregnancy, then tends to fall again during the last few weeks of pregnancy. There is an increase in plasma volume and interstitial fluid. These volume changes may greatly affect volumes of distribution and clearances of medications. Plasma levels of drugs known to have narrow therapeutic indices should be monitored frequently during the course of pregnancy.

The first trimester is the period of maximal differentiation of embryonic tissue and is therefore the period during which drug exposure is most likely to cause structural malformations. Following this period, fetal susceptibility to teratogens is low. Drugs administered during the last two trimesters, however, may nevertheless affect the fetus by causing functional malformations, intrauterine growth retardation (IUGR), fetal addiction or by producing unwanted pharmacological effects.

Administration of medications near term is associated with another hazard, because the fetus relies primarily on maternal tissues for drug elimination. After birth, the infant must use its own metabolic processes to eliminate drugs. These pathways are not fully developed in the neonate; therefore, any medication which had crossed the placenta may have a greatly prolonged fetal action.

Controlled prospective studies of drug use in pregnancy are few; most associations of maternal drug exposure and fetal effect have been established using case reports or retrospective data. Relationships are often difficult to identify because of the numerous variables associated with each report. These include maternal dose, duration of therapy, stage of fetal development (ie, different effects occur at different stages), concomitant exposure to other potential teratogens and genetic predisposition of the mother and fetus. An additional confusing factor is that not all women exposed to a known teratogenic agent have children with malformations; for many agents, the frequency may be less than 1%. Because of all of the confounding variables it is probably most prudent for a pregnant woman who has been exposed or is contemplating exposure to a known teratogen to seek professional teratogen counseling.

The following table presents information available on drugs which are known to cause, or which have the potential to cause unwanted fetal effects, or which should be used with caution in the pregnant patient because of her altered physiology.

The table begins on page 150.

Drug Use and Pregnancy

DRUG	NATURE OF EFFECT
ALCOHOL	
Alcohol	Alcohol consumption during pregnancy should be avoided as consumption of even small amounts can cause adverse fetal effects. As little as 2 ounces of absolute alcohol consumed twice weekly has been associated with an increased frequency of spontaneous abortion, and as little as 1 ounce taken daily has been associated with infants with decreased birth weights. Chronic heavy alcohol consumption by the pregnant woman is associated with the "fetal alcohol syndrome" which consists of IUGR, postnatal growth deficiency, developmental delay, mental retardation, craniofacial anomalies, microcephaly and maxillary hypoplasia. Cleft lip and cardiac and renal anomalies are also seen. A neonatal withdrawal syndrome consisting of irritability, tremor, spontaneous seizures, opisthotonos, abdominal distention, CNS depression and hypoglycemia has also been identified[1-6]
ANALGESICS AND ANTIPYRETICS	
Aspirin	Aspirin is known to cross the placenta and, after delivery, to be eliminated slowly by the neonate. Maternal ingestion is associated with a decrease in factor XII, an increase in prothrombin time, platelet dysfunction and bleeding in the neonate. Neonatal clotting may be affected by as little as 650 mg taken 2 weeks before delivery. An increased length of gestation, which may be due to aspirin's antiprostaglandin effect, and an increased rate of perinatal mortality has been seen in long-term salicylate users[1-3,7]
Indomethacin	Indomethacin used for the prevention of premature delivery and for the control of uterine activity at term has been associated with persistent fetal circulation. This effect is presumably due to its antiprostaglandin activity[8]
Narcotic Analgesics	Narcotic analgesics produce significant neonatal respiratory depression when given to mothers

Continued

Drug Use and Pregnancy

DRUG	NATURE OF EFFECT
	during delivery. Maternal addiction is associated with IUGR, premature labor and toxemia. Infants born to addicted mothers often exhibit withdrawal symptoms including irritability, tremulousness, vomiting and seizures [1,2,4,7]
ANTICOAGULANTS	
Warfarin	Warfarin and related anticoagulants are known to produce the "fetal warfarin syndrome" when ingested during pregnancy. First trimester exposure produces nasal hypoplasia, stippled epiphyses and possible mental retardation. Hydrocephalus, microcephaly, optic atrophy and mental retardation may be due to exposure in the latter trimesters. In addition, prenatal use of warfarin produces an increased risk of fetal hemorrhage, especially at delivery [1-5,9]
Heparin	Heparin, a large molecule which does not cross the placenta, has been advocated as the anticoagulant of choice during pregnancy. A large retrospective study evaluating the maternal and fetal risk of anticoagulant therapy during pregnancy suggests that heparin may not be a safe alternative. Heparin use during pregnancy was associated with a high rate of maternal hemorrhage as well as an almost 33% rate of stillbirth or prematurity [10]
ANTICONVULSANTS	
Phenobarbital	Phenobarbital use during pregnancy has been associated with neonatal withdrawal (see Barbiturates). It is an inducer of fetal liver enzymes and therefore has been used for both the prevention and the treatment of neonatal hyperbilirubinemia. Enzyme induction is associated with an increased rate of steroid metabolism and altered vitamin D metabolism. Neonatal hypocalcemia and coagulopathies, due to a decrease in vitamin K dependent clotting factors, have been seen with antenatal phenobarbital use. Phenobarbital has been implicated as a teratogen causing cleft lip, congenital heart disease and microcephaly, but there are insufficient data to be conclusive [1,3]

Continued

Drug Use and Pregnancy

DRUG	NATURE OF EFFECT
Phenytoin	Phenytoin use has been reported to cause a twofold increase in the prevalence of congenital defects in offspring of mothers who received it during pregnancy. The "fetal hydantoin syndrome" consists of IUGR, microcephaly, mental retardation, broad depressed nasal bridge, and nail and/or distal phalangeal hypoplasia. Features of the syndrome have been reported in up to 30% of exposed newborns[1-3,5]
Primidone	Primidone, used alone and in combination therapy during pregnancy, has been associated with neonates with cleft palates, hypoplasia of distal phalanges and nails, fragile primary teeth and stunted length. A post-partum withdrawal syndrome has also been reported[1]
Trimethadione	Trimethadione when used during pregnancy is associated with a fetal syndrome consisting of mild mental retardation, V-shaped eyebrows, speech difficulties, palatal anomalies, abnormal ears and epicanthi. In addition, there seems to be an increased prevalence of spontaneous abortion when trimethadione is used during pregnancy[1-5]
Valproic Acid	Valproic acid has been shown to cross the placenta and achieve significant levels in the fetus. One report of a woman who received it from the second week of gestation through term implicates it as a teratogen. Her infant exhibited dysmorphic facies, abnormal skeletal development and cardiac anomalies and died at 19 days of age[11,12]
ANTIHISTAMINES	Despite reports implicating both **meclizine** and **Bendectin®** (**doxylamine** and **pyridoxine**) as teratogens, large scale studies have shown no association between either of these agents (or the previous formulation of Bendectin® which also included **dicyclomine**) and fetal malformation[1,2,9] **Diphenhydramine** has been implicated by retrospective data to be a cause of cleft lip and/or palate in the neonate. Such data, however, are not conclusive[1,4]

Continued

Drug Use and Pregnancy

DRUG	NATURE OF EFFECT
ANTI-INFECTIVE AGENTS	
Chloramphenicol	Chloramphenicol crosses the placenta, is toxic to the newborn and therefore poses a theoretical hazard when given to the pregnant woman near term. Incomplete development of neonatal hepatic enzyme systems allow toxic levels to accumulate causing refusal to suck, irregular respirations, flaccidity, ashen-gray color, hypothermia and circulatory collapse. However, no toxic effects have been observed in newborns whose mothers have received up to 1 g every 2 hours of chloramphenicol during labor[1-3,7,13]
Metronidazole	Metronidazole has been shown in a large multicenter study to produce a 99% cure rate of trichomonal vaginitis during pregnancy with no apparent adverse effects to the neonate, as measured by frequency of abortion, prematurity and Apgar score. The overall prevalence of congenital anomalies was within expected levels, but was higher in those treated in the first trimester[14]
Plasmodicides	**Chloroquine,** when given in doses appropriate for malaria prophylaxis, has not been associated with adverse fetal effects. Larger anti-inflammatory doses, however, have resulted in spontaneous abortion and fetal retinal and vestibular damage.[1,5,7] **Quinine** possesses a significant oxytocic action on the gravid uterus which becomes more pronounced as pregnancy proceeds; toxic levels of quinine are associated with abortion. Fetal toxicity is manifested as deafness[1,5,7]
Streptomycin	Streptomycin and dihydrostreptomycin have been reported to cause congenital hearing loss and deafness when given to pregnant women for the treatment of tuberculosis. Insufficient data are available on the use of other aminoglycosides during pregnancy, but they may pose the same risks[1,2,4,5,13]
Sulfonamides	Sulfonamides given during the last trimester of pregnancy may predispose the newborn to kernicterus. These drugs rapidly cross the placenta and compete with bilirubin for albumin binding Continued

Drug Use and Pregnancy

DRUG	NATURE OF EFFECT

sites. After delivery, the placental route of elimination is no longer available and elevated free bilirubin may cross into the neonatal CNS. Although this effect has been associated only with the use of long-acting sulfonamides, it may be wise to avoid all sulfonamide use near term[1,4,7,9,13]

Tetracyclines

Tetracycline use during pregnancy is associated with a significant risk of hepatic injury to the pregnant woman, especially when given intravenously in high doses for the treatment of pyelonephritis. In addition, it affects fetal bone and primary tooth development. These effects may also occur with other tetracyclines[1,2,5,7,9,13]

ANTINEOPLASTIC AGENTS

These agents are used therapeutically to inhibit the growth of rapidly proliferating cells and should be considered to be teratogens. Morphologically normal infants, however, have been born to mothers who received such diverse chemotherapy as **mechlorethamine, thio-tepa** or **azathioprine** during pregnancy[2,4]

Use of the folate antagonists, **aminopterin** and **methotrexate,** during the first trimester has resulted in infants with multiple skeletal anomalies. **Busulfan** therapy of leukemia during pregnancy has been reported to cause IUGR and multiple malformations. Maternal **chlorambucil** use has been associated with congenital absence of one kidney and ureter. **Cyclophosphamide** use has been associated with defects in the extremities[2,4]

CARDIOVASCULAR DRUGS

Diazoxide

Diazoxide is known to cross the placenta, but when given intravenously it seems to have little effect on the fetal cardiovascular system. It relaxes uterine smooth muscle and is a potent inhibitor of labor. The most significant effect of its use in toxemia is severe maternal hypotension and concomitant fetal bradycardia. Fetal hyperglycemia may also be produced. Chronic oral administration has been associated with newborn alopecia, hypertrichosis lanuginosa and decreased bone age[1,4]

Continued

Drug Use and Pregnancy

DRUG	NATURE OF EFFECT
Digoxin	Digoxin readily crosses the placenta and is preferentially concentrated in the fetal heart during the second half of pregnancy. Amniotic fluid digoxin levels, which slightly exceed fetal plasma levels, have been used to monitor the fetus. Maternal digoxin levels should be monitored frequently, because they tend to fall during the course of the pregnancy as the volume of distribution rises with the growth of the fetal compartment[1,7]
Disopyramide	Disopyramide use during pregnancy has been associated with the initiation of uterine contractions which subsided when the drug was discontinued[1]
Propranolol	Propranolol use throughout pregnancy is associated with a significant risk of IUGR, prolonged bradycardia and hypoglycemia. Respiratory depression has been reported in neonates whose mothers received intravenous propranolol immediately before cesarean section. Similar effects may be expected with prenatal use of other beta-adrenergic blockers[1,3,4,7]
Reserpine	Reserpine, when given to mothers within 24 hours of delivery, produces edema of the nasal mucosa in the neonate. This effect is especially significant because the newborn infant is an obligate nose breather. Lethargy, hypothermia and bradycardia have also been reported in infants whose mothers received antenatal reserpine. **Methyldopa** appears to be a safe and effective antihypertensive for use in pregnancy[1,4,7,9]
CORTICOSTEROIDS	Chronic corticosteroid or **corticotropin** therapy during pregnancy is associated with approximately a 1% rate of cleft palate in the offspring. This risk is considered to be minor if withdrawal of steroid therapy would compromise the mother. Sporadic cases of neonatal adrenal insufficiency have been reported after long-term prenatal steroid therapy; therefore, all infants born to such mothers should be observed for signs of addisonism. High-dose **betamethasone** therapy has been shown experimentally to decrease the risk of newborn respiratory distress syndrome in infants born before 34 weeks gestation; such treatment in women who are hypertensive, however, is associated with a higher frequency of fetal death *in utero*[1,3-5,7]

Continued

Drug Use and Pregnancy

DRUG	NATURE OF EFFECT
DIURETICS	Initiation of diuretic therapy should be undertaken with great caution in the pregnant patient, especially in the treatment of pre-eclampsia toxemia. Diuretics can cause a decrease in maternal intravascular volume and consequently diminish uteroplacental perfusion. This effect is most rapid and severe with **loop diuretics.** Pre-eclampsia and toxemia are states of decreased intravascular volume which are aggravated by further diuretic-induced volume depletion, thus compromising fetal oxygenation. **Thiazide diuretics** are known to cross the placenta and their maternal use has been associated with neonatal thrombocytopenia[1,2,4,7,9,16]
GASTROINTESTINAL DRUGS	
Cimetidine	Cimetidine has been associated in one case report with a transient increase in liver function tests (bilirubin, SGOT and SGPT) in an infant whose mother received cimetidine in the third trimester. The association is clouded by the fact that she also received aluminum, magnesium and calcium antacids as well as a phenobarbital-belladonna alkaloid mixture during this period[17]
HORMONES AND SYNTHETIC SUBSTITUTES	
Androgens	Androgen use during pregnancy is associated with masculinization of the female fetus (labial fusion and clitoral hypertrophy). The male fetus does not appear to be adversely affected, but may have genital development somewhat advanced for his gestational age[2-5]
Clomiphene	Clomiphene is used to induce ovulation. Retrospective studies of pregnancies after clomiphene induction show a slightly increased prevalence of severe congenital malformations. Whether these anomalies are due to clomiphene or to the subfertility which made its use necessary has not been established. A twofold increase in the frequency of trisomy 21 among offspring and a significantly higher prevalence of aneuploidy in abortuses conceived after induced ovulation has been reported[1,2]

Continued

Drug Use and Pregnancy

DRUG	NATURE OF EFFECT
Diethylstilbestrol	Diethylstilbestrol used in pregnant women to prevent threatened abortion has been associated with a significantly increased risk of vaginal adenosis, clear cell vaginal adenocarcinoma and upper genital tract anomalies in female offspring. Male offspring of treated mothers have an increased prevalence of penile and genital tract abnormalities and abnormal sperm formation. These effects are usually not identified until late in the second decade of life. Their frequency is highest in those exposed before the ninth week of gestation[1-3,5]
Sulfonylureas	Sulfonylurea use during pregnancy is associated with an increased rate of perinatal mortality and prolonged neonatal hypoglycemia. Pregnant diabetics should be carefully controlled on **insulin** to avoid these effects[1,4,7]
Synthetic Progestogens	Synthetic progestogens (**norethindrone, norethynodrel** and **ethisterone**) have been shown to cause masculinization of the female fetus. The risk of such malformation is decreased by the use of natural agents or their esters (eg, **medroxyprogesterone**). In addition, an increased prevalence of hypospadias has been reported in males prenatally exposed to both natural and synthetic progestogens[1-3,5,18]
Thyroid and Antithyroid Agents	Exogenous thyroid hormone appears to cross the placenta poorly and to have little, if any, effect on the fetus. Antithyroid drugs (**propylthiouracil, methimazole** and **iodine**) are known to produce hypothyroidism and compensatory hypertrophic goiter in the neonate when given to the pregnant woman. Goiters associated with iodide exposures have been large enough to obstruct the trachea and to interfere with delivery.[1,2,7] Goiters produced after thionamide exposure are usually not as large and diminish with time; cretinism may be avoided by careful control of the mother's disease with a minimum maintenance dose. Signs of neonatal hypothyroidism usually disappear within 2–6 weeks after birth. In addition, methimazole use has been associated with an ulcer-like midline scalp defect in 5 infants after *in utero* exposure[2,3,7]

Continued

Drug Use and Pregnancy

DRUG	NATURE OF EFFECT
Radioactive Iodine	Radioactive iodine should not be used in pregnancy, because after 10 weeks gestation the fetal thyroid actively concentrates iodine; any radioactive iodine ingested by the mother will cross the placenta and destroy fetal thyroid tissue[2,3]
PSYCHOTHERAPEUTIC AGENTS	
Lithium	Lithium use during pregnancy is associated with an increased prevalence of congenital heart disease, cardiovascular and CNS anomalies. Symptoms of lithium toxicity, including respiratory distress, cyanosis, hypotonia and hypothermia, have been seen in infants of women whose lithium plasma concentration were in the therapeutic range. Isolated cases of fetal goiter and nephrogenic diabetes insipidus have also been reported in children of women on chronic lithium therapy during pregnancy. Should a woman requiring lithium become pregnant, it is recommended that her plasma level be kept below 1 mEq/L and that she avoid a low sodium diet and diuretics. Levels should be monitored frequently, because clearance of lithium increases during the course of pregnancy and then drops to prepregnancy levels shortly before delivery[1,3-5,7,21]
Phenothiazines	Phenothiazine use during pregnancy has not been implicated as a cause of fetal malformations. Their maternal use, however, has been associated with prolonged extrapyramidal effects, jaundice and sedation followed by motor excitement and agitation in the newborn[1-4,7]
Tricyclic Antidepressants	Tricyclic antidepressants given immediately before delivery have been reported to cause neonatal tachycardia, myoclonus, respiratory distress and heart failure. Withdrawal symptoms have been observed in infants of mothers treated with **imipramine**[1,4]
SEDATIVES AND HYPNOTICS	High doses of any sedative-hypnotic close to or during delivery may result in neonatal CNS and respiratory depression.

Continued

Drug Use and Pregnancy

DRUG	NATURE OF EFFECT
Barbiturates	Barbiturate addiction during pregnancy may lead to neonatal withdrawal symptoms which consist of tremulousness, increased crying, irritability, increased tone and hyperphagia. These acute symptoms may last for 4-6 months, even with **phenobarbital** treatment; subsequent impaired mental development may be seen[3,4]
Bromide	Bromide consumed chronically during pregnancy may be associated with intoxication of the neonate. Such an infant may exhibit either hypertonus, difficulty feeding and a high-pitched cry, or lethargy, hypotonus, and neurodepression. These symptoms are usually reversible, but peritoneal dialysis may be required[3]
Chlordiazepoxide	Chlordiazepoxide use during the first 42 days of pregnancy reportedly caused an increased prevalence of neonatal CNS abnormalities in one study. Other large cooperative studies, however, have shown no association of its use with congenital malformations or poor mental outcomes[2,3,19]
Diazepam	Diazepam use during the first trimester of pregnancy has been associated with a fourfold increase in the prevalence of neonatal oral clefts over the control population. A withdrawal syndrome consisting of tremulousness, hypertonia and hyperreflexia has been seen in infants of mothers who took 10-15 mg of diazepam daily during the third trimester of pregnancy[1-4]
Inhalation Anesthetics	Inhalation anesthetic use during labor is associated with CNS and respiratory depression in the neonate. In addition, a two- to fourfold increase in the rate of spontaneous abortion in pregnant women chronically exposed to inhalation anesthetics (eg, operating room and dental personnel) has been reported[2,4,23]
Meprobamate	Meprobamate use, especially in the first trimester, is associated with an increased frequency of severe congenital anomalies, particularly congenital heart disease[19]

Continued

Drug Use and Pregnancy

DRUG	NATURE OF EFFECT
SYMPATHOMIMETIC AGENTS	
	The treatment of hypotension during pregnancy with sympathomimetic agents is complicated by the fact that the uterine vasculature is supplied solely with alpha-adrenergic receptors and is maximally dilated under basal conditions. Pure alpha-adrenergic agents significantly constrict uterine vessels and decrease blood flow, thereby compromising the fetus. Beta-adrenergic agents cause peripheral vasodilation and tend to shunt blood away from the uterus and also may cause fetal compromise. Volume expanding agents seem to be the most prudent treatment for sudden hypotension in the pregnant patient. Use of sympathomimetics for treatment of nasal congestion may be associated with an increase in fetal activity and fetal tachycardia. Sympathomimetics should be avoided in patients with hypertension or toxemia or in situations where there is poor fetal reserve.[1,7]
Amphetamines	**Amphetamine** and **dextroamphetamine** use during pregnancy for the treatment of narcolepsy or for weight reduction has been associated with an increased prevalence of congenital malformations, especially biliary atresia, cardiovascular anomalies and oral clefts.[1,2,9]
MISCELLANEOUS AGENTS	
Caffeine	Caffeine consumption in excess of 600 mg/day (equivalent to about 6 cups of coffee) is associated with an increased prevalence of spontaneous abortion and stillbirth. Consumption of 300 mg daily has not been associated with fetal anomalies.[1,4,7]
Local Anesthetics	Local anesthetics have been associated with fetal and neonatal depression following maternal use during labor. Fetal bradycardia may occur after as many as 25% of paracervical blocks.[3,4,7]
Oxytocin	Oxytocin given for induction of labor may cause an increased prevalence of neonatal jaundice. Such use has also resulted in tetanic uterine contractions causing decreased uterine blood flow and fetal distress. The use of **ergonovine** and **ergotamine** before delivery carries the same risk.[1,4]

Continued

Drug Use and Pregnancy

DRUG	NATURE OF EFFECT
Penicillamine	Penicillamine in the treatment of pregnant women with Wilson's disease has not been shown to have deleterious fetal effects. Its use for the treatment of cystinuria and rheumatoid arthritis during pregnancy, however, has been associated with fetal connective tissue defects. It has been hypothesized that the penicillamine chelates with the excess copper in Wilson's disease and protects the fetus[2,20]
Smoking	Smoking during pregnancy is associated with increased rates of IUGR, prematurity, spontaneous abortion, neonatal and postnatal deaths and placenta previa. Such conditions are seen particularly in women who are regular smokers of more than 10 cigarettes/day. Tobacco chewing during pregnancy is also associated with a greatly increased rate of stillbirth, IUGR and prematurity[1-3,5,7,22]
Theophylline	Theophylline toxicity (jitteriness, irritability, tachycardia and vomiting), which usually resolves within 48 hours of birth, can be seen in infants exposed to this drug *in utero*[1,3,7]
Vaginal Spermicides	Vaginal spermicide use has been associated with major congenital anomalies in one large retrospective analysis. The association, however, is tentative. No one syndrome of malformation was identified; actual use of spermicide by the mother was not verified; and the prevalence of major anomalies was only 2.2% in the study group, a rate well within that expected for major malformations in the United States[24]
Vaccines	Live viruses (**rubella, measles, smallpox, mumps**) are known to readily cross the placenta and may infect the fetus. **Rubella** virus has been isolated from the abortus of a mother who received the vaccine after becoming pregnant. The absolute risk of congenital rubella after vaccination during pregnancy, however, appears to be low. **Smallpox** vaccination during the first trimester has been associated with an increased prevalence of abortion, fatal vaccinia in the fetus and congenital vaccinia. The risk of killed or inactivated vaccines appears to be minimal[5,7,15]

Continued

Drug Use and Pregnancy

DRUG	NATURE OF EFFECT
Vitamins	The recommended daily allowances of all vitamins are increased during pregnancy. These increases take into account the higher caloric requirements of the pregnant woman as well as the storage and growth requirements of the fetus. Vitamin toxicity has been reported with the use of excessive doses of fat-soluble vitamins during pregnancy. **Vitamin A** excess has been associated with a variety of congenital anomalies including neural tube defects, early epiphyseal closure, growth retardation and urinary tract anomalies.[1,2,4,7] **Vitamin D** excess has been reported to cause an idiopathic hypercalcemic syndrome including cardiovascular malformation, abnormal bone mineralization, elfin facies, mental retardation, hypercalcemia and nephrocalcinosis.[1,3,7] High dose **menadione** (vitamin K_3) therapy in a mother immediately before delivery can cause neonatal red cell hemolysis, hyperbilirubinemia and kernicterus[7]

References

1. Berkowitz RL, Coustan DR, Mochizuki TK, eds. Handbook for prescribing medications during pregnancy. Boston: Little, Brown, 1981.

2. Golbus MS. Teratology for the obstetrician: current status. Obstet Gynecol 1980;55:269-77.

3. Hill RM, Stern L. Drugs in pregnancy: effects on the fetus and newborn. Drugs 1979;17:182-97.

4. Pagliaro LA, Levin RH. Teratogenesis. In: Pagliaro LA, Levin RH, eds. Problems in pediatric drug therapy. Hamilton, IL: Drug Intelligence Publications, 1979:3-48.

5. Shepard TH. Teratogenic drugs and therapeutic agents. In: Shirkey HC, ed. Pediatric therapy, 6th ed. St. Louis: CV Mosby, 1980:94-109.

6. Anon. Surgeon General's advisory on alcohol and pregnancy. FDA Drug Bull 1981;11:9-10.

7. Shirkey HC, Ericson AJ. Adverse reactions to drugs —their relation to growth and development. In: Shirkey HC, ed. Pediatric therapy, 6th ed. St. Louis: CV Mosby, 1980:110-51.

8. Csaba IF, Sulyok E, Ertl T. Relationship of maternal treatment with indomethacin to persistence of fetal circulation syndrome. J Pediatr 1978;92:484.

9. Walters WAW, Humphrey MD. Common medical disorders in pregnancy and their treatment. Drugs 1980;19:455-63.

10. Hall JG, Pauli RM, Wilson KM. Maternal and fetal sequelae of anticoagulation during pregnancy. Am J Med 1980;68:122-40.

11. Dalens B, Raynaud E-J, Gaulme J. Teratogenicity of valproic acid. J Pediatr 1980;97:332-3.

12. Dickinson RG, Harland RC, Lynn RK et al. Transmission of valproic acid (Depakene) across the placenta: half-life of the drug in mother and baby. J Pediatr 1979;94:832-5.

13. Weinstein AJ. Treatment of bacterial infections in pregnancy. Drugs 1979;17:56-65.

14. Peterson WF, Stauch JE, Ryder CD. Metronidazole in pregnancy. Am J Obstet Gynecol 1966;94:343-9.

15. Anon. Safety of immunizing agents in pregnancy. Med Lett Drugs Ther 1970;12:23-4.

16. Bear RA, Erenrich N. Essential hypertension and pregnancy. Can Med Assoc J 1978;118:936-93.

17. Glade G, Saccar CL, Pereira GR. Cimetidine in pregnancy: apparent transient liver impairment in the newborn. Am J Dis Child 1980;134:87-8.

18. Aarskog D. Maternal progestins as a possible cause of hypospadias. N Engl J Med 1979;300:75-8.

19. Milkovich L, van den Berg BJ. Effects of prenatal meprobamate and chlordiazepoxide hydrochloride on human embryonic and fetal development. N Engl J Med 1974;291:1268-71.

20. Lyle WH. Penicillamine in pregnancy. Lancet 1978;1:606-7.

21. Mizrahi EM, Hobbs JF, Goldsmith DI. Nephrogenic diabetes insipidus in transplacental lithium intoxication. J Pediatr 1979;94:493-5.

22. Krishna K. Tobacco chewing in pregnancy. Br J Obstet Gynaecol 1978;85:726-8.

23. Anon. Nitrous oxide hazards. FDA Drug Bull 1980;10:15-6.

24. Jick H, Walker AM, Rothman KJ et al. Vaginal spermicides and congenital disorders. JAMA 1981;245:1329-32.

10 GERIATRIC DRUG USE

GERIATRIC DRUG THERAPY IS BECOMING AN IMPORTANT SPECIALTY area, due to several factors. Among these are the increasing numbers of elderly, particularly those over 80 years; the elderly use more medications than other age groups; the elderly make significant medication errors; and the prevalence of adverse drug reactions is greatest in the elderly.[1-3] It is important, therefore, that health professionals consider that the elderly may react to drugs differently than other adults and may require altered drug regimens.

Researchers have begun to examine why the elderly may react differently to drugs. Alterations in the physiological and pharmacological characteristics described below have been suggested as explanations for drug effects seen in the elderly. See references 4–9 for a more detailed discussion.

Absorption. There is a decrease in gastric secretions, acidity, peristalsis, the number of microvilli, splanchnic blood flow and gastric emptying with aging,[10,11] all of which suggest altered absorption of orally administered drugs in elderly patients. However, a number of studies indicate that the quantity or extent of absorbed drug is *not* affected by age, probably because most drug absorption is passive and primarily dependent on concentration gradients.[4,5] Because of an age-related decrease in intestinal perfusion, it has been hypothesized that the rate of oral drug absorption might be slowed.[9] From a limited number of studies of a few drugs, this hypothesis does not appear to be true.

Cardiac output and regional blood flow decrease with age and in some chronic diseases affecting the elderly. The decreased blood flow may alter the rate or quantity of intramuscular and subcutaneous drug absorption; however, there are no data for most drugs.

Distribution. Body weight generally decreases and body composition changes with age; these factors can alter the volume of distribution (V_d) of drugs in the elderly. Total body water and lean body mass decrease, while body fat increases in proportion to total body weight. The percent of body weight contributed by fat changes from 18% and 33% in young men and women, respectively, to 36% and 45% in their elderly counterparts.[12] Therefore, elderly patients are particularly susceptible to overdosage from drugs which should be dosed on lean body weight (LBW). Theoretically, highly lipid soluble drugs may have an increased V_d and a prolonged effect. Conversely, highly water soluble drugs may have a decreased V_d, and at least transiently increased plasma levels and effect.[7]

Cardiac output decreases approximately 1% per year after age 20[13] and there is some evidence that blood is preferentially shunted to the brain, heart and muscles and away from the liver and kidneys.[7] These changes could explain the slowed elimination of some drugs and the heightened sensitivity to others (eg, CNS drugs).

Protein Binding. The proportion of albumin among total plasma proteins decreases with age and with some chronic diseases.[14] Serum albumin can be significantly decreased despite a normal total serum protein value. One study showed a drop in serum albumin from 3.97 g/dl in those less than 40 years to 3.58 g/dl in those older than 80 years.[15] This phenomenon could alter the percentage of free drug available for pharmacological effect and elimination. The net effect on clearance varies depending on whether metabolism or elimination is also altered. There is also some evidence that the elderly may have a greater potential for protein displacement drug interactions.[16]

Metabolism. Liver size and hepatic blood flow decrease with age. It has been estimated that hepatic blood flow decreases 40% from age 25 to 65 years.[10] Metabolism of drugs with high hepatic extraction ratios depends to a large part on liver blood flow,[17] and several of these drugs show decreased clearances in the elderly. Age may affect oxidation by microsomal enzyme systems more than genetically determined acetylation and other oxidative metabolic processes.[18] Several studies show a large intersubject variation in metabolic rate which is unexplained by age. Continued study into the role of aging in hepatic drug metabolism is needed before more definitive explanations can be made.

Renal. The effect of aging on the renal disposition of drugs is probably the most completely understood and important aspect of geriatric drug therapy. Glomerular filtration and tubular secretion both decrease significantly with age and renal blood flow decreases about 1% per year.[19] Creatinine clearance decreases approximately 35% between ages 20 and 90 in patients without evidence of renal disease.[19] In addition, dehydration, congestive heart failure and renal disease can decrease organ function further. Because creatinine production also decreases with age, serum creatinine may be normal despite a significant decrease in renal function. It is therefore recommended that creatinine clearance be measured or estimated using a method which incorporates age and weight[20,21] when adjusting doses of renally excreted drugs in the elderly. Plasma levels of potentially toxic, renally excreted drugs should be closely monitored even if the drug has not been specifically studied in the elderly.

Pharmacodynamic Factors. Heightened drug effects which have not been explained by altered pharmacokinetic variables have been hypothesized to be caused by changed tissue sensitivity, altered homeostasis or complications of chronic diseases seen in the elderly.[6] More research is needed, especially in quantitatively comparing the changes seen in the elderly with younger adult populations.

Other. Although cigarette smoking has been shown to induce metabolism of some drugs in young patients, this phenomenon may not be as pronounced in the elderly.[4] Some heretofore unexplained interpatient variations of kinetic data may be explained by smoking history; unfortunately, many studies do not include smoking data.

Nutritional intake can be diminished in the elderly and can lead to nutritional and vitamin deficiencies.[22,23] The nutritional status of the elderly may be important in their handling of some drugs.[24]

Use of the Table. The table which follows provides pharmacologic and pharmacokinetic data for drugs which have been studied in the elderly. Some conflicting data may be due to health status of the elderly; status is not always stated, methods of classification vary, and degree of ambulation may differ. When a dosage change is recommended due to decreased renal function, consult specific drug literature or general references such as reference number 25.

The following abbreviations are used in the table:

> (E) —elderly; ages vary for different studies, but uniformly older than 50 years
>
> (Y) —young; uniformly younger than 50 years, usually in 20–30 year range
>
> Cl —plasma clearance
>
> Cl_{cr} —creatinine clearance
>
> Cr_s —serum creatinine
>
> LBW—lean body weight
>
> $t_{1/2}$ —half-life
>
> V_d —volume of distribution

The table begins on page 167.

⊙

Geriatric Drug Use

DRUG	CLINICAL FINDINGS AND MANAGEMENT	DRUG-SPECIFIC DATA
ALCOHOL	Increased blood levels in (E) correlated with decreased V_d; rate of elimination is no different in (Y) vs (E).[26] The (E) should be especially cautioned not to ingest alcohol with other sedative-hypnotics	Peak alcohol level after infusion: 155 mg/dl (Y) vs 176 mg/dl (E)[26] V_d: 35 L (Y) vs 32 L (E)[26]
ANALGESICS AND ANTIPYRETICS		
Acetaminophen	There are large interpatient variations; alteration of dose is not necessary	No difference in extent or rate of PO absorption or V_d in (Y) vs (E)[27] $t_{1/2}$: 1.8 hr (Y) vs 2.2 hr (E)[27,28] Cl: 0.34 L/hr/kg (Y) vs 0.25 L/hr/kg (E)[27]
Aspirin	Single-dose studies indicate no dosage alteration needed for analgesia; more study is needed in anti-inflammatory doses. Monitor carefully for dose-related toxicities; plasma levels may be helpful in (E) with hearing impairment	No difference in extent or rate of PO absorption (Y) vs (E)[29-31] $t_{1/2}$: 2.4 hr (Y) vs 3.7 hr (E)[30] V_d: 3.8 L (Y) vs 5.5 L (E)[30] Tinnitus is not a reliable symptom of toxicity in patients with hearing loss[32]
Meperidine and Morphine	The (E) may have increased sensitivity to narcotic analgesics and require lower doses to achieve pain	Morphine: $t_{1/2}$: 3 hr (Y) vs 4.5 hr (E)

Continued

Geriatric Drug Use

DRUG	CLINICAL FINDINGS AND MANAGEMENT	DRUG-SPECIFIC DATA
	relief.[4] The (E) may have increased potential for side effects such as respiratory depression, because of decreased protein binding and initially higher plasma levels.[33,34] Monitor for respiratory depression, especially with IV doses in (E) with lung disease	V_d: 3.2 L/kg (Y) vs 4.7 L/kg (E) Cl: 14.7 ml/min/kg (Y) vs 12.4 ml/min/kg (E)[35]
Phenylbutazone	Sodium retention and ulcerogenic potential are especially undesirable in (E); avoid or use with caution in (E)	No difference in extent or rate of PO absorption or V_d (Y) vs (E)[27] $t_{1/2}$: somewhat increased in (E),[27] possibly due to decreased serum albumin and drug binding[16]
ANTICHOLINERGICS	The (E) appear to be more sensitive,[4] and many other drugs (E) take have anticholinergic properties. Monitor for confusion, nightmares, urinary hesitancy and retention, and constipation which can lead to fecal impaction	
ANTICOAGULANTS		
Heparin	Age does not increase risk of minor bleeding, but evidence is inconclusive with respect to risk of major bleeding. Women of all ages found to have higher risk of bleeding than men of all ages.[36] Limit anticoagulant treatment in (E) to conditions in which anticoagulants have demonstrated clinical benefit. Dose conservatively; monitor frequently for evidence of bleeding	

Continued

Geriatric Drug Use

DRUG	CLINICAL FINDINGS AND MANAGEMENT	DRUG-SPECIFIC DATA
Warfarin	Two studies[37,38] show increased frequency of bleeding with age, while one study[39] showed no correlation. Difference is probably result of how bleeding was categorized. The (E) and especially (E) women are probably at higher risk of bleeding while on anti-coagulants. Dose of warfarin to achieve same degree of anticoagulation found to be 40% lower in (E), indicating increased sensitivity.[41,42] Recent study failed to show increased sensitivity.[43]	No difference in V_d, Cl, $t_{1/2}$, degree or affinity of protein binding in (Y) vs (E). Increased sensitivity may be due to dietary deficiency and/or altered kinetics of vitamin K in (E)[40]
ANTICONVULSANTS		
Phenytoin	Increased Cl in (E) correlated with decreased serum albumin and phenytoin binding.[44] Overdosage and underdosage possible in (E) due to increased free phenytoin. Monitor carefully for dose-related toxicities and seizure activity, especially in patients with low serum albumin; toxic levels may often result from 350 mg/day in (E).[45] Obtain free phenytoin levels, if possible	Cl: 26 ml/hr/kg (Y) vs 42 ml/hr/kg (E)[44] Total phenytoin plasma levels increase with age[46]
ANTI-INFECTIVE AGENTS		
Aminoglycosides	Potential exists for overdosage and accumulation because (E) have decreased lean body weight and decreased renal Cl of drug. Dose conservatively based on LBW; use established dosage regimens after determining estimated or actual Cl_{cr}. Monitor and adjust	Kanamycin: $t_{1/2}$: 107 min (Y) vs 282 min (E) despite comparable Cr_s[47]

Geriatric Drug Use

DRUG	CLINICAL FINDINGS AND MANAGEMENT	DRUG-SPECIFIC DATA
Amoxicillin and Ampicillin	regimen using plasma aminoglycoside levels. Consider audiometry and vestibular function monitoring, especially in (E) with severe renal or hearing impairment	
	Both drugs have high therapeutic indices; therefore, dosage reduction is considered only in moderate to severe renal impairment	Amoxicillin: $t_{1/2}$: 1 hr (Y) vs 2.7 hr (E)[48]
		Ampicillin: No difference in extent or rate of PO absorption or V_d[49]
Isoniazid	No need to alter dosage regimen unless (E) can be identified as a "slow acetylator". Increased risk of hepatitis with age, especially age group 50–64 years.[50] Routine prophylaxis with isoniazid for recent PPD converters older than 35 yr is not recommended unless additional risk factors for TB are present[52]	$t_{1/2}$: 1.68 hr (Y) vs 6.7 hr (E)[49] CI: 0.18 L/hr/kg (Y) vs 0.08 L/hr/kg (E)[49] $t_{1/2}$: no difference in (Y) vs (E) although both groups had fast and slow acetylators[18,51]
Penicillin G	Because of its high therapeutic index, dosage reduction is considered only in moderate to severe renal impairment	No difference in rate of absorption from IM injection of procaine penicillin G in (Y) vs (E)[53]
Sulfamethizole	Dosage reduction is necessary in moderate to severe renal impairment; consider alternate drug. Maintain adequate fluid intake	No difference in extent or rate of PO absorption or V_d in (Y) vs (E)

Continued

Geriatric Drug Use

DRUG	CLINICAL FINDINGS AND MANAGEMENT	DRUG-SPECIFIC DATA
		Renal Cl: 145 ml/min/1.73 M² (Y) vs 60 ml/min/1.73 M² (E)[27]
Tetracyclines	Dosage alteration probably not necessary; consider **doxycycline** or non-tetracycline in severe renal impairment	No difference in extent or rate of PO tetracycline absorption in (E) with achlorhydria.
		Rate of elimination slower in (E) probably due to decreased renal Cl[54]
CARDIAC DRUGS **Digoxin**	Higher prevalence of side effects in (E), probably due to improper dosing and electrolyte imbalance in most cases; no evidence that (E) myocardium is more sensitive. Avoid loading method of digitalization in CHF when possible; try to digitalize with maintenance dosing and treat CHF acutely with diuretics. Dose conservatively using LBW and estimated or measured Cl$_{cr}$ (see Digoxin monograph). Maintain adequate serum potassium. Monitor usual parameters for toxicity, especially CNS symptoms such as listlessness, agitation and pseudohallucinations.[4] Periodically review the need for continued therapy, because some evidence suggests digoxin withdrawal may not result in cardiac decompensation in certain (E).[55,56]	No difference in extent of PO absorption, although rate of absorption is somewhat slower in (E)
		t$_{1/2}$: 36.8 hr (range 24–53 hr) (Y) vs 70 hr (range 24–129 hr) (E). Note large interpatient variation despite normal Cr$_s$ in all patients[57]
		V$_d$: No difference in (Y) vs (E)[57]
		Cl: 106.2 ml/min (Y) vs 37.4 ml/min (E)[57]
		Cl: 83 ml/min/1.73 M² (Y) vs 53 ml/min/1.73 M² (E)[58]

Continued

Geriatric Drug Use

DRUG	CLINICAL FINDINGS AND MANAGEMENT	DRUG-SPECIFIC DATA
Lidocaine	The (E) have increased prevalence of certain side effects, probably related to underlying cardiac disease.[4] Prolonged $t_{1/2}$ with unchanged Cl, related to increased V_d in (E). Cl is significantly decreased in patients with CHF or liver disease.[60] A nomogram has been developed to aid in dosing of these patients.[60] Because of wide interpatient variation in data, plasma levels are helpful in monitoring	$t_{1/2}$: 1.3 hr (Y) vs 2.3 hr (E)[59] V_d: 0.9 L/kg (Y) vs 1.6 L/kg (E)[59] Cl: No difference (Y) vs (E)[59] Cl: 0.7 L/min (all healthy) vs 0.443 L/min (CHF) vs 0.419 L/min (liver disease)[60]
Propranolol	Serious side effects such as complete heart block, pulmonary edema and profound bradycardia are more common in (E).[61] CNS symptoms of disorientation, visual hallucinations and psychosis have been reported in (E).[62-64] Higher plasma levels in (E) thought to be the result of decreased hepatic extraction and metabolism.[65] The (E) seem to have a decreased sensitivity to the drug which may be related to reduced β-adrenoreceptor responsiveness.[66] The (E) appear to be less sensitive to propranolol-induced bradycardia during exercise;[4] therefore, be wary of using this as an endpoint in dosing	Single IV dose: $t_{1/2}$: 152 min (Y) vs 254 min (E)[65] V_d: No difference (Y) vs (E)[65,67] Cl: 13.2 ml/min/kg (Y) vs 7.8 ml/min/kg (E)[65]
	Plasma levels are higher in nonsmokers than smokers, but the difference is less in (E) than (Y)[67,69] Dose conservatively, especially initially	Multiple PO dosing: (E) plasma levels 3.1 times higher than (Y); no difference found in plasma levels and quantity absorbed in extremely healthy (E)[68]

Continued

Geriatric Drug Use

DRUG	CLINICAL FINDINGS AND MANAGEMENT	DRUG-SPECIFIC DATA
Quinidine	The (E) may be predisposed to toxicity because of prolonged elimination; optimal dosing may require less frequent administration in (E).[70] Plasma levels may be helpful in establishing optimal dosing regimen	$t_{1/2}$: 7.3 hr (Y) vs 9.7 hr (E) V_d and % bound: no difference in (Y) vs (E) Cl: 4.0 ml/min/kg (Y) vs 2.6 ml/min/kg (E)[70]
DIURETICS	The (E) have a high prevalence of hypokalemia and other side effects.[71,72] Maintain adequate serum potassium and hydration. Monitor for symptoms of glucose intolerance and postural hypotension. Periodically re-evaluate the need for continued therapy	Fasting blood sugar increases an average 9.6 mg/dl after 2 yr of diuretic therapy in (E), which correlates with the degree of hypokalemia[73] Diuretics can be withdrawn in certain (E) without deleterious effect[74]
HORMONES AND SYNTHETIC SUBSTITUTES		
Insulin	Dose and monitor insulin therapy as in (Y).	No altered kinetics in (E)[4]
Sulfonylureas	The (E) have a higher prevalence of hypoglycemia precipitated by sulfonylureas than (Y)[75]	Unbound tolbutamide is 25% higher in (E), because of lower serum albumin[76]

Continued

Geriatric Drug Use

DRUG	CLINICAL FINDINGS AND MANAGEMENT	DRUG-SPECIFIC DATA
HYPOTENSIVE AGENTS	Although some caution is needed, treatment of systolic and diastolic hypertension in (E) appears to be indicated, because the risk of cardiovascular morbidity and mortality in general is reduced with treatment.[6,77] Postural hypotension is greater in (E)[78]	
PSYCHOTHERAPEUTIC AGENTS		
Lithium	The (E) may have a higher prevalence of side effects and demonstrate more fluctuation in lithium levels; up to 50% lowering of initial dose has been recommended in (E) with further dosage adjustment based on plasma levels[79]	
Phenothiazines	The (E) can be more sensitive to sedative, anticholinergic, cardiac, extrapyramidal and autonomic side effects.[4,80] Use these agents only with established diagnosis and then start with small dose and increase slowly. Consider using a short-acting benzodiazepine if sedation is the objective	Frequency of choreiform side effects is 6 times higher in (E)[80]
Tricyclic Antidepressants	Increased side effects in (E), especially cardiotoxicity and confusion;[81] may be explained by altered kinetics and underlying cardiac status. Wait longer to assess therapeutic effect and adjust dosage in (E) because of prolonged $t_{1/2}$. Maximum recommended **amitriptyline** dose in those over 65 yr is 100 mg/day.[81]	Imipramine: $t_{1/2}$: 19 hr (Y) vs 34 hr (E) Desipramine: $t_{1/2}$: 23 hr (Y) vs 75 hr (E)[81]

Continued

Geriatric Drug Use

DRUG	CLINICAL FINDINGS AND MANAGEMENT	DRUG-SPECIFIC DATA
	Monitor for excessive anticholinergic effects such as urinary hesitancy and retention and constipation. Maintain adequate hydration	
SEDATIVES AND HYPNOTICS		
Barbiturates	The (E) have shown both prolonged CNS depression and a paradoxical CNS stimulation which can present as restlessness, agitation and psychosis.[4] Avoid using as sedatives in (E). A short-acting benzodiazepine is recommended, if a sedative-hypnotic is indicated	
Benzodiazepines	With all benzodiazepines, periodically assess the need for continued therapy. Short-acting agents such as oxazepam are preferred in (E)[7]	
Chlordiazepoxide	Frequency of drowsiness higher in (E), especially non-smokers.[82,83] Use small initial dose and monitor for signs of accumulation	$t_{1/2}$: 10 hr (Y) vs 18 hr (E) V_d: 0.4 L/kg (Y) vs 0.5 L/kg (E) Cl: 0.6 ml/min/kg (Y) vs 0.3 ml/min/kg (E) No difference in plasma protein binding[84]
Diazepam	Frequency of drowsiness is higher in (E).[82,85] May take	$t_{1/2}$: 20 hr (Y) vs 90 hr (E)

Continued

Geriatric Drug Use

DRUG	CLINICAL FINDINGS AND MANAGEMENT	DRUG-SPECIFIC DATA
	longer to achieve steady-state levels and effect in (E), especially (E) women, because of increased V_d	V_d: 0.7 L/kg (Y) vs 1.7 L/kg (E)[86]
Flurazepam	Increased prevalence of dose-related residual drowsiness in (E).[88] Start with 15 mg as initial dose in (E)	V_d: 1.2 L/kg (Y) men vs 1.7 L/kg (E) men, 1.7 L/kg (Y) women vs 3.0 L/kg (E) women[87]
Lorazepam	Accumulation and side effects in (E) less likely than with long-acting benzodiazepines	$t_{1/2}$: 14.3 hr (Y) vs 15.9 hr (E) V_d: 1.1 L/kg (Y) vs 1 L/kg (E) Cl: 0.99 ml/min/kg (Y) vs 0.78 ml/min/kg (E)[89]
Nitrazepam	Healthy (E) demonstrated poorer psychomotor performance than (Y), despite unchanged kinetics.[90] Hospitalized (E) with various diseases had prolonged $t_{1/2}$.[91] Start with lower initial dose than (Y)	$t_{1/2}$: 24.2 hr (Y) vs 39.6 hr (E) V_d: 2.4 L/kg (Y) vs 4.8 L/kg (E)[91]
Oxazepam	Accumulation and side effects less likely than with long-acting benzodiazepines; may be agent of choice, especially in (E) with liver disease[7]	$t_{1/2}$: 5.1 hr (Y) vs 5.6 hr (E) V_d: 0.6 L/kg (Y) vs 0.8 L/kg (E)

Continued

Geriatric Drug Use

DRUG	CLINICAL FINDINGS AND MANAGEMENT	DRUG-SPECIFIC DATA
MISCELLANEOUS AGENTS		
Cimetidine	Severe confusion has been reported in (E).[94] Determine or estimate Cl_{cr} and reduce dose appropriately[95]	Cl: 113 ml/min (Y) vs 136 ml/min (E)[92] Cl: not significantly different (Y) vs (E)[93] Cl decreased in (E)[95]
Iron	There appears to be no age-related difference in iron absorption. Red cell uptake of iron appears to be diminished in (E) because of decreased erythropoiesis. This may explain "resistant" iron deficiency anemia in (E)	No difference between (Y) and (E) in mucosal iron uptake, mucosal transfer and retention Utilization of retained iron: 91% (Y) vs 66% (E)[96]
Levodopa	Postural hypotension may be more common in women over 70 yr[97] and patients over 70 yr with a history of myocardial infarction.[98] Paradoxical behavioral reactions have been described which include depression, paranoid ideations, disorientation or increased alertness and improvement in depression[99]	
Theophylline	The (E) appear to have somewhat increased frequency of side effects, especially arrhythmias, if underlying cardiovascular disease is present; but, it is not known if (E) are inherently more sensitive to other effects[4]	No difference in extent or rate of PO absorption or V_d between (Y) and (E) $t_{1/2}$: 5.9 hr (Y) smokers vs 7.6 hr (Y) Continued

Geriatric Drug Use

DRUG	CLINICAL FINDINGS AND MANAGEMENT	DRUG-SPECIFIC DATA
	Cigarette smoking appears to increase Cl of theophylline and decrease frequency of side effects, although this effect is less pronounced in (E).[100,101] Presence of CHF or liver disease decreases Cl and requires lowering of dose[102,103]	nonsmokers, 5.9 hr (E) smokers vs 8 hr (E) nonsmokers Cl: 55% higher in (Y) smokers than (Y) nonsmokers; 40% higher in (E) smokers than (E) nonsmokers[101]
VITAMINS	The possibility of vitamin deficiencies should be explored in (E) and therapy monitored for efficacy	Vitamin B_6, B_{12}, niacin, folate and thiamine deficiencies were documented in 39% of (E) patients despite oral vitamin supplementation; deficiencies were corrected with intramuscular vitamin administration.[104] (E) absorbed riboflavin, vitamin B_6 and pantothenate from yeast (natural source) as well as (Y), but did not absorb natural folates as well as (Y); synthetic folates proved an absorbable source for (E)[105]

References

1. Haynes SG, Feinleib M, eds. Second conference on the epidemiology of aging. Bethesda, MD: National Institutes of Health, 1980. (NIH publication no. 80-969).

2. Vestal RE. Drugs and the elderly. National Institute on Aging Science Writer Seminar Series. Bethesda, MD: National Institutes of Health, 1979. (NIH publication no. 79-1449).

3. Schwartz D, Wang M, Zeitz L et al. Medication errors made by elderly, chronically ill patients. Am J Public Health 1962;52:2018-29.

4. Vestal RE. Drug use in the elderly: a review of problems and special considerations. Drugs 1978;16:358-82.

5. Crooks J, O'Malley K, Stevenson IH. Pharmacokinetics in the elderly. Clin Pharmacokinet 1976;1:280-96.

6. O'Malley K, Judge TG, Crooks J. Geriatric clinical pharmacology and therapeutics. In: Avery GS, ed. Drug treatment. New York: ADIS Press, 1980:158-81.

7. Schumacher GE. Using pharmacokinetics in drug therapy VII: pharmacokinetic factors influencing drug therapy in the aged. Am J Hosp Pharm 1980;37:559-62.

8. Richey DP, Bender AD. Pharmacokinetic consequences of aging. Annu Rev Pharmacol Toxicol 1977;17:49-65.

9. Ritschel WA. Disposition of drugs in geriatric patients. Pharm Int 1980;1:226-30.

10. Geokas MC, Haverback BJ. The aging gastrointestinal tract. Am J Surg 1969;117:881-92.

11. Bender AD. Effect of age on intestinal absorption: implications for drug absorption in the elderly. J Am Geriatr Soc 1968;16:1331-9.

12. Novak LP. Aging, total body potassium, fat-free mass, and cell mass in males and females between ages 18 and 85 years. J Gerontol 1972;27:438-43.

13. Bender AD. The effect of increasing age on the distribution of peripheral blood flow in man. J Am Geriatr Soc 1965;13:192-8.

14. Cammarata RJ, Rodnan GP, Fennell RH. Serum anti-gamma-globulin and antinuclear factors in the aged. JAMA 1967;199:455-8.

15. Greenblatt DJ. Reduced serum albumin concentration in the elderly: a report from the Boston collaborative drug surveillance program. J Am Geriatr Soc 1979;27:20-2.

16. Wallace S, Whiting B, Runcie J. Factors affecting drug binding in plasma of elderly patients. Br J Clin Pharmacol 1976;3:327-30.

17. Nies AS, Shand DG, Wilkinson GR. Altered hepatic blood flow and drug disposition. Clin Pharmacokinet 1976;1:135-55.

18. Farah F, Taylor W, Rawlins MD et al. Hepatic drug acetylation and oxidation: effects of aging in man. Br Med J 1977;2:155-6.

19. Rowe JW, Andres R, Tobin JD et al. The effect of age on creatinine clearance in men: a cross-sectional and longitudinal study. J Gerontol 1975;31:155-63.

20. Siersbaek-Nielsen K, Hansen JM, Kampmann J et al. Rapid evaluation of creatinine clearance. Lancet 1971;1:1133-4.

21. Cockcroft DW, Gault MH. Prediction of creatinine clearance from serum creatinine. Nephron 1976;16:31-41.

22. Todhunter EN, Darby WJ. Guidelines for maintaining adequate nutrition in old age. Geriatrics 1978;33:49-56.

23. Krehl WA. The influence of nutritional environment on aging. Geriatrics 1974;29:65-76.

24. Smithard DJ, Langman MJS. Drug metabolism in the elderly. Br Med J 1977;3:520-1.

25. Bennett WM, Muther RS, Parker RA et al. Drug therapy in renal failure: dosing guidelines for adults. Ann Intern Med 1980;93:62-89, 286-325.

26. Vestal RE, McGuire EA, Tobin JD et al. Aging and ethanol metabolism. Clin Pharmacol Ther 1977;21:343-54.

27. Triggs EJ, Nation RL, Long A et al. Pharmacokinetics in the elderly. Eur J Clin Pharmacol 1975;8:55-62.

28. Briant RH, Dorrington RE, Cleal J et al. The rate of acetaminophen metabolism in the elderly and the young. J Am Geriatr Soc 1976;24:359-61.

29. Salem SAM, Stevenson IH. Absorption kinetics of aspirin and quinine in elderly subjects. Br J Clin Pharmacol 1977;4:397P.

30. Cuny G, Royer RJ, Mur JM et al. Pharmacokinetics of salicylates in elderly. Gerontology 1979;25:49-55.

31. Castleden CM, Volans CN, Raymond K. The effects of ageing on drug absorption from the gut. Age Ageing 1977;6:138-43.

32. Mongan E, Kelly P, Nies K et al. Tinnitus as an indication of therapeutic serum salicylate levels. JAMA 1973;226:142-5.

33. Mather LE, Tucker GT, Pflug AE et al. Meperidine kinetics in man. Clin Pharmacol Ther 1975;17:21-30.

34. Berkowitz BA, Ngai SH, Yang JC et al. The disposition of morphine in surgical patients. Clin Phamacol Ther 1975;17:629-35.

35. Stanski DR, Greenblatt DJ, Lowenstein E. Kinetics of intravenous and intramuscular morphine. Clin Pharmacol Ther 1978;24:52-9.

36. Walker AM, Jick H. Predictors of bleeding during heparin therapy. JAMA 1980;244:1209-12.

37. Coon WW, Willis PW. Hemorrhagic complications of anticoagulant therapy. Arch Intern Med 1974;133:386-92.

38. Husted S, Andreasen F. Problems encountered in long-term treatment with anticoagulants. Acta Med Scand 1976;200:379-84.

39. Forfar JC. A 7-year analysis of haemorrhage in patients on long-term anticoagulant treatment. Br Heart J 1979;42:128-32.

40. Shepherd AMM, Hewick DS, Moreland TA et al. Age as a determinant of sensitivity to warfarin. Br J Clin Pharmacol 1977;4:315-20.

41. O'Malley K, Stevenson IH, Ward CA et al. Determinants of anticoagulant control in patients receiving warfarin. Br J Clin Pharmacol 1977;4:309-14.

42. Husted S, Andreasen F. The influence of age on the response to anticoagulants. Br J Clin Pharmacol 1977;4:559-65.

43. Jones BR, Baran A, Reidenberg MM. Evaluating patients' warfarin requirements. J Am Geriatr Soc 1980;28:10-12.

44. Hayes MJ, Langman MJS, Short AH. Changes in drug metabolism with increasing age: 2. phenytoin clearance and protein binding. Br J Clin Pharmacol 1975;2:73-9.

45. Lambie DC, Caird FI. Phenytoin dosage in the elderly. Age Ageing 1977;6:133-7.

46. Houghton GW, Richens A, Leighton M. Effect of age, height, weight and sex on serum phenytoin concentration in epileptic patients. Br J Clin Pharmacol 1975;2:251-6.

47. Kristensen M, Hansen JM, Kampmann J et al. Drug elimination and renal function. J Clin Pharmacol 1974;14:307-8.

48. Ball P, Barford T, Gilbert J et al. Prolonged serum elimination half-life of amoxycillin in the elderly. J Antimicrob Chemother 1978;4:385-6.

49. Triggs EJ, Johnson JM, Learoyd B. Absorption and disposition of ampicillin in the elderly. Eur J Clin Pharmacol 1980;18:195-8.

50. Kopanoff DE, Snider DE, Caras GJ. Isoniazid-related hepatitis. Am Rev Respir Dis 1978;117:991-1001.

51. Gobert C, Houin G, Abengres E et al. Pharmacokinetics of isoniazid in the elderly. Br J Clin Pharmacol 1980;10:167-8.

52. American Thoracic Society. Preventive therapy of tuberculous infection. Am Rev Respir Dis 1974;110:371-4.

53. Leikola E, Vartia KO.On penicillin levels in young and geriatric subjects. J Gerontol 1957;12:48-52.

54. Kramer PA, Chapron DJ, Benson J et al. Tetracycline absorption in elderly patients with achlorhydria. Clin Pharmacol Ther 1978;23:467-72.

55. Whiting B, Wandless I, Sumner DJ et al. Computer-assisted review of digoxin therapy in the elderly. Br Heart J 1978;40:8-13.

56. Dall JLC. Maintenance digoxin in elderly patients. Br Med J 1970;2:705-6.

57. Cusack B, Kelly J, O'Malley K et al. Digoxin in the elderly: pharmacokinetic consequences of old age. Clin Pharmacol Ther 1979;25:772-6.

58. Ewy GA, Kapadia GG, Yao L et al. Digoxin metabolism in the elderly. Circulation 1969;39:449-53.

59. Nation RL, Triggs EJ, Selig M. Lignocaine kinetics in cardiac patients and aged subjects. Br J Clin Pharmacol 1977;4:439-48.

60. Thomson PD, Melmon KL, Richardson JA et al. Lidocaine pharmacokinetics in advanced heart failure, liver disease, and renal failure in humans. Ann Intern Med 1973;78:499-508.

61. Greenblatt DJ, Koch-Weser J. Adverse reactions to propranolol in hospitalized medical patients: a report from the Boston collaborative drug surveillance program. Am Heart J 1973;86:478-84.

62. Whitlock FA, Bonfield AR. Propranolol psychosis. Med J Aust 1980;1:184-5.

63. Kurland ML. Organic brain syndrome with propranolol. N Engl J Med 1979;300:366.

64. Fleminger R. Visual hallucinations and illusions with propranolol. Br Med J 1978;1:1182.

65. Castleden CM, George CF. The effect of ageing on the hepatic clearance of propranolol. Br J Clin Pharmacol 1979;7:49-54.

66. Vestal RE, Wood AJJ, Shand DG. Reduced beta-adrenoreceptor sensitivity in the elderly. Clin Res 1978;26:488A.

67. Vestal RE, Wood AJJ, Branch RA et al. Effects of age and cigarette smoking on propranolol disposition. Clin Pharmacol Ther 1979;26:8-11.

68. Schneider RE, Bishop H, Yates RA et al. Effect of age on plasma propranolol levels. Br J Clin Pharmacol 1980;10:169-70.

69. Wood AJJ, Vestal RE, Branch RA et al. Age related effects of smoking on elimination of propranolol antipyrine and indocyanine green. Clin Res 1978;26:14A.

70. Ochs HR, Greenblatt DJ, Woo E et al. Reduced quinidine clearance in elderly persons. Am J Cardiol 1978;42:481-5.

71. Hamdy RC, Tovey J, Perera N. Hypokalaemia and diuretics. Br Med J 1980;1:1187.

72. Williamson J, Chopin JM. Adverse reactions to prescribed drugs in the elderly: a multicentre investigation. Age Ageing 1980;9:73-80.

73. Amery A, Berthaux P, Bulpitt C et al. Glucose intolerance during diuretic therapy. Lancet 1978;1:681-3.

74. Burr ML, King S, Davies HEF et al. The effects of discontinuing long-term diuretic therapy in the elderly. Age Ageing 1977;6:38-45.

75. Seltzer HS. Drug-induced hypoglycemia. Diabetes 1972;21:955-66.

76. Miller AK, Adir J, Vestal RE. Tolbutamide binding to plasma proteins of young and old human subjects. J Pharm Sci 1978;67:1192-3.

77. Dyer AR, Stamler J, Shekelle RB et al. Hypertension in the elderly. Med Clin N Am 1977;61:513-29.

78. Caird FI, Andrews GR, Kennedy RD. Effect of posture on blood pressure in the elderly. Br Heart J 1973;35:527-30.

79. Hewick DS, Newbury P, Hopwood S et al. Age as a factor affecting lithium therapy. Br J Clin Pharmacol 1977;4:201-5.

80. Salzman C, Shader RI, van der Kolk BA. Clinical psychopharmacology and the elderly patient. NY State J Med 1976;76:71-7.

81. Nies A, Robinson DS, Friedman MJ et al. Relationship between age and tricyclic antidepressant plasma levels. Am J Psychiatry 1977;134:790-3.

82. Boston Collaborative Drug Surveillance Program. Clinical depression of the central nervous system due to diazepam and chlordiazepoxide in relation to cigarette smoking and age. N Engl J Med 1973;288:277-80.

83. Roberts RK, Wilkinson GR, Branch RA et al. Effect of age and parenchymal liver disease on the disposition and elimination of chlordiazepoxide (Librium). Gastroenterology 1978;75:479-85.

84. Shader RI, Greenblatt DJ, Harmatz JS et al. Absorption and disposition of chlordiazepoxide in young and elderly male volunteers. J Clin Pharmacol 1977;17:709-18.

85. Reidenberg MM, Levy M, Warner H et al. Relationship between diazepam dose, plasma level, age and central nervous system depression. Clin Pharmacol Ther 1978;23:371-4.

86. Klotz U, Avant GR, Hoyumpa A et al. The effects of age and liver disease on the disposition and elimination of diazepam in adult man. J Clin Invest 1975;55:347-59.

87. Greenblatt DJ, Allen MD, Locniskar A et al. Age, sex, and diazepam kinetics. Clin Pharmacol Ther 1979;25:227.

88. Greenblatt DJ, Allen MD, Shader RI. Toxicity of high-dose flurazepam in the elderly. Clin Phamacol Ther 1977;21:355-61.

89. Greenblatt DJ, Allen MD, Locniskar A et al. Lorazepam kinetics in the elderly. Clin Pharmacol Ther 1979;25:227.

90. Castleden CM, George CF, Marcer D et al. Increased sensitivity to nitrazepam in old age. Br Med J 1977;1:10-2.

91. Iisalo E, Kangas L, Ruikka I. Pharmacokinetics of nitrazepam in young volunteers and aged patients. Br J Clin Pharmacol 1977;4:646P-7P.

92. Shull HJ, Wilkinson GR, Johnson R et al. Normal disposition of oxazepam in acute viral hepatitis and cirrhosis. Ann Intern Med 1976;84:420-5.

93. Greenblatt DJ, Divoll M, Harmatz JS et al. Oxazepam kinetics: effects of age and sex. J Pharmacol Exp Ther 1980;215:86-91.

94. McMillan M, Ambis D, Siegel J. Cimetidine and mental confusion. N Engl J Med 1978;298:284-5.

95. Redolfi A, Borgogelli E, Lodola E. Blood level of cimetidine in relation to age. Eur J Clin Pharmacol 1979;15:257-61.

96. Marx JJM. Normal iron absorption and decreased red cell iron uptake in the aged. Blood 1979;53:204-11.

97. Grad B, Wener J, Rosenberg G et al. Effects of levodopa therapy in patients with parkinson's disease: statistical evidence for reduced tolerance to levodopa in the elderly. J Am Geriatr Soc 1974;22:489-94.

98. Wener J, Rosenberg G, Grad B et al. Cardiovascular effects of levodopa in aged versus younger patients with parkinson's disease. J Am Geriatr Soc 1976;24:185-8.

99. Riklan M. An L-dopa paradox: bipolar behavioral alterations. J Am Geriatr Soc 1972;20:572-5.

100. Pfeifer HJ, Greenblatt DJ. Clinical toxicity of theophylline in relation to cigarette smoking. Chest 1978;73:455-9.

101. Cusack B, Kelly JG, Lavan J et al. Theophylline kinetics in relation to age: the importance of smoking. Br J Clin Pharmacol 1980;10:109-14.

102. Anon. IV dosage guidelines for theophylline products. FDA Drug Bull 1980;10:4-6.

103. Murphy J, Ward E. Letter to the editor. N Engl J Med 1980;303:760-1.

104. Baker H, Frank O, Jaslow SP. Oral versus intramuscular vitamin supplementation for hypovitaminosis in the elderly. J Am Geriatr Soc 1980;28:42-5.

105. Baker H, Jaslow SP, Frank O. Severe impairment of dietary folate utilization in the elderly. J Am Geriatr Soc 1980;26:218-21.

11 IMMUNIZATION

General Recommendations on Immunization[1]

Introduction. Certain basic principles underlie the immunization practices recommended for infants, children, and adults. Most of these principles depend on scientific knowledge about active and passive immunization. Others represent judgments of public health officials and specialists in clinical and preventive medicine. Thus, recommendations on immunization practices represent a balancing of scientific evidence of benefits and risks in order to achieve optimal levels of protection against infectious or communicable diseases.

Multiple-Dose Vaccines. Some vaccines must be given in more than 1 dose for full protection. In recommending the times and intervals for multiple doses, risks from disease and the objective of inducing satisfactory clinical immunity have been taken into account. Intervals between doses that are longer than those recommended do not usually lead to a reduction in final antibody levels. Therefore, it is not necessary to restart an interrupted series of vaccinations or to add extra doses.

Simultaneous Administration of Certain Vaccines. Experimental evidence and extensive clinical experience are strengthening the scientific basis for giving certain vaccines at the same time. Most of the widely used antigens can safely and effectively be given simultaneously. This knowledge is particularly helpful when circumstances call for giving several vaccines at the same time—such as imminent exposure to several infectious diseases, preparation for foreign travel, or uncertainty that the patient will return for future vaccinations.

In general, inactivated vaccines can be administered simultaneously at separate sites. It should be noted, however, that when vaccines commonly associated with local or systemic side effects—such as cholera, typhoid, and plague vaccines—are given simultaneously, the side effects theoretically could be accentuated. Generally, persons known to experience such side effects should be given these vaccines on separate occasions.

An inactivated vaccine and a live, attenuated-virus vaccine can be administered simultaneously at separate sites, with the precautions that apply to the individual vaccines.

Previously it has been recommended that individual live-virus vaccines be given at least 1 month apart whenever possible. The reason for this was the theoretical concern that more frequent or severe side effects as well as diminished antibody responses might otherwise result. Field observations indicate, however, that simultaneous administration of the most widely used live-virus vaccines has not resulted in impaired antibody response or increased rates of adverse reactions.

Observation of children indicates that antibody responses to trivalent oral polio vaccine (TOPV) given simultaneously with licensed combination measles-mumps-rubella vaccine are comparable to those obtained when the same vaccines are given at different times. It is reasonable to expect equivalently good immunologic responses when other licensed, combination, live attenuated-virus vaccines or their component antigens are given simultaneously with TOPV.

Direct evidence on the response to simultaneous administration of diphtheria and tetanus toxoid and pertussis vaccine (DTP), TOPV, and measles-mumps-rubella vaccines is lacking. However, field experience and antibody data regarding simultaneous administration of either DTP and measles vaccine or DTP and TOPV indicate that the protective response is satisfactory and that the frequency of side effects is not increased. Therefore, simultaneous administration of all of these antigens is feasible, particularly if there is doubt that the recipient will return to receive further doses of vaccine.

There is no evidence to indicate that simultaneous administration of individual measles, mumps, or rubella antigens at different sites will yield different results from administration of the combined vaccines in a single site.

Simultaneous administration of pneumococcal polysaccharide vaccine and whole-virus influenza vaccine has been found to give satisfactory antibody response without increasing the frequency of side effects. Although not yet studied, simultaneous administration of the pneumococcal vaccine and split-virus influenza vaccine may also be expected to yield satisfactory results.

Hypersensitivity to Vaccine Components. Vaccine antigens produced in systems or with substrates that contain allergenic substances—for example, those antigens derived from growing microorganisms in the embryonated eggs of chickens or ducks—may cause hypersensitivity reactions. These may possibly include anaphylaxis, when the final vaccine contains a significant amount of the allergen. Such antigens include those grown in eggs and used against typhus, rabies (duck embryo vaccine), and yellow fever. Vaccines with such characteristics should not be given to persons known to be hypersensitive to components of the substrates. Contrary to this generalization, influenza vaccine antigens, although prepared from viruses grown in embryonated eggs, are highly purified during preparation and have only very rarely been reported to be associated with hypersensitivity reactions. Screening persons by history of ability to eat eggs without adverse effects is a reasonable way to identify those possibly at risk from influenza vaccination. Individuals with anaphylactic hypersensitivity to eggs should not be given influenza vaccine. This would include persons who, upon ingestion of eggs, develop swelling of the lips or tongue or who experience acute respiratory distress or collapse.

Live-virus vaccines prepared by growing viruses in cell cultures are essentially devoid of potentially allergenic substances related to host tissue. No severe hypersensitivity reactions have been reported with the live, attenuated measles, mumps, or rubella vaccines prepared from viruses grown in cell cultures. These vaccines can be given safely regardless of a history of allergy to eggs or egg protein.

Vaccines, such as cholera, DTP, plague, and typhoid, that are derived from organisms grown in simple bacteriologic media, are frequently associated with local, and occasionally systemic, side effects, but they do not appear to be allergenic *per se*. They should not be given, however, to individuals who have experienced any serious side effects from them.

Some vaccines contain preservatives or trace amounts of antibiotics to which patients may be hypersensitive. Those giving vaccines should review carefully the information provided with the package insert before deciding whether the rare patients with known hypersensitivity to such preservatives or antibiotics can be vaccinated safely.

Altered Immunity. Virus replication after administration of live, attenuated-virus vaccines may be enhanced in persons with immune deficiency diseases, and in those with suppressed capability for immune response, as occurs with leukemia, lymphoma, generalized malignancy, or therapy with corticosteroids, alkylating agents, antimetabolites, or radiation. Patients with such conditions should not be given live, attenuated-virus vaccines. Similarly, individuals residing in the household of a susceptible immunocompromised individual should not receive TOPV because vaccine viruses are excreted by the recipient of the vaccine and are communicable to other persons.

Severe Febrile Illnesses. Vaccination of persons with severe febrile illnesses should generally be deferred until these persons have recovered. This precaution is to avoid superimposing adverse side effects from the vaccine on the underlying illness or mistakenly identifying a manifestation of the underlying illness as having been caused by the vaccine. The presence of minor illnesses such as mild upper-respiratory infections should not preclude vaccination.

Live Vaccines and Pregnancy. On grounds of a theoretical risk to the developing fetus, live, attenuated-virus vaccines are not generally given to pregnant women or to those likely to become pregnant within 3 months after vaccination. With some of these antigens, particularly rubella, measles, and mumps vaccines, pregnancy is a contraindication to the vaccination. With TOPV and yellow fever vaccine, however, vaccine should be given if there is a substantial risk of exposure to natural infection. There is no convincing evidence of risk to the fetus from vaccination of pregnant women with inactivated viral vaccines, bacterial vaccines, or toxoids.

Recent Administration of Immune Serum Globulin or Hyperimmune Globulin. Passively acquired antibody can interfere with the response to live, attenuated-virus vaccines. Therefore, administration of such vaccines should be deferred until approximately 3 months after passive immunization. By the same token, immunoglobulins should not be administered for at least 2 weeks after a vaccine has been given, if possible. Inactivated vaccines are sometimes administered concurrently with passive antibody to induce active immunity, as is done for postexposure rabies prophylaxis.

Reporting Adverse Reactions. All vaccines have been reported to cause some adverse effects. These range from minor local reactions to severe systemic illness such as paralysis associated with TOPV. To improve knowledge about adverse effects, all severe reactions should be evaluated and reported in detail to local or state health officials and to the manufacturer.

Recommended Schedule for Active Immunization
of Normal Infants and Children*

RECOMMENDED AGE	VACCINE(S)	COMMENTS
2 months	DTP,[a] TOPV[b]	Can be initiated earlier in areas of high endemicity
4 months	DTP, TOPV	2-month interval desired for TOPV to avoid interference
6 months	DTP, (TOPV)	TOPV optional for areas where polio might be imported (e.g., some areas of the Southwest U.S.)
8–12 months	c	
12 months	Tuberculin Test[d]	May be given simultaneously with MMR at 15 months (see text*)
15 months	Measles, Mumps, Rubella (MMR)[e]	MMR preferred
18 months	DTP, TOPV	Consider as part of primary series—DTP essential
4–6 years[f]	DTP, TOPV	
14–16 years	Td[g]	Repeat every 10 years for lifetime

* American Academy of Pediatrics. Report of the committee on infectious diseases (the red book). 19th ed. Evanston, IL: AAP, 1982, reproduced with permission.
   a. **DTP**–Diphtheria and tetanus toxoids with pertussis vaccine.
   b. **TOPV**–Oral, attenuated poliovirus vaccine contains poliovirus types 1, 2, and 3.
   c. The Advisory Committee on Immunization Practices, Centers for Disease Control, recently revised its recommendation on poliomyelitis prevention (see reference 6); it
Continued

recommends that the three TOPV doses in the primary series be given as follows: the first dose at 6-12 weeks of age; the second dose given six to eight weeks later, and the third dose at least six weeks after that (customarily at 8-12 months of age).

d. **Tuberculin test**–Mantoux (intradermal PPD) preferred. Frequency of tests depends on local epidemiology. The Committee recommends annual or biennial testing unless local circumstances dictate less frequent or no testing (see Tuberculosis* for complete discussion).

e. **MMR**–Live measles, mumps, and rubella viruses in a combined vaccine (see text* for discussion of single vaccines versus combination).

f. Up to the seventh birthday.

g. **Td**–Adult tetanus toxoid (full dose) and diphtheria toxoid (reduced dose) in combination.

For all products used, consult manufacturer's brochure for instructions for storage, handling, and administration. Biologics prepared by different manufacturers may vary, and those of the same manufacturer may change from time to time. The package insert should be followed for a specific product.

For detailed vaccination information, consult the following references:

References

1. ACIP,** Centers for Disease Control. General recommendations on immunization. Morb Mortal Wkly Rep 1980;29:76,81-83.

2. American Academy of Pediatrics. Report of the committee on infectious diseases (the red book). 19th ed. Evanston, IL: AAP, 1982.

3. ACIP,** Centers for Disease Control. Rubella vaccine. Morb Mortal Wkly Rep 1978;27:451-454,459.

4. ACIP,** Centers for Disease Control. Measles prevention. Morb Mortal Wkly Rep 1978;27:427-430, 435-437.

5. ACIP,** Centers for Disease Control. BCG vaccines. Morb Mortal Wkly Rep 1979;28:241-244.

6. ACIP,** Centers for Disease Control. Poliomyelitis prevention. Morb Mortal Wkly Rep 1982;31:22-26, 31-34.

7. ACIP,** Centers for Disease Control. Mumps vaccine. Morb Mortal Wkly Rep 1980;29:87-88, 93-94.

8. ACIP,** Centers for Disease Control. Rubella prevention. Morb Mortal Wkly Rep 1981;30:37-42,47.

9. Committee on Infectious Diseases of the American Academy of Pediatrics. Revised recommendations on rubella vaccine. Pediatrics 1980;65:1182-1184.

**Advisory Committee on Immunization Practices

12 *LABORATORY INDICES*

THE FOLLOWING TABLES LIST SOME COMMON CLINICAL LABORATORY TESTS and include normal values, the major disease states likely to alter values, and drugs which may alter the test results by producing a false value through interference (I) or by altering the result through a pharmacologic or toxic effect (P). The reader should refer to the reference sources listed at the end of this chapter as well as other comprehensive sources for further information.

Normal laboratory value ranges vary from institution to institution, depending upon individual differences in laboratory equipment, methods and personnel. Standard International (SI) units are included in the tables whenever possible for those institutions which utilize this notation. The following abbreviations are used in the table:

(B)	blood
(S)	serum
(I)	test interference
(P)	pharmacologic/toxic effect
arb	arbitrary
s	seconds
hr	hour
mU/ml	milliunits per milliliter
U/ml	units per milliliter
IU/L	international units per liter
mEq/L	milliequivalents per liter
nmol/L	nanomoles per liter
μmol/L	micromoles per liter
mmol/L	millimoles per liter
kPa	$k \times pascal = 10^3$ newton/M^2

Blood Chemistry

TEST AND ALTERATION	NORMAL RANGE	NORMAL RANGE IN SI UNITS
Albumin (S)—see Protein		
Aldolase (S)	1.3–8.2 mU/ml	12–75 nmol·s⁻¹/L

Aldolase (S) — **Aldolase (S)** 1.3–8.2 mU/ml 12–75 nmol·s^{-1}/L
Elevated by myocardial infarction, hemolytic anemia, muscular dystrophies, myopathies, acute hepatitis, malignant neoplasms, hemolysis, severe muscular exertion, ethanol (P), clofibrate (P), aminocaproic acid (P)

Ammonia (B) 80–110 mcg/dl 47–65 μmol/L
Elevated by liver failure or liver bypass, acetazolamide (P), am-

Continued

Blood Chemistry

TEST AND ALTERATION	NORMAL RANGE	NORMAL RANGE IN SI UNITS

monium chloride (P), asparaginase (P), diuretics (P), hyperalimentation therapy (P)
Decreased by kanamycin (P), lactulose (P), neomycin (P), all orally

Amylase (S)   4–25 U/ml   4–25 arb units
Elevated by acute pancreatitis, pancreatic duct obstruction, salivary gland disease, alcohol (P), drugs (eg, diuretics, corticosteroids) causing pancreatitis (P), narcotics (P), cholangiography (P)
Decreased by severe liver damage or marked destruction of pancreas

Bilirubin (S)

Direct (Conjugated)	0–0.2 mg/dl	up to 3 μmol/L
Indirect (Unconjugated)	0.2–0.8 mg/dl	up to 14 μmol/L
Total	0.2–1.0 mg/dl	up to 17 μmol/L

Elevated by hepatocellular damage, biliary duct obstructions, fasting, hemolytic disease; indirect also high in hemolytic disease, deficiency of glucuronyl transferase; drugs causing hepatocellular damage (P), dextran 75 (I), iodine-containing contrast media (P), iron dextran (I), rifampin (P)
Decreased by alcohol and barbiturates in infants (P)

Blood Urea Nitrogen—see Urea Nitrogen

Calcium (S)   8.5–10.5 mg/dl   2.1–2.6 mmol/L
Elevated by hyperparathyroidism, bone destruction, bone tumor, sarcoidosis, excess vitamin D intake (P)
Decreased by hypoparathyroidism, chronic renal disease, malabsorption, hypoalbuminemia

Carbon Dioxide (S)

Content	24–30 mEq/L	24–30 mmol/L
Pressure (pCO$_2$)	35–45 mm Hg	

Elevated by metabolic alkalosis, respiratory acidosis, chronic obstructive lung disease (with decreased pO$_2$)
Decreased by metabolic acidosis, respiratory alkalosis

Ceruloplasmin (S)   27–37 mg/dl   1.8–2.5 μmol/L
Elevated by pregnancy, some malignant neoplasms, hepatic cirrhosis, infection, rheumatoid arthritis, estrogens (P), oral contraceptives (P), phenytoin (P)
Decreased by Wilson's disease, nephrosis

Chloride (S)   100–106 mEq/L   100–106 mmol/L
Elevated by hyperchloremic acidosis, hyperparathyroidism, nephrosis, respiratory alkalosis, renal insufficiency, dehydration, acetazolamide (P), mafenide (P)
Decreased by vomiting, diarrhea, metabolic alkalosis, diabetic ketoacidosis, most diuretics (P)

Cholesterol (S)   120–220 mg/dl   3.1–5.7 mmol/L
Elevated by hypothyroidism, idiopathic hypercholesterolemia, nephrosis, obstructive liver disease, oral contraceptives (P), phenothiazines (P), miconazole (P)

Continued

Blood Chemistry

TEST AND ALTERATION	NORMAL RANGE	NORMAL RANGE IN SI UNITS

Decreased by severe hepatocellular damage, hyperthyroidism, pernicious anemia, malnutrition, niacin (P), cholestyramine (P), clofibrate (P), neomycin (P), thyroid analogues (P), aminosalicylic acid (P)

Creatine Phosphokinase [CPK] (S)

Males	5–55 mU/ml	0.08–0.91 μmol · s^{-1}/L
Females	5–35 mU/ml	0.08–0.58 μmol · s^{-1}/L

Elevated by necrosis or acute damage to striated muscle (myocardial infarction, muscle trauma, status epilepticus, postoperative state), brain infarction, strenuous exercise, IM injection of drugs (P), chronic alcoholism (P), clofibrate (P)

Creatinine (S)   0.6–1.5 mg/dl   60–130 μmol/L

Elevated by impaired renal function, urinary tract obstruction, eating meat, nephrotoxic drugs (P), cefoxitin (I), cefORanide (I)

Globulin—see Protein

Glucose, Fasting (B)   70–110 mg/dl   3.9–5.6 mmol/L

Elevated by diabetes mellitus, stress, acute pancreatitis, hyperthyroidism, diazoxide (P), epinephrine (P), corticosteroids (P), diuretics (P), estrogens (P), phenytoin (P)
Decreased by adrenal insufficiency, hyperinsulinism, hypopituitarism, alcohol (P), monoamine oxidase inhibitors (P), propranolol (P), clofibrate (P)

Iron (S)   50–150 mcg/dl   9.0–26.9 μmol/L

Elevated by hemochromatosis, hemosiderosis, pernicious anemia, hemolysis, oral contraceptives (P), iron dextran (for 3 weeks with some methods only) (I), chloramphenicol (P)
Decreased in iron deficiency anemia, anemias of chronic diseases (rheumatoid arthritis, systemic lupus erythematosus, uremia), nephrosis

Lactic Dehydrogenase [LDH] (S) (Wacker)   60–120 U/ml   1.0–2.0 μmol · s^{-1}/L

Elevated by tissue necrosis, acute myocardial infarction, myopathies, cardiovascular surgery, hepatitis, hemolytic anemia, hemolysis

Magnesium (S)   1.5–2.0 mEq/L   0.8–1.3 mmol/L

Elevated by renal failure, diabetic coma, hypothyroidism, magnesium-containing laxatives or antacids (P)
Decreased by diarrhea, malabsorption, alcoholism, hyperthyroidism, parathyroid disease, hepatic disease, aminoglycosides (P), amphotericin B (P), diuretics (P), calcium salts (P)

Oxygen Tension [pO$_2$] (B)   75–100 mm Hg   10.0–13.3 kPa

Decreased by pulmonary edema, pulmonary embolism (with normal or decreased pCO$_2$), COPD, hypoventilation (with increased pCO$_2$)

pH (B)   7.35–7.45

Elevated by hypokalemia, severe vomiting, metabolic alkalosis ac-

Continued

Blood Chemistry

TEST AND ALTERATION	NORMAL RANGE	NORMAL RANGE IN SI UNITS

companied by acute or chronic acidosis or respiratory alkalosis due to hyperventilation or sodium bicarbonate administration (P)
Decreased by hypoxia, diabetic ketoacidosis, severe diarrhea, metabolic acidosis, renal failure or insufficiency, ammonium chloride (P), acetazolamide (P), mafenide (P)

Phosphatase, Acid, Total (S) (Bessey-Lowry)

Males	0.13-0.63 U/ml	36-175 nmol $\cdot$ s^{-1}/L
Females	0.01-0.56 U/ml	2.8-156 nmol $\cdot$ s^{-1}/L

Elevated by carcinoma of prostate with metastases, hyperparathyroidism, Paget's disease

Phosphatase, Alkaline (S)   13-39 IU/L   0.22-0.65 μmol $\cdot$ s^{-1}/L
Up to 13 U/dl (King Armstrong)

Elevated by bone fractures, osteoblastic bone disease, some malignant neoplasms, some renal disease, pregnancy, obstructive liver disease, drugs inducing hepatic disease (P), some IV albumin (I), anticonvulsants (P)
Decreased by hypothyroidism, pernicious anemia, excessive vitamin D intake (P), clofibrate (P)

Phosphorus, Inorganic (S)   3.0-4.5 mg/dl   1.0-1.5 mmol/L
Elevated by hypoparathyroidism, hypervitaminosis D, bone disease, renal insufficiency
Decreased by hyperparathyroidism, vitamin D deficiency, malabsorption syndrome, chronic alcoholism, severe burns, phosphate-binding antacids (eg, aluminum hydroxide) (P)

Potassium (S)   3.5-5.0 mEq/L   3.5-5.0 mmol/L
Elevated by adrenal insufficiency, renal insufficiency, hemolysis, severe metabolic acidosis, diabetic ketoacidosis, antineoplastics (P), potassium salts of penicillin in large doses (P), amiloride (P), spironolactone (P), triamterene (P), succinylcholine (P), potassium salts (P)
Decreased by inadequate potassium, excessive fluid loss, malabsorption, hyperaldosteronism, renal tubular damage, starvation, amphotericin B (P), corticosteroids (P), carbenicillin (P), potassium-depleting diuretics (P), insulin (P), sodium polystyrene sulfonate (P), mafenide (P)

Protein (S)

Total	6.0-8.5 g/dl	60-85 g/L
Albumin	3.5-5.0 g/dl	35-50 g/L
Globulin	2.3-3.5 g/dl	23-35 g/L
Transferrin	200-400 mg/dl	2.0-4.0 g/L

Albumin: *Elevated* by dehydration, shock, hemoconcentration, anabolic hormones (P)
Decreased by malnutrition, malabsorption, nephrosis, hepatic insufficiency, neoplastic disease, leukemia, overhydration, severe burns
Globulin: *Elevated* by liver and biliary cirrhosis, hemochromatosis, acute infection, neoplastic disease
Decreased by malnutrition, agammaglobulinemia
Transferrin: *Elevated* by iron deficiency, pregnancy, estrogens (P), oral contraceptives (P)

Blood Chemistry

TEST AND ALTERATION	NORMAL RANGE	NORMAL RANGE IN SI UNITS

Decreased by malnutrition, nephrotic syndrome, inflammatory processes, chronic liver disease, asparaginase (P), corticosteroids (P)

Sodium (S)   135–145 mEq/L   135–145 mmol/L
Elevated by dehydration, hyperadrenocorticism, CNS trauma, corticosteroids (P), large doses of sodium-containing drugs (P)
Decreased in adrenal insufficiency, renal insufficiency, trauma, drug-induced inappropriate ADH (P)

Thyroxine [T₄] (S) (RIA)   4–12 mcg/dl   52–154 nmol/L
Elevated by hyperthyroidism, elevation of thyroxine-binding proteins, estrogens (P), oral contraceptives (P), methadone (P)
Decreased by hypothyroidism, hypothyroidism treated with liothyronine (T₃), decrease of thyroxine-binding proteins, corticosteroids (P), phenytoin (P), large doses of salicylate (P), anabolic steroids (P), asparaginase (P), danazol (P)

Transaminase [SGOT] (S)   10–40 U/ml $0.08\text{–}0.32\ \mu\text{mol} \cdot \text{s}^{-1}/\text{L}$
Elevated by acute myocardial infarction, alcoholism, liver disease, acute infections, muscle trauma, acute pancreatitis, IM injection of drugs (P), drugs inducing hepatocellular damage (P)
Decreased by pyridoxine deficiency

Transferrin—see Protein

Urea Nitrogen [BUN] (S)   8–25 mg/dl   2.9–8.9 mmol/L
Elevated by impaired renal function, increased protein catabolism, tetracycline (P), drugs (eg, amphotericin B, aminoglycosides, guanethidine, ganglionic blocking agents) that impair renal function or renal blood flow (P)
Decreased by severe liver damage, inadequate diet, pregnancy

Uric Acid (S)   3.0–7.0 mg/dl   0.18–0.42 mmol/L
Elevated by gout, renal failure, leukemia, increased destruction of nucleoproteins, diuretics (P), salicylates in small doses (P), ethambutol (P), diazoxide (P)
Decreased by iodine-containing contrast media (P), phenylbutazone (P), acetohexamide (P), probenecid (P), sulfinpyrazone (P), guaifenesin (P)

Hematology

TEST	NORMAL RANGE	NORMAL RANGE IN SI UNITS
Bleeding Time	1-4 min (Duke) 1-6 min (Ivy) 3-9 min (Simplate)	
Counts, Blood		
Erythrocytes Males:	$4.8-6.4 \times 10^6$/cu mm	$4.8-6.4 \times 10^6$/µl
Females:	$4.2-5.4 \times 10^6$/cu mm	$4.2-5.4 \times 10^6$/µl
Leukocytes, Total	$4.3-10.8 \times 10^3$/cu mm	$4.8-10.8 \times 10^3$/µl
Basophils	0-1%	
Eosinophils	1-3%	
Lymphocytes	20-40%	
Monocytes	4-8%	
Myelocytes	0%	
Neutrophils		
Bands	0%	
Segmented	40-60%	
Platelets	$200-400 \times 10^3$/cu mm	$200-400 \times 10^3$/µl
Erythrocyte Sedimentation Rate [ESR] Males:	0-10 mm/hr (Wintrobe) 0-13 mm/hr (Westergren)	
Females:	0-15 mm/hr (Wintrobe) 0-20 mm/hr (Westergren)	
Hematocrit Males:	45-52%	0.45-0.52
[PCV] Females:	37-48%	0.37-0.48
Hemoglobin Males:	13-18 g/dl	8.1-11.2 mmol/L
Females:	12-16 g/dl	7.4-9.9 mmol/L
Partial Thromboplastin Time, Activated [APTT]	25-37 s	
Prothrombin Time [PT]	75-100% of control value	
Red Cell Indices		
Diameter	5.5-8.8 µm	
Mean Corpuscular Volume (MCV)	80-94 cu µm	
Mean Corpuscular Hemoglobin (MCH)	27-32 pg	
Mean Corpuscular Hemoglobin Concentration (MCHC)	32-36%	

Renal and Urine Indices

TEST	NORMAL RANGE	NORMAL RANGE IN SI UNITS
Catecholamines		
Epinephrine	<20 mcg/24 hr	<109 nmol/24 hr
Norepinephrine	<100 mcg/24 hr	<590 nmol/24 hr
Creatinine Clearance	105–150 ml/min per 1.73 M^2 of body surface	
Osmolality	500–850 mOsm/kg	
pH	4.6–8.0 (average 6)	
Phenolsulfonphthalein [PSP]		
Fifteen minutes	at least 25% excreted	
Two hours	at least 60% excreted	
Protein		
Qualitative	0	
Quantitative	0–0.1 g/24 hr	
Specific Gravity	1.003–1.030	
Urinalysis		
Bacterial Count		
Contamination	Less than 10^3 colonies/ml	
Infection	Greater than 10^5 colonies/ml	
Ketones		
Qualitative	0	
Microscopic Exam	Up to 1–2 RBC, WBC, epithelial cells/HPF; occasional hyaline cast/LPF	

References

1. Eastham RD. Biochemical values in clinical medicine. 6th ed. Chicago: Year Book, 1978.
2. Friedman RB, Anderson RE, Entine SM et al. Effects of diseases on clinical laboratory tests. Clin Chem 1980;26:1D-476D.
3. Hansten PD. Drug interactions. 4th ed. Philadelphia: Lea and Febiger, 1979:301-491.
4. Krupp MA, Chatton MJ, eds. Current medical diagnosis and treatment 1981. Los Altos, CA: Lange Medical Publ., 1981:1035-1049.
5. Scully RE, McNeely BU, Galdabini JJ. Case records of the Massachusetts General Hospital: normal reference laboratory values. N Engl J Med 1980;302:37-48.
6. Tietz NW. Fundamentals of clinical chemistry. 2nd ed. Philadelphia: WB Saunders, 1976.
7. Wallach J. Interpretation of diagnostic tests. 3rd ed. Boston: Little, Brown, 1978.
8. Young DS, Pestaner LC, Gibberman V. Effects of drugs on clinical laboratory tests. Clin Chem 1975;21:1D-432D.

13 *MEDICAL EMERGENCIES*

Outline of Drug Therapy

THE THERAPEUTIC APPROACHES, DRUGS AND ADULT DOSES given below have been compiled from somewhat divergent and conflicting sources of information (see references). In addition, some recommendations have been made based upon the authors' experience, and suggestions from specialists and researchers in the field. As a result, the therapeutic concepts and dosages contained herein may differ from those advocated by specific practitioners and institutions.

Anaphylaxis

AN ANAPHYLACTIC REACTION is an *urgent* medical problem which can prove fatal. Although the onset of symptoms can vary from minutes to hours, most reactions will occur within 5–30 minutes following ingestion or parenteral administration of an antigen. Symptoms may progress from extreme apprehension and cutaneous reactions to more severe systemic manifestations, such as severe respiratory distress and/or profound shock. Reactions include the following: conjunctivitis; gastrointestinal edema (nausea, vomiting, diarrhea); cutaneous reactions (urticaria, pruritus, angioedema); rhinitis, laryngeal edema, and bronchospasm (coughing, wheezing, dyspnea, cyanosis); vascular collapse, cardiac arrhythmias, and cardiac arrest.

Definitive Therapy (see also Adjunctive Therapy). *Adult doses only are given in this section.*

1a. Treatment of anaphylaxis is always initiated with *immediate* **Epinephrine HCl (aqueous), SC or IM, 0.3–0.5 mg** (0.3–0.5 ml of 1:1000), may repeat q 5–20 minutes.

   or, for nonresponding or severe reactions
   Epinephrine HCl, IV slow push, 0.2–0.5 mg (0.2–0.5 ml of 1:1000 diluted to 10 ml with saline, or 2–5 ml of 1:10,000), may repeat q 5–20 minutes.

b. Patient should be in recumbent position with legs elevated, patent airway established and oxygen given; if applicable, a tourniquet should be placed proximal to the antigen injection site (remove temporarily q 10–15 minutes), and give

Epinephrine HCl, infiltrate 0.1–0.3 mg (0.1–0.3 ml of 1:1000) at injection site.

2. *Bronchospasm* (without shock) not responding to epinephrine therapy may require
Aminophylline, IV slow infusion, 250–500 mg (10–20 ml of 25 mg/ml solution in 500 ml fluid, infusion rate not to exceed 50 mg/minute); may begin continuous infusion if necessary—see theophylline monograph in Drug Reviews Section.

3a. *Hypotension* not responding to epinephrine may be overcome by the use of fluids (see 3b.) and vasopressor agents; for example **Dopamine HCl, IV slow infusion,** adjust rate to response (400 mg in 500 ml NS or D5W = 800 mcg/ml).

or
Norepinephrine Bitartrate, IV infusion, adjust rate to maintain a systolic blood pressure of about 90–100 mm Hg (2 ml of 0.2% solution in 500 ml D5W = 4 mcg base/ml).

b. *Hypovolemia* may be the underlying cause of hypotension, and this requires rapid expansion of the intravascular fluid volume with **saline, plasma, albumin, hetastarch, or whole blood** until the central venous pressure is 15 cm H_2O (constant CVP monitoring is required).

Adjunctive Therapy. *Adult doses only are given in this section.*

1. To prevent further cutaneous reactions, give **Diphenhydramine HCl, PO, IM or slow IV, 25–50 mg,** may repeat q 6 hours.

2. To prevent prolonged antigen-antibody reactions, give **Hydrocortisone Phosphate/Succinate, IV, 100 mg,** may repeat q 6 hours (may administer after the initial epinephrine injection). *This is controversial, however.*

3. To treat cardiac arrest, see the following section.

References

1. Austen KF. Systemic anaphylaxis in the human being. N Engl J Med 1974;291:661-4.
2. Kelly JF, Patterson R. The treatment of anaphylaxis. Ration Drug Ther 1973;7(11):1-5.
3. Kelly JF, Patterson R. Anaphylaxis—course, mechanisms and treatment. JAMA 1974;227:1431-6.
4. Lockey RF, Bukantz SC. Allergic emergencies. Med Clin North Am 1974;58:147-56.
5. MacFarlane MD, McCarron MM. Anaphylactic shock and anaphylactoid reaction—analysis of 62 cases. Drug Intell Clin Pharm 1973;7:394-407.
6. Parker CW. Drug allergy. N Engl J Med 1975;292:511-4, 732-6, 957-60.
7. Plaut M, Lichtenstein LM. Treatment of immediate hypersensitivity reactions to drugs. Ration Drug Ther 1974;8(7):1-6.

Cardiac Arrest

A CARDIAC ARREST IS A MEDICAL EMERGENCY requiring a systematic approach. Early recognition (unconsciousness, apnea, no pulse) must be followed by prompt, effective application of Basic Cardiac Life Support (BCLS) techniques to sustain the patient until Advanced Cardiac Life Support (ACLS) capabilities are available. With ACLS capabilities, a definitive treatment plan can then be attempted.

Thus, management of cardiac arrest is a four-step approach:

Diagnosis
Emergency Treatment (BCLS)
Definitive Therapy (ACLS)
Postresuscitation Care

Diagnosis
Verify that respiration and perfusion have ceased:

1. Loss of consciousness.

2. Loss of functional ventilation (apnea).

3. Loss of functional perfusion (no pulse).

Emergency Treatment (BCLS)
The findings listed above are sufficient to justify the immediate application of BCLS techniques listed below. The goal of BCLS is to rapidly and effectively reperfuse the CNS with oxygenated blood. It is well-recognized that either delays in initiating BCLS or providing ineffective BCLS can result in irreversible hypoxic brain damage in an otherwise "successful" resuscitation.

1. Summon help and resuscitation equipment.

2. If witnessed arrest:
   a. Defibrillate with 200–300 joules of direct current shock if a defibrillator is immediately available, or
   b. Deliver sharp precordial blow.

3. If no response to above, or if an unwitnessed arrest, start artificial ventilation:
   a. Establish an adequate airway.
   b. Ventilate by mouth-to-mouth, mouth-to-nose, mouth-to-tube or bag-valve-mask techniques.
   c. The first few ventilations should be rapid (hyperventilation), then decrease rate to approximately 12 per minute.

4. Begin artificial perfusion via external chest compressions:
   a. Position patient supine on firm surface.
   b. Ensure proper placement of hands on sternum.
   c. Depress sternum at rate of 60 cycles per minute (50% of cycle should be compression).

Definitive Therapy (ACLS). *Adult doses only are given in this section.*
Initiate attempts by trained personnel to maintain a patent airway, establish an intravenous route for administration of fluids and drugs, establish an electrocardiographic diagnosis, and apply specific treatments to correct a recognized electrical and/or mechanical abnormality.

Definitive therapy can be divided into **General Therapy** — modalities to be considered in all cases of cardiac arrest before a specific electrical abnormality has been identified; and **Specific Therapy** — modalities designed for specific electrocardiographic or mechanical abnormalities.

General Therapy

Management of Acidosis. Severe acidosis can develop within 5 minutes after cardiac arrest and will continue unless BCLS is provided. Acidosis is due primarily to a respiratory component and, to a lesser extent, a metabolic component.

1. *Respiratory acidosis:*
    a. Etiology: Accumulation of CO_2 secondary to hypoventilation.
    b. Treatment: Adequate ventilation; *no* role for sodium bicarbonate.

2. *Metabolic acidosis:*
    a. Etiology: Slow accumulation of lactic acid secondary to anaerobic metabolism within hypoperfused (hypoxic) tissues.
    b. Treatment: Adequate perfusion of oxygenated blood will delay development of significant lactic acidosis. However, in patients with unwitnessed cardiac arrest, sodium bicarbonate may be necessary to overcome pre-existing metabolic acidosis. Therefore:

    If unwitnessed arrest and ABG's not available: **Sodium Bicarbonate, IV slow push, 1 mEq/kg initially** empirically, then not more than **44.6–50 mEq** (50 ml of 7.5% or 8.4% solution) q 10 minutes.

    If unwitnessed arrest and ABG's available: **Sodium Bicarbonate, IV slow push, 1 mEq/kg initially,** then future doses calculated on basis of base deficit:

$$NaHCO_3 \text{ Dose in mEq} =$$
$$\text{Base Deficit in mEq/L} \times 0.2 \times \text{Body Weight in kg}$$

    If witnessed arrest: Do not administer sodium bicarbonate without a reasonable determination of acid-base status as noted above. Inappropriate sodium bicarbonate may produce hypernatremia, hyperosmolality and alkalosis.

Epinephrine—Empiric Use. Epinephrine is often given empirically at the start of definitive therapy, even before an ECG diagnosis has been made. The basis for this empiric use is epinephrine's complex cardiovascular actions (positive inotropic and chronotropic effects and peripheral vasoconstriction), which may enhance automaticity and subsequent perfusion pressures in bradycardia or asystole. If the heart is fibrillating, epinephrine may facilitate effective defibrillation and subsequent resumption of an adequate coronary artery perfusion gradient. Thus, the following may be appropriate:

Epinephrine HCl, IV slow push, 0.5–1 mg (5–10 ml of 1:10,000 solution, or 0.5–1 ml of 1:1000 diluted to 10 ml with saline).

Specific Therapy

In order to simplify the pharmacologic management of cardiopulmonary arrest, disturbances of cardiac activity associated with cardiac arrest may be grouped into three major categories, each of which can be approached in a logical, reproducible manner: ventricular tachydysrhythmias, asystole and electromechanical dissociation.

Ventricular Tachydysrhythmias. Considered in this category, and treated in the same way, are ventricular fibrillation, ventricular flutter, and ventricular tachycardia when associated with ineffective cardiac output.

1. *Electrical defibrillation, 200–300 joules delivered.*

2. Epinephrine HCl, IV slow push, 0.5–1 mg (5–10 ml of 1:10,000 solution) is commonly stated to be an effective adjunct for successful defibrillation, especially when ventricular fibrillation is monitored as "fine" fibrillatory waves. There are no scientific data to support this concept; thus, epinephrine is not recommended as an aid to defibrillation.

3. In intractable ventricular tachydysrhythmias or when there is repeated reversion to tachydysrhythmias following electrical defibrillation, an irritable focus in the myocardium may be the source of persistent tachydysrhythmias and an antidysrhythmic drug is indicated. (If digitalis toxicity is suspected, see item 7).
   Lidocaine HCl, IV slow push, 50–100 mg (1 mg/kg) (2.5–5 ml of 2% or 5–10 ml of 1% solution), may repeat q 3–5 minutes to total of 300 mg.

   If response occurs to loading dose, then *maintenance*:
   Lidocaine HCl, IV infusion, 1–4 mg/minute (20–50 mcg/kg/minute) (10 ml of 20% in 500 ml D_5W = 4 mg/ml).

4. If lidocaine fails to maintain electrical stability, then:
   Bretylium Tosylate, IV rapid push, 500 mg (5 mg/kg) (50 mg/ml, 10 ml vial), may repeat with 10 mg/kg q 15 minutes to total of 30 mg/kg. Note that bretylium frequently has a slow onset of action (> 10 minutes). While waiting for this effect, one could administer procainamide HCl (see item 5) in an attempt to gain control of the dysrhythmia rapidly. The important point to recognize is that once primary therapy fails, second-line agents are not predictably effective. Should procainamide fail to suppress tachydysrhythmias, the slower acting bretylium will already have been administered. Should procainamide be effective, then subsequent doses of bretylium will not be necessary.

5. If lidocaine- and bretylium-resistant dysrhythmias persist, or if one elects to administer procainamide concurrently with bretylium, then:
   Procainamide HCl, IV slow push, 500 mg (5 ml of 100 mg/ml vial,

or 1 ml of 500 mg/ml vial), may repeat in 5 minutes to total of 1 g.

Note that this rate is greater than the commonly reported 25–50 mg/minute; however, this is a life-threatening dysrhythmia and delays in drug administration may prove ineffective.

6. If lidocaine, bretylium and procainamide resistant dysrhythmias persist, then:
   Propranolol HCl, IV slow push, 1 mg over 1 minute (1 mg/ml amp), may repeat q 5 minutes to total of 0.1 mg/kg.

7. If all of above fail, or if digitalis toxicity is suspected, consider:
   Magnesium Sulfate, IV slow push, 1 g (8 mEq) over 1 minute (2 ml of 50% solution), may repeat after 5 minutes if no response.

Asystole. Considered in this category, and treated in the same way, are asystole, complete heart block, slow ventricular focus, sinus bradycardia and agonal rhythm. In dealing with any of these dysrhythmias (except asystole), transvenous pacing is probably the best long-term approach, but is generally not readily available. Thus, drugs are used to enhance or initiate cardiac activity, at least until transvenous equipment is available.

It is important to note that true asystole, unless the result of excessive vagal tone (bradyasystole event), is frequently associated with irreversible cardiac damage.

1. Treatment of asystole should be initiated with:
   Atropine Sulfate, IV push, 0.5–1 mg (5–10 ml of 0.1 mg/ml solution), may repeat with 0.5–1 mg q 5 minutes to total of 4 mg.

2. For asystole failing to respond to atropine, then:
   Epinephrine HCl, IV push, 0.5–1 mg (5–10 ml of 1:10,000), may repeat after 5 minutes.

3. For bradydysrhythmias (sinus bradycardia, AV block) failing to respond to the above, then:
   Isoproterenol HCl, IV push, 0.02–0.04 mg (1–2 ml of 1:50,000 solution which is 1 ml of 1:5000 diluted with 9 ml of saline), may repeat q 3–5 minutes. If isoproterenol is effective, then *maintenance:*
   Isoproterenol HCl, IV infusion, beginning with 1–2 mcg/minute, titrated to response (5 ml of 1:5000 in 250 ml D_5W = 4 mcg/ml).

Electromechanical Dissociation. Considered in this category are ineffective cardiac output (hypotension) in face of ECG evidence of electrical myocardial activity, hypotension secondary to inadequate peripheral vasoconstriction, volume depletion or cardiac tamponade.

1. Rapidly assess volume status—if depleted, fluid challenge with crystalloid (normal saline or lactated Ringer's injection).

2. If volume is adequate and no evidence of tamponade, then consider cardiac sympathomimetics for vasoconstricting and inotropic/chronotropic effects. Begin with:
   Dopamine HCl, IV infusion, 5 mcg/kg/minute initially, increasing prn to maximum of 20 mcg/kg/minute, adjusting rate to

keep systolic blood pressure between 90–100 mm Hg (400 mg in 500 ml D$_5$W = 800 mcg/ml).

3. If dopamine fails, then:
   Norepinephrine Bitartrate, IV infusion, 8 mcg/minute initially, changing prn to keep systolic blood pressure between 90–100 mm Hg [8 ml of 0.1% solution (1 mg/ml) in 500 ml D$_5$W = 16 mcg/ml].

4. If norepinephrine fails, then:
   Calcium Chloride, IV slow push, 0.5–1 g
      (5–10 ml of 10% solution = 6.8–13.6 mEq), *or:*
   Calcium Gluconate, IV slow push, 1–2 g
      (10–20 ml of 10% solution = 4.7–9.4 mEq), *or:*
   Calcium Gluceptate, IV slow push, 1.1–2.2 g
      (5–10 ml = 4.5–9 mEq).

Note that calcium administration in the therapy of elec-tromechanical dissociation has not been shown to be effective and, in fact, may be harmful. Therefore, its use should be confined to situations in which more acceptable therapy has failed.

Postresuscitation Care

Patients who have been successfully resuscitated are at great risk of experiencing subsequent events. Thus, if the patient is not already in an intensive care setting with constant monitoring, readily available resuscitation equipment and skilled nursing staff, transport the patient to such an area as soon as possible. The cause of the initial episode must be sought and corrected if possible.

Special Considerations/Precautions

Systemic circulation times are grossly prolonged during external chest compression. Remember to allow *at least* 45–60 seconds between the time of peripheral injection of pharmacologic agents and anticipated response.

Intracardiac injections of drugs play no role in modern manage-ment of cardiopulmonary arrest. Drugs do not work within the chambers of the heart, but rather at the cellular level after delivery via the coronary circulation. Stopping BCLS to attempt intracar-diac injections only serves to interrupt vital CNS perfusion.

Be aware of the possible physical incompatibilities of sodium bicarbonate and catecholamines. In addition, sodium bicarbonate and calcium containing solutions may form a precipitate if in-fused at the same time in the same IV line.

References

1. Anon. Standards and guidelines for cardiopulmonary resuscitation (CPR) and emergency cardiac care (ECC). JAMA 1980;244:453-509.

2. Bishop RL, Weisfeldt ML. Sodium bicarbonate administration during cardiac arrest. JAMA 1976;235:506-9.

3. Goldberg AH. Cardiopulmonary arrest. N Engl J Med 1974;290:381-5.

4. Greenblatt DJ, Gross PL, Bolognini V. Pharmacotherapy of cardiopulmonary arrest. Am J Hosp Pharm 1978;33:579-83.

5. Mattar JA, Weil MH, Shubin H et al. Cardiac arrest in the critically ill. II. Hyperosmolal states following cardiac arrest. Am J Med 1974;56:162-8.

6. Redding JS, ed. Second Wolf Creek conference on CPR. Crit Care Med 1981;9:357-435.

Poisoning

General Information. Management of the poisoned patient involves procedures designed to prevent the absorption, minimize the toxicity and hasten elimination of the suspected contaminant. The prompt employment of appropriate emergency management procedures can often prevent unnecessary morbidity and mortality.

A regional poison information center is a practitioner's best source of definitive treatment information and should be consulted in all poisonings, regardless of the apparent simplicity of the case. Contact the regional poison information center in your area to learn of their staffing, resources and capabilities before a need for their services arises. Well-qualified regional centers are certified by the American Association of Poison Control Centers.

In all cases, every attempt should be made to accurately identify the contaminant, estimate the quantity involved and determine the time which has expired since the exposure. These data plus patient-specific parameters such as age, weight, sex and underlying medical conditions or drug use will assist you and the regional poison information center in designing an appropriate therapeutic plan for the patient.

The techniques described below are intended for the initial management of the poisoned patient using materials which should be readily available.

Topical Exposures.

1. Irrigate affected areas with a copious amount of water; use soap only if a stubborn, oily substance is the contaminant. Skin should be gently washed, not scrubbed, and special attention should be paid to the hair, skin folds, umbilicus and other areas where the contaminant might be trapped.

2. If the patient's clothing has been contaminated, remove them during the irrigation and either destroy them or clean them before the patient is allowed to wear them again. Clothing can interfere with the irrigation process and can serve as a reservoir of toxic material.

3. Do not attempt to "neutralize" the contaminant with another chemical (eg, acids and alkalis). Attempts at neutralization waste valuable time, are of no benefit and may be harmful.

4. Do not cover the affected area with emollients. These may trap unremoved contaminant against the skin. Severely damaged skin may be temporarily covered with a light, dry dressing.

5. Protect yourself from contamination. Gloves, aprons or a change of clothes may be necessary.

6. After the irrigation is complete, contact a regional poison information center for definitive treatment information.

Eye Exposure.

1. *Immediately* irrigate the eye; damage can occur within

seconds. The stream of water from the tap or a pitcher should strike the patient on the forehead, temple or bridge of the nose and then flow into the eye.

2. The eyelids should be held open during the irrigation. Small children may resist having their eyelids held open and may have to be restrained by being wrapped in a blanket or towel.

3. The irrigation should continue for at least 15 minutes (by the clock) to ensure adequate removal of the contaminant and normalization of the conjunctival pH. Body temperature water or saline may be substituted for tap water as the irrigation proceeds, but only if they can be obtained without interrupting the irrigation.

4. After the irrigation is complete, contact a regional poison information center for definitive treatment information.

Inhalation Exposures.
1. Remove the patient from the contaminated area, regardless of its apparent safety. Carbon monoxide, a common inhaled toxin, cannot be detected by sight, smell or taste.

2. Institute artificial respiration, if necessary, and provide supplementary hydrated oxygen if available and needed.

3. Protect yourself from contamination at all times.

4. Contact a regional poison information center for definitive treatment information.

Ingestions.
1. Remove any remaining contaminant from inside and around the mouth of the patient.

2. Give a small amount of water to clear the mouth and esophagus.

3. Contact a regional poison information center for definitive treatment information.

4. In many cases, it will not be necessary to take further steps. The following information can be utilized if additional care is recommended by the regional poison center.

Induction of Emesis
a. Do not induce emesis if the patient has evidence of CNS depression, seizures, loss of gag reflex or if the patient has ingested a caustic substance. Emesis following hydrocarbon ingestions remains controversial and must be evaluated on an individual case basis.

b. Induce emesis only with syrup of ipecac. Salt water, mustard water, other "home remedies" or gagging have no place in the management of the poisoned patient. These techniques are only marginally effective and can be dangerous.

c. The usual initial dose of **syrup of ipecac is 30 ml in persons over 5 years of age, 15 ml in children 1–5 years old** and **10 ml in children between 6 months and one year of age.**

d. Give the patient additional water to drink: 4 to 8 oz in children, 8 to 16 oz in adults. This distends the stomach and may improve the efficiency of the emesis. Do not give milk, because it may delay the action of syrup of ipecac. Activated charcoal should not be given until after ipecac-induced emesis has occurred.

e. Emesis usually occurs within 15–20 minutes. If 30 minutes have passed without emesis, it may be necessary to give an additional dose of syrup of ipecac and more water.

f. When emesis occurs, the risk of aspiration is minimized if the patient's head is lower than his hips. With a small child, this can be accomplished by having the child lie face down across the lap of an adult.

g. Have the patient vomit into a bowl or other container so that the vomitus can be inspected for the presence of the contaminant.

Activated Charcoal

a. Doses range from 30 to 120 g. Activated charcoal must be dispersed in a liquid like water or 70% sorbitol before administration. Gentle encouragement may be needed to make children swallow the charcoal. Having the child take the liquid through a drinking straw from an opaque container is sometimes helpful.

b. Activated charcoal is usually followed by the administration of a cathartic.

c. Alert the patient that charcoal will cause the stools to turn black.

Cathartics

a. Cathartics hasten elimination of unabsorbed drug and charcoal-adsorbed drug.

b. The most commonly used cathartics and their doses are:
  • **Magnesium sulfate (Epsom salts)** or **sodium sulfate (Glauber's salt), 250 mg/kg** given as 20% solutions. Solutions of these salts taste bad and some patients may reject them.

  • **Citrate of magnesia, 300–600 ml in adults; 4 ml/kg in children.** Although better tasting than the sulfate salts, the major limitation of this agent is the volume of fluid consumed.

References

1. Anon. Ipecac syrup and activated charcoal for treatment of poisoning in children. Med Lett Drugs Ther 1979;21:70-2.

2. Dabbous IA, Bergman AB, Robertson WO. The ineffectiveness of mechanically induced vomiting. J Pediatr 1965;66:952-4.

3. Rumack BH. Management of acute poisoning and overdose. In: Rumack BH, Temple AR, eds. Management of the poisoned patient. Princeton: Science Press, 1977;250-80.

4. Temple AR, Mancini RE. Management of poisoning. In: Yaffe SJ, ed. Pediatric pharmacology: therapeutic principles in practice. New York: Grune and Stratton, 1980;391-406.

Status Epilepticus

STATUS EPILEPTICUS IS DEFINED AS SEIZURES of sufficient duration or frequency to produce an enduring epileptic condition. Thus, status epilepticus is a serious neurological emergency which requires immediate recognition and prompt treatment to reduce morbidity and mortality.

Although status epilepticus can be subdivided into two major categories, convulsive and nonconvulsive status, the approach below deals only with generalized convulsive status. This type of status occurs most commonly, is most serious in terms of morbidity and mortality, and presents the greatest possibility for therapeutic error.

There is limited agreement on the most appropriate treatment regimen for convulsive status epilepticus, because there are no controlled studies from which objective data can be obtained. These guidelines present an approach which, if followed, will result in adequate control for most patients while minimizing drug toxicity.

The emergency treatment of generalized convulsive status epilepticus centers on four major approaches:

Protection From Physical Harm
Airway Maintenance
Drug Therapy
Identification and Treatment
of Precipitating Factors

Protection from Physical Harm.

1. If patient is on the ground or floor, move potentially harmful objects.

2. If patient is on a bed and side rails are available, they should be raised and padded.

3. A padded tongue blade or similar device can be inserted carefully between the teeth to decrease trauma to tongue, teeth and lips. Never force a tongue blade; insert during interictal period only.

Airway Maintenance

1. Position patient properly to decrease aspiration.

2. Insert soft plastic airway during interictal period.

3. Suction secretions.

4. Intubate if necessary (nasotracheal; orotracheal if interictal).

Drug Therapy. *Adult doses only are given in this section.* If a rapidly identifiable and treatable cause for seizure activity can be found (see the section Identification and Treatment of Specific Precipitating Factors below), general pharmacologic management of the seizure may be unnecessary. However, when such an etiology cannot be identified, drug therapy should be considered.

The principle goal of pharmacologic treatment of convulsive status is to quickly control the seizure state by administering a rapid-acting anticonvulsant. This is followed by the administration of an adequate loading dose of a long-acting anticonvulsant to initiate maintenance therapy.

1. For inital control, administer the following rapid-acting anticonvulsant:
   Diazepam, IV slow push (5 mg/minute), 5–10 mg initially (1–2 ml of 5 mg/ml solution), may repeat, if necessary, at 5 minute intervals to a total of 30 mg. If diazepam is effective, consider initiating long-term control with a second agent (phenytoin or phenobarbital).

2. If initial control is not successful with diazepam, then add:
   Phenytoin Sodium, IV slow push (50 mg/minute), 15 mg/kg (using 50 mg/ml solution). If seizure control is established, then begin maintenance therapy with phenytoin.

3. If seizure control is not established by completion of infusion, then add:
   Phenobarbital Sodium, IV slow push (100 mg/minute), 5 mg/kg (using 130 mg/ml solution). If seizure control is established with phenobarbital, then begin maintenance therapy with phenobarbital. If seizure control is not established within 20 minutes of completing infusion, may repeat dose.

For patients who continue to have seizures despite full therapeutic doses of the above drugs, the following alternatives can be attempted.

1. **Paraldehyde, IM, 0.1–0.15 ml/kg,** may repeat in 2 hours.

2. **Lidocaine HCl, IV slow push (50 mg/minute), 2–3 mg/kg** (using 20 mg/ml solution). This agent is not approved for status epilepticus, but has demonstrated effectiveness in refractory cases.

3. **General Anesthesia.** Very little information is available as to proper agent, monitoring or duration.

4. **Neuromuscular Blocking Agents.** These agents suppress neuromuscular evidence of seizure activity, but do not prevent or attenuate continued cerebral seizure activity; they should only be used with continuous EEG monitoring.

Identification and Treatment of Specific Precipitating Factors

Generalized convulsive status epilepticus occurs primarily in patients with a known seizure disorder and a specific, identifiable precipitating factor. Although most cases of generalized seizures can be temporarily controlled with drugs, it is important to simultaneously attempt to determine the presence of a treatable precipitating factor.

The following list of precipitating factors, although not complete, should be considered. This list follows on page 206.

1. Anticonvulsant drug withdrawal.

2. Drug withdrawal states (sedatives, rarely alcohol).

3. Metabolic abnormalities (hypoxia, hypoglycemia, hyponatremia, etc.).

4. Febrile state.

5. Drug toxicity (isoniazid, theophylline, tricyclic antidepressants).

6. Recent CNS diagnostic procedures.

7. New CNS lesions (infarction, tumor, encephalitis, meningitis, etc.).

Special Considerations/Precautions

Only patients who present with active seizure activity should be treated vigorously. The aggressive use of diazepam or phenobarbital in a patient who has stopped convulsing sedates the patient and interferes with the subsequent work-up.

Generalized seizures in pediatric patients present special problems, not only with respect to recognition of precipitating factors, but also with treatment. Practitioners who deal with pediatric seizure patients should refer to specific reviews of these special problems.

References

1. Browne TR. Drug therapy reviews: drug therapy of status epilepticus. Am J Hosp Pharm 1978;35:915-22.
2. Celesia GG. Modern concepts of status epilepticus. JAMA 1976;235:1571-4.
3. Cranford RE, Leppik IE, Patrick B et al. Intravenous phenytoin in acute treatment of seizures. Neurology 1979;29:1474-9.
4. Nicol CF. Status epilepticus. JAMA 1975;234:419-20.
5. Tharp BR. Recent progress in epilepsy—diagnostic procedures and treatment. Calif Med 1973;119:19-48.
6. Wilder BJ, Ramsay RE, Willmore LJ et al. Efficacy of intravenous phenytoin in the treatment of status epilepticus: kinetics of central nervous system penetration. Ann Neurol 1977;1:511-8.
7. Delagado-Escueta AV, Wasterlain C, Treiman DM et al. Management of status epilepticus. N Engl J Med 1982;306:1337-40.

The following is a cross-reference index of the generic and proprietary drug names used throughout the Medical Emergencies chapter.

Generic-Proprietary Name Index

Aminophylline—Generic
Atropine Sulfate—Generic
Bretylium Tosylate—Bretylol®
Calcium Chloride—Generic
Calcium Gluceptate—Generic
Calcium Gluconate—Generic
Diazepam—Valium®
Diphenhydramine HCl—Benadryl®, Various
Dopamine HCl—Intropin®
Epinephrine HCl—Adrenalin®, Various
Hetastarch—Hespan®
Hydrocortisone Phosphate/Succinate—
    Hydrocortone®/Solu-Cortef®
Isoproterenol HCl—Isuprel®
Lidocaine HCl—Xylocaine®, Various
Norepinephrine Bitartrate—Levophed®
Paraldehyde—Generic
Phenobarbital Sodium—Generic
Phenytoin Sodium—Dilantin®, Various
Procainamide HCl—Pronestyl®, Various
Propranolol HCl—Inderal®
Sodium Bicarbonate—Generic

14 NUTRITIONAL ASSESSMENT AND PARENTERAL NUTRITION

NUTRITIONAL STATUS IS A MAJOR DETERMINANT of patients' morbidity and mortality. Morbidity increases with malnutrition as manifested by depressed cell-mediated immunity and impaired wound healing.[1,2] Conditions that indicate a possible need for nutritional support include inadequate oral nutrition for longer than 7 days, recent body weight loss greater than 10%, an illness lasting more than 3 weeks, recent major surgery, a lymphocyte count of less than 1500/cu mm, serum albumin less than 3.5 g/dl and impaired cellular immunity demonstrated by anergy with skin testing.

Whenever possible, maintenance rather than repletion should be the primary objective of nutritional support. Early implementation promotes the preservation of lean body mass which is synthesized at a slower rate than adipose tissue when energy balance is exceeded.[3]

Initial Assessment

NUTRITIONAL ASSESSMENT OF THE PATIENT aids in diagnosing malnutrition and determining its degree of severity, so that a proper regimen for nutritional support can be formulated. The patient's physical and dietary history should be obtained to establish baseline data. Clinical parameters for assessing the patient's nutritional status can be most effectively evaluated through the use of an assessment form (Table 1). Because a patient's nutritional status is best reflected by body protein,[4] nutritional assessment should focus on the protein compartments. Protein compartments are classified into two types: somatic (muscle protein) and visceral (all other protein).

Somatic Protein Assessment Parameters
Percent Ideal Body Weight. The simplest initial measurement of a patient's nutritional status is body weight expressed as

Table 1. Nutritional Assessment

NAME: DATE:	STANDARD	DEPLETION		
		Mild 90 %	Moderate 60 - 90 %	Severe < 60 %
1. FAT STORES $\dfrac{TSF}{Standard\ TSF} \times 100 =$				
2. SOMATIC PROTEIN (Marasmus) Triceps Skinfold (TSF) mm =	M 12.5 F 16.5	11.3 14.9	11.3–7.5 14.9–9.9	< 7.5 < 9.9
% Ideal Body Weight $\dfrac{ABW}{IBW} \times 100 =$				
Mid-Upper Arm Circumference (MUAC) cm =	M 29.3 F 28.5	26.3 25.7	26.3–17.6 25.7–17.1	< 17.6 < 17.1
Mid-Upper Arm Muscle Circumference MUAC (cm)-[0.314 × TSF (mm)] =	M 25.3 F 23.2	22.8 20.9	22.8–15.2 20.9–13.9	< 15.2 < 13.9
Urinary Creatinine mg/24 hours =				
Creatinine/Height Index $\dfrac{UCr}{IUCr\ for\ height} \times 100 =$				
3. VISCERAL PROTEIN (Kwashiorkor) Serum Albumin g/dl =	3.5–5.0	3.5–3	3–2.5	< 2.5
Total Iron Binding Capacity mcg				
Serum Transferrin mg (0.8 × TIBC mcg/dl) − 43 =	200–400	200–180	180–160	< 160
Total Lymphocyte/cu mm $\dfrac{WBC/cu\ mm\ \times\ \%\ Lymphocytes}{100}$	1800–3000	1800–1500	1500–900	< 900
CELLULAR IMMUNITY mm Candida albicans Mumps PPD Tetanus Toxoid Trichophyton	15	15–10	10–5	< 5–0
DIAGNOSIS		Mild	Moderate	Severe
Kwashiorkor	ICDA # 267			
Marasmus	ICDA # 268			
Mixed Marasmus - Kwashiorkor	ICDA # 269.9			

Abbreviations:

ABW	—	Actual body weight
IBW	—	Ideal body weight
IUCr	—	Ideal urinary creatinine
MUAC	—	Mid-upper arm circumference
TIBC	—	Total iron binding capacity
TSF	—	Triceps skin fold
UCr	—	Urinary creatinine

a percentage of ideal body weight (see Body Measurements chapter):

$$\text{Percent Ideal Body Weight} = \frac{\text{Actual Body Weight}}{\text{Ideal Body Weight}} \times 100$$

Creatinine/Height Index. Creatinine/height index (CHI), when accurately obtained, is a more sensitive indicator of somatic protein and nutritional status than percent ideal body weight.[5]

Creatinine, a product of muscle metabolism, is normally excreted in urine at a constant rate proportional to the amount of skeletal muscle and lean body mass catabolized. CHI is calculated from a 24-hour urinary creatinine measurement and the ideal urinary creatinine value found in Table 2, using the following formula:

$$\text{CHI} = \frac{\text{Actual Urinary Creatinine}}{\text{Ideal Urinary Creatinine for Height}} \times 100$$

It is important that the sample be an aliquot drawn from a 24-hour collection of urine rather than a random sample. Creatinine is then assayed using standard creatinine clearance test methods.

Table 2. Ideal Urinary Creatinine[a]

MALES[b]		FEMALES[c]	
Height (cm)	Ideal Creatinine (mg/24 hr)	Height (cm)	Ideal Creatinine (mg/24 hr)
157.5	1288	147.3	830
160.0	1325	149.9	851
162.6	1359	152.4	875
165.1	1386	154.9	900
167.6	1426	157.5	925
170.2	1467	160.0	949
172.7	1513	162.6	977
175.3	1555	165.1	1006
177.8	1596	167.6	1044
180.3	1642	170.2	1076
182.9	1691	172.7	1109
185.4	1739	175.3	1141
188.0	1785	177.8	1174
190.5	1831	180.3	1206
193.0	1891	182.9	1240

a. From Blackburn GL, Bistrian BR, Maini BS et al. Nutritional and metabolic assessment of the hospitalized patient. J Parenter Enter Nutr 1977;1:11-22, reproduced with permission.
b. Creatinine coefficient (men) = 23 mg/kg of ideal body weight.
c. Creatinine coefficient (women) = 18 mg/kg of ideal body weight.

Certain limitations should be understood in using CHI as an indicator of malnutrition. Patients sometimes excrete amounts of creatinine and nitrogen that vary with different diets or conditions of illness or stress. Administration of corticosteroids, androgens or nitrofuran derivatives is reported to increase urinary levels of creatinine, whereas thiazides are reported to decrease levels.[6]

Anthropometric Measurements. Anthropometric measurements should be taken on the mid-upper portion of the nondominant arm by trained personnel. Detailed procedures and methods of measurement are available.[7,8] Triceps skin fold (TSF) measurement with calipers is compared to the standards in Table 1 to give a reasonable estimate of subcutaneous fat reserves.[4] Both TSF and mid-upper arm circumference (MUAC), obtained with a metric tape measure, can be used to derive the mid-upper arm muscle circumference (MUAMC) by the formula:[4]

$$\text{MUAMC} = \text{MUAC (cm)} - [0.314 \times \text{TSF (mm)}]$$

Visceral Protein Assessment Parameters

The status of visceral protein reflects the patient's ability to respond to stress by means such as immunocompetence and wound healing. This is determined by measurements of serum albumin, serum transferrin and total lymphocytes.[8] Serum albumin and transferrin levels usually decrease after trauma or surgery; however, consistent hypoalbuminemia for a period of at least 1 week may indicate a degree of malnutrition.[8] Serum albumin is unreliable as an assessment parameter in patients with hepatic or renal disease, or severe burns (see Laboratory Indices chapter).

Transferrin, having a shorter half-life (7 days) than albumin (14 days), more rapidly reflects nutritional depletion.[8] Direct radial immune diffusion is the preferred laboratory method of measuring serum transferrin levels;[9] however, when this method is unavailable, transferrin levels may be calculated from total iron binding capacity (TIBC) by the formula:

$$Transferrin = (0.8 \times TIBC) - 43$$

Laboratory values must be interpreted carefully as serum transferrin is elevated by iron deficiency and certain other conditions (see Laboratory Indices chapter). Serum transferrin values indicative of varying degrees of depletion are given in Table 1.

Cell Mediated Immunity. Skin test data have been the most widely utilized parameters for assessment of the effect of nutritional depletion on cellular immunity.[10] Skin test antigens are injected intradermally and the response is measured after 24–48 hours. A diameter of induration greater than 5 mm to any one of the antigens listed below (Table 3) indicates an immune response. A lack of response to all of the antigens indicates anergy and possible malnutrition. However, other possible causes of anergy include shock, infection, trauma, burns, therapeutic immunosuppression and old age. The response values indicating degrees of nutritional depletion are designated in Table 1.

Table 3. Skin Testing for Anergy[8,11]

ANTIGEN	DILUTION	INJECT
Candida albicans	1:100	0.1 ml (1 PNU)
Mumps	Undiluted	0.1 ml
PPD	5 t.u.	0.1 ml
Tetanus Toxoid	1:5	0.1 ml
Trichophyton	1:500	0.1 ml

Diagnoses of Malnutrition. Utilizing any or all of the parameters discussed, an initial or screening assessment can be done to establish the degree of malnutrition and need for nutritional support, if any. Diagnoses of malnutrition can be made using the International Classification of Diseases (Adapted for Use in the U.S.) categories of kwashiorkor (ICDA #267), marasmus (ICDA #268) or combined elements of both (ICDA #269.9).

Kwashiorkor is a protein deficit characterized by depletion of visceral protein, but with adequate reserves of fat and somatic muscle mass. Marasmus is a prolonged and gradual depletion of somatic muscle mass and fat reserves due to deficiencies of both protein and calories. In this diagnosis, visceral proteins may not be depleted; however, assessment parameters show depletion of somatic protein. An impaired immune system can be detected by the anergic response to skin tests in malnourished patients with either kwashiorkor or marasmus. The gravest diagnosis is a combination of elements of both kwashiorkor and marasmus. It is manifested by depressed levels of all assessment parameters.

Maintenance Assessment

THE INITIAL OR DIAGNOSTIC ASSESSMENT should be made prior to beginning a nutritional support regimen. Periodic reassessment of the patient, using some or all of the previously mentioned parameters, provides a means of objectively evaluating the efficacy of the nutritional support. Additional parameters to consider during this stage of assessment are nitrogen balance and body weight.

Nitrogen Balance

Nitrogen balance determinations can indicate the extent to which exogenous protein is being utilized and can serve as a method for evaluating the efficacy of nutritional support selected for the patient. Because nitrogen balance data is subject to daily errors of collection and other variables, it should be used only as a relative index of daily change and not of absolute depletion or improvement. Nitrogen balance is calculated for a 24-hour period using the following formulas:[8]

Nitrogen Balance = Total Nitrogen In − Total Nitrogen Out

Total nitrogen output by Kjeldahl analysis is the most accurate method of estimating nitrogen balance; however, it is not available in many institutions. Estimation of urinary urea nitrogen is a reasonable alternative and is summarized as follows:

$$\text{Nitrogen Balance} = \frac{\text{Protein Intake (g)}}{6.25} - [\text{Urinary Urea Nitrogen (g)} + 4]$$

Urinary urea nitrogen (UUN) is usually reported as a mg/dl value; therefore, to derive the amount in grams for use in the above formula, the value must be multiplied by the total 24-hour volume of urine output. The urine sample sent to the laboratory must be an aliquot drawn from an accurate 24-hour urine collection. The factor "4" is added as an empirical number to account for nonurinary nitrogen, such as that excreted in feces, sweat and other normal losses. Excessive nitrogen losses that cannot be measured, such as nitrogen lost in exudates from severe burns or in dialysate fluids, render nitrogen balance data less reliable.

Positive nitrogen balance can indicate a retention of nitrogen both as newly synthesized body protein tissue and as nitrogen retained in body fluids. Because only synthesized protein is of interest, elevations in BUN should be subtracted from total nitrogen balance. This calculation is summarized:

$$\text{Corrected Nitrogen Balance} =$$
$$\text{Nitrogen Balance} - \text{BUN Increment (g)}$$

To derive the BUN increment above normal in grams, the total body water volume of the patient must be considered. If the actual volume cannot be established for the patient, body water can be assumed to be 55% of total body weight (0.55 L/kg).[12] A BUN of 10 mg/dl above baseline in a 70 kg patient represents a BUN increment of 3.85 g (70 kg × 0.55 L/kg × 100 mg/L = 3.85 g).

Body Weight

The weight difference between tissue and body water is indistinguishable unless water balance can be measured. Body weight gain alone is therefore not a reliable maintenance assessment parameter. It is known, however, that weight gain in excess of 250 g/day is undesirable because patients cannot synthesize tissue at a greater rate.[13] Despite its shortcomings as a monitoring parameter, body weight should nevertheless be measured throughout the support regimen at the same time each day as an index of progress. Intake and output should be considered in the interpretation of body weight changes.

Nutrient Requirements

Caloric Requirements

Depending upon the nutritional status and clinical condition of the patient, daily caloric requirements can be calculated as a multiple of the patient's basal energy expenditure (BEE). BEE is the amount of energy required to maintain basic metabolic functions in the resting state and can be derived from the Harris-Benedict formulas:[15]

$$\text{BEE (Men): } 66 + (13.7 \times \text{wt in kg}) + (5 \times \text{ht in cm})$$
$$- (6.8 \times \text{age in yr})$$
$$\text{BEE (Women): } 655 + (9.6 \times \text{wt in kg}) + (1.8 \times \text{ht in cm})$$
$$- (4.7 \times \text{age in yr})$$

Trauma increases energy and protein requirements, and the nutritional support regimen should be adjusted accordingly.[14] Based on the amount of urinary urea nitrogen excreted per 24 hours, the severity of catabolism in stress conditions can be determined. Caloric requirements can then be estimated as a multiple of BEE as follows:[15]

Table 4. Caloric Requirements During Catabolism

24-HOUR UUN	DEGREE OF NET CATABOLISM	CALORIC REQUIREMENTS
0–5 g	1° (normal)	1.0 × BEE
5–10 g	2° (mild)	1.5 × BEE
10–15 g	3° (moderate)	1.75 × BEE
> 15 g	4° (severe)	2.0 × BEE

Sepsis increases oxygen consumption, and presumably energy consumption, about 7% with each degree F of fever.[16] Alternative methods of estimating caloric requirements are also available.[17]

In estimating the calories to be provided by each calorigenic substrate, yields may be considered as: dextrose, 3.4 kcal/g; fat, 9 kcal/g; and protein, 4 kcal/g. Calories provided by protein should be considered only when calculating their percentage share of the total caloric input. Protein calories should not be relied upon in meeting total energy requirements, because protein should be utilized for the preservation or synthesis of lean body mass.

Protein Requirements

The normal adult protein requirement is suggested to be about 0.6–0.8 g/kg/day.[18] This requirement may be doubled in severely ill or traumatized patients. For optimal synthesis of protein, concurrent provision of nonprotein calories must be sufficient. The optimal ratio of nonprotein calories to nitrogen for efficient nitrogen retention and nitrogen balance has been reported to be anywhere from 150:1 to 450:1.[19] This ratio is presumably not constant, but varies with the metabolic state of the patient.

Parenteral Nutrition

WHENEVER POSSIBLE, THE ENTERAL ROUTE should be used. The parenteral or intravenous (IV) route of nutrition should be reserved for patients who cannot be adequately maintained by the GI tract or who are in need of bowel rest. It is beyond the scope of this chapter to discuss enteral nutrition, and the remainder of this discussion will focus on parenteral nutrition.

Route of Intravenous Administration

Parenteral nutrition may be administered by either of two routes of access: the peripheral veins or larger central veins. The peripheral route is indicated for those patients who require only short-term supplementation or supplementation in addition to enteral support, or for those in whom the risks of central venous administration are too great. Peripheral veins are predisposed to thrombophlebitis, particularly when the osmolarity of the solution exceeds 600 mOsm/L. Therefore, it is recommended that formulas for peripheral administration not exceed final concentrations of 5% dextrose and 2.75% amino acids (AA) plus electrolyte and vitamin additives. Addition of small amounts of hydrocortisone (5 mg/L) and heparin (1000 units/L) to dextrose and AA solutions have been reported to prevent thrombophlebitis;[23] however, this should not be considered a routine practice. Concurrent administration of IV fat emulsion, which is a concentrated, iso-osmotic calorie source, is vital to increase the caloric content of a peripheral regimen.

Considering the IV caloric solutions that are available and the limitations of daily fluid requirements, the nutritional needs of the malnourished or hypermetabolic patient are difficult to achieve via peripheral vein. The concentrated, hyperosmolar solutions required by such patients *must* be administered into a large central vein, such as the superior vena cava where rapid dilution occurs. Such infusion requires surgical implantation of a catheter and subsequent monitoring. For such techniques and procedures the reader is referred elsewhere.[20-22]

Parenteral Nutrients

There are no known qualitative differences between the substrates required for parenteral nutrition and the basic components of a normal diet: water, carbohydrate, fat, protein, electrolytes, vitamins and trace elements.

Water. The average healthy adult can tolerate a fluid infusion volume of about 5 L/day. The patient who is fluid restricted might be limited to an intake of 2 L/day or less. This may be the deciding factor in selecting a hypertonic concentrated solution for infusion through a large central vein rather than a more dilute solution for peripheral administration.

Carbohydrate. The usual carbohydrate substrate recommended for parenteral nutrition is dextrose. The concentration of dextrose should be determined by the osmotic limitation of the administration route and the nonprotein calorie to nitrogen ratio required for the patient. The concentrations of available dextrose solutions with their corresponding caloric concentrations and osmolarities are as follows:

Table 5. IV Dextrose Solutions

CONCENTRATION	kcal/L	mOsm/L
5%	170	252
10%	340	505
20%	680	1010
40%	1360	2020
50%	1700	2520
60%	2040	3030
70%	2380	3530

When not precluded by osmotic or metabolic limitations, about $2/3$ of the caloric goal should be provided by dextrose calories.[17] On a calorie for calorie basis, carbohydrate is more efficient than fat in sparing body protein during hypocaloric feedings; however, both dextrose and fat are recommended as nonprotein caloric components of parenteral nutrition.

Fat. Fat is valued as a parenteral substrate for 3 major reasons: (1) it is a concentrated source of calories in an isotonic medium which makes it useful for peripheral administration; (2) it is a source of essential fatty acids (EFA) required for prevention or treatment of EFA deficiency, which may develop during extensive parenteral nutrition with dextrose;[24] and (3) it is a useful substitute for carbohydrate when dextrose calories must be limited due to glucose intolerance or excessive respiratory load. Metabolism of fat results in an increase in heat production, a decrease in respiratory quotient (RQ) and an increase in oxygen consumption. The RQ of fat is 0.7 versus 1 for carbohydrate.[25]

Having a lower RQ, fat produces less CO_2 for a given number of calories, thereby minimizing the respiratory effort required to eliminate CO_2.

Fat is available as emulsions of 10 or 20% soybean oil (Intralipid®, Travamulsion®) or safflower oil (Liposyn®). Clinical studies have not shown any major advantages of one over the other. The major differences in these products are their fatty acid contents which are summarized as follows:

Table 6. IV Fat Emulsions

FATTY ACID	SOYBEAN OIL		SAFFLOWER OIL
	INTRALIPID®	TRAVAMULSION®	
Linoleic Acid*	54%	56%	77%
Linolenic Acid	8%	6%	0.1%
Oleic Acid	26%	23%	13%
Palmitic Acid	9%	11%	7%
Stearic Acid	2.5%	0%	2.5%
Other	0.5%	4%	0.4%

*Linoleic acid is the only fatty acid "essential" to man.[24]

The caloric density of 10% fat emulsions is 1.1 kcal/ml of which 1 kcal is supplied by lipid and 0.1 kcal by glycerol (carbohydrate); the 20% emulsion has a caloric density of 2 kcal/ml, of which 0.1 kcal/ml is glycerol. The average particle size (0.5 microns) is the same in both concentrations, and both are nearly iso-osmotic: 10% = 280 mOsm/L; 20% = 330 mOsm/L. Although the manufacturers recommend not to exceed 60% of total calories as fat, some researchers advocate the use of fat as 80% of daily nonprotein calories when peripheral IV regimens are used.[26] For further information on dosage, administration and precautions of fat emulsion, the product literature should be consulted.

Protein. The protein or amino acid nitrogen available for IV infusion can be derived from either protein hydrolysate or crystalline AA solutions. Hydrolysate solutions are considered inferior to AA solutions[27] and, although still commercially available, they are no longer used in many institutions.

Various brands and concentrations of AA solutions are available for infusion. The profile of amino acids differs in each, and therefore their nitrogen contents are not equivalent. A comparison of popular brands and concentrations are summarized in Table 7. Most central venous parenteral nutrition formulas involve the combination of equal volumes of crystalline AA and 50% dextrose. In some situations, a higher nonprotein calorie to nitrogen ratio may be desired. Under these circumstances, 70% dextrose can be used. The nonprotein calorie to nitrogen ratios that result with each formula are included in Table 7. It is generally recommended that 5–5.5% AA be used in regimens for maintenance or repletion of slightly catabolic patients. Furthermore, the lower osmolarity of this concentration when mixed with an equal volume of a lower concentration of dextrose (eg, 10%) makes it more suitable for peripheral administration than the 7–10% AA

Table 7. Amino Acid Solutions Comparison Chart

AA SOLUTION AND CONCENTRATION	AVAILABLE VOLUME	TOTAL ESSENTIAL AA (g/dl)	TOTAL N (g/dl)	NONPROTEIN CAL: N RATIO WHEN MIXED WITH 500 ml D50W	D70W	Na⁺	K⁺	Mg⁺⁺	Cl⁻	Ac⁻	PO₄	OSMOLARITY (mOsm/L)
For TPN												
Aminosyn® 5%	(250 ml) 500 ml (1000 ml)	2.35	0.79	215:1	301:1	-	5.4	-	-	60	-	500
Travasol® 5.5%	500 ml	2.15	0.92	185:1	259:1	-	-	-	22	35	-	520
(with Electrolytes)						70	60	10	70	100	30	850
Aminosyn® 7%	500 ml	3.3	1.1	155:1	216:1	-	5.4	-	-	88	-	700
(with Electrolytes)						70	66	10	96	124	30	1013
Veinamine® 8%	500 ml	2.8	1.33	128:1	179:1	40	30	6	50	50	-	950
Aminosyn® 8.5%	500 ml	4.0	1.34	127:1	178:1	-	5.4	-	35	90	-	850
(with Electrolytes)						70	66	10	98	142	30	1160
Travasol® 8.5%	500 ml	3.3	1.43	119:1	166:1	-	-	-	34	52	-	860
(with Electrolytes)						70	60	10	70	135	30	1160
Freamine® III 8.5%	500 ml	4.2	1.26	135:1	189:1	10	-	-	2	74	10	810 Continued

Table 7. Amino Acid Solutions Comparison Chart

AA SOLUTION AND CONCENTRATION	AVAILABLE VOLUME	TOTAL ESSENTIAL AA (g/dl)	TOTAL N (g/dl)	NONPROTEIN CAL:N RATIO WHEN MIXED WITH 500 ml		ELECTROLYTES (mEq/L)						OSMOLARITY (mOsm/L)
				D50W	D70W	Na$^+$	K$^+$	Mg^{++}	Cl$^-$	Ac$^-$	PO$_4$	
Aminosyn® 10%	500 ml	4.7	1.57	108:1	152:1	–	5.4	–	–	148	–	1000
Travasol® 10%	250 ml	4.5	1.7	200:1	280:1	–	–	–	40	87	–	1060
	500 ml	4.5	1.7	100:1	140:1	–	–	–	40	87	–	1060
	1000 ml	4.5	1.7	–	–	–	–	–	40	87	–	1060
For Protein Sparing												
Aminosyn® 3.5% M	1000 ml	1.6	0.55	–	–	40	18.4	3	40	68	–	460
3.5% Travasol® M	500 ml 1000 ml	1.4	0.6	–	–	25	15	5	25	54	8	450
For Renal Failure												
Aminosyn® RF	300 ml	4.2	0.8	–	500:1	–	5.4	–	–	105	–	475
Nephramine® 5.4%	250 ml	5.4	0.6	–	745:1	6	–	–	–	44	–	440

solutions. Higher concentrations of AA (eg, 7–10%) are more suited for maintenance or repletion of patients who are in greater need of protein.

Special Amino Acid Formulas

Protein Sparing. It has been demonstrated than an isotonic infusion of 3.5% AA with no dextrose conserves endogenous nitrogen more efficiently than the traditional 5% dextrose infusion without nitrogen provision.[28] For a limited infusion of no more than 1 week's duration in patients who are not severely catabolic, isotonic amino acid infusions merit consideration.

Renal Failure. The objective of parenteral nutrition in patients with renal failure is to provide sufficient amino acids and calories for protein synthesis without exceeding the renal capacity for excretion of fluid and metabolic wastes. Two formulas which contain primarily essential amino acids have been developed for this purpose and are commercially available as Aminosyn® RF and Nephramine®. There are many special considerations in the nutritional support of renal patients and the reader is referred elsewhere for guidelines.[20,29]

Hepatic Failure. Treatment of patients in hepatic failure in whom muscle breakdown contributes to hepatic encephalopathy require a special amino acid formula with relatively greater amounts of branched chain amino acids (leucine, isoleucine and valine) and smaller amounts of the more hepatotoxic aromatic amino acids (phenylalanine, methionine, tyrosine and tryptophan). Such a formula is currently being investigated.[30]

Electrolytes. Electrolyte provision should be based on close monitoring of patients' laboratory values. Average daily requirements are summarized in Table 8 which follows on page 220.

Table 8. Electrolytes and Requirements

ELECTROLYTES	AVERAGE DAILY[20,29] TPN REQUIREMENT	DOSAGE FORMS	COMMENTS
Cations: Sodium	60–150 mEq	Sodium chloride concentrate (4 mEq/ml) Sodium acetate (2 mEq/ml) Sodium phosphate (4 mEq Na^+/ml)	Requirements during parenteral nutrition should not differ from normal fluid therapy requirements unless there is excessive sodium loss; lactate and bicarbonate should not be used
Potassium	40–240 mEq	Potassium chloride (2 mEq/ml) Potassium acetate (2 mEq/ml) Potassium phosphate (4.4 mEq K^+/ml)	Requirements are related to glucose metabolism and therefore increase with higher concentrations of dextrose infused
Magnesium	10–45 mEq	Magnesium sulfate (4 mEq/ml)	Requirements increase with anabolism; however, with less variation than does potassium
Calcium	3–30 mEq	Calcium gluconate 10% (4.5 mEq/10 ml) Calcium chloride 10% (13 mEq/10 ml)	Calcium requirements increase only slightly during parenteral nutrition. Calcium may be combined in solution with phosphate, but should be well diluted before mixing. Concentration should be kept under 5 mEq of calcium and 40 mmol of phosphorus in each liter
Anions: Phosphate	10 mmol/1000 kcal	Potassium phosphate (3 mmol P/ml—Abbott) Sodium phosphate (3 mmol P/ml—Abbott) (other concentrations vary according to manufacturer)	Requirements increase with anabolism. Safe empirical dosing guidelines should be developed taking into account the amount of sodium or potassium in solution as well as the amount of phosphate

Acetate and Chloride: The amount of acetate and chloride contained in each amino acid solution varies (see Table 7). To avoid acid/base disturbances, keep the ratio of sodium to chloride in the formula close to 1:1.[29] This guideline should not replace the monitoring of serum electrolytes to determine electrolyte requirements

Vitamins. Vitamin requirements for parenteral nutrition have not been adequately defined. MVI-12® is the commercially available product that most closely resembles the multivitamin formulation suggested for parenteral nutrition programs.[31] It is available as 2 separate vials, both of which are given once daily. Exceeding the recommended dosage may result in toxicity which is known to occur with excesses of the fat soluble vitamins A and D. Because water soluble vitamins are excreted rapidly after IV administration and no toxic effects are known, supplementation with 2 ml/L of B complex with C (Berocca C®) is recommended.

Vitamin K is available parenterally as phytonadione and 2–4 mg should be given weekly by IM or SC administration;[31] IV use should be avoided if possible. See the Phytonadione drug monograph, page 608.

Table 9. IV Multivitamins

	MVI-12® (per 5 ml vial)		Berocca C® (per 2 ml)	
Vial 1:	Ascorbic Acid (C)	100 mg	Ascorbic Acid (C)	100 mg
	Vitamin A	3300 IU	Thiamine (B_1)	10 mg
	Vitamin D	200 IU	Riboflavin (B_2)	10 mg
	Vitamin E	10 IU	Pantothenic Acid	20 mg
	Thiamine (B_1)	3 mg	Niacin	80 mg
	Riboflavin (B_2)	3.6 mg	Pyridoxine (B_6)	20 mg
	Pantothenic Acid	15 mg	Biotin	200 mcg
	Niacinamide	40 mg		
	Pyridoxine (B_6)	4 mg		
Vial 2:	Biotin	60 mcg		
	Folic Acid	400 mcg		
	Cyanocobalamin (B_{12})	5 mcg		

Trace Elements. Solutions of *individual* trace elements are commercially available in the following concentrations:

Table 10. IV Trace Elements

	MANUFACTURER AND CONCENTRATION	
ELEMENT	ABBOTT	IMS
Zinc	1 mg/ml (Zinc chloride)	4 mg/ml (Zinc sulfate)
Copper	0.4 mg/ml (Cupric chloride)	1 mg/ml (Copper sulfate)
Chromium	4 mcg/ml (Chromic sulfate)	10 mcg/ml (Chromic chloride)
Manganese	0.1 mg/ml (Manganese chloride)	0.5 mg/ml (Manganese sulfate)

Solutions of *multiple* trace elements have recently been made commercially available. One such formulation is MTE®-4 which provides:

ELEMENT	CONCENTRATION
Zinc	1 mg/ml (Zinc sulfate)
Copper	0.4 mg/ml (Copper sulfate)
Chromium	4 mcg/ml (Chromic chloride)
Manganese	0.1 mg/ml (Manganese sulfate)

Daily dosage is suggested in the table below and guidelines for use are suggested in reference 32. Although selenium deficiency has been reported during long-term total parenteral nutrition (TPN),[33] selenium requirements during TPN are yet to be defined.

Table 11. Daily IV Intake of Trace Elements[a]

	PEDIATRIC PATIENTS, mcg/kg[b]	STABLE ADULT	ADULT IN ACUTE CATABOLIC STATE[c]	STABLE ADULT WITH INTESTINAL LOSSES[c]
Zinc	300[d] 100[e]	2.5–4.0 mg	Additional 2.0 mg	Add 12.2 mg/L small-bowel fluid lost; 17.1 mg/kg of stool or ileostomy output[f]
Copper	20	0.5–1.5 mg	—	
Chromium	0.14–0.2	10–15 mcg	—	20 mcg[g]
Manganese	2–10	0.15–0.8 mg	—	

a. From American Medical Association Department of Foods and Nutrition. Guidelines for essential trace element preparations for parenteral use: a statement by an expert panel. JAMA 1979;241:2051-4, reproduced with permission.

b. Limited data are available for infants weighing less than 1,500 g. Their requirements may be more than the recommendations because of their low body reserves and increased requirements for growth.

c. Frequent monitoring of plasma levels in these patients is essential to provide proper dosage.

d. Premature infants (weight less than 1,500 g) up to 3 kg of body weight. Thereafter, the recommendations for full-term infants apply.

e. Full-term infants and children up to 5 years old. Thereafter, the recommendations for adults apply, up to a maximum dosage of 4 mg/day.

f. Values derived by mathematical fitting of balance data from a 71-patient-week study in 24 patients.

g. Mean from balance study.

Iron. Iron deficiency can occur in patients deprived of iron during long-term TPN. Iron for parenteral use is available as iron dextran. At least one study has concluded that iron dextran can be safely added to TPN solutions,[34] but dosing recommendations by this route have not been established. Methods of IV and IM administration are given in the Iron Dextran drug monograph.

Insulin. Insulin may be added to parenteral formulas of high dextrose concentration to control hyperglycemia and glycosuria, if necessary. Guidelines for dosage are empirical and 10–50 units of regular insulin may be added to each liter of solution. Standardized admixture procedures should be used to minimize variations of insulin activity due to adsorption loss. Other alternatives to control hyperglycemia and glycosuria should be investigated before insulin is employed.[20]

Monitoring the Patient

PARENTERAL NUTRITION offers a potential for many metabolic complications as summarized in Table 12. Most of these can be avoided by proper precautions and close monitoring of the patient. Laboratory parameters for patient monitoring are summarized in Table 13; more complete discussions are found in references 20–22 and 29.

Table 12. Parenteral Nutrition: Metabolic Complications and Management

COMPLICATION	FREQUENT CAUSES	TREATMENT(S)
Hyponatremia	Excessive GI or urinary sodium losses Water intoxication Inadequate sodium intake	Increase sodium concentration in TPN solution based on patient's requirements Limit free water intake to treat water intoxication
Hypokalemia	Excessive GI or urinary potassium losses Deficit of potassium in TPN solution Large glucose infusion	Increase potassium concentration in TPN solution based on patient's requirements
Hypomagnesemia	Insufficient magnesium in TPN solution Excessive GI or renal losses	Increase magnesium in TPN solution In an emergency, a magnesium sulfate solution may be given
Hypophosphatemia	Usually due to inadequate inorganic phosphate in TPN solution (concentrated glucose infusion may precipitate syndrome)	Add phosphate to TPN solution
Hypoglycemia	Usually due to abrupt interruption of TPN solution infusion	Immediately begin appropriate dextrose infusion and monitor blood glucose and potassium
Hyperglycemia	Insufficient insulin for relatively high glucose infusion	Give insulin Reduce rate of glucose infusion
Elevated BUN— Azotemia	Dehydration Calorie:nitrogen imbalance Peptides Renal dysfunction	Correct dehydration Give insulin if hyperglycemia present Increase nonprotein calories to achieve

Continued

Table 12. Parenteral Nutrition:
Metabolic Complications and Management

COMPLICATION	FREQUENT CAUSES	TREATMENT(S)
		calorie:nitrogen ratio of about 185:1
Hyperammonemia	Hepatic dysfunction Excess free ammonia Insufficient arginine	Slow infusion rate Discontinue infusion
Metabolic Acidosis	Excessive renal or GI losses of base Infusion of preformed hydrogen ion Inadequate amount of base-producing substance in TPN solution to neutralize acid products of amino acid degradation	Increase acetate in TPN solution Improve balance between cationic and anionic amino acids in TPN solution
Osmotic Diuresis	Failure to recognize initial hyperglycemia and increased glucose in urine	Reduce infusion rate Give insulin to correct hyperglycemia Give 5% dextrose and ¼ to ½ strength normal saline rather than TPN solution to correct dehydration Continue to monitor blood glucose, sodium, and potassium
Essential Fatty Acid Deficiency	Insufficient provision of fat during TPN	Daily provision of fat

Table 13. Routine Patient Monitoring Parameters[a]

PARAMETER	FREQUENCY
Urinary glucose and specific gravity	Every voided specimen until stable, then every shift
Vital signs, weight, intake & output	Daily
Serum glucose, electrolytes, BUN	Daily until stable, then twice weekly
Serum protein	Initially, then once weekly
Hemoglobin, WBCs, platelets	Twice weekly
Magnesium, calcium, phosphorus	Weekly
Prothrombin time	Weekly
Blood ammonia	Weekly (in renal and hepatic patients)

a. Frequency should be increased in critically ill patients.

References

1. Irvin TT. Effects of malnutrition and hyperalimentation on wound healing. Surg Gynecol Obstet 1978;146:33-7.

2. Bistrian BR, Blackburn GL, Scrimshaw NS et al. Cellular immunity in semistarved states in hospitalized adults. Am J Clin Nutr 1975;28:1148-55.

3. Elwyn DH. Nutritional requirements of adult surgical patients. Crit Care Med 1980;8:9-19.

4. Bistrian BR, Blackburn GL, Hallowell E et al. Protein status of general surgical patients. JAMA 1974;230:858-60.

5. Bistrian BR, Blackburn GL, Sherman M et al. Therapeutic index of nutritional depletion in hospitalized patients. Surg Gynecol Obstet 1975;141:512-6.

6. Martin EW, ed. Hazards of medication. Philadelphia: JB Lippincott, 1971:200.

7. Butterworth CE, Blackburn GL. Hospital malnutrition and how to assess the nutritional status of a patient. Nutrition Today 1975;10:8-18.

8. Blackburn GL, Bistrian BR, Maini BS et al. Nutritional and metabolic assessment of the hospitalized patient. J Parenter Enter Nutr 1977;1:11-22.

9. Rowlands BJ, Jensen T, Dudrick SJ. Comparison of two methods of measurement of serum transferrin (abstract). J Parenter Enter Nutr 1979;3:504.

10. Miller CL. Immunological assays as measurements of nutritional status: a review. J Parenter Enter Nutr 1978;2:554-63.

11. Borut TC, Ank BJ, Gard SE et al. Tetanus toxoid skin test in children: correlation with in vitro lymphocyte stimulation and monocyte chemotaxis. J Pediatr 1980;97:567-73.

12. Kinney JM, Moore FD. Surgical metabolism in metabolism of body fluids. In: Zimmerman LM, Levine R, eds. Physiologic principles of surgery. 2nd ed. Philadelphia: WB Saunders, 1964:136-60.

13. Kinney JM, Long CL, Gump FE et al. Tissue composition of weight loss in surgical patients. Ann Surg 1968;168:459-74.

14. Bistrian BR. A simple technique to estimate severity of stress. Surg Gynecol Obstet 1979;148:675-8.

15. Rutten P, Blackburn GL, Flatt JP et al. Determination of optimal hyperalimentation infusion rate. J Surg Res 1975;18:477-83.

16. Kinney JM. Energy requirements for parenteral nutrition. In: Fischer JE, ed. Total parenteral nutrition. Boston: Little, Brown, 1976:135-70.

17. Wilmore DW. The metabolic management of the critically ill. New York: Plenum, 1977.

18. Munro HN. Nutritional requirements in health. Crit Care Med 1979;8:2-8.

19. Chen W-J, Ohashi E, Kasai M. Amino acid metabolism in parenteral nutrition: with special reference to the calorie:nitrogen ratio and the blood urea nitrogen level. Metabolism 1974;23:1117-23.

20. Grant JP. Handbook of total parenteral nutrition. Philadelphia: WB Saunders, 1980.

21. Goldfarb IW, Yates AP. Total parenteral nutrition: concepts and methods. Pittsburgh: Synapse, 1978.

22. Anon. Insights into parenteral nutrition. Deerfield, IL: Travenol Laboratories, 1977.

23. Isaacs JW, Millikan WJ, Stackhouse J et al. Parenteral nutrition of adults with a 900 milliosmolar solution via peripheral veins. Am J Clin Nutr 1977;30:552-9.

24. Kellenberger TA, Johnson TA, Zaske DE. Essential fatty acid deficiency: a consequence of fat-free total parenteral nutrition. Am J Hosp Pharm 1979;36:230-4.

25. Askanazi J, Rosenbaum SH, Hyman AI et al. Respiratory changes induced by the large glucose loads of total parenteral nutrition. JAMA 1980;243:1444-7.

26. Jeejeebhoy KN, Anderson GH, Sanderson I et al. Total parenteral nutrition: nutrient needs and technical tips (part 1). Mod Med Can 1974;29(9).

27. Long CL, Zikria BA, Kinney JM et al. Comparison of fibrin hydrolysates and crystalline amino acid solutions in parenteral nutrition. Am J Clin Nutr 1974;27:163-74.

28. Blackburn GL, Flatt JP, Clowes GHA et al. Peripheral intravenous feeding with isotonic amino acid solutions. Am J Surg 1973;125:447-54.

29. Fischer JE, ed. Total parenteral nutrition. Boston: Little, Brown, 1976.

30. Fischer JE, Yoshimura N, Aguirre A et al. Plasma amino acids in patients with hepatic encephalopathy: effects of amino acid infusions. Am J Surg 1974;127:40-7.

31. American Medical Association Department of Foods and Nutrition. Multivitamin preparations for parenteral use: a statement by the nutrition advisory group. J Parenter Enter Nutr 1979;3:258-62.

32. American Medical Association Department of Foods and Nutrition. Guidelines for essential trace element preparations for parenteral use: a statement by an expert panel. JAMA 1979;241:2051-4.

33. Van Rij AM, McKenzie JM, Thomson DC et al. Selenium supplementation in total parenteral nutrition. J Parenter Enter Nutr 1981;5:120-4.

34. Peters ML, Maher M, Brennan MF. Minimal IV iron requirements in TPN (abstract). J Parenter Enter Nutr 1980;4:601.

15 *PHARMACOGENETICS*

PHARMACOGENETICS IS THE STUDY of altered drug effects attributable to individual genetic differences. The following table is a synopsis of the best studied pharmacogenetic conditions. The table is divided into two parts. The first part lists conditions in which an altered drug response is the primary, and often only, feature. Such conditions are usually due to a single abnormal enzyme, which has usually only one different amino acid from the normal enzyme.

The second part of the table lists genetic conditions which result in physical or biochemical variations in the individual. These variations have a significance beyond an abnormal drug response. Often, multiple organ systems are involved.

There is evidence that genetic differences account for the wide variability in distribution, metabolism and dosage requirements of many drugs in normal subjects. This variability is often transmitted in more complex ways than the conditions in the table. In addition, environmental factors, diet, age, disease states and many other factors can interact with genetic conditions to alter drug metabolism.[1]

For further information on specific conditions, consult the references cited. Drugs that may cause hemolysis in patients with G6PD deficiency and related conditions are found in Drug-Induced Blood Dyscrasias, page 62.

Genetic Conditions in Which Abnormal Drug Response is a Primary Feature

CONDITION	DRUGS	FREQUENCY	CLINICAL SIGNIFICANCE	ENZYME	TRANS-MISSION	REFERENCES
Glucose-6-Phosphate Dehydrogenase (G6PD) Deficiency (over 80 variants)	See Drug-Induced Blood Dyscrasias Chapter	13% of American black males; 1% of American black females; occurs at various rates in whites of Mediterranean origin[5,6]	Hemolysis, primarily in hemizygous males and homozygous females; self-limiting and less severe in blacks (A⁻ variant)	Glucose-6-phosphate dehydrogenase	X-linked incomplete codominant	1-10
6-Phosphogluconic Dehydrogenase Deficiency	Same as G6PD	Very rare	Hemolysis	6-phosphogluconic dehydrogenase	Unknown	7,11,12
Glutathione Reductase Deficiency	Same as G6PD	Very rare	Hemolysis, thrombocytopenia, pancytopenia	Glutathione reductase	Autosomal dominant	7,11,12
Glutathione Synthetase Deficiency	Same as G6PD	Very rare	Hemolysis	Glutathione synthetase	Unknown	7,11,12

Continued

Genetic Conditions in Which Abnormal Drug Response is a Primary Feature

CONDITION	DRUGS	FREQUENCY	CLINICAL SIGNIFICANCE	ENZYME	TRANS-MISSION	REFERENCES
Hemoglobin H	Same as G6PD	1 in 300 births in Bangkok	Hemolysis	Hemoglobin composed of 4β chains	Autosomal recessive	1,2,4,11
Hemoglobin Zurich	Same as G6PD	Two small pedigrees	Hemolysis	One amino acid difference in β chain of hemoglobin	Autosomal dominant	1,4,11
Slow Acetylator	**Isoniazid, Hydralazine, Procainamide, Sulfamethazine, Dapsone, Phenelzine**	50% of American blacks and whites; 20% of American Indians; 13% of Japanese; 5% of Eskimos	Slow acetylators are more prone to peripheral neuritis with INH and may be predisposed to SLE with INH, hydralazine and procainamide; slow acetylators on INH and phenytoin are prone to toxicity; rapid acetylators may be more prone to INH hepatitis	Liver N-acetyl transferase	Autosomal recessive	1–4,9,11, 13,17

Continued

Genetic Conditions in Which Abnormal Drug Response is a Primary Feature

CONDITION	DRUGS	FREQUENCY	CLINICAL SIGNIFICANCE	ENZYME	TRANSMISSION	REFERENCES
Atypical pseudocholinesterase (Dibucaine Resistant, Fluoride Resistant and "Silent")	**Succinylcholine**	1 in 2500 Europeans homozygous, 3% heterozygous for dibucaine resistant variant; 1.5% of southern Eskimos homozygous for "silent"	Homozygotes have prolonged paralysis after usual doses of succinylcholine; check phenotype in patients with a family history prior to surgery	Plasma pseudocholinesterase	Autosomal recessive	1-4,8,9,11, 12,17,18
Atypical pseudocholinesterase, C5+ (Cynthiana)	**Succinylcholine**	One family	Resistant to succinylcholine because of rapid hydrolysis rate secondary to excessive amount of enzyme in blood	Plasma pseudocholinesterase	Unknown	3,11
Methemoglobin Reductase Deficiency	**Nitroglycerin, Amyl Nitrite, Nitrites, Nitrates, Sulfas, G6PD Drugs**	1 in 100 are heterozygous carriers	Homozygotes have cyanosis at birth; heterozygotes may be affected by drugs	NADH-methemoglobin reductase	Autosomal recessive	1-4,8,9,11

Continued

Genetic Conditions in Which Abnormal Drug Response is a Primary Feature

CONDITION	DRUGS	FREQUENCY	CLINICAL SIGNIFICANCE	ENZYME	TRANSMISSION	REFERENCES
Phenacetin-Induced Methemoglobinemia	**Phenacetin**	One small pedigree	Abnormal phenacetin metabolism to toxic compound, causing methemoglobinemia and hemolysis	? Hepatic dealkylase	Autosomal recessive	1,4,9,11
Parahydroxylation Deficiency	**Phenytoin**	One small pedigree	Defect in ability to parahydroxylate phenytoin, resulting in high plasma levels and toxicity	? Mixed function oxidase in liver	Autosomal or X-linked dominant	1,4,11
Acatalasia	**Hydrogen Peroxide**	Mainly Japanese, Koreans, Swiss, Germans and Israelis. Up to 1% in areas of Japan	Defect in ability to catalyze breakdown of hydrogen peroxide to oxygen; some patients develop spontaneous oral ulcerations	Erythrocyte (and usually tissue) catalase	Autosomal recessive	1,3,4

Continued

Genetic Conditions in Which Abnormal Drug Response is a Primary Feature

CONDITION	DRUGS	FREQUENCY	CLINICAL SIGNIFICANCE	ENZYME	TRANS-MISSION	REFERENCES
Warfarin Resistance (Coumarin Resistance)	**Warfarin**	Two large pedigrees	Decreased effectiveness of warfarin; high doses needed; increased sensitivity to antidotal effect of vitamin K	? Altered receptor or enzyme in liver with increased affinity for vitamin K	Autosomal dominant	1,4,8,11
Bishydroxycoumarin (Dicumarol) Sensitivity	**Dicumarol**	One small pedigree	Very long half-life of dicumarol; patients susceptible to increased bleeding while on drug	? Mixed-function oxidase in liver that hydroxylates dicumarol	Unknown	1,4,11
Hepatic Porphyria (3 variants)	**Barbiturates, Drugs having Allyl Group,** and possibly **Sulfas** and **Chloroquine**	1.5 per 100,000 in Sweden and Australia have acute intermittent variant; 1% of white South Africans have porphyria cutanea tarda	Precipitation of porphyria attacks	Abnormally increased synthesis of porphyrins	? Autosomal dominant	2,8,9,11

Continued

Genetic Conditions in Which Abnormal Drug Response is a Primary Feature

CONDITION	DRUGS	FREQUENCY	CLINICAL SIGNIFICANCE	ENZYME	TRANS-MISSION	REFERENCES
Inability to Taste Phenyl-thiourea	**Phenylthio-urea (Phenyl-thiocarbamide)**	More than 50% of US popula-tion	Athyrotic cretins and those with nodular goiter tend to be nontasters; those with diffuse toxic goiter and cigarette smokers tend to be tasters	Unknown	Autosomal recessive	1,2,8

Genetic Conditions in Which Abnormal Drug Response is a Secondary Feature

CONDITION	DRUGS	FREQUENCY	CLINICAL SIGNIFICANCE	ABNORMAL FEATURE	TRANS- MISSION	REFERENCES
Angle Closure Glaucoma	**Atropine, Scopolamine, Mydriatics**	1 in 4,000; rare in blacks	Use of the agents may precipitate angle closure in persons over 30 yr	Narrow angle of an- terior cham- ber of eye	Dominant, possibly with incom- plete pene- trance; pos- sibly multifac- torial	2,11,19
Chronic Simple Glaucoma and Associated Pressor Re- sponse	**Corticosteroids** (topically to eye)	1% of popula- tion has chronic simple glaucoma; 5% homozygous for pressor response	Increased intraocular pres- sure after instilla- tion of steroids in eye of those with pressor response	? Trabecular meshwork system of eye	? Dominant (disease); ? recessive (pressor re- sponse)	4,19
Variations in Eye Color	**Mydriatics (Parasympa- tholytics** and **Sympatho- mimetics)**	—	Response varies with amount of eye pigmentation; re- peated doses or higher concentra- tions needed in dark eyes, espe- cially with sym- pathomimetics	Not applica- ble	Not completely understood	19–21

Continued

Genetic Conditions in Which Abnormal Drug Response is a Secondary Feature

CONDITION	DRUGS	FREQUENCY	CLINICAL SIGNIFICANCE	ABNORMAL FEATURE	TRANS-MISSION	REFERENCES
Idiopathic Hypertrophic Subaortic Stenosis	**Digitalis Glycosides, Inotropic Catecholamines, Nitrites**	Rather common	Cardiac output decreases paradoxically; digitalis glycosides should not be given	Musculature around heart valve	Autosomal dominant	11,12
Malignant Hyperthermia	**Potent Inhalation Anesthetics, Muscle Relaxants** and possibly **Lidocaine** and **Mepivicaine**	1 in 20,000 anesthetized patients	Hyperthermia, often with muscle rigidity; affected patients should not receive general anesthesia, but may receive neuroleptanalgesia; 65% mortality if inadequately treated; **dantrolene** injection is treatment	Slow calcium uptake by sarcoplasmic reticulum of muscle	Autosomal dominant	1,4,23–25
Vitamin D-Dependent Rickets	**Vitamin D**	Unknown	Rickets that respond to 3,000–7,000 U/day or more of calciferol or ergocalciferol	Deficiency of enzyme that hydroxylates 25-dihydroxycholecalciferol	Autosomal recessive	26

Continued

Genetic Conditions in Which Abnormal Drug Response is a Secondary Feature

CONDITION	DRUGS	CLINICAL SIGNIFICANCE	ABNORMAL FEATURE	TRANS-MISSION	FREQUENCY	REFERENCES
Familial Dysautonomia (Riley-Day Syndrome)	**Histamine, Methacholine, Norepinephrine**	Exaggerated response to autonomic drugs; usual flare response to intradermal histamine absent	Autonomic abnormalities; lack of tear production; insensitivity to pain	Autosomal recessive	Most often in Eastern European Jews	9,11,27
Lesch-Nyhan Syndrome	**Azathioprine, Mercaptopurine, Thioguanine**[a]	Drugs ineffective or less effective because they are not metabolized to active metabolite(s)	Hypoxanthine-guanine phosphoribosyl transferase deficiency	X-linked recessive	Rare	3,11,12,27
Crigler-Najjar Syndrome (2 variants)	**Salicylates, Acetaminophen, Chloral Hydrate, Trichloroethanol, Tetrahydrocortisone, Menthol**	Homozygotes have severe icterus at birth and exhibit decreased conjugation of drugs as glucuronides	Liver glucuronyl transferase deficiency	Autosomal recessive (severe form); autosomal dominant (less severe form)	Rare	2,3,9,11,12

Continued

Genetic Conditions in Which Abnormal Drug Response is a Secondary Feature

CONDITION	DRUGS	FREQUENCY	CLINICAL SIGNIFICANCE	ABNORMAL FEATURE	TRANS-MISSION	REFERENCES
Down's Syndrome (Mongolism)	**Atropine, Mydriatics**	1.5% of births overall; 1 in 50 of mothers over 45 yr, 1 in 2500 in 18 year old mothers	Increased ocular response to atropine and other mydriatics	Multiple somatic and mental abnormalities	Complex	2,12,21

a. The metabolism of allopurinol to its nucleotide is also deficient in this condition; however, its efficacy in treating hyperuricemia in these patients is undiminished. It is, in fact, the most effective drug in these patients.[28]

References

1. Vesell ES. Pharmacogenetics: multiple interactions between genes and environment as determinants of drug response. Am J Med 1979;66:183-7.

2. Kalow W. Pharmacogenetics: heredity and the response to drugs. Philadelphia: WB Saunders, 1962.

3. Stanbury JB, Wyngaarden JB, Fredrickson DS, eds. The metabolic basis of inherited disease, 3rd ed. New York: McGraw-Hill, 1972.

4. Vesell ES. Pharmacogenetics. Biochem Pharmacol 1975;24:445-50.

5. Marks PA, Banks J. Drug-induced hemolytic anemias associated with glucose-6-phosphate dehydrogenase deficiency: a genetically heterogeneous trait. Ann N Y Acad Sci 1965;123:198-206.

6. Kirkman HN. Glucose-6-phosphate dehydrogenase variants and drug-induced hemolysis. Ann N Y Acad Sci 1968;151:753-64.

7. Wintrobe MM, ed. Clinical hematology, 6th ed. Philadelphia: Lea and Febiger, 1967.

8. Goldstein A, Aronow L, Kalman SM. Principles of drug action: the basis of pharmacology, 2nd ed. New York: John Wiley and Sons, 1974.

9. WHO Scientific Group. Pharmacogenetics: report of a WHO scientific group. Geneva: World Health Organization, 1973. (Technical report series number 524).

10. Desforges JF. Current concepts in genetics: genetic implications of G-6-PD deficiency. N Engl J Med 1976;294:1438-40.

11. La Du BN. Pharmacogenetics: defective enzymes in relation to reactions to drugs. Annu Rev Med 1972;23:453-68.

12. Cohen SN, Weber WW. Pharmacogenetics. Pediatr Clin North Am 1972;19:21-36.

13. Reidenberg MM, Drayer DE, Levy M et al. Polymorphic acetylation of procainamide in man. Clin Pharmacol Ther 1975;17:722-30.

14. Henningsen NC, Cederberg A, Hanson A et al. Effects of long-term treatment with procaine amide. Acta Med Scand 1975;198:475-82.

15. Mitchell JR, Thorgeirsson UP, Black M et al. Increased incidence of isoniazid hepatitis in rapid acetylators: possible relation to hydrazine metabolites. Clin Pharmacol Ther 1975;18:70-9.

16. Perry HM. Late toxicity due to hydralazine resembling systemic lupus erythematosus or rheumatoid arthritis. Am J Med 1973;54:58-72.

17. La Du BN. Pharmacogenetics. Med Clin North Am 1969;53:839-55.

18. Gutsche BB, Scott EM, Wright RC. Hereditary deficiency of pseudocholinesterase in Eskimos. Nature (London) 1967;215:322-3.

19. Sorsby A, ed. Modern ophthalmology, 2nd ed. Philadelphia: JB Lippincott, 1972.

20. Keeney AH. Ocular examination: basis and technique. Saint Louis: CV Mosby, 1970.

21. Stern C. Principles of human genetics, 3rd ed. San Francisco: WH Freeman, 1973.

22. Hurst JW, Logue RB, eds. The heart. New York: McGraw-Hill, 1966.

23. Britt BA. Malignant hyperthermia: a pharmacogenetic disease of skeletal and cardiac muscle. N Engl J Med 1974;290:1140-1.

24. Ryan JF, Donlon JV, Malt RA et al. Cardiopulmonary bypass in the treatment of malignant hyperthermia. N Engl J Med 1974;290:1121-2.

25. Anon. Dantrolene sodium approved for malignant hyperthermia. FDA Drug Bull 1979;9:27.

26. Anon. New developments in the pharmacology of vitamin D. Med Lett Drugs Ther 1974;16:15-6.

27. Riley CM. Familial dysautonomia. Adv Pediatr 1957;9:157-90.

28. Nyhan WL. Personal communication. San Diego: May 5, 1976.

16 SCHEDULES OF CONTROLLED DRUGS

Schedules of Controlled Drugs[a]

SCHEDULE I—All nonresearch use forbidden.
Narcotics
Heroin and many nonmarketed synthetic narcotics
Hallucinogens
LSD
MDA, STP, DMT, DET, mescaline, peyote, bufotenine, ibogaine, psilocybin
Marihuana, tetrahydrocannabinols

SCHEDULE II—No telephoned prescriptions; no refills.
Narcotics
Opium
Opium alkaloids and derived phenanthrene alkaloids: Morphine, codeine, hydromorphone (Dilaudid®), oxymorphone (Numorphan®), oxycodone (dihydrohydroxycodeinone, a component of Percodan®)
Designated synthetic drugs: Meperidine (Demerol®), anileridine (Leritine®), methadone (Dolophine®), levorphanol (Levo-Dromoran®), phenazocine (Prinadol®)
Stimulants
Coca leaves and cocaine
Amphetamine
Dextroamphetamine
Methamphetamine
Phenmetrazine (Preludin®)
Methylphenidate (Ritalin®)
Above in mixtures with other controlled or uncontrolled drugs (eg, Eskatrol®)
Depressants
Amobarbital
Pentobarbital
Secobarbital
Mixtures of above (eg, Tuinal®)
Methaqualone
Phencyclidine (PCP)

SCHEDULE III—Prescription must be rewritten after 6 months or 5 refills.

Continued

Schedules of Controlled Drugs[a]

Narcotics: The following opiates in combination with one or more active nonnarcotic ingredients, provided the amount does not exceed that shown:

Codeine and dihydrocodeine: Not to exceed 1800 mg/dl or 90 mg/tablet or other dose unit

Dihydrocodeinone (hydrocodone and in Hycodan®): Not to exceed 300 mg/dl or 15 mg/tablet

Opium: 500 mg/dl, or 25 mg/5 ml, or other dosage unit (paregoric)

Narcotic antagonist

Nalorphine

Depressants

Schedule II barbiturates in mixtures with noncontrolled drugs or in suppository dose form

Butabarbital (Butisol®)

Glutethimide (Doriden®)

Methyprylon (Noludar®)

Stimulants

Benzphetamine (Didrex®)

Chlorphentermine (Pre-Sate®)

Mazindol (Sanorex®)

Phendimetrazine

SCHEDULE IV—Prescription must be rewritten after 6 months or 5 refills. Differs from Schedule III in penalties for illegal possession.

Narcotics

Pentazocine (Talwin®)

Propoxyphene (Darvon®)

Stimulants

Diethylpropion (Tenuate®)

Fenfluramine (Pondimin®)

Phentermine

Depressants

Benzodiazepines:

Alprazolam (Xanax®)

Chlordiazepoxide (Librium®)

Clonazepam (Clonopin®)

Clorazepate (Tranxene®)

Diazepam (Valium®)

Flurazepam (Dalmane®)

Halazepam (Paxipam®)

Lorazepam (Ativan®)

Oxazepam (Serax®)

Prazepam (Verstran®)

Temazepam (Restoril®)

Triazolam (Halcion®)

Chloral hydrate

Ethchlorvynol (Placidyl®)

Ethinamate (Valmid®)

Continued

Schedules of Controlled Drugs[a]

Meprobamate
Mephobarbital (Mebaral®)
Paraldehyde
Phenobarbital

SCHEDULE V—As any other nonnarcotic prescription drug; may also be dispensed without prescription unless additional state regulations apply.
Narcotics
Diphenoxylate (not more than 2.5 mg and not less than 0.025 mg of atropine per dosage unit, as in Lomotil®)
Loperamide (Imodium®)
The following drugs in combination with other active, non-narcotic ingredients and provided the amount per 100 ml or 100 g does not exceed that shown:
Codeine: 200 mg
Dihydrocodeine: 100 mg
Ethylmorphine: 100 mg

---

a. Meyers FH, Jawetz E, Goldfien A. Review of medical pharmacology. 7th ed. Los Altos, CA: Lange Medical Publications, 1980, reproduced with permission. For a complete listing, see Drug Enforcement Administration. Controlled substances inventory list. Washington, DC: Drug Enforcement Administration, January 1979.

17 *DRUG REVIEWS*

Introduction

THE DRUG REVIEWS SECTION PROVIDES INFORMATION on over 350 drugs having widespread usage and/or therapeutic importance. In general, combination products are not listed. Information on drugs is presented in three formats: monographs, mini-monographs and comparison charts. The monograph format (described below) is utilized for most drugs. The mini-monograph is used for investigational and recently marketed drugs for which only limited information is available, drugs for which a prototype drug monograph appears and for drugs of lesser importance within a drug class. Comparison charts are used to present information on members of the same chemical class (eg, thiazide diuretics) or different drugs within the same therapeutic class (eg, diuretics). Comparison charts are also used to contrast specific properties of related agents (eg, antiplatelet effects, electrophysiologic properties) and to present information on non-therapeutic agents (eg, glucose testing systems).

Monographs and charts are categorized and grouped according to the American Hospital Formulary Service (AHFS) Pharmacologic-Therapeutic Classification System.[a] All drugs are arranged alphabetically by generic name within each category. Comparison charts are located immediately following the monographs to which they relate. References for each major AHFS category (eg, 8:00, 92:00) are found immediately following the last monograph of that category. The user will find that the easiest method to gain access to information on a particular drug is to use the index at the end of the book.

Monograph Format

The following is a description of the monograph format. The absence of any heading for a given drug indicates that such information was either unavailable at the time of writing or that the information available was not considered to be applicable to the drug or clinical situation.

Common brand names are given directly across from the generic name. This is for identification purposes only and is not meant to imply that the brand name products listed are superior to other brand name or generic products. "Various" indicates the availability of numerous brand or generic products.

Pharmacology. A description of the chemistry, major mechanism(s) of action and human pharmacology of specific clinical applications, when appropriate, are included.

Administration and Adult Dose. Route of administration and dosage ranges are given for the most common uses of the drug. Doses correspond to those given in the manufacturer's product information or in standard reference sources unless specifically referenced otherwise.

Dosage Individualization. Any known specific guidelines for dosing alterations that are needed in various disease states and patient subgroups are presented. Changes in pharmacokinetic parameters occurring in these disease states are presented in Pharmacokinetics and Biopharmaceutics rather than under this heading.

Pediatric Dose. Dosages correspond to those given in the product information or in Shirkey's *Pediatric Therapy* unless specifically referenced otherwise. When a dosage based on body surface area is given, the body surface area nomogram found in Body Measurements (Chapter 3) may be utilized.

Dosage Forms. The most commonly used dosage forms and strengths are listed. Combination products are generally not listed. See the abbreviations list on page 244 for dosage form abbreviations.

Patient Instructions. Key information that should be given to the patient when prescribing or dispensing the drug is presented in order to optimize efficacious, safe and compliant use. When instructions pertain to an entire drug category, the reader is referred to **Class Instructions** which appear at the beginning of the drug category.

Pharmacokinetics and Biopharmaceutics

Onset and Duration. The onset, peak and duration of the pharmacologic and/or therapeutic effect are listed when appropriate.

Plasma Levels. The therapeutic and/or toxic plasma levels are given when a correlation has been made between these concentrations and the effects of the drug.

Fate. The fate of the drug in the body is traced. Absorption, bioavailability, distribution, metabolism and excretion are discussed and alterations in disease states are mentioned. The pharmacokinetic data given in this section may be affected by variables in the study design and among patients.

$t_{1/2}$. The range and/or average distribution (α phase) and elimination (β phase) half-life of the drug, obtained from the best sources available are listed. Many studies only measure half-lives in a small number of normal subjects and often these do not apply to diseased patients. Changes in half-life due to the disease state or age group of the patient are given when these are known.

Adverse Reactions. This section is intended to be a brief list limited to reactions that are important due to their frequency or seriousness. Some indication of the frequency of the reaction and its relationship to dosage is made.

Contraindications. Absolute contraindications are given as they are found in the manufacturer's product information. In general, a person should not be given a drug to which he is allergic or hypersensitive; therefore, "hypersensitivity" is not listed as a contraindication in each monograph.

Precautions. Cautions against the use of a drug in various groups of patients and/or disease states are listed, together with any cross-sensitivities with other drugs. Unusual drug interactions which are not included in Drug Interactions (Chapter 7) are listed here. The word "pregnancy" appearing alone means that insufficient data have been accumulated to ensure drug safety in pregnancy; also refer to the Drugs and Pregnancy Chapter.

Parameters to Monitor. The clinical signs and laboratory tests that should be monitored in order to ensure safe and efficacious therapy are listed. The frequency with which such signs should be monitored may also be given; however, in most cases, the optimal frequency has not been determined and is dependent upon the condition of the patient and other variables.

Notes. Under this heading, miscellaneous information is presented that relates to the physicochemical properties, handling, relative cost, distinguishing characteristics, therapeutic usefulness and relative efficacy of the drug. Occasionally, information on similar drugs is also provided.

Abbreviations

The following are the abbreviations used in the drug monographs:

Cap capsule
Chew chewable
Cl clearance
Cl$_{cr}$ creatinine clearance
Crm cream
Cr$_s$ serum creatinine
    concentration
Drp drops
EC enteric coated
Elxr elixir
Gran granules
Hyp hypodermic
IM intramuscular(ly)
Inhal inhalation
Inj injection
IP intraperitoneal(ly)
IT intrathecal(ly)
IV intravenous(ly)

Lot lotion
Oint ointment
Ophth ophthalmic
PO oral(ly)
PR rectal(ly)
Pwdr powder
SC subcutaneous(ly)
SL sublingual(ly)
Soln solution
SR sustained-release
Supp suppository
Susp suspension
Tab tablet
Top topical(ly)
U units
Vag vaginal(ly)
V$_d$ apparent volume of
    distribution

Limitations

It should be noted that the information in the Drug Reviews section is not exhaustive; rather an attempt has been made to provide the most important aspects relating to each drug's use. For medicolegal purposes, the reader should become familiar with the manufacturer's product information or other comprehensive drug information sources.

General References

The general references listed below are recommended as good sources of further information. Additional general review articles and books are listed at the beginning of each drug category. These also contain information on the drugs listed in that category or on the disease state(s) for which these drugs are indicated.

General Prescribing Information

Martindale: the extra pharmacopoeia. 28th ed. London: The Pharmaceutical Press, 1982.

Facts and comparisons. St. Louis: Facts and Comparisons, Inc, Division of J.B. Lippincott, 1947-82.

American Society of Hospital Pharmacists. American hospital formulary service. Washington, DC: American Society of Hospital Pharmacists, 1959-82.

Pharmacology/Pharmacotherapy

Avery GS, ed. Drug treatment: principles and practice of clinical pharmacology and therapeutics. 2nd ed. Sydney: ADIS Press, 1980.

Gilman AG, Goodman LS, Gilman A, eds. Goodman and Gilman's the pharmacological basis of therapeutics. 6th ed. New York: Macmillan, 1980.

Kucers A, Bennett N McK. The use of antibiotics: a comprehensive review with clinical emphasis. 3rd ed. Philadelphia: JB Lippincott, 1979.

American Pharmaceutical Association. Handbook of nonprescription drugs. 7th ed. Washington, DC: American Pharmaceutical Association, 1982.

Pediatric Therapy

Biller JA, Yeager AM, eds. The Harriet Lane handbook. 9th ed. Chicago: Year Book Medical Publishers, 1981.

Pagliaro LA, Levin RH, eds. Problems in pediatric drug therapy. Hamilton, IL: Drug Intelligence Publications, 1979.

Shirkey HC, ed. Pediatric therapy. 6th ed. Saint Louis: CV Mosby, 1980.

Patient Instructions

Maudlin RK, Young LY. Drug consultation guide. Hamilton, IL: Drug Intelligence Publications, 1982.

United States Pharmacopeial Convention. United States Pharmacopeia dispensing information. Rockville, MD: The United States Pharmacopeial Convention, 1983.

American Society of Hospital Pharmacists. The medication teaching manual. 2nd ed. Washington, DC: American Society of Hospital Pharmacists, 1980.

Pharmacokinetic Parameters/Dosage Individualization

Anderson RJ, Schrier RW, eds. Clinical use of drugs in patients with kidney and liver disease. 2nd ed. Philadelphia: WB Saunders, 1981.

Benet LZ, Sheiner LB. Design and optimization of dosage regimens; pharmacokinetic data. In: Gilman AG, Goodman LS, Gilman A, eds. Goodman and Gilman's the pharmacological basis of therapeutics. 6th ed. New York: Macmillan, 1980.

Bennett WM, Muther RS, Parker RA et al. Drug therapy in renal failure: dosing guidelines for adults (2 parts). Ann Intern Med 1980;93:62-89, 286-325.

Evans WE, Schentag JJ, Jusko WJ, eds. Applied pharmacokinetics: principles of therapeutic drug monitoring. San Francisco: Applied Therapeutics, 1980.

Rowland M, Tozer TN. Clinical pharmacokinetics: concepts and applications. Philadelphia: Lea and Febiger, 1980.

Williams RL, Mamelok RD. Hepatic disease and drug pharmacokinetics. Clin Pharmacokinet 1980;5:528-47.

Winter ME, Katcher BS, Koda-Kimble MA, eds. Basic clinical pharmacokinetics. San Francisco: Applied Therapeutics, 1980.

Adverse Reactions/Drug Interactions

Ascione FJ, ed. Evaluation of drug interactions. 2nd ed. Washington, DC: American Pharmaceutical Association, 1976 and Supplement, 1978.

Davies DM, ed. Textbook of adverse drug reactions. 2nd ed. New York: Oxford University Press, 1981.

Dukes MNG, ed. Meyler's side effects of drugs. 9th ed. Amsterdam: Excerpta Medica, 1980 and Annuals.

Hansten PD. Drug interactions. 4th ed. Philadelphia: Lea and Febiger, 1979.

Swanson M, Cook R. Drugs, chemicals and blood dyscrasias. Hamilton, IL: Drug Intelligence Publications, 1977.

Zimmerman HJ. Hepatotoxicity: the adverse effects of drugs and other chemicals on the liver. New York: Appleton-Century-Crofts, 1978.

Compatibility and Stability

Trissel LA. Handbook on injectable drugs. 2nd ed. Washington, DC: American Society of Hospital Pharmacists, 1980.

4:00 ANTIHISTAMINE DRUGS

General References: 1–4

Class Instructions. This drug may cause drowsiness, dry mouth and, on occasion, dizziness. Until the degree of drowsiness is known, caution should be used when driving, operating machinery or performing other tasks requiring mental alertness. Alcohol should be consumed in small amounts until tolerance to taking both drugs together is determined. Use other drugs which cause drowsiness with caution.

Chlorpheniramine Maleate

Chlor-Trimeton®, Isoclor®, Various

Pharmacology. A competitive antagonist of histamine at the H_1 histamine receptor. Also has anticholinergic and transient sedative effects when used intermittently.

Administration and Adult Dose. PO for acute allergic reactions 12 mg in 2–3 divided doses. **PO for seasonal allergic rhinitis** (effectiveness is maximized if given continuously just prior to the pollen season) 4 mg hs (2 mg in children) initially, increasing gradually over 10 days as tolerated to 24 mg/day (12 mg/day in children) in 2–3 divided doses and maintain until end of season.[5] **IV as adjunctive treatment in anaphylaxis** 10–20 mg; **IM or IV for allergic reactions to blood or plasma** 10–20 mg, to maximum of 40 mg/day.

Pediatric Dose. PO 0.35 mg/kg/day. **PO for seasonal allergic rhinitis** 1–2 mg tid up to 12 mg/day titrated as above. SR not recommended.

Dosage Forms. SR Cap 8, 12 mg (see Notes); **Syrup** 2 mg/5 ml; **Chew Tab** 2 mg; **Tab** 4 mg; **Inj** 10 mg/ml (IM, SC, IV), 100 mg/ml (IM, SC only).

Patient Instructions. Effectively suppresses seasonal allergic rhinitis only when taken continuously. See also Class Instructions.

Pharmacokinetics and Biopharmaceutics. *Onset and Duration.* Onset 0.5–1 hr; duration of suppression of wheal and flare response (IgE mediated) to skin tests with allergenic extract 2 days.[6]
   Fate. Well absorbed from GI tract[7] (see Notes); rapidly and extensively metabolized to N-dealkylated and unidentified metabolites. Small amount excreted unchanged in urine.[8]
   $t_{1/2}$. (Adults) 30 hr; (children) 16 hr.[9]

Adverse Reactions. Drowsiness, dry mouth, dizziness and irritability occur frequently with intermittent therapy; however, most patients develop tolerance to these side effects during continuous therapy, particularly if dose is increased slowly.

Contraindications. Newborn and premature infants; manufacturer states contraindicated in asthma; however, this was not supported in a controlled study,[10] except during prolonged acute asthma symptoms (ie, status asthmaticus).[1] Avoid in patients with narrow angle glaucoma, symptomatic prostatic hypertrophy, bladder neck obstruction, intestinal stasis and pyloroduodenal obstruction.

Precautions. Use with caution in the elderly.

Parameters to Monitor. In seasonal allergic rhinitis, observe for sneezing, rhinorrhea, itchy nose and conjunctivitis.

Notes. Not effective for nasal stuffiness. Belongs to alkylamine class; however, chemical structure does not relate to efficacy or side effects. Inexpensive generic formulations available, but bioavailability has not been documented for many products. SR formulations offer no advantage over syrup or plain, uncoated tablets, because the drug is eliminated slowly;[1] Isoclor® is the only SR brand with documented bioavailability.

Cyproheptadine Hydrochloride   Periactin®, Various

Pharmacology. See Chlorpheniramine. Also has antiserotonin activity.[11]

Administration and Adult Dose. PO 4–20 mg/day, usually 4 mg tid-qid, to maximum of 0.5 mg/kg/day.

Pediatric Dose. PO 0.25 mg/kg/day, usually; (2–6 yr) 2 mg bid-tid, to maximum of 12 mg/day; (7–14 yr) 4 mg bid-tid, to maximum of 16 mg/day.

Dosage Forms. Syrup 2 mg/5 ml; Tab 4 mg.

Patient Instructions. See Class Instructions.

Pharmacokinetics and Biopharmaceutics. Fate. About 70% excreted in urine, primarily as a conjugate of glucuronic acid; the remainder is excreted in feces.[12]

Adverse Reactions. See Chlorpheniramine.

Contraindications. See Chlorpheniramine.

Precautions. See Chlorpheniramine.

Notes. May have potential as an inhibitor of ACTH release in patients with Cushing's disease due to its antiserotonin activity;[11] long-term use of cyproheptadine and human growth hormone enhances growth of children with hypopituitarism.[13] Effective for appetite stimulation[14] and cold urticaria. Ineffective as an antipruritic.

Diphenhydramine Hydrochloride   Benadryl®, Various

Pharmacology. See Chlorpheniramine.

Administration and Adult Dose. PO as an antihistamine 50 mg tid-qid (see $t_{1/2}$); PO for motion sickness 50 mg 30 min before exposure, ac and hs; Deep IM or IV as an antihistamine, for adjunctive treatment for anaphylaxis or for extrapyramidal reactions 50 mg, to maximum of 400 mg/day.

Dosage Individualization. Increase dosing interval by 1½–2 times in moderate to severe renal impairment.[15]

Pediatric Dose. PO (over 9 kg) 5 mg/kg/day, usually 12.5–25 mg tid-qid, to maximum of 300 mg/day; Deep IM or IV 5 mg/kg/day, in 4 divided doses, to maximum of 300 mg/day.

Dosage Forms. Cap 25, 50 mg; Elxr 12.5 mg/5 ml; Syrup 12.5, 13.3 mg/5 ml; Tab 25, 50 mg; Inj 10, 50 mg/ml.

Patient Instructions. See Class Instructions.

Pharmacokinetics and Biopharmaceutics. *Onset and Duration.*
Onset 1 hr; duration 4–6 hr.[16] Wheal and flare suppression lasts up to 1.9
days.[6]
 Plasma Levels. Frequency of sedation is increased over 50 ng/ml.[17]
 Fate. As a result of first-pass metabolism, oral bioavailability averages
43%; a single 50 mg oral dose in adults produces plasma concentrations
between 25–50 ng/ml in most cases.[17] Less than 4% excreted unchanged in
urine.[18]
 $t_{1/2}$. Estimated to be 3–4 hr;[17] however, wheal and flare reaction is suppressed for about 2 days.[6] Thus, duration of effect does not appear related
to plasma levels and qid dosing appears unnecessary.

Adverse Reactions. See Chlorpheniramine.

Contraindications. See Chlorpheniramine.

Precautions. See Chlorpheniramine.

Notes. Ethanolamine class; **dimenhydrinate** (Dramamine®), used for motion sickness, is the chlorotheophylline salt of diphenhydramine; by weight
100 mg dimenhydrinate is about equal to 50 mg diphenhydramine. Because
of low degree of efficacy for pruritus and relatively weak suppression of IgE-
mediated skin tests, this drug is not the antihistamine of choice except for
extrapyramidal reactions.

Hydroxyzine Hydrochloride   Atarax®
Hydroxyzine Pamoate   Vistaril®

Pharmacology. A competitive antagonist of histamine at the H_1 histamine receptor. Also has antiemetic effects. Claims of antianxiety properties
have not been substantiated by well-designed studies.

Administration and Adult Dose. PO for pruritus 25–75 mg tid-qid prn.
PO for seasonal allergic rhinitis (effectiveness is maximized if given continuously just prior to the pollen season) 25 mg (10 mg for children) initially
q hs until no sedation in morning, then increase dose q 2–3 days, to maximum of 150 mg/day (25–75 mg/day for children) in 2–3 divided doses and
maintain until end of season. Reduce dose by 1/3 or more if sedation persists. Dose may be increased, if tolerated, for symptoms during peak of
pollen season.[1,19] **IM for sedation pre- and post-general anesthesia** 50–100
mg, **IM for nausea and vomiting, and pre- and postoperative adjunctive
medication** 25–100 mg. **Not for SC or IV use.**

Pediatric Dose. **PO for pruritus** (under 6 yr) 50 mg/day in 2–3 divided
doses; (over 6 yr) 50–100 mg in divided doses; **PO for seasonal allergic
rhinitis** titrate as above. **IM for pre- and postoperative sedation** 0.6 mg/kg. **IM
for nausea and vomiting and pre- and postoperative adjunctive medication**
1.1 mg/kg.

Dosage Forms. **Cap** (as pamoate) 25, 50, 100 mg; **Susp** (as pamoate) 25
mg/5 ml; **Syrup** (as HCl) 10 mg/5 ml; **Tab** (as HCl) 10, 25, 50, 100 mg; **Inj** (as
HCl) 25, 50 mg/ml (IM only).

Patient Instructions. See Chlorpheniramine.

Pharmacokinetics and Biopharmaceutics. *Onset and Duration.* Onset 15–30 min after oral administration. Duration of suppression of wheal and flare response to allergenic extract skin tests is 4 days.[6,20]

$t_{1/2}$. 3 hr;[21] however, plasma half-life is not related to pharmacologic effect.

Adverse Reactions. Transient drowsiness frequently and dry mouth on occasion when taken intermittently. Most patients develop tolerance to these effects when the drug is taken continuously, particularly if the dose is slowly increased over 7–10 days.

Contraindications. Early pregnancy; SC or intra-arterial use of injectable solution.

Precautions. Potentiation of other CNS depressants may require a dosage reduction. Use with caution in the elderly.

Parameters to Monitor. See Chlorpheniramine.

Notes. Piperazine class. Suppresses wheal and flare response to the greatest degree and for the longest duration of all antihistamines.[6,20]

References, 4:00 Antihistamine Drugs

1. Hendeles L, Weinberger M, Wong L. Medical management of noninfectious rhinitis. Am J Hosp Pharm 1980;37:1496-504.

2. Anon. Choice of antihistamines. Med Lett Drugs Ther 1971;13:102-4.

3. Anon. Antihistamines. Fed Regist 1976;41:38379-96.

4. Cirillo VJ, Tempero KF. Pharmacology and therapeutic use of antihistamines. Am J Hosp Pharm 1976;33:1200-7.

5. Wong L, Hendeles L, Weinberger M. Pharmacologic prophylaxis of allergic rhinitis: relative efficacy of hydroxyzine and chlorpheniramine. J Allergy Clin Immunol 1981;67:223-8.

6. Cook TJ, MacQueen DM, Wittig HJ et al. Degree and duration of skin test suppression and side effects with antihistamines. J Allergy Clin Immunol 1973;51:71-7.

7. Hanna S, Tang A. GLC determination of chlorpheniramine in human plasma. J Pharm Sci 1974;63:1954-7.

8. Peets EA, Jackson M, Symchowicz S. Metabolism of chlorpheniramine maleate in man. J Pharmacol Exp Ther 1972;180:464-74.

9. Chiou WL, Athanikar NK, Huang S-M. Long half-life of chlorpheniramine. N Engl J Med 1979;300:501. Letter.

10. Karlin JM. The use of antihistamines in asthma. Ann Allergy 1972;30:342-7.

11. Krieger DT, Amorosa L, Linick F. Cyproheptadine-induced remission of Cushing's disease. N Engl J Med 1975;293:893-6.

12. Hintze KL, Wold JS, Fischer LJ. Disposition of cyproheptadine in rats, mice, and humans and identification of a stable epoxide metabolite. Drug Metab Dispos 1975;3:1-9.

13. Kenien AG, Zeidner DL, Pang SJ et al. The effect of cyproheptadine and human growth hormone on adrenocortical function in children with hypopituitarism. J Pediatr 1978;92:491-4.

14. Anon. Cyproheptadine as an appetite stimulant. Drug Ther Bull 1970;8:71-2.

15. Bennett WM, Muther RS, Parker RA et al. Drug therapy in renal failure: dosing guidelines for adults. Ann Intern Med 1980;93:286-325.

16. Gilman AG, Goodman LS, Gilman A, eds. Goodman and Gilman's the pharmacological basis of therapeutics, 6th ed. New York: Macmillan, 1980.

17. Carruthers SG, Shoeman DW, Hignite CE et al. Correlation between plasma diphenhydramine level and sedative and antihistamine effects. Clin Pharmacol Ther 1978;23:375-82.

18. Albert KS, Hallmark MR, Sakman E et al. Pharmacokinetics of diphenhydramine in man. J Pharmacokinet Biopharm 1975;3:159-70.

19. Schaaf L, Hendeles L, Weinberger M. Suppression of seasonal allergic rhinitis symptoms with daily hydroxyzine. J Allergy Clin Immunol 1979;63:129-33.

20. Cook TJ, Leifer KN, Cohan R et al. Suppression of histamine-induced pruritus by three antihistaminic drugs. J Allergy Clin Immunol 1975;55:180-5.

21. Fouda HG, Hobbs DC, Stambaugh JE. Sensitive assay for determination of hydroxyzine in plasma and its human pharmacokinetics. J Pharm Sci 1979;68:1456-8.

8:00 ANTI-INFECTIVE AGENTS

For **Antimicrobial Drugs of Choice,** see the Table on the following pages.

8:00 ANTI-INFECTIVE AGENTS

Antimicrobial Drugs of Choice*†

INFECTING ORGANISM	DRUG OF FIRST CHOICE	ALTERNATIVE DRUGS
GRAM-POSITIVE COCCI		
Staphylococcus aureus		
Nonpenicillinase-producing	Penicillin G or V[1]	A cephalosporin;[2,3] clindamycin; vancomycin
Penicillinase-producing	A penicillinase-resistant penicillin[4]	A cephalosporin;[2,3] vancomycin; clindamycin
Streptococcus pyogenes (Group A) and Groups C and G	Penicillin G or V[1]	An erythromycin;[5] a cephalosporin;[2,3] clindamycin
Streptococcus, Group B	Penicillin G[1] or ampicillin	Vancomycin; an erythromycin; a cephalosporin[2,3]
Streptococcus, viridans group[6]	Penicillin G[1] with or without streptomycin	A cephalosporin;[2,3] vancomycin
Streptococcus bovis[6]	Penicillin G[1]	A cephalosporin;[2,3] vancomycin
Streptococcus, Enterococcus group		
Endocarditis[6] or other severe infection	Ampicillin or penicillin G with gentamicin or streptomycin	Vancomycin with gentamicin or streptomycin
Uncomplicated urinary tract infection[7]	Ampicillin or amoxicillin	Nitrofurantoin

Continued

Antimicrobial Drugs of Choice*†

INFECTING ORGANISM	DRUG OF FIRST CHOICE	ALTERNATIVE DRUGS
Streptococcus, anaerobic	Penicillin G[1]	Clindamycin; a tetracycline;[8] an erythromycin;[9] chloramphenicol;[10] a cephalosporin[2,3]
*Streptococcus pneumoniae (pneumococcus)	Penicillin G or V[1,11]	An erythromycin;[5,11] a cephalosporin;[2,3] chloramphenicol;[10,11] vancomycin
GRAM-NEGATIVE COCCI		
*Neisseria gonorrhoeae[12]	A tetracycline[8] or penicillin G or amoxicillin	Ampicillin; spectinomycin; cefoxitin;[2] cefotaxime;[2] moxalactam;[2,9] an erythromycin
Neisseria meningitidis[13]	Penicillin G	Chloramphenicol;[10] a sulfonamide[14]
GRAM-POSITIVE BACILLI		
Bacillus anthracis (anthrax)	Penicillin G	An erythromycin;[9] a tetracycline[8]
Clostridium perfringens (welchii)[15]	Penicillin G	Chloramphenicol;[10] clindamycin; metronidazole; a tetracycline[8]
Clostridium tetani[16]	Penicillin G	A tetracycline[8]
Clostridium difficile	Vancomycin	Metronidazole
Corynebacterium diphtheriae[17]	An erythromycin	Penicillin G
Listeria monocytogenes	Ampicillin[9] or penicillin G with or without gentamicin[9]	A tetracycline[8]

Continued

Antimicrobial Drugs of Choice*†

INFECTING ORGANISM	DRUG OF FIRST CHOICE	ALTERNATIVE DRUGS
ENTERIC GRAM-NEGATIVE BACILLI		
Bacteroides		
Oropharyngeal strains	Penicillin G	Clindamycin; an erythromycin;[9] a tetracycline;[8] metronidazole
Gastrointestinal strains	Clindamycin[18]	Metronidazole;[18] cefoxitin;[2] chloramphenicol;[10,18] mezlocillin or piperacillin; moxalactam;[2] cefotaxime;[2,9] minocycline[8]
Enterobacter	Gentamicin[19] or tobramycin[19]	Cefotaxime[2] or moxalactam;[2] carbenicillin, ticarcillin, mezlocillin, or piperacillin; amikacin; cefamandole;[2] chloramphenicol;[10] a tetracycline;[8] trimethoprim-sulfamethoxazole; trimethoprim
Escherichia coli[20]	Gentamicin[21] or tobramycin[21]	Ampicillin; carbenicillin, ticarcillin, mezlocillin, or piperacillin; a cephalosporin;[2,3] amikacin; a tetracycline;[8] trimethoprim-sulfamethoxazole; chloramphenicol[10]
Klebsiella pneumoniae[20]	Gentamicin[22] or tobramycin[22]	A cephalosporin;[2,3] amikacin; a tetracycline;[8] trimethoprim-sulfamethoxazole; chloramphenicol;[10] mezlocillin or piperacillin
Proteus mirabilis[20]	Ampicillin[23]	A cephalosporin;[2,3] gentamicin or tobramycin; carbenicillin, ticarcillin, mezlocillin, or

Continued

Antimicrobial Drugs of Choice*[†]

INFECTING ORGANISM	DRUG OF FIRST CHOICE	ALTERNATIVE DRUGS
		piperacillin; amikacin; trimethoprim-sulfamethoxazole; chloramphenicol[10]
*Proteus, indole-positive (including Providencia rettgeri, Morganella morganii, and Proteus vulgaris)	Gentamicin[19] or tobramycin[19]	Cefotaxime[2] or moxalactam;[2] carbenicillin, ticarcillin, mezlocillin, or piperacillin; amikacin; a tetracycline;[8,9] trimethoprim-sulfamethoxazole; chloramphenicol;[10] cefoxitin[2]
*Providencia stuartii	Amikacin	Cefotaxime[2] or moxalactam;[2] gentamicin or tobramycin; carbenicillin, ticarcillin, mezlocillin, or piperacillin; trimethoprim-sulfamethoxazole; chloramphenicol;[10] cefoxitin[2] or cefamandole[2]
*Salmonella typhi[24]	Chloramphenicol[10]	Ampicillin; amoxicillin;[9] trimethoprim-sulfamethoxazole[9]
*other Salmonella[25]	Ampicillin or amoxicillin[9]	Chloramphenicol;[10] trimethoprim-sulfamethoxazole[9]
*Serratia	Gentamicin[19] or amikacin[19]	Cefotaxime[2,9] or moxalactam;[2] trimethoprim-sulfamethoxazole;[9] carbenicillin,[9] ticarcillin, mezlocillin, or piperacillin;[9] cefoxitin[2,9]
*Shigella	Trimethoprim-sulfamethoxazole	Chloramphenicol;[10] a tetracycline;[8] ampicillin

Continued

Continued

Antimicrobial Drugs of Choice*†

INFECTING ORGANISM	DRUG OF FIRST CHOICE	ALTERNATIVE DRUGS
OTHER GRAM-NEGATIVE BACILLI		
*Acinetobacter (Mima, Herellea)	Gentamicin[9] or tobramycin[9]	Kanamycin; amikacin; minocycline;[8] doxycycline;[8] carbenicillin, ticarcillin, mezlocillin,[9] or piperacillin; trimethoprim-sulfamethoxazole[9]
Bordetella pertussis (whooping cough)	An erythromycin	Trimethoprim-sulfamethoxazole[9]
*Brucella (brucellosis)	A tetracycline[8] with or without streptomycin	Chloramphenicol[10] with or without streptomycin; trimethoprim-sulfamethoxazole[9]
Calymmatobacterium granulomatis (granuloma inguinale)	A tetracycline[8]	Streptomycin
Campylobacter fetus, jejuni	An erythromycin[9]	A tetracycline;[8] gentamicin;[9] chloramphenicol[10]
*Francisella tularensis (tularemia)	Streptomycin	A tetracycline;[8] chloramphenicol[10]
Fusobacterium	Penicillin G	Metronidazole; clindamycin; chloramphenicol[10]
Gardnerella (Haemophilus) vaginalis	Metronidazole[9]	Ampicillin

Antimicrobial Drugs of Choice*†

INFECTING ORGANISM	DRUG OF FIRST CHOICE	ALTERNATIVE DRUGS
*Haemophilus ducreyi (chancroid)	Trimethoprim-sulfamethoxazole[9]	A tetracycline;[8] streptomycin; an erythromycin;[9] cephalothin[9]
*Haemophilus influenzae Meningitis, epiglottitis, arthritis, and other serious infections	Chloramphenicol plus ampicillin initially[2b]	Moxalactam;[2] trimethoprim-sulfamethoxazole[9]
Other infections	Ampicillin or amoxicillin	Trimethoprim-sulfamethoxazole; a sulfonamide; cefaclor;[2] cefamandole;[2] cefotaxime;[2] moxalactam;[2] a tetracycline[8]
Legionella micdadei (L. pittsburgensis)	An erythromycin[9] with or without rifampin[9,27]	
Legionella pneumophila	An erythromycin[9] with or without rifampin[9,27]	
Leptotrichia buccalis (Vincent's infection)	Penicillin G	A tetracycline;[8] an erythromycin[9]
Pasteurella multocida	Penicillin G	A tetracycline[8]
*Pseudomonas aeruginosa Urinary tract infection	Carbenicillin or ticarcillin	Mezlocillin or piperacillin; tobramycin; gentamicin; amikacin; a polymyxin
*Other infections[28]	Tobramycin or gentamicin with carbenicillin, ticarcillin, mezlocillin, or piperacillin	Amikacin with carbenicillin, ticarcillin, mezlocillin, or piperacillin

Continued

Antimicrobial Drugs of Choice*†

INFECTING ORGANISM	DRUG OF FIRST CHOICE	ALTERNATIVE DRUGS
Pseudomonas (Actinobacillus) *mallei* (glanders)	Streptomycin with a tetracycline[8,9]	Streptomycin with chloramphenicol[10]
Pseudomonas pseudomallei (melioidosis)	Trimethoprim-sulfamethoxazole[9]	A tetracycline[8,9] with or without chloramphenicol;[10,29] a sulfonamide[9]
Pseudomonas cepacia	Trimethoprim-sulfamethoxazole[9]	Chloramphenicol[10]
Spirillum minor (rat bite fever)	Penicillin G	A tetracycline;[8,9] streptomycin
Streptobacillus moniliformis (rat bite fever; Haverhill fever)	Penicillin G	A tetracycline;[8,9] streptomycin
Vibrio cholerae (cholera)[30]	A tetracycline[8]	Trimethoprim-sulfamethoxazole[9]
Yersinia pestis (plague)	Streptomycin	A tetracycline;[8,9] chloramphenicol[10]
ACID FAST BACILLI *Mycobacterium tuberculosis*[31]	Isoniazid with rifampin[32]	Ethambutol; streptomycin; pyrazinamide; para-aminosalicylic acid (PAS); cycloserine;[10] ethionamide;[10] kanamycin;[9,10] capreomycin[10]
Mycobacterium kansasii[31]	Isoniazid with rifampin with or without ethambutol	Streptomycin;[10] ethionamide;[10] cycloserine[10]
Mycobacterium avium-intracellulare-scrofulaceum complex[31]	Isoniazid, rifampin, ethambutol, and streptomycin[10]	Capreomycin;[10] ethionamide;[10] cycloserine;[10] clofazimine[33]

Continued

Antimicrobial Drugs of Choice*†

INFECTING ORGANISM	DRUG OF FIRST CHOICE	ALTERNATIVE DRUGS
Mycobacterium fortuitum[31]	Amikacin[9,10] and doxycycline[8,9]	Rifampin; an erythromycin
Mycobacterium marinum (balnei)[34]	Minocycline[8,9]	Trimethoprim-sulfamethoxazole; rifampin; cycloserine[10]
Mycobacterium leprae (leprosy)	Dapsone[10] with rifampin with or without clofazimine[33]	Acedapsone;[10,33] ethionamide;[10] prothionamide[33]
ACTINOMYCETES *Actinomyces israelii* (actinomycosis)	Penicillin G	A tetracycline[8]
Nocardia	Trisulfapyrimidines	Trimethoprim-sulfamethoxazole;[9] trisulfapyrimidines with minocycline[9] or ampicillin[9] or erythromycin;[9,10] cycloserine[9,10]
CHLAMYDIAE *Chlamydia psittaci* (psittacosis; ornithosis)	A tetracycline[8]	Chloramphenicol[10]
Chlamydia trachomatis Trachoma	A tetracycline[8] (topical plus oral)	A sulfonamide (topical plus oral)
Inclusion conjunctivitis	An erythromycin	A tetracycline;[8] a sulfonamide
Pneumonia	An erythromycin	A sulfonamide
Urethritis	A tetracycline[8]	An erythromycin
Lymphogranuloma venereum	A tetracycline[8]	An erythromycin; a sulfonamide

Continued

Antimicrobial Drugs of Choice*†

INFECTING ORGANISM	DRUG OF FIRST CHOICE	ALTERNATIVE DRUGS
FUNGI		
Aspergillus	Amphotericin B[10]	No dependable alternative
Blastomyces dermatitidis	Amphotericin B[10]	Ketoconazole[9]
Candida species[35]	Amphotericin B[10] with or without flucytosine[10,36]	Ketoconazole; nystatin (oral or topical); miconazole (topical); clotrimazole (topical)
Chromomycosis	Flucytosine[9]	Ketoconazole
Coccidioides immitis	Amphotericin B[10]	Ketoconazole; miconazole
Cryptococcus neoformans	Amphotericin B[10,37] with or without flucytosine[10,36]	Ketoconazole;[9] miconazole
Dermatophytes (tinea)	Clotrimazole (topical) or miconazole (topical)	Tolnaftate (topical); haloprogin (topical); griseofulvin;[10] ketoconazole[9]
Histoplasma capsulatum	Amphotericin B[10]	Ketoconazole
Mucor	Amphotericin B[10]	No dependable alternative
Paracoccidioides brasiliensis	Amphotericin B[10]	Ketoconazole; a sulfonamide; miconazole
Sporothrix schenckii	An iodide[38]	Amphotericin B[10]

Continued

Antimicrobial Drugs of Choice*†

INFECTING ORGANISM	DRUG OF FIRST CHOICE	ALTERNATIVE DRUGS
MYCOPLASMA		
Mycoplasma pneumoniae	An erythromycin or a tetracycline[8]	
Ureaplasma urealyticum	An erythromycin	A tetracycline[8]
PNEUMOCYSTIS CARINII	Trimethoprim-sulfamethoxazole	Pentamidine[10,33]
RICKETTSIA Rocky Mountain spotted fever, endemic typhus (murine), tick bite fever, trench fever, typhus, scrub typhus, Q fever	A tetracycline[8]	Chloramphenicol[10]
SPIROCHETES		
Borrelia recurrentis (relapsing fever)	A tetracycline[8]	Penicillin G
Leptospira	Penicillin G	A tetracycline[8,9]
Treponema pallidum (syphilis)	Penicillin G[1]	A tetracycline;[8] an erythromycin
Treponema pertenue (yaws)	Penicillin G	A tetracycline[8]
VIRUSES *Herpes simplex* Keratitis	Trifluridine (topical)	Vidarabine (topical); idoxuridine (topical)

Continued

Antimicrobial Drugs of Choice*†

INFECTING ORGANISM	DRUG OF FIRST CHOICE	ALTERNATIVE DRUGS
Encephalitis	Vidarabine	Acyclovir[33]
Influenza A[39]	Amantadine	No alternative

*Because resistance may be a problem, susceptibility tests should be performed.

†From Med Lett Drugs Ther 1982;24;21-8, reproduced with permission.

1. Penicillin V is preferred for oral treatment of infections caused by nonpenicillinase-producing staphylococci and other gram-positive cocci, but is ineffective for gonorrhea. For initial therapy of severe infections, crystalline penicillin G, administered parenterally, is first choice. For somewhat longer action in less severe infections due to Group A streptococci, pneumococci, gonococci, or *Treponema pallidum*, procaine penicillin G, an intramuscular formulation, is administered once or twice daily. Benzathine penicillin G, a slowly absorbed intramuscular preparation, is usually given in a single monthly injection for prophylaxis of rheumatic fever, once for treatment of Group A streptococcal pharyngitis, and once or more for treatment of syphilis outside of the central nervous system.

2. The cephalosporins have been used as alternatives to penicillins in patients allergic to penicillins, but such patients may also have allergic reactions to cephalosporins.

3. For parenteral treatment of staphylococcal infections, cephalothin, cephapirin, or cefazolin can be used; for staphylococcal endocarditis, some Medical Letter consultants prefer cephalothin or cephapirin. For oral therapy, cephalexin or cephradine is preferred. Cefamandole, cefoxitin, cefotaxime, and moxalactam have greater activity against enteric gram-negative bacilli than other cephalosporins. Cefoxitin, cefotaxime, and moxalactam are active against many strains of *Bacteroides fragilis*. The activity of all currently available (February 1982) cephalosporins against *Pseudomonas aeruginosa* is poor or inconsistent.

4. For oral use against penicillinase-producing staphylococci, cloxacillin or dicloxacillin is preferred; for severe infections, a parenteral formulation of methicillin, nafcillin, or oxacillin should be used. Neither ampicillin, amoxicillin, bacampicillin, cyclacillin, carbenicillin, ticarcillin, mezlocillin, nor piperacillin is effective against penicillinase-producing staphylococci. Occasional strains of coagulase-positive staphylococci may be resistant to penicillinase-resistant penicillins, and these strains are usually also resistant to cephalosporins; infections due to these resistant strains are treated with vancomycin, with or without either rifampin or gentamicin.

5. Occasional strains of Group A streptococci and pneumococci may be resistant to erythromycins.

6. In endocarditis, disk sensitivity testing may not provide adequate information; dilution tests for susceptibility should be used to assess bactericidal as well as inhibitory end points. Peak bactericidal activity of the serum against the patient's own organism should be present at a serum dilution of at least 1:8.

7. Routine antimicrobial susceptibility tests may be misleading. Ampicillin is often effective in urinary tract infections, while streptomycin, kanamycin, or gentamicin alone is not.

8. Tetracycline hydrochloride is preferred for most indications. Doxycycline is recommended for uremic patients with infections outside the urinary tract for which a tetracycline is indicated. Tetracyclines are generally not recommended for pregnant women, infants, or children eight years old or younger. Continued

9. Not approved for this indication by the U.S. Food and Drug Administration.

10. Because of the frequency of serious adverse effects, this drug should be used only for severe infections when less hazardous drugs are ineffective.

11. In patients allergic to penicillin, an erythromycin is preferred for respiratory infections, and chloramphenicol is recommended for meningitis. Rare strains of *Streptococcus pneumoniae* may be resistant to penicillin; these strains are susceptible to vancomycin.

12. Since many strains of gonococci are relatively resistant to penicillin G, ampicillin, or amoxicillin, large doses together with probenecid are prescribed for single-dose treatment of uncomplicated infection; pelvic inflammatory disease and disseminated gonococcal infection are treated with multiple doses. Some strains of gonococci produce penicillinase and are totally resistant to penicillin G, ampicillin, or amoxicillin; these strains may also be resistant to tetracycline, and should be treated with spectinomycin. Rare strains resistant to spectinomycin should be treated with cefoxitin, cefotaxime, or moxalactam. Penicillin V, benzathine penicillin G, and penicillinase-resistant penicillins should not be used for gonococcal infection.

13. Rifampin is recommended for prophylaxis in close contacts of patients infected by sulfonamide-resistant organisms. Minocycline may also be effective for such prophylaxis but frequently causes vomiting and vertigo. An oral sulfonamide is recommended for prophylaxis in close contacts of patients known to be infected by sulfonamide-sensitive organisms.

14. Sulfonamide-resistant strains are frequent in the USA and sulfonamides should be used only when susceptibility is established by susceptibility tests.

15. Debridement is primary. Large doses of penicillin G are required. Hyperbaric oxygen therapy may be a useful adjunct to surgical debridement in management of the spreading, necrotic type.

16. For prophylaxis, tetanus toxoid and, in some patients, tetanus immune globulin (human) are required.

17. Antitoxin is primary; antimicrobials are used only to halt further toxin production and to prevent the carrier state.

18. When infection is in the central nervous system, either intravenous metronidazole or chloramphenicol is recommended.

19. In severely ill patients Medical Letter consultants would add carbenicillin, ticarcillin, mezlocillin, or piperacillin (but see footnote 28), or cefotaxime or moxalactam.

20. For an acute, uncomplicated urinary tract infection, before the infecting organism is known, the drug of first choice is one of the oral soluble sulfonamides, such as sulfisoxazole, or ampicillin or amoxicillin. Trimethoprim or trimethoprim-sulfamethoxazole may also be useful for treatment of urinary tract infections caused by susceptible organisms.

21. In severely ill patients Medical Letter consultants would add ampicillin, carbenicillin, ticarcillin, mezlocillin, piperacillin, or a cephalosporin, but see footnote 28.

22. In severely ill patients Medical Letter consultants would add a cephalosporin.

23. Large doses (6 grams or more daily) are usually necessary for systemic infections. In severely ill patients some Medical Letter consultants would add gentamicin or tobramycin.

24. Ampicillin or amoxicillin may be effective in milder cases. Ampicillin is the drug of choice for *S. typhi* carriers.

25. Most cases of *Salmonella* gastroenteritis subside spontaneously without antimicrobial therapy.

26. Some strains of *H. influenzae* are resistant to ampicillin and rare strains are resistant to chloramphenicol. Chloramphenicol (100 mg/kg/day IV) plus ampicillin should be used for initial treatment of meningitis, epiglottitis, or arthritis in children more than two months old until the organism is identified and its antimicrobial susceptibility is determined. Ampicillin is preferred by most Medical Letter consultants for treatment of organisms known to be susceptible.

27. Rifampin should be added only for patients who do not respond to erythromycin alone.

28. Neither gentamicin, tobramycin, nor amikacin should be mixed in the same bottle with carbenicillin, ticarcillin, mezlocillin, or piperacillin for intravenous administration.

Continued

29. Seriously ill patients should be treated with both tetracycline and chloramphenicol.

30. Antibiotic therapy is an adjunct to and not a substitute for prompt fluid and electrolyte replacement.

31. Susceptibility tests should be performed by appropriate reference laboratories but antituberculosis drugs may be effective *in vivo* even when *in vitro* tests show resistance. Some isolates may require vigorous chemotherapy using multiple drugs.

32. Rifampin should be used concurrently with other drugs to prevent emergence of resistance. It is always included in treatment regimens for isoniazid-resistant organisms and is generally used together with isoniazid in the treatment of cavitary and far advanced pulmonary tuberculosis as well as for extrapulmonary tuberculosis.

33. An investigational drug in the USA.

34. Most infections are self-limited without drug treatment.

35. Amphotericin B administered intravenously is first choice for systemic candidal infections, although some Medical Letter consultants recommend concurrent use of flucytosine and amphotericin B. Ketoconazole administered orally is the drug of choice for chronic mucocutaneous candidiasis and may prove to be useful in systemic infections. For gastrointestinal infections, oral nystatin may be sufficient. Topical miconazole, clotrimazole, or nystatin can be used for skin or vaginal infections.

36. Some strains may be resistant to flucytosine, or resistance may emerge during treatment.

37. In some patients with meningitis who do not respond to intravenous amphotericin B, intraventricular or intrathecal administration of amphotericin B may be helpful.

38. Lymphocutaneous form only.

39. Uncomplicated influenza usually needs no treatment.

Immunobiologic Agents and Antiparasitic Drugs Available from CDC*

THE CENTERS FOR DISEASE CONTROL (CDC) DISTRIBUTE 4 special immunobiologic agents and 13 drugs for parasitic diseases through the Immunobiologics Services, Biologic Products Division, Bureau of Laboratories, and through the Parasitic Disease Drug Service and the Quarantine Division, Bureau of Epidemiology (Tables 1 and 2) in Atlanta, GA. CDC will dispense an immunobiologic agent or drug to a requesting physician for administration to a patient whose situation or condition calls for its use. Appropriate information regarding indications/contraindications, dosages, routes and frequency of administration, expected adverse reactions, toxicity and other general data are included in the package inserts with all licensed products.

In addition to the supplies of immunobiologics and drugs maintained at CDC in Atlanta, emergency supplies of 5 products are available at CDC quarantine stations located at airports in 10 major U.S. cities.† These 5 products are botulinal equine antitoxin (ABE), diphtheria equine antitoxin, vaccinia immune globulin (VIG), pentamidine isethionate, and varicella-zoster immune globulin (VZIG). These products can be requested by calling CDC or, in the case of VZIG, one of the regional distribution centers listed in Table 3.

Nonemergency requests for immunobiologics such as anthrax vaccine, botulinal toxoid, eastern equine encephalitis vaccine, tularemia vaccine, and Venezuelan equine encephalitis vaccine may be made by writing or calling Immunobiologics Services, Biological Products Division, Monday through Friday 8 AM to 4:30 PM (eastern time) at (404) 329-3356; and for drugs for parasitic diseases by calling Parasitic Disease Drug Service, Parasitic Diseases Division, Monday through Friday 8 AM to 4:30 PM (eastern time) at (404) 329-3670 or by writing to this division at 1600 Clifton Rd., Bldg. 6, Room 161, Atlanta, GA 30333.

*From Morbid Mortal Wkly Rep 1980;29:129-30 and 1982;31:275-6.
†Although CDC should be contacted first, the names of these cities are Boston, MA; New York City, NY; Houston, TX; Seattle, WA; Washington, D.C.; Los Angeles, CA; San Francisco, CA; Miami, FL; Chicago, IL; and New Orleans, LA.

Table 1. Drugs for Parasitic Diseases Available from CDC

DRUGS	INDICATIONS
Pentamidine Isethionate (Lomidine®)	Pneumocystosis, African trypanosomiasis
Niridazole (Ambilhar®)	Dracunculiasis, schistosomiasis
Sodium Antimony Gluconate (Pentostam®)	Leishmaniasis
Bayer 205 (Suramin)	African trypanosomiasis, onchocerciasis
Melarsoprol (Mel B®)	African trypanosomiasis
Bayer 2502 (Lampit®)	American trypanosomiasis
Diloxanide Furoate (Furamide ®)	Amebiasis
Dehydroemetine	Amebiasis
Bithionol	Paragonimiasis, *Fasciola hepatica*
Sodium Antimony Dimercaptosuccinate (Astiban®)	Schistosomiasis
Metrifonate (Bilarcil®)	Schistosomiasis
Quinine Dihydrochloride (parenteral)	Pernicious malaria
Chloroquine Hydrochloride (parenteral)	Pernicious malaria

Table 2. Products Available at CDC Quarantine Stations and Telephone Numbers to Call to Order, January 1980

PRODUCT	TELEPHONE NUMBER	
	Monday-Friday 8 AM to 4:30 PM	After working hours holidays and weekends
Botulinal Equine Antitoxin (ABE)	(404) 329-3753	(404) 329-3644
Diphtheria Equine Antitoxin	(404) 329-3091	(404) 329-3644
Vaccinia Immune Globulin (VIG)	(404) 329-2562	(404) 329-3644
Pentamidine Isethionate and Other Parasitic Drugs	(404) 329-3670	(404) 329-2888

Table 3. VZIG Regional Distribution Centers

Massachusetts: Mass. Public Health Biologic Laboratories, 375 South Street, Jamaica Plain, MA 02130, (617) 522-3700

Maine: American Red Cross Blood Services, Northeast Region, 812 Huntington Avenue, Boston, MA 02115, (617) 731-2130 ext. 146

Connecticut: American Red Cross Blood Services, Connecticut Region, 209 Farmington Avenue, Farmington, CT 06032, (203) 677-4531, (203) 677-4538 (night)

Vermont, New Hampshire: American Red Cross Blood Services, Vermont-New Hampshire Region, 32 North Prospect Street, Burlington, VT 05402, (802) 658-6400

Rhode Island: Rhode Island Blood Center, 551 North Main Street, Providence, RI 02917, (401) 863-8366

New Jersey, New York: The Greater New York Blood Program, 150 Amsterdam Avenue, New York, NY 10023, (212) 570-3067, (212) 570-3068 (night)

Delaware, Pennsylvania: American Red Cross, Penn-Jersey Region, 23rd & Chestnut Streets, Philadelphia, PA 19103, (215) 299-4114

Maryland, Virginia, West Virginia, Washington, DC: American Red Cross Blood Services, Washington Region, 2025 E Street N.W., Washington, DC 20006, (202) 857-2021

Alabama, Georgia, Mississippi, North Carolina, South Carolina, Puerto Rico: American Red Cross Blood Services, Atlanta Region, 1925 Monroe Drive N.E., Atlanta, GA 30324, (404) 881-9800 ext. 244, (404) 881-6752 (night)

Florida: South Florida Blood Service, P.O. Box 420100, Miami, FL 33142, (305) 326-8888

Indiana, Michigan, Ohio: American Red Cross Blood Services, Southeastern Michigan Region, 100 Mack Avenue, P.O. Box 351, Detroit, MI 48232, (313) 949-2715

Iowa, Minnesota, North Dakota, South Dakota, Wisconsin, Northern Illinois (Chicago): The Blood Center of S.E. Wisconsin, 1701 Wisconsin Avenue, Milwaukee, WS 53233, (414) 933-5003

Arkansas, Kansas, Kentucky, Missouri, Southern Illinois, Tennessee, Nebraska: American Red Cross, Missouri/Illinois Regional Blood Services, 4050 Lindell Boulevard, St. Louis, MO 63108, (314) 658-2000

Louisiana, Oklahoma, Texas: Gulf Coast Region Blood Center, 1400 La Concha, Houston, TX 77054, (713) 791-6250

Arizona, Colorado, New Mexico: United Blood Services, P.O. Box 25445, Albuquerque, NM 87125, (505) 247-9831

Hawaii, Southern California: American Red Cross Blood Services, L.A. - Orange Counties Region, 1130 South Vermont Avenue, Los Angeles, CA 90006, (213) 739-5620

Nevada, Utah, Wyoming, Northern California: American Red Cross Blood Services, Central California Region, 333 McKendrie Street, San Jose, CA 95110, (408) 292-6242, (408) 292-1626 (night)

Alaska, Idaho, Montana, Oregon, Washington: Puget Sound Blood Center, Terry at Madison, Seattle, WA 98104, (206) 292-6525

Canada: Canadian Red Cross Blood Transfusion Service, National Office, 95 Wellesley Street East, Toronto, Ontario (416) 923-6692

All other countries: American Red Cross Blood Services, Northeast Region, 60 Kendrick Street, Needham, MA 02194, (617) 449-0773

8:08 ANTHELMINTICS

General References: 1-4, 344

Class Instructions. Purgation, enemas or special dietary restrictions are unnecessary with this drug, which may be taken with food or beverages. To avoid reinfestation with pinworms, the perianal area should be washed thoroughly each morning. Nightclothes, undergarments and bedclothes should be changed and washed daily. Wash hands and under fingernails thoroughly after bowel movements and before eating. Treat all family members simultaneously and clean bedroom and bathroom floors thoroughly at the end of the course of treatment. In order to demonstrate a cure, no eggs must be found in the anal area at least 5 weeks after the end of treatment.

Mebendazole

Vermox®

Pharmacology. Inhibits glucose uptake in the parasite with no effect on blood sugar concentrations in the host.

Administration and Adult Dose. PO for pinworms 100 mg in single dose, repeat in 2 weeks. PO for roundworms, whipworms and hookworms 100 mg bid for 3 days; if infestation persists 3 weeks later, repeat treatment.

Pediatric Dose. PO (over 2 yr) same as adult dose.

Dosage Forms. Chew Tab 100 mg

Patient Instructions. Chew tablets before swallowing. See also Class Instructions.

Pharmacokinetics and Biopharmaceutics. Fate. Almost all eliminated unchanged in the feces, but up to 10% may be recovered in the urine 24 to 48 hr after a dose, primarily as the decarboxylated metabolite.[5]

Adverse Reactions. Occasional abdominal pain and diarrhea in cases of massive infestation and expulsion of worms.

Precautions. Pregnancy.

Parameters to Monitor. When treating whipworm, a stool sample for egg count should be taken 3 weeks after treatment to detect frequent (about 30%) persistent infestation requiring retreatment.[6,7]

Notes. This is the agent of choice for whipworm, producing about 70% cure-rate with single treatment; 90–100% cure-rate with roundworms, hookworms and pinworms.[8,9] Particularly useful in mixed infestations.[3] Nonstaining.

Piperazine Citrate

Antepar® Citrate, Various

Pharmacology. Paralyzes the parasite by blocking response of the neuromuscular junction to acetylcholine, allowing the worm to be expelled by peristalsis.

Administration and Adult Dose. PO for pinworms 65 mg/kg/day to maximum of 2.5 g/day in single daily dose for 7–8 days; may repeat in 7 days. PO for roundworms 75 mg/kg/day to maximum of 3.5 g/day for 2 days. Doses are expressed as hexahydrate equivalent.

Pediatric Dose. PO for pinworms 1 g/M^2/day, in a single dose for 7 days. **PO for roundworms** 2 g/M^2/day in a single dose for 2 days.

Dosage Forms. **Syrup** 100 mg/ml; **Tab** 500 mg; **Wafer** 500 mg (strengths expressed as hexahydrate equivalent).

Patient Instructions. See Class Instructions.

Pharmacokinetics and Biopharmaceutics. *Fate.* 15-75% absorbed and excreted in the urine as changed and unchanged drug.[10]

Adverse Reactions. Rare, except with excessive doses. Nausea, vomiting, diarrhea, headache; other neurological disturbances including vertigo, incoordination, weakness, seizures and coma may occur, especially with pre-existing CNS disorders and impaired renal function.[11]

Precautions. Pregnancy. Use with caution in patients with impaired renal or hepatic function or convulsive disorders.[11]

Notes. Virtually 100% effective for pinworms and roundworms; no significant effect on hookworms, tapeworms or whipworms. Nonstaining. No clinical differences among salt forms.[12,13]

Pyrantel Pamoate   Antiminth®

Pharmacology. A depolarizing neuromuscular blocker that produces spastic paralysis of the parasite with no similar effects on the host after oral use.

Administration and Adult Dose. **PO for roundworms and pinworms** 11 mg/kg, to maximum of 1 g in single dose; **for pinworms** repeat after 2 week interval. Doses are expressed as base equivalent. **PO for hookworms** (investigational) 11 mg/kg/day for 3 days—80–95% effective.[3]

Pediatric Dose. PO (over 1 yr) same as adult dose in mg/kg.

Dosage Forms. **Susp** 50 mg/ml (strength expressed as base equivalent).

Patient Instructions. See Class Instructions.

Pharmacokinetics and Biopharmaceutics. *Fate.* Slight oral absorption with peak plasma levels of 50–130 ng/ml reached within 1–3 hr after a 11 mg/kg dose. Less than 15% of dose is excreted in the urine as parent drug and metabolites.[14]

Adverse Reactions. Rare, nausea, vomiting, headaches and transient SGOT elevations.[14,15]

Precautions. Pregnancy. Use with caution in patients with impaired liver function.

Notes. Virtually 100% effective for pinworms and roundworms; ineffective for whipworm and *Strongyloides*.

Pyrvinium Pamoate   Povan®

Pharmacology. A cyanine dye which interferes with the absorption of exogenous glucose in intestinal helminths.

Administration and Adult Dose. PO for pinworms 5 mg/kg, to maximum of 350 mg in single dose, repeat in 2 weeks. Doses are expressed as base equivalent.

Pediatric Dose. PO (over 10 kg) same as adult dose in mg/kg.

Dosage Forms. Susp 10 mg/ml; Tab 50 mg (strengths expressed as base equivalent).

Patient Instructions. Swallow whole tablets immediately, to avoid staining teeth. This drug discolors stools and vomitus bright red; the suspension stains if it is spilled. See also Class Instructions.

Pharmacokinetics and Biopharmaceutics. *Fate.* Excreted via feces with no detectable absorption.[16]

Adverse Reactions. Rare, but nausea, vomiting and diarrhea may occur after large doses, especially with suspension.[17]

Precautions. Pregnancy. Use with caution in patients with impaired renal or hepatic function.

Notes. Use restricted to treatment of pinworms; virtually 100% effective. Tablets may be less effective than the suspension.[17]

8:12 ANTIBIOTICS

8:12.02 AMINOGLYCOSIDES

General References: 18–27

Aminoglycosides   Various

Pharmacology. Aminocyclitol derivatives which have bactericidal activity against Gram-negative aerobic bacteria via attachment to the 30S and 50S ribosomal subunit; anaerobic bacteria are universally resistant, because aminoglycoside transport into cells is oxygen-dependent.[18,19,25] Dibasic cations (eg, magnesium and calcium) and acidic conditions inhibit their action.[28] Their spectrum is similar, although streptomycin and kanamycin have no utility against some Gram-negative bacteria, especially *Pseudomonas aeruginosa*. Some Gram-positive organisms (eg, streptococci) are relatively resistant to all aminoglycosides; this may be overcome by addition of inhibitors of cell wall synthesis (eg, penicillins).[25] Most resistance among Gram-negative organisms is due to transferable R-factor mediated enzymatic inactivation.[18,19,25]

Administration and Adult Dose. IM or IV by slow intermittent infusion over 30–60 min, although 15 min infusions are safe. With gentamicin there are some data to indicate that injection over 3–5 min does not increase the risk of toxicity.[29] Continuous IV infusion has been used to maintain constant suprainhibitory plasma concentrations, primarily in granulocytopenic patients. Toxicity is probably more frequent and the value of this method relative to intermittent administration has not been established.[27,30] Irrigation of vascularized areas dosage should not exceed usual parenteral dose. Intrathecal or Intraventricular administration is usually necessary to achieve therapeutic CSF levels. See Aminoglycosides Dosage Comparison Chart.

Dosage Individualization. Individualization is critical because these agents have a very low therapeutic index. Use of ideal body weight (IBW) for determining the mg/kg dose appears to be more accurate than dosing on the basis of total body weight (TBW). In morbid obesity, dosage may best be based on IBW + 0.4 (TBW − IBW).[31] Initial and periodic peak and trough plasma drug levels should be determined, even in patients with normal renal function, because dosage requirements can vary widely[30,32] (this is unnecessary in less serious infections in patients without significant renal impairment)—see both Aminoglycosides Comparison Charts.

In renal impairment, use the following guidelines:[33]

1. Select loading dose in mg/kg (ideal body weight) to provide peak plasma levels in the range listed below for the desired aminoglycoside.

AMINOGLYCOSIDE	USUAL LOADING DOSES	EXPECTED PEAK PLASMA LEVELS
Tobramycin	1.5–2 mg/kg	4–10 mcg/ml
Gentamicin		
Amikacin	5–7.5 mg/kg	15–30 mcg/ml
Kanamycin		

2. Select maintenance dose (as percentage of chosen loading dose) to continue peak plasma levels indicated above, according to desired dosing interval and the patient's corrected creatinine clearance.

Percentage of Loading Dose Required For Dosage Interval Selected

Cl_{cr} (ML/MIN)	HALF-LIFE[a](HR)	8 HR	12 HR	24 HR
90	3.1	84%	–	–
80	3.4	80	91%	–
70	3.9	76	88	–
60	4.5	71	84	–
50	5.3	65	79	–
40	6.5	57	72	92%
30	8.4	48	63	86
25	9.9	43	57	81
20	11.9	37	50	75
17	13.6	33	46	70
15	15.1	31	42	67
12	17.9	27	37	61
10[b]	20.4	24	34	56
7	25.9	19	28	47
5	31.5	16	23	41
2	46.8	11	16	30
0	69.3	8	11	21

a. Alternatively, one-half of the chosen loading dose may be given at an interval approximately equal to the estimated half-life.

b. Dosing for patients with Cl_{cr} less than 10 ml/min should be assisted by measured plasma levels.

c. From reference 33, reproduced with permission.

These guidelines serve only to rapidly approximate the correct dosage; factors other than renal function and body weight affect aminoglycoside pharmacokinetics.[27,30]

Pediatric Dose. See Aminoglycosides Dosage Comparison Chart.

Dosage Forms. See Aminoglycosides Dosage Comparison Chart.

Patient Instructions. Report any dizziness or sensations of ringing or fullness in the ears.

Pharmacokinetics and Biopharmaceutics. *Plasma Levels.* See Aminoglycosides Plasma Levels Comparison Chart.

Fate. Absorption after oral or rectal administration is about 0.2–2%; absorption across denuded skin may reach 5%. Irrigation of vascularized areas (eg, peritoneal cavitity,[34] pleural space, joint spaces and deep soft tissue wounds) results in absorption approximating IM use. IM administration is followed by rapid and complete absorption, with peak plasma levels occurring after 0.5–1.5 hr. IV infusions over 0.5–1 hr produce plasma levels similar to equal IM doses. Binding of aminoglycosides to plasma proteins is negligible (0–30%).[20,27,30] These agents distribute rapidly into the extracellular fluid compartment with a V_d of about 0.2–0.3 L/kg which is increased by fever, edema, ascites, fluid overload and in neonates.[18-20] Aminoglycosides accumulate markedly in some lean tissues, especially the renal cortex, to levels many times those found in the plasma.[19] This is a slow process, reaching steady-state after 1–3 weeks of therapy. Concentrations in most other tissues and fluids reach 50–100% of plasma concentration; distribution into fatty tissues is about 40% that of lean tissues. Levels in the CSF of patients with meningitis generally do not exceed 25% of plasma levels, except in neonates;[18-20] penetration into the eye is inadequate for treatment of intraocular infections. Penetration into lung tissues is usually less than 40%,[20] and large doses may be necessary to optimally treat pneumonias with relatively insensitive organisms (eg, *Pseudomonas aeruginosa*). Penetration of systemic aminoglycosides into the peritoneal cavity of patients with peritonitis is therapeutically adequate.[35]

Elimination is via glomerular filtration of unchanged drug.[20] During the first few days of therapy, excretion in the urine is delayed, despite rapid disappearance from plasma. The mechanism of this delay is unknown, although it appears to be related to slow distribution into peripheral lean tissue compartments. After discontinuation, low levels of aminoglycoside can be detected in the urine for several days.[20,27,30,36]

$t_{1/2}$. α phase 5–15 min; β phase (adults) about 1.5–3 hr (average 2) with normal renal function (1.5–9 hr in neonates less than 1 week and 3 hr in older infants); may be more variable in certain groups (eg, obstetric[37] and burn patients) despite normal renal function; 50–70 hr in anuria. γ phase (redistribution from lean tissue into, and elimination from, the extracellular and intravascular spaces) 60–350 hr (usually 150–200). β phase half-life is most important for use in dosage individualization while the γ phase may account for the gradual rise of plasma levels and apparent increase in half-life with continued therapy, despite stable renal function.[20,27,30,36]

Adverse Reactions. Nephrotoxicity involving the proximal tubules and ranging from frequent (2–20%), mild reversible renal insufficiency to very rare, acute nonoliguric renal failure; most often seen in patients with pre-existing renal impairment. The appearance of casts,[38] tubular enzymes or beta$_2$-microglobulin in the urine precedes clinical nephrotoxicity.[23] Depletion of magnesium and other minerals due to increased renal excretion occurs.[39] Infrequent, but usually permanent, vestibular damage is reported, usually in association with streptomycin or high doses of other aminoglycosides in renal impairment. Subclinical vestibular disturbances can be detected in 40% or more of patients receiving aminoglycosides.[18,40] Deafness, beginning as high-tone auditory impairment, is rare except with systemic neomycin and may be preceded by evidence of vestibular damage. Early auditory damage can be detected only by sequential audiometric examination, because hearing loss in conversational frequencies is a sign of advanced auditory impairment. Furthermore, early auditory damage is not as apparent in the elderly or others with pre-existing high-tone deficits.[40] Oral aminoglycosides, primarily neomycin, have been associated with a sprue-like malabsorption syndrome.[18] Neuromuscular blockade with respiratory failure is rare, except in predisposed patients—see Precautions. Significant differences in the frequency of toxicity of amikacin, gentamicin, kanamycin and tobramycin have not been clearly demonstrated, although recent studies suggest that tobramycin is the least nephrotoxic.[41,42] However, the clinical significance of this difference is not clear because most nephrotoxic events are minor, asymptomatic and rapidly reversible if the drug is carefully dosed and monitored. The body of experimental data clearly indicates that tobramycin is much less nephrotoxic and ototoxic *in animals* than are the other agents.[19] See Aminoglycosides Plasma Levels Comparison Chart.

Precautions.   Pregnancy; pre-existing renal impairment; vestibular or auditory impairment; myasthenia gravis, hypocalcemia, postoperative or other conditions which depress neuromuscular transmission; history of aminoglycoside hypersensitivity reactions. See Drug Interactions chapter.

Parameters to Monitor.   Renal function tests before and every 2–3 days during therapy. In patients with pre-existing renal, auditory or vestibular impairment or in patients who receive prolonged, high-dose therapy, obtain baseline and weekly audiograms, and check for tinnitus or vertigo daily, if possible. In neonates or other patients with rapidly changing renal function, obtain plasma drug concentrations initially and every 2–3 days until stable. See Dosage Individualization.

Notes.   Of the available aminoglycosides, gentamicin, tobramycin and amikacin are the most clinically useful.[18,19,21,22,25] **Streptomycin** use is largely restricted to the treatment of enterococcal endocarditis (in combination with penicillin G), tuberculosis, brucellosis, plague and tularemia. **Neomycin** is much more toxic than the other aminoglycosides when given parenterally; it is restricted to oral use for gut sterilization and topical use for minor infections. Rising resistance among Gram-negative organisms, especially *Pseudomonas aeruginosa,* has limited the use of **kanamycin.** **Tobramycin** is roughly equivalent to gentamicin therapeutically, although it is about 2–4 times more active against *Pseudomonas aeruginosa* than is gentamicin, and it is active against about 50% of gentamicin-resistant *Pseudomonas aeruginosa.*[26] The prevalence of **gentamicin** resistance varies considerably among institutions, and strains highly resistant to gentamicin are usually resistant to tobramycin. **Amikacin** has the lowest overall rate of resistance of all aminoglycosides.[22] Many institutions prefer to reserve amikacin for the treatment of infections with organisms resistant to other aminoglycosides, to prevent development of resistance to this drug. Whether such restriction will delay the emergence of resistance is unclear.[22] The relative merits of the gentamicin derivatives, **netilmicin** and **sisomicin**, are undetermined at present.[18,43,44]

Aminoglycosides Dosage Comparison Chart

DRUG	DOSAGE FORMS	ADULT DOSE	PEDIATRIC DOSE
Gentamicin Sulfate Garamycin® Various	Inj 10, 40 mg/ml IT Inj 2 mg/ml	IM or IV 5–6 mg/kg/day in 3 equally divided doses q 8 hr	IM or IV (neonates) 5–6 mg/kg/day in 3 equally divided doses q 8 hr
	Ophth Oint 3 mg/g Ophth Soln 3 mg/ml	IM or IV for less serious infections[a] 3–5 mg/kg/day in 3 equally divided doses q 8 hr	IM or IV (infants over 1 week) 7.5 mg/kg/day in 3 equally divided doses q 8 hr
Tobramycin Sulfate Nebcin®	Inj 10, 40 mg/ml	IT 4–8 mg q 18–24 hr	IM or IV (children) 6–7.5 mg/kg/day in 3 equally divided doses q 8 hr IT 1–2 mg q 18–24 hr
Amikacin Sulfate Amikin®	Inj 50, 250 mg/ml	IM or IV 15–20 mg/kg/day in 2–3 equally divided doses IT 5–20 mg/day	IM or IV (neonates) 10 mg/kg loading dose, then 7.5 mg/kg q 12 hr IM or IV (children) same as adult mg/kg dose
Kanamycin Sulfate Kantrex® Various	Cap 500 mg Inj 37.5, 250, 333 mg/ml	PO 4–8 g/day in 2–4 divided doses IM or IV same as Amikacin IT same as Amikacin	PO (infants) 50 mg/kg/day in 2–4 divided doses IM or IV same as adult mg/kg dose

Continued

Aminoglycosides Dosage Comparison Chart

DRUG	DOSAGE FORMS	ADULT DOSE	PEDIATRIC DOSE
Streptomycin Sulfate Various	Inj 400, 500 mg, 1, 5 g	IM 15–25 mg/kg/day (usually 1–2 g/day) in 2 equally divided doses q 12 hr IM for TB 1 g q week	IM (neonates) 20–30 mg/kg/day in 2 equally divided doses q 12 hr IM (children) 20–40 mg/kg/day in 2 equally divided doses q 12 hr
Neomycin Sulfate Mycifradin® Various	Soln 25 mg/ml Tab 500 mg Inj 500 mg Crm 5 mg/g Oint 5 mg/g	PO 2–8 g/day in 2–4 divided doses	PO (neonates) 10–50 mg/kg/day in 4 divided doses PO (infants and children) 50–100 mg/kg/day in 4 divided doses
Netilmicin Sulfate Netromycin®	Inj 10, 25, 100 mg/ml	IM or IV 3[a]–6.5 mg/kg/day in 2–3 equally divided doses q 8–12 hr	IM or IV (neonates) 4–6.5 mg/kg/day in 2 equally divided doses q 12 hr. IM or IV (infants and children) 5.5–8 mg/kg/day in 2–3 equally divided doses q 8–12 hr
Sisomicin Sulfate Siseptin® (Miles)	Inj-Investigational	IM or IV 4 mg/kg/day in 2–3 equally divided doses[b]	—

a. For uncomplicated UTI or mild soft tissue infection.
b. These doses conform to those used in published clinical trials.

Aminoglycosides Plasma Levels Comparison Chart

DRUG	USUAL THERAPEUTIC PLASMA LEVELS (MCG/ML)		USUAL TOXIC PLASMA LEVELS [b] (MCG/ML)		RELATIVE NEPHROTOXICITY[c]	RELATIVE OTOTOXICITY[c]	
	PEAK[a]	TROUGH	PEAK	TROUGH		COCHLEAR	VESTIBULAR
Gentamicin Sulfate Garamycin® Various	5–8	1–2	10–12	2–3	+ +	+	+ +
Tobramycin Sulfate Nebcin®	5–8	1–2	10–12	2–3	+	+	+ / + +
Amikacin Sulfate Amikin®	20–30	5–10	35	10	+ +	+ +	+
Kanamycin Sulfate Kantrex® Various	20–30	5–10	35	10	+ +	+ +	+
Streptomycin Sulfate Various	15–20	5	40–50	5	+	+	+ + +

Continued

Aminoglycosides Plasma Levels Comparison Chart

DRUG	USUAL THERAPEUTIC PLASMA LEVELS (MCG/ML) PEAK[a]	TROUGH	USUAL TOXIC PLASMA LEVELS [b] (MCG/ML) PEAK	TROUGH	RELATIVE NEPHROTOXICITY[c]	RELATIVE OTOTOXICITY[c] COCHLEAR	VESTIBULAR
Neomycin Sulfate Mycifradin® Various	—	—	—	—	+ + +	+ + + +	+
Netilmicin Sulfate Netromycin® (Schering)	7–9	1–2	—	—	+/+ +	+	+ +
Sisomicin Sulfate Siseptin® (Miles)	4–6	1	—	—	+/+ +	+	+ +

a. As seen after a 30 min IV infusion or approximately 1 hr after IM administration of a usual adult dose. Uncomplicated UTI may be treated with smaller doses that produce much lower plasma levels; however, serious infections, such as Gram-negative bacteremia or pneumonia may require doses and plasma levels approaching the range associated with frequent toxicity.

b. Specific peak and/or trough plasma drug levels have only been loosely related to the rate of nephrotoxicity and ototoxicity and may reflect a general overdosage. However, based on available evidence, it is recommended that these plasma levels not be exceeded. See references 27 and 30.

c. There is considerable disagreement as to the relative frequency of these adverse reactions because of differences in evaluation methods and criteria. Based on references 18, 19, 27, 36, 40-46.

8:12.04 ANTIFUNGAL ANTIBIOTICS

General References: 18, 47-51

Amphotericin B

Fungizone®

Pharmacology. A polyene which preferentially binds to fungal cytoplasmic membrane sterols (chiefly ergosterol), increasing the permeability of the membrane. Binds somewhat to human cytoplasmic sterols (chiefly cholesterol), which accounts for a portion of amphotericin's toxicity.

Administration and Adult Dose. IV **initial test dose** 1 mg by slow infusion advocated by some sources;[47,49] **otherwise IV** 250 mcg/kg/day initially in a single dose, and increased by daily increments of 250 mcg/kg/day, or faster if tolerated, to maximum of 1.5 mg/kg/day or every other day (usually 50 mg/day, except in severe infections). Lower doses have been used successfully,[47] but their use is controversial. **Recommended infusion concentration** is 10 mg/dl of D5W administered over 2-6 hr. Do not mix with electrolyte solutions; protection from light unnecessary if infused in less than 24 hr from time of preparation.[52,53] **Intrathecally** 500 mcg in 5 ml CSF 2-3 times a week, or 300 mcg/day in D5W or D10W[54] infused over 1 hr.[50] **Bladder Irrigation:** 15-50 mg/day in sterile water at 5 mg/dl concentration.[55]

Dosage Individualization. No dosage alteration necessary with impaired renal function,[56] although further impairment may occur as a result of the amphotericin.

Pediatric Dose. IV same as adult dose in mg/kg.

Dosage Forms. **Inj** 5 mg/ml (when reconstituted); **Top Crm** 30 mg/g; **Top Lot** 30 mg/ml; **Top Oint** 30 mg/g.

Patient Instructions. Patient should be forewarned of expected immediate reactions to infusion. Topical preparations may stain clothes.

Pharmacokinetics and Biopharmaceutics. *Fate.* Poor oral and IM absorption. 370-650 mcg/kg/day infused IV over 4-6 hr produces levels of 1.8-3.5 mcg/ml 1 hr after infusion; concentrations of 0.5-1.5 mcg/ml remain 20 hr after infusion discontinued;[57] plasma concentrations are not directly proportional to dose and tend to plateau at doses exceeding 50 mg. With usual doses, trough concentrations on alternate day or daily administration schedules are not significantly different; peaks are generally higher on alternate day schedule. Plasma concentrations represent less than 10% of administered dose;[58] greater than 95% bound to plasma beta lipoprotein;[18] V_d is about 4 L/kg.[59] Does not diffuse well into body cavities, eye or CSF. Appears to be stored in the body, very slowly released, metabolized and slowly excreted by the kidneys with 3-5% as active drug. No metabolites have been specifically identified. Despite slow elimination, plasma concentrations do not increase after repeated administration or in the presence of impaired renal function. When therapy is discontinued, amphotericin and metabolites continue to appear in the urine for 7-8 weeks.[58]

$t_{1/2}$. About 24-48 hr initially, with a terminal phase $t_{1/2}$ of about 15 days;[59] probably not changed with renal impairment.

Adverse Reactions. Very common during infusion period: fever, chills, headache, anorexia, nausea, vomiting, malaise, pain at infusion site. Severity of reactions may be reduced by premedication with aspirin, corticosteroids, antiemetics and addition of phosphate buffer and heparin to solution.[60] Prolonged administration times (greater than 6 hr) may produce more immediate reactions.[58] IV meperidine HCl 50 mg rapidly terminates shaking chills in some patients in whom spontaneous disappearance does not occur when the infusion is stopped.[61] With repeated administration: thrombophlebitis, normocytic, normochromic anemia, impaired renal function with distal tubular acidosis, isosthenuria, hypokalemia and hypomagnesemia frequently occur, and are generally reversible, although permanent renal impairment may result, especially if total dose exceeds 4–5 g.[60] Potassium supplementation is usually necessary and administration of an alkalinizing potassium salt (bicarbonate, gluconate, etc.) is often useful in preventing the occurrence of hypokalemic acidosis. Mannitol does not appear to provide any protection against renal damage.[18,60] Rapid infusion has been carried out safely,[60,62] but may produce cardiovascular collapse.[49] Intrathecal administration can produce peripheral nerve pain, paresthesias, nerve palsies, paraplegia, convulsions and chemical meningitis;[49,54] bladder irrigations containing amphotericin have produced no reported toxicity.[55]

Precautions. Impaired renal function. Safety of use during pregnancy not established despite reports of safe use.[63]

Parameters to Monitor. BUN, serum creatinine or creatinine clearance should be monitored before therapy and at least weekly during therapy; hematocrit, serum potassium and magnesium need monitoring periodically. Some sources consider temporary drug discontinuation if renal function becomes severely impaired due to the amphotericin (serum creatinine greater than 3.5 mg/dl); however, other sources do not.[64]

Notes. Amphotericin B is very water insoluble; commercial product is a colloidal dispersion in bile salts, buffered with sodium phosphate. Store powder in refrigerator, protect from light. Reconstitute with sterile water for injection *without* a bacteriostatic agent; reconstituted drug is stable for 1 week under refrigeration. The drug is probably removed by in-line filters of less than 1 micron pore size, despite contrary claims; therefore, filtration is not recommended.[65] Due to serious common toxicities, use only when clearly indicated. Necessary dosages and duration of therapy are very inexactly known.[47]

Clotrimazole   Lotrimin®, Mycelex®

Clotrimazole is an imidazole antifungal agent which has failed to be useful for systemic infections due to GI and liver toxicity and poor oral bioavailability. Also, it is a potent inducer of the microsomal enzyme system. A topical cream (10 mg/g) is equal to other antifungal creams in the treatment of *Candida* or dermatophyte skin infections. A 100 mg vaginal tablet (Gyne-Lotrimin®, Mycelex-G®) used once a day for 7 days is similar in efficacy to miconazole or 14 days of nystatin for vulvovaginal candidiasis.[66] Troches of 10 mg are used 5 times/day orally to treat or prevent orotracheal candidiasis.

Flucytosine   Ancobon®

Pharmacology. A fluorinated cytosine analogue that appears to be deaminated to the cytoxic antimetabolite fluorouracil by cytosine deaminase, an enzyme present in fungal, but not human cells. However, a very small amount of fluorouracil may be produced in some recipients, which may account for some of the drug's toxicity.[47]

Administration and Adult Dose. PO 50–150 mg/kg/day in 4 divided doses; in all cases the use of higher doses has been suggested in order to prevent the emergence of resistance. With severe infections such as meningitis, even higher doses (250 mg/kg/day) have been suggested.[67]

Dosage Individualization. Dosage must be reduced in the presence of impaired renal function.[47,56] An approximate reduction can be determined by dosing at intervals in hours equal to 4 times the Cr_s in mg/dl. Alternative regimens involving reduced dosage at 6 hr dosing intervals have been recommended.[68] In patients on maintenance hemodialysis q 48–72 hr, may give 20–50 mg/kg after each dialysis.[47,56,69] May give normal doses to patients with liver disease; however, see Adverse Reactions.

Pediatric Dose. PO same as adult dose in mg/kg.

Dosage Forms. Cap 250, 500 mg.

Patient Instructions. Take the capsules required for a single dose over a 15 min period with food, to minimize stomach upset. Close follow-up with the physician is essential.

Pharmacokinetics and Biopharmaceutics. *Plasma Levels.* Toxicity most likely over 100 mcg/ml.[47,67] See also Precautions.
   Fate. Rapidly and well absorbed (about 90%) with peak about 1–2 hr after administration of a 500 mg dose to adults averaging 8–12 mcg/ml[69] in patients with normal renal function. Insignificant binding to plasma proteins;[56] V_d is 0.7 L/kg.[69] Widely distributed throughout the body, including the CSF and eye.[51] Eliminated almost entirely (average 90%) in the urine by glomerular filtration of unchanged drug, with urine levels many times greater than plasma levels.[47,48,69]
   $t_{1/2}$. 3–8 hr (average 6); up to 100 hr or greater with renal impairment.[56,69]

Adverse Reactions. Occasional nausea, vomiting, diarrhea, bone marrow depression and elevated liver function tests (usually asymptomatic and rapidly reversible).[47,67]

Precautions. Pregnancy. With severe renal impairment, elimination is highly variable and monitoring of plasma levels is recommended, keeping peak concentrations between 50–75 mcg/ml;[47] impaired hepatic function; hematologic disorders.

Parameters to Monitor. Before, and frequently during therapy, monitor BUN, serum creatinine, creatinine clearance, full hematology and liver function tests. See also Precautions.

Notes. Certain fungi may develop resistance to the drug during therapy. Flucytosine may be synergistic with amphotericin B, depending on the organism involved. Some preliminary results have been encouraging, although amphotericin B can increase the toxicity of flucytosine by increasing its cellular penetration and impairing its elimination secondary to nephrotoxicity.[18,47,51] Duration of therapy must be guided by severity of infection and response to therapy. An IV preparation has been studied in clinical trials and appears to be similar to the oral form in efficacy and toxicity.[70]

Griseofulvin, Micronized

Fulvicin-U/F®,
Grifulvin V®, Grisactin®

Pharmacology. A fungistatic agent concentrated in sensitive organisms and impairing fungal growth by an unknown mechanism which appears to affect mitosis. Very active against most dermatophytes (ringworm fungi); little activity against other yeasts or fungi.

Administration and Adult Dose. PO 500 mg–1 g/day in single or 2–4 divided doses; larger doses (2 g/day) may be used initially for severe infections. Symptomatic relief usually appears within several days. Lesions of skin not involving the palms, soles or nails usually require 3 weeks of therapy; infections of the palms or soles require 4–8 weeks of therapy; infections of the nails may require 6–12 months of therapy. Continue therapy until lesions clear.[71] See also Notes.

Dosage Individualization. No dosage reduction required for patients with renal disease.

Pediatric Dose. PO 10 mg/kg/day (300 mg/M^2/day) in a single or 2–4 divided doses; larger doses (600 mg/M^2/day) may be used initially for severe infections.

Dosage Forms. Cap 125, 250 mg; Susp 25 mg/ml; Tab 125, 250, 500 mg.

Patient Instructions. Taking dose at noon may increase absorption.

Pharmacokinetics and Biopharmaceutics. *Fate.* Considerable individual variation in absorption is experienced with all dosage forms, with an average of 50% absorbed in fasted patients. Fatty meals may increase rate but not extent of absorption.[72] Only 25% of nonmicronized products absorbed. Absorption takes place over 30–40 hr; dissolution of drug appears rate-limiting;[73] 1 g orally in fasted adults produces peak plasma levels at 4–8 hr of 1–2 mcg/ml. Widely distributed with multicompartment kinetics and a V_d of 1–2 L/kg.[48] Appears in stratum corneum within 8 hr after a single oral dose, due to transport in sweat and other transepidermal fluids.[72] Most of absorbed drug is metabolized by liver to 6-demethylgriseofulvin which is excreted in the urine; about 0.1% appears in the urine as unchanged drug.[72-74]

$t_{1/2}$. Difficult to estimate after oral administration due to prolonged absorption. 9–21 hr (average 17.5 hr) after IV administration.[73]

Adverse Reactions. Headache, nausea and vomiting occasionally occur; may exacerbate acute intermittent porphyria; rare photosensitivity reactions, peripheral neuritis and leukopenia.

Contraindications. Porphyria, hepatocellular failure.

Precautions. Pregnancy. See Drug Interactions chapter.

Parameters to Monitor. Occasional hematologic, hepatic and renal function tests if long-term therapy.

Notes. A preparation of griseofulvin dispersed in polyethylene glycol (PEG) 6000 (Gris-PEG®) is much more completely and somewhat more rapidly absorbed and is administered at one-half of the usual griseofulvin dose.[72,75]

Ketoconazole   Nizoral®

Ketoconazole is an imidazole antifungal agent, similar to miconazole; however, it is water soluble and well absorbed from the GI tract. It is highly effective for superficial and mucocutaneous mycoses and moderately effective for some systemic mycoses. Adverse reactions include nausea, pruritus, frequent elevated liver function tests and occasional hepatotoxicity. PO dosage is 200–400 mg/day. It is supplied as a 200 mg tablet.[76]

Miconazole
Miconazole Nitrate

Monistat IV®
Monistat-Derm®, Monistat® 7

Pharmacology. A water-insoluble imidazole derivative having primarily fungistatic action. It appears to increase the permeability of the cell membrane by inhibiting ergosterol synthesis,[77] and appears to interfere with membrane transport of nutrients and toxins.[51,78]

Administration and Adult Dose. IV (as miconazole base) usually 1.2–2.4 g/day, but may range from 200 mg–3.6 g/day (depending on organism), in 3 divided doses at 8 hr intervals. Dilute in at least 200 ml of NS or D5W and infuse over 30–60 min if given by peripheral vein. Can be given by central venous catheter in 50–100 ml of solution over 15–30 min.[78] **Intrathecal for meningitis** (as miconazole) 10–20 mg/day or every other day. **Bladder irrigation** (as miconazole) 200 mg diluted and instilled 2–4 times daily.[79] **Intravaginally for candidiasis** (as miconazole nitrate) one applicatorful each evening for 7 days.

Dosage Individualization. No alteration of dosage is required for patients with renal failure or during hemodialysis.[51]

Pediatric Dose. IV (over 1 yr) 20–40 mg/kg/day (usually 15 mg/kg twice daily).

Dosage Forms. **Inj** 10 mg/ml; **Top Crm** 20 mg/g; **Top Lot** 20 mg/ml; **Vag Crm** 20 mg/g.

Pharmacokinetics and Biopharmaceutics. *Fate.* Topical or vaginal absorption is negligible. Oral absorption about 25–50%.[51,79] IV 522 mg given over 15 min to healthy adults produces average concentrations of 6.0, 1.9, 0.44 and 0.19 mcg/ml at 15 min, 1, 4 and 8 hr, respectively.[78] Distribution appears to follow a 3-compartment model with V_d of 1500 L and 800 L in adults with normal and impaired renal function, respectively. Very poor CSF penetration (usually 5–20% of plasma levels).[51,78] Extensively metabolized by liver microsomes via oxidative dealkylation, breakdown of the imidazole ring and other pathways. About 50% of an IV dose is eliminated in the feces, 25% of which is active. About 20% of a dose is excreted in the urine, but less than 1% in an active form.[51,78]

$t_{1/2}$. About 24 hr; unchanged by renal impairment.[80]

Adverse Reactions. Frequent phlebitis (about 40% of patients).[81] Nausea, vomiting, fever, chills and pruritus occur in about 10–15% of patients in the first few hours after infusion. A dose-related, slowly reversible anemia and thrombocytosis occurs in 30–40% of patients. Aggregation of erythrocytes and rouleaux formation on blood smear is almost universal, interfering with blood smear preparation and may persist for days to months after drug discontinuation. Some patients develop elevated plasma triglyceride levels with an unusual (gamma 2) electrophoretic pattern; this has been attributed to the vehicle and may persist for several months after therapy is discontinued. Hyponatremia may occur; close attention to serum sodium concentration may avert this problem. Rapid infusions (less than 15 min duration) may produce cardiac arrhythmias. Significant renal or hepatic toxicity have not been observed. Intrathecal doses are generally well tolerated, but may produce arachnoiditis. Topical, vaginal and bladder applications have produced no major adverse effects.[51,78,79,81]

Precautions. Pregnancy. (IV use) impaired liver function; pre-existing anemia or hyponatremia.

Parameters to Monitor. (IV use) hematocrit and serum sodium concentration periodically; signs of vein irritation daily.

Notes. IV product is supplied as a colloidal dispersion in polyethylene glycol 40 castor oil. In early reports, IV miconazole was extremely phlebitogenic (about 70% of patients);[79] elimination of the acetic acid/sodium acetate buffer from the vehicle in 1975 has reduced the frequency of phlebitis.[51,81] Miconazole is a second-line drug for the treatment of systemic fungal infections, because its efficacy in these infections is either inferior to other agents or inadequately established.[18,78] Very effective topically and vaginally for local fungal infections.[18]

Nystatin   Mycostatin®, Nilstat®

Pharmacology. A polyene antifungal agent, similar to amphotericin B, that is too toxic for parenteral use and is used only for superficial infections.

Administration and Adult Dose.   **PO Susp for oral candidiasis** 400,000–600,000 U qid, continue for at least 48 hr after oral symptoms have cleared and cultures have returned to normal. **PO Tab for GI candidiasis** 500,000–1,000,000 U tid; **Vag Tab** 100,000 U/day or bid for 2 weeks.

Pediatric Dose. **PO Susp** (premature and newborn) 100,000 U qid; **PO Susp** (older infants and children) 1,000,000–2,000,000 U/day in 4 divided doses.

Dosage Forms. **Susp** 100,000 U/ml; **Tab** 500,000 U; **Top Crm** 100,000 U/g; **Top Oint** 100,000 U/g; **Top Pwdr** 100,000 U/g; **Vag Tab** 100,000 U.

Patient Instructions. Retain suspension in mouth as long as possible when treating oral candidiasis. Retain vaginal tablet as long as possible when treating vaginal candidiasis.

Pharmacokinetics and Biopharmaceutics. *Fate.* Negligible oral absorption; not absorbed through intact skin or mucous membranes.

Adverse Reactions. Too toxic for parenteral use. Oral, vaginal and topical routes are virtually nontoxic. Rare topical sensitization.

Notes. The vaginal tablet has been successfully used in place of the oral suspension to treat oral candidiasis; its slow dissolution allows prolonged oral contact.[18]

8:12.06 CEPHALOSPORINS

General References: 18, 82–88

Cefamandole Naftate   Mandol®

Cefamandole is a "second-generation" cephalosporin, distinguished from cefazolin and other "first-generation" agents by greater resistance to β-lactamases. It has improved activity against many Gram-negative bacteria, most notably *Haemophilus influenzae* (including ampicillin-resistant strains), *Escherichia coli*, *Proteus* sp. and many *Enterobacter* sp. Gram-positive activity is equivalent to, or less than, first-generation agents. Adverse effects are similar to cefazolin, but also include a disulfiram-like interaction with alcohol. Dosage is IM or IV for adults 500 mg–1 g q 4-6 hr, to maximum of 12 g/day. Supplied as Inj 500 mg, 1, 2 g.[89] See Cephalosporins Comparison Chart.

Cefazolin Sodium

Ancef®, Kefzol®

Pharmacology. A broad-spectrum semisynthetic β-lactam antibiotic which inhibits bacterial cell wall synthesis. Resistance is due primarily to bacterial elaboration of β-lactamases which hydrolyze and inactivate the antibiotic. Some bacteria also have outer cell wall layers which are impermeable to the antibiotic.

Administration and Adult Dose. IM or IV 250 mg–1g q 6–12 hr, to maximum of 6 g/day. **IM or IV for surgical prophylaxis** 1 g 30–60 min prior to surgery and 500 mg–1 g q 6–8 hr for 24 hr.

Dosage Individualization. Dosage should be reduced for patients with impaired renal function, although recommendations vary considerably.[82-84,90] With severe renal failure, may give a loading dose followed by 10–25% of the usual daily dose q 24 hr.[83,90] The effect of hemodialysis is variable.[82] No adjustment is necessary for patients with liver disease.

Pediatric Dose. IV (newborn and premature infants) 20 mg/kg q 12 hr. **IM or IV** (over 1 month) 1.25 g/M^2/day or 25–50 mg/kg/day in 3–4 divided doses, to maximum of 100 mg/kg/day.

Dosage Forms. Inj 250, 500 mg, 1, 5, 10 g.

Pharmacokinetics and Biopharmaceutics. *Fate.* 500 mg IM produces a peak concentration of about 30–40 mcg/ml at 30 min; 1 g IV given over 20 min produces a postinfusion concentration of 110–140 mcg/ml.[82-84,90] 75–85% bound to plasma proteins;[84,91] V_d is about 10 L/1.73 M^2. Widely distributed throughout the body with high free levels in many tissues and cavities; CSF concentrations are undetectable or subtherapeutic.[82,84,90] Negligible metabolism, with virtually 100% urinary excretion via filtration and secretion of unchanged drug.[18,82-84,92-95]

$t_{1/2}$. 1.6–2 hr; 20–70 hr with severe renal impairment.[82-84,90]

Adverse Reactions. Infrequent except for various allergic reactions occurring in about 5% of patients. With excessive doses, especially in renal impairment, neurotoxicity may occur manifested as CNS irritation with delirium, seizures and coma which may be fatal.[96] Also, false positive direct Coombs' reactions[83] and very rare coagulopathy[97] have been observed after high doses in uremic patients. Significant nephrotoxicity not reported with cefazolin;[98] generally well tolerated by IM or IV route.[83,90]

Precautions. Use with caution in patients with a history of severe allergic reaction (ie, anaphylaxis, hives, angioneurotic edema) to penicillin;[99] renal impairment. See Drug Interactions chapter.

Parameters to Monitor. Renal function tests initially and repeated periodically if receiving high-dose regimen or nephrotoxic agents concomitantly.

Notes. See Cephalosporins Comparison Chart.

Cefoperazone Sodium

Cefobid®

Cefoperazone is a "third-generation" cephalosporin similar to cefotaxime and moxalactam; however, its activity against *Pseudomonas aeruginosa* is superior, inhibiting 50% of strains at 5–6.2 mcg/ml. The pharmacokinetics of cefoperazone have not been studied completely, but it appears to undergo very significant biliary elimination, producing biliary concentrations exceeding 1 mg/ml. Only 15–30% of the drug is excreted unchanged in the urine. The half-life of the drug is about 2 hr. Early studies have reported frequent diarrhea, perhaps related to biliary elimination, and a disulfiram-like reaction. Dosage for serious infections is IM or IV for adults 1–2 g q 8–12 hr. Supplied as Inj 1, 2 g; refrigerate vials until used.[100] See Cephalosporins Comparison Chart.

Cefotaxime Sodium   Claforan®

Cefotaxime is the first of the "third-generation" cephalosporin derivatives, distinguished from previous agents by markedly increased activity against a variety of Gram-negative organisms, including some potentially useful activity (similar to ticarcillin) against *Pseudomonas aeruginosa.* Gram-positive activity is somewhat inferior to cefazolin. It is extensively metabolized, partially to a generally less active desacetyl derivative. About 20–36% of the drug is eliminated unchanged in the urine with a half-life of 0.8–1.2 hr. Adverse effects are similar to other cephalosporins. Most strains of *Clostridium difficile* are resistant, and cases of pseudomembranous colitis have been observed. Dosage is IV for adults 1–2 g q 6–8 hr, to maximum of 12 g/day. Supplied as Inj 500 mg, 1, 2 g.[101,102] See Cephalosporins Comparison Chart.

Cefoxitin Sodium   Mefoxin®

Cefoxitin is parenteral cephamycin which is structurally and pharmacologically indistinguishable from the cephalosporins. It has greater Gram-negative activity than "first-generation" cephalosporins (eg, cefazolin), especially against *B. fragilis* and other anaerobic organisms, generally due to the greater β-lactamase resistance of cefoxitin. Gram-positive activity is equivalent to, or less than, cefazolin. Adverse effects are similar to cefazolin, except that cefoxitin is very painful on IM injection. Dosage is IV for adults 1–2 g q 6–8 hr, to maximum of 12 g/day.[103] Supplied as Inj 1, 2 g. See Cephalosporins Comparison Chart.

Ceftriaxone Disodium   Rocephin®
(Investigational - Roche)

Ceftriaxone is a parenteral "third-generation" cephalosporin very similar to cefotaxime in structure and activity. It is not metabolized, but 40% of a dose undergoes biliary elimination, while the remainder is excreted unchanged in the urine. The drug has an unusually long half-life of about 8 hr. Adverse effects have not been thoroughly studied, although the drug is very painful when given by IM injection. Suggested dosage from early clinical trials is IV for adults 500 mg–2 g/day as a single dose. Supplied as Inj 500 mg, 1, 2 g.[104,105] See Cephalosporins Comparison Chart.

Cefuroxime Sodium   Zinacef®

Cefuroxime is a cephalosporin having antibacterial activity similar to cefamandole. Cefuroxime is unmetabolized and is excreted almost entirely by the kidneys. It has few adverse effects, similar to other cephalosporins, and appears to be as well tolerated as cefazolin after IM injection. Suggested dosage is IM or IV for adults 750 mg-1.5 g q 8 hr.[106] See Cephalosporins Comparison Chart. Available as Inj 750 mg, 1.5 g.

Moxalactam Disodium   Moxam®

Moxalactam is a 1-oxa-β-lactam that differs structurally from cephalosporins in that the sulfur atom in the dihydrothiazine ring has been replaced by oxygen; however, it shares most pharmacological properties with cephalosporins. It closely resembles cefotaxime in its spectrum and activity, although moxalactam's activity against streptococci and staphylococci is inferior and moxalactam's activity against anaerobic organisms is superior. It is not significantly metabolized, and is primarily eliminated unchanged in the urine with a half-life of about 2-3 hr. Early trials suggest that it may provide effective CSF concentrations for the treatment of meningitis. Adverse reactions are similar to other cephalosporins, although several cases of thrombocytosis, enterococcal superinfection, agranulocytosis and colitis have been reported. A vitamin K-responsive hypoprothrombinemia and bleeding have occurred as has a disulfiram-like interaction with alcohol. Dosage is IM or IV for adults 2-6 g/day in 2-3 divided doses, to maximum of 12 g/day. Supplied as Inj 1, 2 g.[107,108] See Cephalosporins Comparison Chart.

Cephalosporins Comparison Chart[a]

DRUG	DOSAGE FORMS	ADULT DOSE	PEAK PLASMA LEVELS (MCG/ML)[b]	PERCENT PROTEIN BOUND	HALF-LIFE (HOURS) NORMAL	HALF-LIFE (HOURS) ANURIC	PERCENT UNCHANGED IN URINE[c]	COMMENTS
Cefazolin Sodium Ancef® Kefzol®	Inj 250, 500 mg, 1, 5, 10 g	IM or IV 250 mg -1 g q 6-12 hr	50-75	75-85	1.5-2.0	20-70	85-95	See monograph
Cephalothin Sodium Keflin®	Inj 1, 2, 4, 20 g	IV 500 mg-1 g q 4-6 hr; IM not recommended	15-20	65-80	0.5-0.85	2-2.9	60-70	Spectrum similar to cefazolin
Cephradine Anspor® Velosef®	Cap 250, 500 mg Susp 125, 250 mg/5 ml Tab 1 g Inj 250, 500 mg, 1, 2, 4g	PO 250 mg-1 g q 6 hr; IM or IV 500 mg -1 g q 4-6 hr	30 (PO) 10-12 (IM)	5-20	0.7-0.9	↑	80-95	Oral form comparable to cephalexin; spectrum similar to cefazolin
Cephapirin Sodium Cephadyl®	Inj 1, 2, 4, 20 g	IM or IV 500 mg -1 g q 4-6 hr	15-25	45-50	0.3-0.7	1.5-2.4	60	Very similar to cephalothin
Cephalexin Keflex®	Cap 250, 500 mg Drp 100 mg/ml Susp 125, 250 mg/5 ml Tab 1 g	PO 250 mg-1 g q 6 hr	32-39	5-15	0.5-1.0	20-40	85-95	Oral absorption is almost complete; spectrum similar to cefazolin

Continued

Cephalosporins Comparison Chart[a]

DRUG	DOSAGE FORMS	ADULT DOSE	PEAK PLASMA LEVELS (MCG/ML) [b]	PERCENT PROTEIN BOUND	HALF-LIFE (HOURS) NORMAL	HALF-LIFE (HOURS) ANURIC	PERCENT UNCHANGED IN URINE[c]	COMMENTS
Cefamandole Naftate Mandol®	Inj 500 mg, 1, 2 g	IM or IV 500 mg–1 g q 4–8 hr	20–35	67–74	0.7–1.2	11–18	65–85	See monograph
Cefoxitin Sodium Mefoxin®	Inj 1, 2 g	IV 1–2 g q 6–8 hr	22–24	65–80	0.7–1	20	85–90	See monograph
Cefadroxil Duricef® Ultracef®	Cap 500 mg Susp 125, 250, 500 mg/5 ml Tab 1 g	PO 500 mg– 1 g q 12–24 hr	28–33	20	1–2	15–20	90	Spectrum similar to cefazolin
Cefaclor Ceclor®	Cap 250, 500 mg Susp 125, 250 mg/5 ml	PO 250 mg– 1 g q 6–8 hr	25	22–26	0.5–1	2.3–2.8	60–85	Spectrum similar to cefazolin, but includes ampi-cillin-resistant *H. influenzae*
Ceftazidime Fortaz® Various	Inj	IM or IV 1–3 g q 8–12 hr	145	<5	1.5	25–34	70	Broad spectrum with good activity against *Pseudomonas* and *Serratia*. Investigational

Continued

Cephalosporins Comparison Chart[a]

DRUG	DOSAGE FORMS	ADULT DOSE	PEAK PLASMA LEVELS (MCG/ML) [b]	PERCENT PROTEIN BOUND	HALF-LIFE (HOURS) NORMAL	HALF-LIFE (HOURS) ANURIC	PERCENT UNCHANGED IN URINE[c]	COMMENTS
Cefotaxime Sodium Claforan®	Inj 500 mg, 1, 2 g	IM or IV 1–2 g q 6–8 hr	20	30	0.8–1.2	1.4–3.6	20–36	See monograph
Cefuroxime Sodium Zinacef®	Inj 750 mg, 1.5 g	IM or IV 750 mg–1.5 g q 8 hr	40	33	1–1.5	↑	85–95	See monograph
Cefatrizine Briceph® – Bristol	—	PO 250–500 mg q 6 hr	12	58	1.5	?	35–45	Investigational
Moxalactam Disodium Moxam®	Inj 1, 2 g	IM or IV 1–2 g q 8–12 hr	30–53	50	2–3	20–40	60–80	See monograph
Ceftizoxime Sodium Cefizox®	Inj 1, 2 g	IM or IV 1–2 g q 8–12 hr	36	28	1.7–1.8	24–36	85–95	Spectrum similar to cefotaxime

Continued

Cephalosporins Comparison Chart[a]

DRUG	DOSAGE FORMS	ADULT DOSE	PEAK PLASMA LEVELS (MCG/ML) [b]	PERCENT PROTEIN BOUND	HALF-LIFE (HOURS) NORMAL	HALF-LIFE (HOURS) ANURIC	PERCENT UNCHANGED IN URINE[c]	COMMENTS
Cefonicid Sodium Monocid®	Inj 1 g	IM or IV 500 mg– 2 g/day as a single dose	100	98	3.5–4.5	70	98	Spectrum similar to cefamandole, but less Gram + activity
Cefoperazone Sodium Cefobid®	Inj 1, 2 g	IM or IV 1–2 g q 8–12 hr	75	85–95	1.6–2.1	↑ slight	15–30	See monograph
Ceftriaxone Disodium Rocephin® – Roche	Inj	IM or IV 500 mg–2 g/day as a single dose	145	83–96	6.5–8.6	↑	60–65	See monograph; investigational

a. From references 18, 82–86, 88–95, 103, 105, 109–121.

b. Represents peak plasma level after PO or IM 1 g dose in normal adults.

c. Represents amount collected over 8–12 hr period after a parenteral dose, except for ceftizoxime, cefonicid and ceftazidime which are based on a 24 hr collection period and ceftriaxone, which is based on a 48 hr collection period. Those agents with less than 70% urinary recovery are either poorly absorbed (cephaloglycin and cefatrizine), extensively metabolized to less active compounds via desacetylation (cephalothin, cephapirin and cefotaxime), or exhibit extensive biliary elimination (cefoperazone, ceftriaxone and moxalactam).

8:12.08 CHLORAMPHENICOL

General References: 18, 122

Chloramphenicol and Salts

Chloromycetin®,
Various

Pharmacology. A broad-spectrum bacteriostatic antibiotic particularly useful against ampicillin-resistant *Haemophilus influenzae,* salmonella and most anaerobic organisms. Inhibits protein synthesis by binding the 50S ribosomal subunit; may be bactericidal against some bacteria. Resistance occurs due to impermeability of the cell wall or bacterial elaboration of an R-factor mediated acetyltransferase.

Administration and Adult Dose. PO or IV 25–100 mg/kg/day depending on severity, location and organism; divide into 4 doses. **IM not recommended.**

Dosage Individualization. Reduce dose with impaired liver function as guided by plasma levels; no alteration necessary in impaired renal function.[18,123,124]

Pediatric Dose. PO or IV (newborn to 2 weeks) 25 mg/kg/day in 1–4 divided doses; (over 2 weeks) 50 mg/kg/day in 4 divided doses; may double dose for a short time in severe infections. These regimens produce unpredictable levels and plasma level monitoring is recommended.[125-128] **IM not recommended.**

Dosage Forms. **Cap** (as base) 50, 100, 250 mg; **Susp** (as palmitate) 30 mg/ml; **Inj** (as sodium succinate) 250 mg/ml, 1 g (100 mg/ml when reconstituted); **Ophth Oint** 10 mg/g; **Ophth Soln** 5 mg/ml; **Otic Soln** 5 mg/ml; **Top Crm** 10 mg/g (expressed as chloramphenicol base).

Patient Instructions. This drug should be taken with a full glass of water on an empty stomach (1 hr before or 2 hr after meals) for best absorption. Sore throat, fever or oral lesions may be an early sign of a severe, but rare, blood disorder and should be reported immediately.

Pharmacokinetics and Biopharmaceutics. *Plasma Levels.* Levels over 25 mcg/ml are associated with bone marrow depression; over 50–100 mcg/ml with gray syndrome. See Adverse Reactions.

Fate. Well absorbed orally (90–100%), with peak plasma levels averaging 12 mcg/ml after administration of 1 g to normal adults. Suspension (palmitate ester) must be hydrolyzed before absorption; in newborns, infants and children, hydrolysis may be inadequate and absorption delayed and unreliable.[129] 1 g IV produces levels of 5–12 mcg/ml 1 hr after administration to normal adults. In infants and young children, hydrolysis of succinate to the active form may be slow and incomplete.[127] IM administration may produce plasma levels of active drug which are 50% lower than the equivalent oral dose and is therefore not recommended for treating severe infections. The drug attains therapeutic levels in most body cavities, the eye and CSF; it is 50% plasma protein bound; V_d is about 1 L/kg.[130] 90% of an oral dose is eliminated by glucuronidation in the liver followed by excretion in the urine; the remainder is excreted in the urine unchanged.[130] The rate of glucuronidation and renal elimination is greatly reduced in neonates.[129] 6.5–80% of succinate may be excreted unhydrolyzed.[123,127] Urine concentrations may be inadequate to treat UTI, especially in patients with moderately to severely impaired renal function.[131] A small amount (2–4%) of a dose appears in the bile and feces, mostly as the glucuronide.

$t_{1/2}$. 1.5-3 hr in healthy adults; 3.2-4.3 hr in anuria.[124] Extremely prolonged and variable in neonates, infants and young children.[125-127,129] Unpredictable in patients with impaired liver function. Some normal patients and patients with impaired renal function exhibit impaired free drug elimination.[123,130,132]

Adverse Reactions. Plasma levels greater than 25 mcg/ml frequently produce reversible bone marrow depression[18,123] with reticulocytopenia, decreased hemoglobin, increased serum iron and iron-binding globulin saturation, thrombocytopenia and mild leukopenia. The drug inhibits iron uptake by bone marrow and anemic patients do not respond to iron or vitamin B_{12} therapy while receiving chloramphenicol.[134] This anemia most often follows parenteral therapy, large doses, long duration of therapy or impaired drug elimination. Complete recovery usually occurs within 1-2 weeks after drug discontinuation.[128,133] Aplastic anemia is rare (1/40,000-1/100,000), but generally fatal. It is not dose-related and can occur long after a short course of oral or parenteral therapy.[18,122] Fatal cardiovascular-respiratory collapse (gray syndrome) may develop in neonates given excessive doses. This syndrome is associated with plasma levels above 50-100 mcg/ml.[129] A similar syndrome has been reported in children and adults given large overdoses.[18,123]

Contraindications. Trivial infections; uses other than those for which it is indicated (eg, colds, influenza, infections of the throat); prophylactic use.

Precautions. Pregnancy; lactation. Use with caution in patients with liver disease (especially cirrhosis, ascites and jaundice), pre-existing hematologic disorders or patients receiving other bone marrow depressants. May cause hemolytic episodes in patients with G6PD deficiency; observe dosing recommendations closely in neonates and infants. See Drug Interactions and Drug-Induced Blood Dyscrasias chapters.

Parameters to Monitor. CBC, with platelet and reticulocyte counts before and frequently during therapy; serum iron and iron-binding globulin saturation may also be useful. Liver and renal function tests before and occasionally during therapy.

8:12.12 ERYTHROMYCINS

General References: 18, 135-138

Erythromycin and Salts   Various

Pharmacology. A bacteriostatic macrolide antibiotic with a spectrum similar to penicillin G; also active against *Mycoplasma pneumoniae* and *Legionella pneumophila*.[139] Acts by binding to the 50S ribosomal subunit, inhibiting protein synthesis. Gram-positive organisms develop resistance via R-factor mediated alteration of the binding site. Gram-negative organisms are resistant due to cell wall impermeability.

Administration and Adult Dose. See Erythromycins Comparison Chart.

Dosage Individualization. Dosage adjustment is probably unnecessary in renal impairment.[124]

Pediatric Dose. See Erythromycins Comparison Chart

Dosage Forms. See Erythromycins Comparison Chart.

Patient Instructions. This drug should be taken with a full glass of water on an empty stomach (1 hr before or 2 hr after meals) for optimum absorption; refrigerate suspension and suppositories.

Pharmacokinetics and Biopharmaceutics. *Fate.* Oral absorption varies widely with the salt and dosage form (see Erythromycins Comparison Chart), with peak plasma concentrations occurring anywhere from 30 min (suspension) to 4 hr (coated tablet) after administration. However, enteric-coated erythromycin base tablets, stearate tablets and estolate capsules produce equivalent erythromycin plasma levels when administered to fasting subjects. Food or restricted water intake (ie, 20 ml or less) with a dose dramatically lowers the absorption of the stearate form only.[136] V_d is 0.5–0.6 L/kg;[138] 75–90% plasma protein bound.[140] Widely distributed into most tissues, cavities and body fluids except the brain and CSF (even with meningeal inflammation). Partially metabolized in the liver; excreted primarily as unchanged erythromycin with high concentrations in the bile and feces. Only 12–15% of IV dose is excreted unchanged in urine.[18,138]

$t_{1/2}$. About 1–1.5 hr; 5–6 hr in anuric patients, based on minimal data.[18,138]

Adverse Reactions. Occasional GI distress. IM form is very painful, despite local anesthetic (butamben) in product, and may produce sterile abscesses. IV administration frequently produces pain, venous irritation and phlebitis. Rare, but potentially serious, reversible intrahepatic cholestatic jaundice is seen with the estolate and ethylsuccinate forms, usually in adults after 10–14 days of therapy, although it may occur after the first dose if there is a history of previous use. Prodrome includes malaise, nausea, vomiting, fever and abdominal pain (which may be severe and misdiagnosed as acute surgical abdomen). Symptoms resolve in 1–2 weeks, while serum enzymes return to normal over several months.[18,135-137] Transient tinnitus and deafness occur rarely.[141]

Contraindications. IM form contraindicated in patients with hypersensitivity to local anesthetics of the para-aminobenzoic acid type (eg, procaine); hepatic dysfunction (estolate and ethylsuccinate forms).

Precautions. Pregnancy. Use with caution in patients with liver disease (impaired excretion).

Parameters to Monitor. Liver function tests in patients who experience prodromal symptoms (see Adverse Reactions) while receiving estolate or ethylsuccinate form; check daily for vein irritation and phlebitis in patients receiving IV forms.

Notes. Avoid injectable forms if at all possible. Erythromycin is more active in an alkaline environment.[18]

Erythromycins Comparison Chart

DRUG	DOSAGE FORMS	ADULT DOSE	PEDIATRIC DOSE[a]	COMMENTS[b]
Erythromycin Base E-Mycin® Ery-Tab® Ilotycin® Various	EC Cap (beads) 250 mg EC Tab 250, 333, 500 mg Tab (buffered) 250, 500 mg Supp 125 mg	PO 250–500 mg q 6 hr, to maximum of 4 g/day	PO 30–50 mg/kg/day in 4 divided doses; may double if severe infection	Food interferes with absorption except for enteric coated products; highly susceptible to gastric acid hydrolysis; rectal suppository is very irritating—avoid use
Erythromycin Estolate Ilosone®	Cap 125, 250 mg Drp 100 mg/ml Susp 125, 250 mg/5 ml (reconstituted) Chew Tab 125, 250 mg Tab 500 mg	PO 250–500 mg q 6 hr, to maximum of 4 g/day	PO 30–50 mg/kg/day in 4 divided doses	PO well absorbed; unaffected by food and highly resistant to gastric acid hydrolysis; absorbed as propionate ester which predominates in plasma (8:1) and may be less active;[139] rare intrahepatic cholestatic jaundice
Erythromycin Ethylsuccinate E.E.S® Pediamycin® Various	Drp 40 mg/ml Susp 200, 400 mg/5 ml Chew Tab 200 mg Tab (coated) 400 mg Inj (IM only) 50 mg/ml[c]	PO 400 mg q 6 hr, to maximum of 4 g/day; Deep IM 100 mg q 4–8 hr or 5–8 mg/kg/day in divided doses	PO 30–50 mg/kg/day in 4 divided doses; may double if severe infection; IM (over 13.6 kg) 50 mg q 4–6 hr or 12 mg/kg/day in divided doses	Absorbed better than base; intermediate susceptibility to gastric acid hydrolysis. Absorbed as ester which predominates in plasma (3:1) and may be less active. IM very painful—avoid use. Rare intrahepatic cholestatic jaundice

Continued

Erythromycins Comparison Chart

DRUG	DOSAGE FORMS	ADULT DOSE	PEDIATRIC DOSE[a]	COMMENTS[b]
Erythromycin Gluceptate Ilotycin®	Inj (IV only) 250, 500 mg, 1 g	IV 15–20 mg/kg/day in 4 divided doses, to maximum of 4 g/day	IV same as adult dose in 2–4 divided doses; may double in severe infection	Painful; phlebitis frequent; avoid use if possible. Infuse over at least 30 min
Erythromycin Lactobionate Erythrocin®	Inj (IV only) 500 mg, 1 g			
Erythromycin Stearate Erythrocin® Various	Tab (film coated) 125, 250, 500 mg	PO 250–500 mg q 6 hr, to maximum of 4 g/day	PO 30–50 mg/kg/day in 4 divided doses; may double in severe infection	Absorption about equal to ethylsuccinate, although food interferes significantly with absorption. Hydrolyzed to free base before absorption

a. In newborns, limited data are available for erythromycin estolate only, suggesting an oral dose of 40 mg/kg/day in 2–4 divided doses.[137]

b. Despite differences in oral absorption, no clinical studies have shown any salt to be clearly superior in any particular therapeutic use.

c. Contains 2% butamben (butyl aminobenzoate) as a local anesthetic.

8:12.16 THE PENICILLINS

General References: 18, 142–145

Amoxicillin Sodium

Amoxil®, Larotid®, Polymox®

Amoxicillin differs from ampicillin in the presence of a hydroxyl group on the amino side chain. It has activity essentially identical to ampicillin. However, it is completely absorbed, with about 85% bioavailability due to a small first-pass effect. Plasma levels are greater than those seen after equivalent doses of ampicillin; post-absorptive pharmacokinetics are identical to ampicillin. Adverse effects are similar to ampicillin, although diarrhea is much less frequent with amoxicillin. Oral dosage for adults is 250–500 mg q 8 hr, to maximum of 6 g/day (1 g q 4 hr); for children 20–40 mg/kg/day orally in 3 equally divided doses q 8 hr.[146,147] See Ampicillin Derivatives Comparison Chart.

Ampicillin

Various

Pharmacology.   A semisynthetic penicillin having greater activity than penicillin G against Gram-negative organisms; generally less active against Gram-positive organisms, except enterococci. Mechanism of action similar to penicillin G. Inactivated by staphylococcal β-lactamase, as well as β-lactamase producing *H. influenzae*.

Administration and Adult Dose.   **PO for mild to moderate infections** 250–500 mg q 6 hr. **IM or IV for mild to moderate infections** 250–500 mg q 6 hr. **IM or IV for severe infections** (eg, meningitis) 150–200 mg/kg/day to maximum of 8–14 g in 6–8 divided doses. **PO for uncomplicated gonorrhea** 3.5 g taken simultaneously with 1 g probenecid.

Dosage Individualization.   Except when using large doses for severe infections, dosage adjustment is necessary only with Cl_{cr} less than 10–15 ml/min, whereupon the dosing interval may be doubled.[145] Some sources recommend more careful adjustment, however.[148] No adjustment necessary for liver disease.[149]

Pediatric Dose.   **PO** (under 20 kg) 50–100 mg/kg/day in divided doses; **PO** (over 20 kg) or **IV** (over 40 kg) generally same as adult, to maximum of 400 mg/kg/day.

Dosage Forms.   **Cap** 250, 500 mg; **Drp** 100 mg/ml (reconstituted): **Susp** 125, 250, 500 mg/5 ml (reconstituted); **Chew Tab** 125 mg; **Inj** 125, 250, 500 mg, 1, 2, 2.5, 4 g. Strengths are expressed as ampicillin equivalent.

Patient Instructions.   This drug should be taken with a full glass of water on an empty stomach (1 hr before or 2 hr after meals) for best absorption. Refrigerate suspension after reconstitution and discard after 14 days.

Pharmacokinetics and Biopharmaceutics.   *Fate.*   Oral forms are 20–70% (average 50) absorbed in the fasting state; food may significantly delay oral absorption.[142] A 500 mg dose produces a peak of about 2–6 mcg/ml 1-2 hr after oral administration to normal adults.[150-152] 500 mg IM produces a peak of 8 mcg/ml at 1 hr.[148] V_d is about 0.3 L/kg in healthy adults and 0.85 L/kg in cirrhotic adults;[149] 15-25% plasma protein bound.[145] The drug attains therapeutic levels in joints, serosal cavities, and very high levels in the biliary tree (without obstruction), kidney tissue and urine (unless severe renal impairment); therapeutic CSF levels only in the presence of meningitis.[143,144] Approximately 90% of parenteral dose is excreted unchanged in the urine within 24 hr.[143,148]

$t_{1/2}$.   About 1.1-1.3 hr;[143] 2 hr in neonates;[153] 8-20 hr in anuric patients;[143,148] may increase to 1.9 hr in chronic liver disease.[149]

Adverse Reactions. Skin rashes are frequent (7-10%); many of these are erythematous, maculopapular rashes which are 2-3 times more frequent in patients with hyperuricemia taking allopurinol and extremely frequent (50-100%) in patients with mononucleosis and certain lymphomas; many of these rashes are suspected to be nonallergic in nature.[154] Nausea and vomiting occasionally occur after oral administration; diarrhea is frequent and may be preventable with lactobacillus (Lactinex®) pretreatment.[155] Very rarely associated with pseudomembranous colitis[156] and interstitial nephritis.[157] Very large doses can produce hypokalemic metabolic alkalosis[158] or classic penicillin encephalopathy.[18,144] See Penicillin G.

Contraindications. See Penicillin G.

Precautions. Pregnancy. Use caution in patients with impaired renal function, or a history of penicillin or cephalosporin hypersensitivity. See Drug Interactions chapter.

Parameters to Monitor. Initial and periodic renal function tests with prolonged use or high doses.

Notes. Since IV preparation is very unstable in D5W, use within 1 hr of admixture; stable for 24 hr in sterile water or normal saline. Oral suspension stable for 7 days at room temperature and 14 days under refrigeration. See Ampicillin Derivatives Comparison Chart on page 296.

Azlocillin   Azlin®

Azlocillin is a ureidopenicillin with a spectrum similar to mezlocillin and piperacillin. It is less active than the latter agents against most enterobacteracae and anaerobes, but is more active against *Pseudomonas aeruginosa*. Its primary use is in *Pseudomonas* infections, generally with an aminoglycoside for severe infections. Azlocillin is pharmacokinetically similar to mezlocillin and piperacillin, but it exhibits greater dose-dependent kinetics. The half-life is about 1 hour, increasing to 5.9 hours with a Cl_{cr} of less than 10 ml/min. Adverse reactions are similar to mezlocillin and the sodium content is 2.17 mEq/g. Dosage is IV for serious infections 200-300 mg/kg/day given in 4-6 divided doses (usually 3 g q 4 hr) to a maximum of 350 mg/kg/day or 4 g q 4 hr in life-threatening infections. Dosage should be decreased in renal impairment; with a dose of 3 g q 12 hr in anuria. Supplied as Inj 2, 3, 4 g.

Ampicillin Derivatives Comparison Chart

DRUG	DOSAGE FORMS	ADULT DOSE	PEAK PLASMA LEVELS[a] (MCG/ML)	PERCENT BIOAVAILABILITY[b]	PERCENT GI SIDE EFFECTS[c]	COMMENTS
Ampicillin Various **Ampicillin Sodium** Various	Cap 250, 500 mg Chew Tab 125 mg Drp 100 mg/ml (reconstituted) Susp 125, 250, 500 mg/5 ml (reconstituted) Inj 125, 250, 500 mg, 1, 2, 2.5, 4 g	PO 250-500 mg q 6 hr; IM or IV 0.25- 2 g q 6 hr, to maximum of 8- 14 g/day	2-6	30-70	10-20	Recent bioavailability studies have tended to support the higher end of the range
Amoxicillin Amoxil® Larotid® Polymox®	Cap 250, 500 mg Drp 50 mg/ml (reconstituted) Susp 125, 250 mg/5 ml (recon- stituted) Inj (investigational)	PO 250-500 mg q 8 hr, to maximum of 6 g/day	6-8	80-90	4-5	In vitro activity essentially equivalent to ampicillin; small volumes of water lower bioavailability, while food has little effect
Bacampicillin Hydrochloride Spectrobid®	Tab 400 mg (278 mg ampicillin) Susp 125 mg/5 ml (reconstituted)	PO 400-800 mg q 12 hr; PO for gonorrhea 1.6 g plus probenecid 1 g	10-15	80-90	3-6	Essentially equivalent to amoxicillin in efficacy & toxicity; inactive ester of ampi- cillin which is rapidly hydrolyzed in vivo

Continued

Ampicillin Derivatives Comparison Chart

DRUG	DOSAGE FORMS	ADULT DOSE	PEAK PLASMA LEVELS[a] (MCG/ML)	PERCENT BIOAVAILABILITY[b]	PERCENT GI SIDE EFFECTS[c]	COMMENTS
Cyclacillin® Cyclapen®	Susp 125, 250 mg/5 ml (reconstituted) Tab 250, 500 mg	PO 250-500 mg q 6 hr	10-15	50-70	5-10	Very rapidly eliminated ($t_{1/2}$ = 0.5-0.6 hr); inferior in vitro activity
Hetacillin® Versapen® **Hetacillin Potassium** Versapen-K®	Cap (as potassium) 225, 450 mg Drp 112.5 mg/ml (reconstituted) Susp 112.5, 225 mg/5 ml (reconstituted)	PO 225-450 mg q 6 hr; IM or IV 225-450 mg q 6 hr	2-6	50	–	Acetone ester of ampicillin; rapidly hydrolyzed to ampicillin; essentially equivalent to ampicillin

a. Represents peak plasma level after a 500 mg (ampicillin equivalent) oral dose.

b. Maximum theoretical bioavailability is about 90% (ie, about 10% is removed by the liver during the first pass).[151]

c. Diarrhea is the most frequent GI side effect with ampicillin; upper GI side effects (eg, nausea, vomiting, dyspepsia) are less common and equally frequent with ampicillin, amoxicillin and bacampicillin.[142,159,160]

Carbenicillin Disodium   Geopen®, Pyopen®
Carbenicillin Indanyl Sodium   Geocillin®

Pharmacology. A broad-spectrum semisynthetic penicillin with activity similar to ampicillin and increased activity against *Pseudomonas aeruginosa* and indole-positive *Proteus* sp. Synergistic in vitro with aminoglycosides against *Pseudomonas aeruginosa;* used almost exclusively in combination with an aminoglycoside when used for infections outside the urinary tract.

Administration and Adult Dose. PO for UTI due to *Escherichia coli*, *Proteus* sp. and *Enterobacter* sp. (expressed as carbenicillin base) 382-764 mg qid; **PO for UTI** due to *Pseudomonas aeruginosa* and enterococci 764 mg qid. **IV for serious infections outside the urinary tract** due to *Pseudomonas aeruginosa* or anaerobic organisms 400-500 mg/kg/day (30-40 g/day) in divided doses or by continuous infusion; **IV for serious infections outside the urinary tract** due to *Proteus* sp. of *Escherichia coli* 300-400 mg/kg/day (20-30 g/day) in divided doses or by continuous infusion; **IV for serious UTI** due to *Escherichia coli*, *Proteus* sp., *Enterobacter* sp., enterococci or *Pseudomonas aeruginosa* 200 mg/kg/day by continuous infusion. **IM or IV for uncomplicated UTI** 1-2 g q 6 hr. **IM maximum** dose is 40 g/day with not more than 2 g per injection.

Dosage Individualization. Carefully adjust dose in renal impairment or simultaneous renal and hepatic impairment. Recommendations vary considerably; consult literature.[124,161,162] In anuria give no more than 2 g q 8-12 hr after a normal first dose; when liver function is also impaired give only 2 g q 24 hr.

Pediatric Dose. IM or IV for serious infections outside the urinary tract (neonates under 2 kg) 100 mg/kg initially, then 75 mg/kg q 8 hr during first week of life; thereafter, 100 mg/kg q 6 hr. **IM or IV for serious infections outside the urinary tract** (neonates over 2 kg) 100 mg/kg initially, then 75 mg/kg q 6 hr during the first 3 days of life; thereafter 100 mg/kg q 6 hr; **IV for serious infections outside the urinary tract** (infants and children) same mg/kg dose as adult. **IM or IV for UTI** due to *Ps. aeruginosa*, *Enterobacter* sp. or enterococci (infants and children) 50-200 mg/kg/day in divided doses q 4-6 hr; **IM or IV for UTI** due to *Proteus* sp. or *E. coli* (infants and children) 50-100 mg/kg/day in divided doses q 4-6 hr; **PO not recommended.**

Dosage Forms. **Tab** (as indanyl sodium ester) 500 mg (382 mg of carbenicillin base equivalent); **Inj** (as disodium salt) 1, 2, 5, 10 g.

Patient Instructions. Tablets must be taken with a full glass of water on an empty stomach (1 hr before or 2 hr after meals) for best absorption.

Pharmacokinetics and Biopharmaceutics. *Fate.* 30-50% absorbed orally, primarily as indanyl ester which is rapidly hydrolyzed in the blood to produce peak plasma carbenicillin concentrations of approximately 6 mcg/ml at 1 hr after a 382 mg dose administered to normal fasting adults.[163] 1 g IM produces a peak concentration of approximately 15-20 mcg/ml 1 hr after administration.[163] IV doses produce varying levels depending on mode of administration;[145] however, an infusion of 2 g over 30 min produces a plasma concentration of approximately 175 mcg/ml. V_d is about 0.15-0.2 L/kg;[145] about 50% bound to plasma proteins.[143,145,164] Widely distributed in body tissues, cavities and fluids, including significant biliary concentrations, CSF levels 10-20% of plasma level with normal meninges.[143] Virtually 100% of the absorbed dose is excreted unchanged in the urine within 24 hr,[164] producing extremely high urine concentrations after usual doses in patients with normal renal function.

t₁/₂. Approximately 1 hr;[151,164] 10–15 hr in patients with impaired renal function; 20 hr or longer in patients with simultaneous renal and hepatic failure;[143] 1.5–4 hr in neonates (less than 2 weeks);[145] 4–5 hr in premature newborns.[145]

Adverse Reactions. Oral use frequently produces dose-related nausea, diarrhea and occasional flatulence.[163] IV administration may cause pain and phlebitis. Neurotoxicity, manifested by confusion, drowsiness and myoclonus which may progress to seizures; coma has been reported, especially with large parenteral doses in the presence of renal disease. Coagulation abnormalities and bleeding occur, especially with large parenteral doses in the presence of renal disease; however, this is also reported in patients with normal renal function receiving therapeutic doses. Interference with platelet function or a heparin-like anticoagulant effect are possible mechanisms.[18,144,166] Occasionally, asymptomatic elevations of serum transaminases with rare symptomatic anicteric hepatitis occur, which rapidly reverse after drug discontinuation and promptly return upon rechallenge.[144] Hypokalemic metabolic alkalosis has been reported, especially with larger doses.[144,157] High sodium content of parenteral carbenicillin may produce fluid overload and pulmonary edema, especially in patients with impaired cardiac function. Occasionally mild leukopenia is reported.

Contraindications. Tablets in patients with severely impaired renal function (Cl_cr less than 15 ml/min) due to inadequate urinary concentrations.[165] See Penicillin G.

Precautions. Pregnancy. Use caution in patients with history of penicillin or cephalosporin hypersensitivity, impaired renal function or simultaneously impaired renal and hepatic function, impaired cardiac function or pre-existing seizure disorder. Use tablets with caution in pediatric age group. See Drug Interactions chapter.

Parameters to Monitor. Initial renal function tests; during prolonged therapy, periodic assessment of renal, hepatic and hematopoietic function and serum electrolytes.

Notes. Tablets must be used only for UTI due to susceptible strains of *E. coli, Proteus* sp., *Ps. aeruginosa, Enterobacter* sp. and enterococci which are resistant to more conventional therapy. Resistance may develop rapidly during therapy; use maximum doses and check sensitivity of organism at regular intervals. Combination with gentamicin in the treatment of *Ps. aeruginosa* infections may delay emergence of resistance and be synergistic in effect, although its exact significance has not been assessed.[144] Avoid admixture of aminoglycosides and carbenicillin in the same IV solution, as this results in the slow inactivation of the aminoglycoside.[167] Inactivation may also occur in vivo in patients with severe renal impairment. Sodium content is 5.2–6.5 mEq/g.

Cloxacillin Sodium
Cloxapen®, Tegopen®

Pharmacology. A narrow-spectrum semisynthetic penicillin resistant to staphylococcal penicillinase. Otherwise, Gram-positive activity is less than other penicillins and Gram-negative activity is negligible.

Administration and Adult Dose. PO 250–500 mg q 6 hr; 2–4 times higher doses may be used for severe infections (but a parenteral anti-staphylococcal agent is preferred in such cases).

Dosage Individualization. Dosage is unaltered in patients with renal impairment.[124]

Pediatric Dose. (Infants) no data. PO (under 20 kg) 50–100 mg/kg/day in 4 divided doses; 2–4 times higher doses may be used in severe infections. PO (over 20 kg) same as adult dose.

Dosage Forms. Cap 250, 500 mg; Soln 125 mg/5 ml (reconstituted).

Patient Instructions. Oral forms should be taken with a full glass of water on an empty stomach (1 hr before or 2 hr after meals) for best absorption; refrigerate solution.

Pharmacokinetics and Biopharmaceutics. Fate. 50% absorbed orally, with peak of 7–14 mcg/ml at 1 hr after administration of a 500 mg dose.[145] V_d is about 0.14 L/kg.[168] Significant metabolism; 75% of absorbed drug is excreted unchanged in the urine.[168]

$t_{1/2}$. 30 min;[168] 50 min with severe renal impairment.[124]

Adverse Reactions. Allergic reactions are frequent and similar to those occurring with oral penicillin G; cross-reactive with other penicillins. Neurotoxicity (see Penicillin G) may occur with excessive doses, although case reports are lacking.

Contraindications. See Penicillin G.

Precautions. Use caution in patients with a history of penicillin or cephalosporin hypersensitivity reactions. See Drug Interactions chapter.

Notes. For treatment of penicillin G-resistant staphylococcal infections only; see Antistaphylococcal Penicillins Comparison Chart.

Antistaphylococcal Penicillins Comparison Chart

DRUG	DOSAGE FORMS	ADULT DOSE	PERCENT ORAL ABSORPTION[a]	PERCENT PROTEIN BINDING	HALF-LIFE (HOURS) NORMAL	HALF-LIFE (HOURS) ANURIC[b]	PERCENT UNCHANGED IN URINE[c]
Cloxacillin Sodium Cloxapen® Tegopen®	Cap 250, 500 mg Soln 125 mg/5 ml (reconstituted)	PO 250-500 mg q 6 hr; may double in severe infection	50	94	0.5	0.8	75
Dicloxacillin Sodium Dynapen® Various	Cap 125, 250, 500 mg Susp 62.5 mg/5 ml (reconstituted)	PO 250-500 mg q 6 hr; may double in severe infection	74	96	0.7-0.8	1-2	70
Methicillin[d] Sodium Staphcillin® Various	Inj 1, 4, 6 g	IM or IV 1 g q 4-6 hr; may give double or more IV dose in severe infection	–	30-50	0.4-0.5	4	70-75
Nafcillin Sodium Unipen®	Cap 250 mg Soln 250 mg/5 ml (reconstituted) Tab 500 mg Inj 500 mg-1, 2, 4 g	PO 250 mg-1 g q 4-6 hr; IM 500 mg q 4-6 hr; IV 500 mg-1 g q 4 hr	50	90	0.5-1	1.2	30-40[e]

Continued

Antistaphylococcal Penicillins Comparison Chart

DRUG	DOSAGE FORMS	ADULT DOSE	PERCENT ORAL ABSORPTION[a]	PERCENT PROTEIN BINDING	HALF-LIFE (HOURS) NORMAL	HALF-LIFE (HOURS) ANURIC[b]	PERCENT UNCHANGED IN URINE[c]
Oxacillin Sodium Bactocil® Prostaphlin®	Cap 250, 500 mg; Soln 250 mg/5 ml (reconstituted) Inj 250, 500 mg, 1, 2, 4 g	PO 500 mg q 4-6 hr; may double in severe infection; IM or IV 250-500 mg q 4-6 hr; may give double or more IV dose in severe infection	33	90	0.4-0.7	0.5-1	55

a. Some studies indicate much lower values for oral absorption of dicloxacillin and nafcillin. Values shown are the best estimates in the opinion of author.
b. Concomitant renal and hepatic dysfunction can greatly increase half-life with these agents.
c. Represents excretion of unchanged drug in urine after parenteral administration or as percent of absorbed oral dose.
d. Methicillin is associated with a dose-related, apparently allergic, interstitial nephritis which is much more common than with other agents in this chart.
e. Significant biliary excretion with concentrations in bile many times plasma concentrations.

Mezlocillin

Mezlin®

Mezlocillin is a ureidopenicillin with activity similar to carbenicillin, except that it is more active against *Streptococcus faecalis* (similar to ampicillin), indole positive *Proteus, Klebsiella* sp., *Enterobacter* sp. and *Serratia* sp. Its activity against *Pseudomonas aeruginosa* is greater than carbenicillin, similar to ticarcillin. Although it has been used alone in the treatment of *Pseudomonas* infections, there is no evidence that it is better than carbenicillin or ticarcillin as a first-line drug. It has a shorter half-life (1 hr) than carbenicillin, but the half-life is increased little in renal failure until Cl_{cr} falls below 10 ml/min; 60% is excreted in the urine. Adverse reactions are similar to carbenicillin, although it has a much lower sodium load (1.85 mEq/g). Dosage for adults is 200–300 mg/kg/day in 4–6 divided doses; for Cl_{cr} of 10–30 ml/min, reduce dose to 3 g q 4 hr; for Cl_{cr} less than 10 ml/min, use 2 g q 6 hr. Supplied as Inj 1, 2, 3, 4 g vials.[169]

Penicillin G Benzathine

Bicillin® L-A, Permapen®

Pharmacology. A very insoluble suspension of benzathine and penicillin G producing low plasma penicillin levels which limit its use to infections caused by highly susceptible organisms. See Penicillin G.

Administration and Adult Dose. IM only for group A streptococcal upper respiratory infection 1,200,000 U as a single injection. IM for prophylaxis of post-streptococcal rheumatic fever or glomerulonephritis 1,200,000 U once a month or 600,000 U twice a month. IM for early syphilis (less than a year in duration) 2,400,000 U as a single injection. IM for syphilis of more than a year in duration 2,400,000 U weekly for 3 successive weeks,[170] although the adequacy of this regimen has been questioned.[171]

Pediatric Dose. IM only for group A streptococcal upper respiratory infection (under 27 kg) 300,000–600,000 U; (over 27 kg) 900,000 U as a single injection. IM for the prophylaxis of post-streptococcal rheumatic fever or glomerulonephritis 1,200,000 U once a month or 600,000 U twice a month. IM for congenital syphilis with normal CSF (under 2 yr) 50,000 U/kg as a single injection.

Dosage Forms. Inj (IM only) 300,000, 600,000 U/ml.

Pharmacokinetics and Biopharmaceutics. *Fate.* Very slowly absorbed from the injection site; hydrolyzed in the bloodstream to produce penicillin G levels of approximately 30 ng/ml which are maintained for 21–28 days after a 2,400,000 U injection in adults.[172] Distribution and elimination follow the same patterns as penicillin G.[144]

Adverse Reactions. The Jarisch-Herxheimer reaction, an acute febrile reaction presumably due to the release of endotoxin from killed treponemes, frequently occurs in patients treated for early syphilis. The reaction occurs within 24 hr of injection and subsides within 24 hr. Inadvertent intravenous administration of the drug has resulted in cardiac arrest and death.

Contraindications. See Penicillin G.

Precautions. Use caution in patients with history of penicillin or cephalosporin hypersensitivity reaction. Hypersensitivity reactions may be prolonged due to slow drug absorption.

Penicillin G Procaine   Various

Pharmacology.   A relatively insoluble suspension of procaine and penicillin G that dissolves slowly at the site of injection providing prolonged low plasma penicillin levels. See Penicillin G.

Administration and Adult Dose. IM only for early syphilis 600,000 U/day for 8 days. IM for syphilis of more than a year in duration 600,000 U/day for 15 days.[170] IM for uncomplicated gonorrhea 4,800,000 U in at least 2 divided doses injected at different sites during one visit, together with 1 g probenecid orally. IM for gonococcal arthritis 600,000 U q 12 hr for up to 10 days.[173] IM for uncomplicated pneumococcal pneumonia 600,000–1,200,000 U/day.[174]

Pediatric Dose. IM only for congenital syphilis with abnormal CSF, 50,000 U/kg/day for a minimum of 10 days. IM for uncomplicated gonorrhea (less than 45 kg) 100,000 U/kg/day in 2 divided doses, with 25 mg/kg probenecid orally (maximum 1 g).[175]

Dosage Forms.   Inj (IM only) 300,000, 500,000, 600,000 U/ml.

Pharmacokinetics and Biopharmaceutics. *Fate.* Absorbed slowly from the injection site. Hydrolyzed in the plasma to produce peak penicillin G levels of approximately 0.9 mcg/ml 2 hr after the administration of 300,000 U to normal adults; plasma levels fall to 0.13 mcg/ml after 24 hr. Distribution and elimination follow the same patterns as penicillin G.[144]

Adverse Reactions. Similar to penicillin G benzathine. Acute psychotic reactions (known as "pseudoanaphylactic" reactions) and characterized by acute anxiety, hallucinations, confusion and palpitations with or without cardiovascular collapse are reported occasionally. The cause is unknown, although some cases have been documented as being associated with inadvertent IV administration.[176,177] Procaine may also cause some allergic reactions.

Contraindications. See Penicillin G.

Precautions.   Use caution in patients with history of penicillin or cephalosporin hypersensitivity reactions.

Penicillin G Salts   Various

Pharmacology. A β-lactam antibiotic with activity against most Gram-positive organisms and some Gram-negative organisms, notably *Neisseria* sp. Acts by interfering with late stages of bacterial cell wall synthesis; resistance is primarily due to bacterial elaboration of β-lactamases, although some organisms have impermeable outer cell wall layers.

Administration and Adult Dose. PO 250–500 mg (400,000–800,000 U) q 6 hr for mild to moderate infections. IV doses vary, depending on organism, severity and location; consult literature for dose in specific indications.[144] IM not recommended (very painful); use benzathine or procaine salt form as indicated.

Dosage Individualization. With usual oral doses no dosage adjustment is required in patients with impaired renal function; however, in treating more severe infections with larger IV doses, careful adjustment is necessary.[142] In anuric patients, give no more than 3,000,000 U/day.[178]

Pediatric Dose. **PO** (under 12 yr) 25,000–90,000 U/kg/day in 3–6 divided doses; **PO** (over 12 yr) same as adult dose. **IV** consult literature.

Dosage Forms. **Susp/Syrup** (as potassium salt) 200,000, 250,000, 400,000 U/5 ml (reconstituted); **Tab** (as potassium salt) 100,000, 200,000, 250,000, 400,000, 500,000, 800,000 U; **Inj** (as potassium salt) 200,000, 500,000, 1,000,000, 5,000,000, 10,000,000, 20,000,000 U; **Inj** (as sodium salt) 5,000,000 U.

Patient Instructions. This (oral) drug should be taken with a full glass of water on an empty stomach (1 hr before or 2 hr after meals) for best absorption; refrigerate solution.

Pharmacokinetics and Biopharmaceutics. *Fate.* Only 15–30% orally absorbed due to its high susceptibility to gastric acid hydrolysis; peak concentrations of 1.5–2.7 mcg/ml occur 0.5–1 hr after administration of 500 mg.[143] Widely distributed in body tissues, fluids and cavities, with biliary levels up to 10 times plasma levels. 30–60% plasma protein bound.[143,145] Penetration into CSF is poor, even with inflamed meninges; however, large parenteral doses (greater than 20,000,000 U/day) adequately treat meningitis due to susceptible organisms.[143,144] 80–85% of absorbed dose is excreted unchanged in the urine.[145]

$t_{1/2}$. 30–40 min; 7–10 hr in patients with renal failure;[145] 20–30 hr in patients with hepatic and renal failure.[143]

Adverse Reactions. Occasional nausea or diarrhea after usual oral dosages. CNS toxicity may occur with massive IV doses (60,000,000–100,000,000 U/day) or excessive doses in combination with impaired renal function (usually greater than 10,000,000–20,000,000 U/day in anuric patients); characterized by confusion, drowsiness and myoclonus which may progress to convulsions and result in death. Large doses of the sodium salt form may result in hypernatremia and fluid overload with pulmonary edema, especially in patients with impaired renal function or congestive heart failure. Large doses of the potassium salt form may result in hyperkalemia, especially in patients with impaired renal function and with rapid infusions. Occasional positive Coombs' reactions with rare hemolytic anemia have been reported after large IV doses. Interstitial nephritis has been rarely reported following large IV doses.[18,144] Hypersensitivity reactions (primarily rashes) occur with a 5–10% frequency. Most serious hypersensitivity reactions follow injection rather than oral administration.[179]

Contraindications. History of anaphylactic, accelerated (eg, hives) or serum sickness reaction to previous penicillin administration. See Notes.

Precautions. Use caution in patients with a history of penicillin or cephalosporin hypersensitivity reactions, atopic predisposition (eg, asthma), impaired renal function (hence neonates and geriatric patients), impaired cardiac function or pre-existing seizure disorder. See Drug Interactions chapter.

Parameters to Monitor. Initial renal function tests when using high doses. During prolonged high-dose therapy, periodic renal function tests and serum electrolytes.

Notes. 250 mg equals 400,000 U of penicillin G. Penicillin V potassium is preferred to penicillin G potassium for oral administration, due to more complete and reliable absorption.[144,145] Skin testing with penicilloyl-polylysine *and* penicillin G can help determine the likelihood of serious reactions to penicillin in penicillin allergic individuals. However, occasionally a skin-test negative individual may have an anaphylactic reaction to therapeutic doses of penicillin. Desensitization may be attempted (rarely) in patients with life-threatening infections that are likely to be responsive only to penicillin, but this is a dangerous procedure.[18,180,181]

Penicillin V   Various

Pharmacology. A phenoxymethyl derivative of penicillin that is more acid stable than penicillin G. Spectrum and mechanism of action are the same as penicillin G, although penicillin V is 2–4 times less active against sensitive organisms.[18]

Administration and Adult Dose. **PO for mild to moderate infections** 250–500 mg q 6 hr; parenteral penicillin is preferred for more serious infections.

Dosage Individualization. No dosage adjustment is required for patients with impaired renal function with recommended doses.

Pediatric Dose. PO (infants and children under 12 yr) 15–50 mg/kg/day in 3–4 divided doses; (over 12 yr) same as adult dose.

Dosage Forms. **Soln/Susp** 125, 250 mg/5 ml (reconstituted); **Tab** 125, 250, 500 mg.

Patient Instructions. This drug should be taken with a full glass of water on an empty stomach (1 hr before or 2 hr after meals) for best absorption; refrigerate solution after reconstitution.

Pharmacokinetics and Biopharmaceutics. *Fate.* Average oral absorption of potassium salt form is 60%, producing peak plasma levels 2–5 times greater than penicillin G potassium. Probably distributed in the body in a fashion similar to penicillin G, although no data available; 80% plasma protein bound.[143,145] Extensively metabolized (about 50%), with products eliminated primarily in the urine. About 50% of absorbed dose is excreted unchanged.[145]

$t_{1/2}$. 30 min in normal adults;[145] no other data available, although impaired renal function should not greatly prolong half-life unless liver function is simultaneously impaired.

Adverse Reactions. Nausea and diarrhea are infrequent with usual doses. Hypersensitivity reactions similar to those following oral penicillin G occur.

Contraindications. See Penicillin G.

Precautions. Pregnancy. Use caution in patients with history of penicillin or cephalosporin hypersensitivity reaction. See Drug Interactions chapter.

Notes. 250 mg equals approximately 400,000 U of penicillin V base or potassium salt. Potassium salt is more water soluble and probably better absorbed.[145]

Piperacillin Sodium   Pipracil®

Piperacillin is a piperazine penicillin derivative with activity similar to carbenicillin, except that it is more active against *Streptococcus faecalis* (similar to ampicillin), and many Gram-negative bacteria, including

Pseudomonas aeruginosa, Klebsiella sp., *Enterobacter* sp. and *Bacteroides fragilis*. The emergence of resistance during therapy has been observed when piperacillin was used alone in serious infections with *Pseudomonas aeruginosa*. Its pharmacokinetic properties are similar to carbenicillin, although it has a shorter half-life (0.7–1 hr) and greater nonrenal elimination (about 20%). Adverse reactions are similar to carbenicillin, although having a lower sodium content (2 mEq/g) may reduce the risk of sodium overload. Dosage is IV for serious infections in adults 200–300 mg/kg/day in equally divided doses q 4–6 hr. Dosage must be reduced in renal impairment. In anuria may give 4 g q 12 hr. Supplied as Inj 2, 3, 4 g.[169,182-184]

Ticarcillin Disodium   Ticar®

Pharmacology. A semisynthetic penicillin with activity similar to carbenicillin, but 2–4 times as active against *Pseudomonas aeruginosa*, while slightly less active against Gram-positive organisms.

Administration and Adult Dose. IV for serious systemic infections 200–300 mg/kg/day (about 18–24 g/day) in 3–8 divided doses; **IV for complicated UTI** 150–200 mg/kg/day in 4–6 divided doses; **IM or IV for uncomplicated UTI** 50–100 mg/kg/day in divided doses. **IM** maximum dose not more than 2 g per injection.

Dosage Individualization. Carefully adjust dose in renal impairment. In anuria give no more than 2 g q 12 hr after a 3 g loading dose with 3 g after each dialysis; when liver function is also impaired, give only 2 g q 24 hr.

Pediatric Dose. IV for serious systemic infection (neonates under 2 kg) 75 mg/kg q 12 hr for the first week and 75 mg/kg q 8 hr thereafter; (neonates over 2 kg) 75 mg/kg q 8 hr for the first week and 100 mg/kg q 8 hr thereafter.

Dosage Forms. Inj 1, 3, 6 g.

Pharmacokinetics and Biopharmaceutics. *Fate.* Negligible oral absorption. IM 1 g produces a peak plasma level of 22–33 mcg/ml at 0.5–2 hr after administration.[185] IV 2 g infused over 30 min produces a plasma level of about 175 mcg/ml at the end of the infusion.[164] V_d is about 0.2–0.25 L/kg, slightly larger than carbenicillin; about 55–65% bound to plasma proteins.[185] Widely distributed similar to carbenicillin with CSF levels about 6% of simultaneous plasma levels with normal meninges; 39% in patients with meningitis. A total of 90–95% of a dose is recovered in the urine within 24 hr, 10–14% as penicilloic acid and the remainder as unchanged drug.[185]

$t_{1/2}$. 72–77 min in normal adults; 15–16 hr in patients with severely impaired renal function; about 30 hr in patients with simultaneous hepatic and renal failure.[185] In neonates (under 2 kg and less than 7 days of age) 3.5–5.6 hr; infants (1–8 weeks) 1.3–2 hr; children (5–13 yr) 0.9 hr.[185]

Adverse Reactions. Similar to parenteral carbenicillin, although dose-related effects may be less frequent and severe due to lower dosage of ticarcillin.[185] See Carbenicillin Disodium.

Precautions. See Carbenicillin Disodium.

Contraindications. See Penicillin G.

Parameters to Monitor. See Carbenicillin Disodium.

Notes. Efficacy of ticarcillin in most infections is equivalent to carbenicillin. Used almost exclusively in combination with an aminoglycoside for systemic infections. Sodium content is 5.2–6.5 mEq/g.

8:12.24 THE TETRACYCLINES

General References: 186–188

Doxycycline and Salts

Vibramycin®

Pharmacology. Somewhat more active than other tetracyclines against anaerobes and facultative Gram-negative bacilli. See Tetracycline.

Administration and Adult Dose. PO 100 mg q 12 hr for one day, followed by 50–100 mg/day in 1–2 doses; **PO for prophylaxis against travelers' diarrhea** 200 mg en route, then 100 mg daily;[189] **PO for uncomplicated gonorrhea** 200 mg initially and 100 mg hs for 1 day, followed by 100 mg bid for 3 days; **PO for primary and secondary syphilis** 100 mg tid for at least 10 days. **IV** 200 mg in 1–2 divided doses for 1 day, followed by 100–200 mg/day, infused at a concentration of 0.1–1.0 mg/ml over a 1–4 hr period; double maintenance dose in severe infections. **Not for SC or IM use.**

Dosage Individualization. No dosage adjustment necessary in renal impairment.[186]

Pediatric Dose. Not recommended under 8 yr. PO (under 45 kg) 2.2 mg/kg q 12 hr for 1 day followed by 2.2 mg/kg/day in 1–2 divided doses; (over 45 kg) same as adult dose. **IV** (under 45 kg) 4.4 mg/kg in 1–2 divided doses for 1 day followed by 2.2–4.4 mg/kg/day in 1–2 divided doses; (over 45 kg) same as adult dose.

Dosage Forms. Cap (as hyclate) 50, 100, 300 mg; **Susp** (as monohydrate) 25 mg/5 ml (reconstituted); **Syrup** (as calcium) 50 mg/5 ml; **Tab** (as hyclate) 100 mg; **Inj** (as hyclate) 100, 200 mg.

Patient Instructions. This (oral) drug should be taken on an empty stomach, but if stomach upset occurs, it may be taken with food or milk, but not antacids or iron products. Avoid prolonged exposure to direct sunlight while taking this drug.

Pharmacokinetics and Biopharmaceutics. *Onset and Duration.* Duration of protection against travelers' diarrhea is about 1 week after discontinuation.[189]

Fate. Virtually 100% orally absorbed producing a peak of 3 mcg/ml at 2–4 hr after administration of 200 mg dose;[18] antacids and iron may significantly impair oral absorption, although food has little effect.[188] V_d is about 0.7 L/kg; about 60–90% plasma protein bound.[18,187] Widely distributed in the body, penetrating most cavities including CSF (12–20% of plasma levels). About 35–57% is excreted unchanged in the urine in normal adults; remainder is eliminated in feces via intestinal and biliary secretion.[186,190]

$t_{1/2}$. 12–20 hr (average 15) in normal adults; 17–25 hr in severe renal impairment.[190]

Adverse Reactions. IV dosage frequently produces phlebitis. In contrast to other tetracyclines, doxycycline is not significantly antianabolic and will not further increase azotemia in renal failure. Although oral doxycycline causes less alteration of intestinal flora than other tetracyclines, it may cause nausea and diarrhea with equal frequency. Binds to calcium in teeth and bones, which may cause discoloration of teeth in children, especially during growth; although doxycycline has a lower potential for this effect than most other tetracyclines.[18] Occasional phototoxic skin reactions may occur.[18,186]

Contraindications. Severe hepatic dysfunction.

Precautions. Pregnancy. Oral iron lowers plasma levels, even of IV doxycycline, by binding the drug after its secretion into intestine and increasing fecal elimination.[186] See Drug Interactions chapter.

Parameters to Monitor. Check for signs of phlebitis daily during IV use.

Notes. Doxycycline is the tetracycline of choice for extrarenal infection in the presence of renal impairment, although tetracyclines are the drugs of choice for very few infections.[186,188] Each vial contains 480 mg of ascorbic acid per 100 mg of doxycycline hyclate for injection.

Tetracycline and Salts   Various

Pharmacology. A broad-spectrum bacteriostatic antibiotic which inhibits protein synthesis at the 30S ribosomal subunit. Many bacteria have developed resistance by an R-factor mediated enzyme, changes in ribosomal binding characteristics or changes in cell wall permeability.

Administration and Adult Dose. PO 250–500 mg q 6–12 hr, between meals; **IV (not recommended)** 250–500 mg q 12 hr, to maximum of 250 mg q 6 hr. **IM not recommended.**

Pediatric Dose. Not recommended under 8 yr. PO 25–50 mg/kg/day in 2–4 divided doses between meals; **IV (not recommended)** 12 mg/kg/day to maximum of 20 mg/kg/day in 2 divided doses. **IM not recommended.**

Dosage Forms. Cap 100, 250, 500 mg; Susp 125 mg/5 ml; Syrup 125 mg/5 ml; Tab 250, 500 mg; Inj (IM) 100, 250 mg; Inj (IV) 250, 500 mg; Ophth Oint 1%; Ophth Susp 1%; Top Oint 3%. Strengths are expressed as hydrochloride equivalent.

Patient Instructions. This (oral) drug should be taken with a full glass of water on an empty stomach (1 hr before or 2 hr after meals) for best absorption. Do not take within 1 hr of dairy products, antacids (including sodium bicarbonate) or iron products.

Pharmacokinetics and Biopharmaceutics. *Fate.* About 75% absorbed orally; however, marked differences in bioavailability have been documented, although no significant differences in absorption reported among the different salts. IM injections are poorly absorbed, producing peak levels significantly lower than after oral administration. V_d is about 1.5 L/kg; 36–65% plasma protein bound.[18,187] Widely distributed in the body, including significant biliary concentrations and low CSF concentrations. About 60% of the absorbed dose appears unchanged in the urine.[18,186]

$t_{1/2}$. 9–11 hr (average 10); up to 100 hr with severe renal impairment.[186,190]

Adverse Reactions. IM injections are very irritating and painful; IV injections frequently cause phlebitis; oral administration produces bowel flora alterations and GI complaints which are dose-related. Antianabolic effect may produce elevation in BUN, hyperphosphatemia and acidosis in patients with pre-existing renal impairment. Binds to calcium in teeth and bones, which may cause mottling and discoloration of teeth in children, especially with repeated courses during growth;[18,187] this may also occur as a result of in utero administration. Acute, extensive, fatty infiltration of the liver with pancreatitis, acidosis and nonoliguric renal failure has occurred rarely; but, these reactions are more frequently reported after IV administration of large doses (greater than 2 g/day) in the presence of renal impairment, especially in pregnant or malnourished individuals. They are occasionally fatal.[18,186]

Contraindications. Renal impairment.

Precautions. Pregnancy. Use with caution in patients with liver impairment. Do *not* repeat courses in children under 8 yr. See Drug Interactions chapter.

Parameters to Monitor. Initial renal function tests; liver function tests if liver toxicity likely to occur (parenteral administration, high doses and/or pregnancy). Check for signs of phlebitis daily during IV administration.

Notes.   Rarely the drug of choice.[186] Each vial of tetracycline hydrochloride or phosphate complex contains from 250 mg–1+ g of ascorbic acid depending on the manufacturer and the amount of tetracycline.

Tetracyclines Comparison Chart

DRUG	DOSAGE FORMS	ADULT DOSE	PERCENT ORAL ABSORP- TION	AVERAGE HALF-LIFE (HOURS)	PERCENT UNCHANGED IN URINE	COMMENTS
Demeclocycline Hydrochloride Declomycin®	Cap 150 mg Tab (coated) 75, 150, 300 mg	PO 600 mg/day in 2–4 divided doses	66	15	42	Most phototoxic tetracycline; causes nephrogenic diabetes insipidus rarely.
Doxycycline Calcium Doxycycline Hyclate Doxycycline Monohydrate Vibramycin® Various	Cap (as hyclate) 50, 100, 300 mg Susp (as monohydrate) 25 mg/5 ml Syrup (as calcium) 50 mg/5 ml Tab (as hyclate) 100 mg Inj (as hyclate) 100, 200 mg	PO 100 mg q 12 hr for 1 day, then 50–100 mg/day in 1–2 divided doses; IV 200 mg in 1–2 divided doses for 1 day, then 100–200 mg/day	90–100	12–20	35–40	Safest in renal failure due to its lack of accumulation & lack of antianabolic effects
Methacycline Hydrochloride Rondomycin®	Cap 150, 300 mg	PO 300 mg q 12 hr or 150 mg q 6 hr	60	14	60	
Minocycline Hydrochloride Minocin® Vectrin®	Cap 50, 100 mg Susp 50 mg/5 ml Inj (IV only) 100 mg	PO or IV 200 mg initially, then 100 mg q 12 hr	95–100	13–17	5–10	Very frequent transient vestibular toxicity[191]

Continued

Tetracyclines Comparison Chart

DRUG	DOSAGE FORMS	ADULT DOSE	PERCENT ORAL ABSORPTION	AVERAGE HALF-LIFE (HOURS)	PERCENT UNCHANGED IN URINE	COMMENTS
Oxytetracycline **Oxytetracycline Hydrochloride** **Oxytetracycline Calcium** Various	Cap (as HCl) 125, 250 mg Syrup (as calcium) 125 mg/5 ml Tab (coated) 250 mg Inj (IM only) 50, 125 mg/ml Inj (IV only, as HCl) 250, 500 mg	PO 250–500 mg q 6 hr; IM 100–250 mg q 12 hr; IV 250–500 mg q 6–12 hr to a max of 2 g/day	58	9	70	IM preparations contain lidocaine and should not be used IV; IM not recommended
Tetracycline Various **Tetracycline Hydrochloride** Various **Tetracycline PO4 Complex** Tetrex®	Cap (as HCl) 100, 250, 500 mg Cap (as phosphate complex) 250, 500 mg Susp 125 mg/5 ml Syrup 125 mg/5 ml Tab (as HCl) 250, 500 mg Inj (IM only, as HCl) 100, 250 mg Inj (IV only, as HCl) 250, 500 mg	PO 250–500 mg q 6–12 hr; IV 250–500 mg q 6–12 hr to a max of 2 g/day	75	10	60	IM preparations contain procaine and should not be used IV; IM not recommended due to pain and low plasma levels

8:12.28 OTHER ANTIBIOTICS

Clindamycin Salts   Cleocin®

Pharmacology. A semisynthetic 7-chloro, 7-deoxylincomycin derivative which is very active against most Gram-positive organisms except enterococci and *Clostridium difficile*. Gram-negative aerobes are highly resistant, while most anaerobes are very sensitive. Inhibits bacterial protein synthesis by binding to the 50S ribosomal subunit; bactericidal or bacteriostatic depending on the concentration, organism and inoculum.[192]

Administration and Adult Dose. **PO** 150–450 mg q 6 hr; **IM or IV** 600 mg–2.7 g/day in 2–4 divided doses, to maximum of 4.8 g/day. Single IM doses greater than 600 mg not recommended; infuse IV no faster than 30 mg/min. **Top for acne** apply bid.

Dosage Individualization. Dosage adjustment is unnecessary in renal impairment[193,194] or cirrhosis,[195,196] although the effect of acute liver disease is unknown.[195]

Pediatric Dose. **PO** (over 10 kg) 8–25 mg/kg/day in 3–4 divided doses; (under 10 kg) give no less than 37.5 mg q 8 hr; **IM or IV** (over 1 month) 15–40 mg/kg/day in 3–4 divided doses (not less than 300 mg/day in severe infection, regardless of weight).

Dosage Forms. **Cap** (as hydrochloride) 75, 150 mg; **Soln** (as palmitate) 75 mg/5 ml (reconstituted); **Inj** (as phosphate) 150 mg/ml; **Top Soln** (as phosphate) 1%.

Patient Instructions. Report any significant diarrhea immediately. Do *not* refrigerate the reconstituted oral solution, because it will thicken.

Pharmacokinetics and Biopharmaceutics. *Fate.* Absorption is nearly complete and is the same from the capsule or the solution; food may delay, but not decrease, absorption.[18,197] A 500 mg oral dose produces a peak plasma level of 5–6 mcg/ml in 1 hr.[197] A 300 mg IM dose produces a peak level of 5–6 mcg/ml 1–2 hr post-injection.[193,194,198] A 600 mg IV dose infused over 30 min produces a peak plasma level of 10 mcg/ml.[18] The drug is widely distributed throughout the body except the CSF.[194,198] V_d is about 0.6 L/kg; 80–94% plasma protein bound.[195] The palmitate and phosphate esters are absorbed intact and rapidly hydrolyzed to the active base. Unhydrolyzed phosphate ester usually constitutes less than 20% of the total peak plasma level after parenteral clindamycin, but may increase to 40% in patients with impaired renal function.[193] There is significant hepatic metabolism, and excretion of active forms in the bile.[194,198,199] 5–10% of the absorbed dose is recovered as unchanged drug and active metabolites in the urine within 24 hr.[194,195,198]

$t_{1/2}$. 1.5–4 hr (average 2.5);[18,194] unchanged or slightly increased in severe renal disease;[193,194] may be increased or unchanged in liver disease.[195,196]

Adverse Reactions. After oral administration, anorexia, nausea, vomiting, cramps and diarrhea occur frequently.[18,200] Oral, and rarely, parenteral clindamycin may cause severe, sometimes fatal, pseudomembranous colitis (PMC) which may be clinically indistinguishable at onset from non-PMC diarrhea.[18,201] PMC has been reported after topical administration.[202] Clindamycin-associated PMC is secondary to overgrowth of toxin-producing *Clostridium difficile*.[201,203] PMC is terminated in many patients by discontinuing clindamycin immediately; however, if diarrhea is severe or does not improve promptly after discontinuation, treat with van-comycin.[201] The value of corticosteroids, cholestyramine and anti-spasmodics in the management of clindamycin-associated diarrhea and PMC has not been established.[201,204] Antidiarrheals such as diphenoxylate may worsen PMC and should *not* be used.

Precautions. Pregnancy; lactation. Use with caution in neonates under 4 weeks of age, and in patients with liver disease. Discontinue *immediately* if significant diarrhea occurs. Drug accumulation may occur in patients with severe concomitant hepatic and renal dysfunction, however data are lacking.

Parameters to Monitor. Observe for changes in bowel frequency.

Notes. Oral solution is stable for 2 weeks at room temperature following reconstitution; do not refrigerate.

Colistimethate Sodium   Coly-Mycin M®
Colistin Sulfate   Coly-Mycin S®

Pharmacology. A bactericidal cyclic polypeptide, polymyxin E, closely related to polymyxin B. Disrupts osmotic integrity of the cell membrane by detergent action. Spectrum includes Gram-negative aerobes except *Proteus, Serratia* and *Neisseria* sp. Resistance is related to the permeability characteristics of the bacterial cell wall.[18]

Administration and Adult Dose. PO for gastroenteritis (as colistin sulfate) 5–15 mg/kg/day in 3 equally divided doses. IM or IV (as colistimethate sodium) 2.5–5 mg/kg/day in 2-4 equally divided doses or 15 mg/square root of body weight in pounds/day in 2-4 divided doses.[205]

Dosage Individualization. IM or IV dosage must be reduced in patients with impaired renal function, although precise guidelines are not available. One source suggests anuric patients receive 2.5 mg/kg followed by 1.5 mg/kg q 5–7 days.[18] Another suggests 100 mg q 2–4 days.[206] Dosage modification probably unnecessary in liver disease.

Pediatric Dose. All ages including premature infants, same as adult dose.[18]

Dosage Forms. Susp (as colistin sulfate) 25 mg/5 ml (reconstituted); Inj (as colistimethate sodium) 150 mg. Colistimethate is the methane sulfonate salt of colistin.

Patient Instructions. Report any numbness, tingling, weakness or dizziness.

Pharmacokinetics and Biopharmaceutics. *Fate.* Oral doses are not significantly absorbed. IM 2 mg/kg usually produces peak plasma concentrations of 5–13 mcg/ml at 1-2 hr[207] — see Notes. Peak plasma concentrations after IV administration depend on rate of administration; a 3 min injection of 2 mg/kg in adults produces a peak of 18 mcg/ml 10 min post-injection, followed by a rapid fall as the drug distributes in the body; plasma concentrations after 1-2 hr coincide with concentrations found after IM administration.[207] Colistimethate is inactive until hydrolyzed to colistin base; hydrolysis is not complete.[18] Does not diffuse well into cavities, spaces or CSF; not detected in bile. May persist in organ tissues for prolonged periods after plasma clearance is completed; this is apparently a result of an affinity for cell membranes. Eliminated primarily via the kidneys with resulting high urine levels; 65-75% of a parenteral dose is excreted as the active drug within 24 hr.[207]

$t_{1/2}$. Variously reported in the range of 3–8 hr in normal adults; 10–20 hr in patients with renal failure.[124] See Notes.

Adverse Reactions. Parenteral administration, usually of excessive doses, can produce transient neurological disturbances (eg, circumoral paresthesias, tingling of extremities, vertigo, dizziness), depolarizing neuromuscular blockade (which may result in respiratory arrest) and acute tubular necrosis or slowly progressive renal insufficiency. Toxicity is probably equivalent to that produced by polymyxin B in therapeutically equivalent doses.[205]

Precautions. Pregnancy. Use with caution in pre-existing renal impairment, myasthenia gravis and post-operative patients or other patients who may have depressed neuromuscular transmission. See Drug Interactions chapter.

Parameters to Monitor. Obtain renal function tests and observe for neurological disturbances before and frequently during therapy. Plasma levels are recommended in patients with impaired renal function due to unpredictable kinetics. See Notes.

Notes. A second-line drug because it is toxic and relatively ineffective for systemic infections. For IV use, polymyxin B is preferred because it does not require hydrolytic activation.[18] Cross-resistance and cross-allergenicity to polymyxin B should be expected.

Kinetic patterns observed after parenteral administration of colistimethate sodium are complicated by the fact that the commercial product is a mixture of compounds with varying degrees of sulfomethyl substitution. The degree of sulfomethylation confers different degrees of antibacterial activity and different patterns of kinetic behavior upon the parent colistin molecule. The more sulfomethylated derivatives are less active and more rapidly cleared from the plasma by the kidneys. Consequently, kinetic studies have produced widely disparate results and must be interpreted with caution. Also, the results of studies involving colistimethate sodium should not be generalized to other polymyxins.

Polymyxin B Sulfate   Aerosporin®, Various

Pharmacology. See Colistimethate Sodium.

Administration and Adult Dose. IV 1.5–2.5 mg/kg/day in 2 equally divided doses. **IM not recommended,** but if used, administer with local anesthetic using same dosage range as for IV but give in 4–6 equally divided doses. **IT** 5 mg/day in 1 ml sterile saline for 3–4 days, then 5 mg every other day. **Intrabronchial aerosol** 2.5 mg/kg/day in 6 divided doses.[208] **Ophth** 1–3 drops/hr of 0.1–0.25% solution.

Dosage Individualization. Dosage adjustment is necessary with renal impairment, although accurate guidelines are not available. One author suggests 2.5 mg/kg followed by 1 mg/kg q 5–7 days in anuria.[18] See Notes.

Pediatric Dose. IV (infants) 2.5–4 mg/kg/day in 2 equally divided doses; (over 2 yr) same as adult mg/kg dose. **IT** (infants less than 2 yr) 2 mg/day in 0.4 ml sterile saline for 3–4 days, then 2.5 mg every other day; (over 2 yr) same as adult dose.[18]

Dosage Forms. **Inj, Ophth Pwdr** 50 mg (500,000 U).

Patient Instructions. Report any numbness, tingling, weakness or dizziness.

Pharmacokinetics and Biopharmaceutics. *Fate.* Absorption orally and across mucous membranes is stated to be negligible; however, absorption of toxic amounts during wound irrigation has been documented.[209] Its kinetics are poorly characterized and highly variable. Complex interaction of polymyxin B with plasma results in generally low plasma concentrations of active drug after parenteral administration. Widely distributed in the body, highly tissue bound with poor penetration into cavities or CSF and not detected in bile. In contrast to colistimethate sodium, there is a considerable delay in urinary excretion, such that after an IM dose only 0.1% is recovered unchanged in the urine in the first 12 hr; thereafter, approximately 60% is recovered unchanged in the urine.[210]

$t_{1/2}$. Reported as 4.4 hr in normal adults and 35 hr or more in patients with impaired renal function;[211] however, data are inadequate.

Adverse Reactions. IM injections are very painful and should be avoided. Neurologic and nephrotoxic reactions are similar to colistimethate sodium in therapeutically equivalent doses. See Colistimethate Sodium.

Precautions. See Colistimethate Sodium.

Parameters to Monitor. See Colistimethate Sodium.

Notes. Although dosage adjustment guidelines for colistimethate sodium have been said to also apply to polymyxin B,[212] data to support this conclusion are lacking. Cross-resistance and cross-allergenicity with colistin compounds should be expected.

Spectinomycin Dihydrochloride   Trobicin®

Pharmacology. A non-aminoglycoside aminocyclitol active against a variety of bacteria, especially *Neisseria gonorrhoeae*. Acts by inhibiting protein synthesis at the 30S ribosomal subunit.

Administration and Adult Dose. IM for uncomplicated gonorrhea 2 g as a single dose; **IM for disseminated gonorrhea** 2 g bid for 3 days.[213] **Not for IV use.**

Dosage Individualization. No dosage adjustment is necessary in renal impairment with a single dose.

Dosage Forms. Inj 2, 4 g.

Pharmacokinetics and Biopharmaceutics. *Fate.* Poorly absorbed orally. 2 g IM produces a peak concentration of 100–150 mcg/ml 1 hr after administration.[214,215] Minimal protein binding. 70–80% of the dose is excreted in the urine as a microbiologically active form within 48 hr. Urine concentrations may reach 1000 mcg/ml.[214]

$t_{1/2}$. 1.7 hr in normal adults;[214] prolonged in proportion to degree of renal impairment.[215]

Adverse Reactions. Pain at injection site; transient dizziness and nausea noted occasionally after injection. No reports of ototoxicity or nephrotoxicity with normal doses,[214] and when given to volunteers in doses of 2 g qid for 21 days.[216]

Precautions. Pregnancy. Use with caution in infants and children. May mask or delay symptoms of incubating syphilis.

Parameters to Monitor. Serological tests for syphilis should be followed.

Notes. Not effective against syphilis. Should only be used as an alternative agent in penicillin-allergic patients for uncomplicated gonorrhea, when treating infections with gonococci resistant to penicillins or when other agents have failed.[214,217] Spectinomycin resistance is rare and only observed with penicillin-sensitive gonococci.[218] Gonococcal infections of the pharynx respond poorly to spectinomycin.[214]

Vancomycin Hydrochloride   Vancocin®

Pharmacology. Binds irreversibly to cell wall of many Gram-positive cocci and bacilli; inhibits cell wall synthesis in a manner slightly different from β-lactam antimicrobials. Most Gram-negative bacteria are resistant.

Administration and Adult Dose. PO for staphylococcal enterocolitis 2 g/day in 2–4 divided doses. PO for pseudomembranous colitis 125–500 mg q 6 hr for 7–10 days; retreat with a longer course if relapse occurs.[219,220] IV 20–30 mg/kg/day (usually 2 g/day) in 2–4 divided doses as a dilute infusion over 20–30 min. Not for IM use.

Dosage Individualization. Adjust dosage carefully in renal impairment; clearance is directly related to creatinine clearance.[221] Anuric patients on hemodialysis have been given the usual dose q 7–14 days with good results,[221-223] although one source recommends a loading dose of 15 mg/kg followed by 1.9 mg/kg/day.[224] Monitoring of plasma concentrations is recommended. Dosage adjustment is unnecessary in liver disease.

Pediatric Dose. PO or IV (neonate) 12–15 mg/kg/day; (older infants and children) 40 mg/kg/day in 2–4 divided doses.

Dosage Forms. Pwdr 10 g; Inj 500 mg.

Patient Instructions. Report pain at infusion site, dizziness, fullness or ringing in ears, nausea or vomiting.

Pharmacokinetics and Biopharmaceutics. *Plasma Levels.* Toxicity likely with sustained levels over 80 mcg/ml.[224]
   Fate. Oral absorption negligible. Fecal concentrations during therapy with PO 500 mg q 6 hr reach 3 mg/g.[225] 500 mg IV produces plasma levels of 6–10 mcg/ml in 1 hr. V_d is about 1.3 L/kg;[224] 10% plasma protein bound.[221] Widely distributed, except to the CSF. Negligible metabolism or biliary excretion; 80–90% is excreted in the urine unchanged within 24 hr.
   $t_{1/2}$. 6–8 hr;[226] 6–10 days with renal failure.[221-223,227] No change expected with liver disease.

Adverse Reactions. Chills, fever, nausea, phlebitis may occur, especially with direct injection of undiluted drug (not recommended). Rapid infusion may cause transient systolic hypotension.[224,228] Extravasation will cause local tissue necrosis. Ototoxicity (auditory and vestibular) and possibly nephrotoxicity occur with excessive plasma concentrations; usually reversible upon discontinuation. Eosinophilia and urticarial rashes have been reported frequently. Side effects of vancomycin may not be as prevalent today as in the past, perhaps due to changes in the manufacturing process which eliminated some impurities.[229-231]

Precautions. Pregnancy. Use with caution in patients with impaired renal function, pre-existing hearing loss or those receiving other ototoxic or nephrotoxic agents.

Parameters to Monitor. With IV use obtain initial renal function tests and repeat frequently during therapy; serial audiometry should be performed if patient has decreased renal function. With decreased renal function, plasma concentrations should be monitored. Check for signs of phlebitis daily.

Notes. An alternative agent for treatment or prophylaxis of staphylococcal or streptococcal infections when a less toxic agent is inappropriate (eg, penicillin or cephalosporin allergy, or resistant organisms) or has not produced an adequate therapeutic response.

8:16 ANTITUBERCULOSIS AGENTS

(SEE ALSO STREPTOMYCIN 8:12.02)

Ethambutol Hydrochloride   Myambutol®

Pharmacology. A synthetic tuberculostatic which acts by an unknown mechanism, possibly as an RNA antimetabolite; its activity is restricted to mycobacteria. Primary resistance among mycobacteria is rare, but resistance occurs rapidly if used alone.

Administration and Adult Dose. PO for treatment of tuberculosis 25 mg/kg/day as a single daily dose for 3 months, then 15 mg/kg/day for a total of 18–24 months in combination with rifampin or isoniazid.[232] Initial dosage of 25 mg/kg/day is probably unnecessary, however.[233,234]

Dosage Individualization. Dosage should be decreased in severe renal impairment; exact guidelines are not established, but one source recommends 8–10 mg/kg/day in severe renal impairment.[235]

Pediatric Dose. (Over 13 yr) same as adult dose.

Dosage Forms. Tab 100, 400 mg.

Patient Instructions. Report any changes in vision.

Pharmacokinetics and Biopharmaceutics. *Fate.* About 80% absorbed orally with 15 mg/kg producing peak plasma concentrations of 4–6 mcg/ml at 2–4 hr after the dose.[236] The distribution of ethambutol is largely unknown, although low therapeutic concentrations appear in the CSF in the presence of inflamed meninges. Disposition is complex and multicompartmental with a prolonged (5 hr) initial distribution phase.[236] V_d is about 1.5–4 L/kg;[237] 20–30% plasma protein bound.[236] Of the absorbed dose, nearly 100% is recovered in the urine within 24 hr, with 80% as unchanged ethambutol.[237]

$t_{1/2}$. 4–6 hr in normal adults;[236] actual terminal half-life is about 15 hr, but this is not the most important half-life for dosage calculations.[237] In anuric patients, reported half-life values range from 7–32 hr,[237] although the upper end of this range appears most likely.

Adverse Reactions. Optic neuritis is rare with doses less than 25 mg/kg/day, but may be more frequent in the presence of impaired renal function. It appears over several months, usually as blurred vision, color blindness and restriction of visual fields. It is usually completely reversible over weeks to months with prompt drug discontinuation, although defective color vision may persist for prolonged periods and permanent impairment of vision may occur if the drug is not promptly discontinued.[238] Hyperuricemia due to impaired urinary excretion of uric acid may occur.

Contraindications. Optic neuritis.

Precautions. Pregnancy. Use with caution in children under 13 yr and in patients with impaired renal function.

Parameters to Monitor. Initial renal function tests. With prolonged therapy at dosages greater than 15 mg/kg/day, or if pre-existing renal impairment or visual loss, periodic visual acuity and color discrimination testing is advised.

Isoniazid   Various

Pharmacology. A synthetic hydrazine derivative of isonicotinic acid which inhibits the synthesis of mycolic acid, a component of mycobacterial cell wall; it probably has other unknown actions. Activity is limited to mycobacteria; tuberculostatic or tuberculocidal depending on concentration and reproductive rate of the organism. Primary resistance is uncommon, but resistance can develop rapidly if used alone in active tuberculosis; resistance is uncommon in preventive therapy.

Administration and Adult Dose. PO for prophylaxis of tuberculosis 5 mg/kg/day (usually 300 mg) as a single daily dose, to maximum of 300 mg/day, given as a single agent for 1 yr — see Notes. **PO for treatment of tuberculosis** same dose as above, but combine with at least one other antitubercular agent for 18–24 months. Course may be shortened to 12–18 months if isoniazid (INH) is combined with rifampin for the first 6 months.[239] Alternatively, **PO for uncomplicated pulmonary tuberculosis** 5 mg/kg/day with rifampin 600 mg/day for 9–12 months; or use these same doses for 2–8 weeks, followed by INH 15 mg/kg and rifampin 600 mg twice weekly for a total of 9–12 months.[239,240] **IM or IV** (rarely used) same as oral dose.

Dosage Individualization. Acetylator phenotype has not been evaluated as a parameter for dosage individualization; however, some sources recommend a dose of 150–200 mg/day in slow acetylators with renal impairment.[18,241]

Pediatric Dose. PO for prophylaxis of tuberculosis 10 mg/kg/day as a single daily dose, to maximum of 300 mg/day, given as a single agent for 1 year.[240] **PO for treatment of tuberculosis** same dose as above, but combine with at least one other antitubercular agent for 18–24 months. Alternatively, **PO for uncomplicated pulmonary tuberculosis** 10 mg/kg/day with rifampin 15 mg/kg/day (to maximum of 600 mg/day) for 9–12 months; or use these same doses for 2–8 weeks, followed by INH 10 mg/kg and rifampin 15 mg/kg (to maximum of 600 mg) twice weekly for a total of 9–12 months.[240,242]

Dosage Forms. Tab 50, 100, 300 mg; Inj 100 mg/ml.

Patient Instructions. Report any burning, tingling or numbness in the extremities, unusual malaise, fever, dark urine or yellowing of eyes.

Pharmacokinetics and Biopharmaceutics. *Fate.* Rapid and nearly complete oral absorption with peak plasma concentrations of 1–5 mcg/ml 1 hr after a 5 mg/kg dose.[243] Widely distributed in the body tissues including the CSF of normal patients and those with meningitis. V_d is 0.6 L/kg;[241,244] 15% plasma protein bound.[243] Eliminated primarily by acetylation in the liver to inactive metabolites which are excreted in the urine. Specific pattern of elimination depends on acetylator phenotype of the individual.[244] See Pharmacogenetics chapter.

$t_{1/2}$. (Rapid acetylators) 0.5–1.5 hr; (slow acetylators) 2–4 hr. 4 hr with renal impairment;[241,245] increased to 6.7 hr in patients with liver disease.[246]

Adverse Reactions. Pyridoxine-responsive peripheral neuropathy can occur, especially in alcoholics, malnourished patients, slow acetylators and with doses greater than 5 mg/kg/day.[18,232,247] Subclinical hepatitis is frequent (10–20%) and characterized by usually asymptomatic elevation of SGOT and SGPT which may return to normal despite continued therapy; it may be more common with combined INH-rifampin therapy.[248] Clinical hepatitis is rare, but is strikingly related to age (rising to 2–3% in 50–65 year old patients); relationship to fast acetylator phenotype is uncertain.[249,250,267] Rare cases of massive liver atrophy resulting in death usually appear in association with alcoholism or pre-existing liver disease; most severe cases occur within the first 6 months.[249,250] With acute overdosage (usually 6–10 g), INH may produce severe CNS toxicity including stupor and coma followed by seizures, hypotension, cyanosis and occasionally death.[251]

Contraindications. Acute or chronic liver disease, previous INH-associated hepatitis.

Precautions. Pregnancy; lactation. Use with caution in daily users of alcohol, elderly patients and those with a slow acetylator phenotype. See Drug Interactions chapter.

Parameters to Monitor. Question for prodromal signs of hepatitis (fever, malaise, etc.) and signs of peripheral neuropathy (burning, tingling, numbness) monthly during therapy. Baseline and monthly SGOT and SGPT are recommended only in high risk groups (those over 35 yr, daily alcohol users, and those with a history of liver dysfunction);[252] although, they are not predictive of clinical hepatitis.[253]

Notes. It is generally recommended that all patients receive INH for prophylaxis of tuberculosis who have had a positive reaction to intermediate strength Purified Protein Derivative (PPD 5 Tuberculin Units) and who: (1) are household contacts of patients with active tuberculosis; or (2) converted their PPD to positive within the past 12–24 months; or (3) have radiologic evidence of inactive tuberculosis or a history of inadequately treated active tuberculosis; or (4) are receiving prolonged treatment with corticosteroids or immunosuppressants (although the need for prophylaxis in this group has been questioned);[254] or (5) have leukemia, Hodgkin's disease, diabetes mellitus, silicosis or have undergone a subtotal or total gastrectomy.[232] Most sources suggest that the use of INH prophylaxis in patients older than 35 yr should be further restricted due to the increased risk of fatal hepatotoxicity.[252,255,256]

To prevent peripheral neuropathy, adults receiving large doses of INH (10 mg/kg/day or more) and those who are predisposed to peripheral neuritis (eg, alcoholics) should receive **pyridoxine** in a dose of 50 mg/day. Pyridoxine IV in a dose equal to the estimated amount of INH ingested is recommended for acute INH overdose.[251,257]

Rifampin

Rimactane®, Rifadin®

Pharmacology. A synthetic rifamycin B derivative; highly active against mycobacteria, most Gram-positive bacteria and some Gram-negative bacteria, most notably, *Neisseria meningitidis*. Inhibits the action of DNA-dependent RNA polymerase. Primary resistance is uncommon, but resistance can develop rapidly if used alone.

Administration and Adult Dose. PO for treatment of tuberculosis 600 mg/day as a single daily dose in combination with at least one other antitubercular agent — see Isoniazid; PO for the prophylaxis of meningococcal meningitis 600 mg bid for 2 days.[258]

Dosage Individualization. No dosage adjustment is necessary in patients with impaired renal function; accumulation would be expected in patients with hepatic dysfunction or biliary obstruction, but dosage guidelines for use in patients with these conditions are not available.

Pediatric Dose. PO for treatment of tuberculosis (over 5 yr) 15 mg/kg/day as a single daily dose, to maximum of 600 mg/day,[242] in combination with at least one other antitubercular agent; PO for prophylaxis of meningococcal meningitis (less than 1 yr) 5 mg/kg bid for 2 days; (1–12 yr) 10 mg/kg bid, to maximum of 600 mg bid, for 2 days.[258,259]

Dosage Forms. Cap 300 mg.

Patient Instructions. This medication should be taken with a full glass of water on an empty stomach (1 hr before or 2 hr after meals) for best absorption. It is important to take this medication regularly as directed, because inconsistent dosing may increase its toxicity. May cause harmless red-orange discoloration of sweat, saliva, feces and urine.

Pharmacokinetics and Biopharmaceutics. *Fate.* 100% absorbed orally, with a 600 mg dose producing a peak plasma concentration of approximately 10 mcg/ml 1–3 hr after administration.[260] Food delays absorption, but does not affect overall bioavailability.[260,261] First-pass hepatic extraction is substantial, but saturated with doses greater than 300–450 mg; thus, larger doses produce disproportionate plasma levels.[260] Widely distributed throughout the body; however, significant amounts appear in the CSF only in the presence of inflamed meninges.[260,262] About 80% plasma protein bound.[260] Eliminated primarily by deacetylation in the liver to a partially active metabolite which is extensively enterohepatically recirculated, producing very high biliary concentrations.[260,263] About 50–60% of a dose is eventually excreted in the feces.[260] Urinary excretion is variable and appears to increase with the dose. At usual doses, 12–15% is excreted unchanged in the urine;[260] at a dose of 900 mg, 30–40% is recovered unchanged in the urine within 24 hr.[263]

$t_{1/2}$. 1.5–5 hr (average 2.8).[260] Half-life increases with higher doses, but may become shorter over the first few weeks of treatment. It is not changed by renal impairment, but is increased unpredictably by liver disease or biliary obstruction.[246,263]

Adverse Reactions. Adverse reactions are more frequent and severe with intermittent, high-dose administration. GI symptoms are frequent. Acute, reversible renal failure, characterized as tubular damage with interstitial nephritis, sometimes appearing with concomitant hepatic failure has been reported rarely, especially in association with intermittent administration.[18,252] Subclinical hepatitis may be frequent (up to 18%), while clinical hepatitis is rare, but apparently more common with pre-existing liver disease or alcoholism; the effect of INH co-administration on the frequency of hepatitis is unclear.[248] Competition with bile for biliary excretion may produce jaundice, especially with pre-existing liver disease.[264] Intermittent therapy is also associated with thrombocytopenia and a flu-like syndrome (ie, fever, joint pain, muscle cramps).[232] Rifampin affects cellular immunity, impairing skin-test reactivity in about 50% of recipients.[265]

Contraindications. Previous rifampin-associated hepatitis.

Precautions. Pregnancy; lactation. Use with caution in daily users of alcohol and those with pre-existing liver disease. See Drug Interactions chapter.

Parameters to Monitor. Question for prodromal signs of hepatitis (eg, fever, malaise). Baseline and monthly SGOT and SGPT have been recommended, especially for patients with factors predisposing to hepatotoxicity from rifampin (eg, alcoholism, pre-existing liver disease), although they are not predictive of clinical hepatitis in the absence of symptomatology.

Notes. Not useful as a single agent for the treatment or prophylaxis of tuberculosis, or the treatment of meningococcal infection, although it is very useful in the prophylaxis of meningococcal disease in selected high-risk patients (ie, household or intimate contacts of patients with diagnosed meningococcal disease).[258,259]

Second-Line Antituberculars Comparison Chart[a,b]

DRUG	DOSAGE FORMS	ADULT DOSE	HALF-LIFE (HOURS) NORMAL	HALF-LIFE (HOURS) ANURIA	PERCENT UNCHANGED IN URINE	MAJOR ADVERSE EFFECTS
Aminosalicylic Acid Salts[c] Various	Tab 500 mg, 1 g Tab (coated) 500 mg Pwdr 4, 18, 120, 454 g	PO 8-12 g/day in 2-4 divided doses (as the acid)	1	?	20	GI intolerance; hepatitis; lupus-like syndrome
Capreomycin Sulfate Capastat®	Inj 1 g	IM 15-20 mg/kg/day (usually 1 g) for 60-120 days, then 1 g 2-3 days/week	2.5	↑	50-60	Nephrotoxicity; ototoxicity
Cycloserine Seromycin®	Cap 250 mg	PO 15 mg/kg/day (usually 500 mg) in 2 divided doses, to maximum of 1 g/day	10	↑	60-70	CNS (drowsiness, dizziness, headache, depression, rare seizures and psychosis)
Ethionamide Trecator-SC®	Tab 250 mg	PO 10-15 mg/kg/day (usually 500-750 mg) as a single daily dose, to maximum of 1 g/day	3	–	1-5	GI intolerance; hepatitis; CNS (drowsiness, dizziness, headache, depression, rare seizures)

Continued

Second-Line Antituberculars Comparison Chart[a,b]

DRUG	DOSAGE FORMS	ADULT DOSE	HALF-LIFE (HOURS)		PERCENT UNCHANGED IN URINE	MAJOR ADVERSE EFFECTS
			NORMAL	ANURIA		
Kanamycin Sulfate Kantrex®	Inj 37.5, 250, 333 mg/ml	IM 15 mg/kg/day (usually 1 g/day) 5-7 days/week	2-3	80-90	90	Nephrotoxicity; ototoxicity
Pyrazinamide	Tab 500 mg (available only in hospitals)	PO 20-35 mg/kg/day in 3-4 divided doses, to maximum of 3 g/day	9-10	↑	4-14	Hepatitis; hyperuricemia

a. Adapted from references 18, 232, 252, 266.
b. Use only in combination with other effective antituberculars.
c. Potassium salt contains 81%, and sodium salt contains 73% aminosalicylic acid; increase dose accordingly.

8:18 ANTIVIRALS

(SEE ALSO AMANTADINE 92:00)

Acyclovir
Zovirax®

Acyclovir is an antiviral nucleoside analogue which blocks replication of a number of herpesviruses by competing with viral nucleosides for DNA polymerase. It is activated by virus-specific phosphorylating enzymes, but has little activity in cells not containing viruses. Its pharmacokinetics have not been thoroughly studied, although it appears to be about 45% excreted unchanged in the urine and to have a half-life of about 2–4 hr in adults with normal renal function. In experimental and early clinical studies the drug has shown remarkable activity and lack of toxicity. It is much more soluble than vidarabine, requiring much smaller fluid volumes for IV infusion. Dosages in clinical trials have been IV for adults 5 mg/kg or 250 mg/M^2 q 8 hr.[268-271] The topical ointment is useful in mucocutaneous herpes simplex infections in immunocompromised patients.[341] In *initial* episodes of herpes genitalis, the ointment slightly decreases healing time and viral shedding.[342] Available as a 5% ointment and Inj 500 mg vials.

Vidarabine
Vira-A®

Pharmacology. A poorly soluble analogue of adenine deoxyriboside active against DNA viruses, especially members of the herpesvirus family (herpes simplex, varicella-zoster virus and cytomegalovirus). Vidarabine and its major metabolite, arabinosyl hypoxanthine (ara-Hx), are phosphorylated in cells; triphosphate derivatives inhibit both viral (primarily) and cellular DNA polymerase. Vidarabine's mechanism of action may be related to this effect or other actions on the genetic code process.[272,273] Although ara-Hx is about 50 times less active than the parent compound, the two may act synergistically.[18]

Administration and Adult Dose. IV for herpes simplex encephalitis 15 mg/kg/day as a single daily dose infused over 12–24 hr for 10 days. IV suspension must be diluted and administered as a solution containing no more than 700 mg/L (preferably less than 450 mg/L) to avoid precipitation. **Ophth Oint for herpes simplex keratoconjunctivitis** instill ½ inch or 1 cm ribbon (delivers about 1 mg vidarabine) into lower conjunctival sac q 3 hr (5 times/day) for 7–10 days after epithelial healing occurs (as demonstrated by lack of fluorescein dye staining). **IV for treatment of deeper ocular infections and herpes zoster** — see Notes.

Dosage Individualization. Reduce dose in patients with renal failure[18] and hepatitis;[274] see Adverse Reactions.

Pediatric Dose. Same as adult mg/kg dose.

Dosage Forms. Ophth Oint 30 mg/g; Inj (IV only) 200 mg/ml.

Pharmacokinetics and Biopharmaceutics. *Fate.* Peak plasma levels following a 12 hr infusion of 10–15 mg/kg are 0.2–0.4 mcg/ml of vidarabine and 3–8 mcg/ml of ara-Hx. Ophth Oint vidarabine does not penetrate into the anterior chamber of the eye to any measurable extent,[274] although a small amount of ara-Hx is detected in the aqueous humor.[272] IV vidarabine achieves intraocular levels similar to plasma levels.[272] High levels of drug and its metabolite have been found in many tissues. CSF levels are about

50% of plasma, but may be detectable for several days after therapy is stopped.[274] Vidarabine and ara-Hx appear to be concentrated intracellularly, and can be measured in RBCs several weeks after a dose. Plasma levels are similar after single and repeated daily doses. The deamination of vidarabine to its major metabolite, ara-Hx, appears to occur rapidly in the liver. 60% excreted in urine, primarily as ara-Hx, within 24 hr.[272,274]

$t_{1/2}$. 1.5–3.3 hr in adults based on limited data.[272,274]

Adverse Reactions. (Ophth Oint) generally without significant toxicity; reported reactions are difficult to distinguish from symptoms of the underlying ophthalmologic disorder (eg, irritation).[274] (IV) nausea and vomiting occur in about 10% of patients. When administered to patients with chronic hepatitis B, unexplained tremor, jitteriness and rare myoclonus have appeared at usual doses; this is reversible upon drug discontinuation.[274] This syndrome, plus weight loss and erythroid megaloblastosis, have been observed in patients without liver disease given more than 20 mg/kg/day. Severe thrombocytopenia, leukopenia and severe encephalopathy (hallucinations, psychosis, abnormal EEG) can occur with doses greater than 30 mg/kg/day.[268,274] Encephalopathy has been frequent in renal failure patients given usual doses.[18] CHF and cerebral edema may be exacerbated by the high fluid volume required to administer the drug.

Precautions. Pregnancy (teratogenic in some animals).[272] CHF, cerebral edema (ie, CNS trauma or infection), liver disease, renal failure.

Parameters to Monitor. Fluorescein dye staining and distant visual acuity to assess therapy for herpes simplex keratoconjunctivitis. (IV) monitor fluid status closely in patients with CHF, cerebral edema or renal failure. Check mental status, CBC and platelets frequently during therapy in patients with liver disease or renal failure, or in patients receiving high doses.

Notes. Ophthalmic vidarabine is effective in patients who have not responded to IDUR,[272] and is superior to IDUR in promoting optimal healing of herpes simplex keratoconjunctivitis.[268,274] Ophthalmic ointment is ineffective in herpes genitalis or labialis (herpes simplex type 2) and deeper ocular herpes infections (eg, keratouveitis).[18,274] IV supplied as a suspension which must be diluted before use. Dissolution may be hastened if the diluent is warmed to 37–38 °C before the drug is added. IV is well tolerated in usual doses, without the alopecia, mucositis and common bone marrow toxicity of the other antiviral nucleosides, cytarabine and idoxuridine (IDUR). IM usage may produce tenderness and inflammation at the injection site and slow absorption; IM administration is not recommended.[275] Although vidarabine is not as potent an antiviral agent in vitro as IDUR or cytarabine, it is preferred because of its much higher therapeutic index with systemic use. IV 20 mg/kg/day for 7 days has been somewhat successful in treating deeper ocular infections. IV 10 mg/kg/day for 5–7 days appears useful for herpes zoster infection (shingles, due to varicella-zoster virus) in immunosuppressed patients.[268,274,275] Vidarabine is ineffective in patients infected with cytomegalovirus, hepatitis B or smallpox.[18,268,272,274] Patients who are already in coma from herpes simplex encephalitis do not benefit from vidarabine therapy; therefore, it is imperative to begin therapy as soon as possible after the diagnosis is established.[272,276]

8:24 SULFONAMIDES

General References: 277, 278

Sulfamethoxazole and Trimethoprim

Bactrim®,
Septra®, Various

Pharmacology. A combination which provides sequential and synergistic inhibition of bacterial folic acid synthesis. Sulfamethoxazole (SMZ) acts similarly to other sulfonamides (see Sulfisoxazole) while trimethoprim (TMP) acts at a later step to inhibit the enzymatic reduction of dihydrofolic acid to tetrahydrofolic acid. TMP binds selectively to bacterial dihydrofolic acid reductase (50,000 times more avidly than to the comparable human enzyme). The combination is active against many bacteria except anaerobes, *Ps. aeruginosa* and many *S. faecalis*. It is also highly active and effective against the protozoa, *Pneumocystis carinii*. The most important determinant of efficacy is usually the level of susceptibility to TMP. The basic mechanisms of resistance to SMZ and TMP are similar to sulfisoxazole, although resistance is very uncommon with the combination.[277,278]

Administration and Adult Dose. PO for UTI 800 mg of SMZ and 160 mg of TMP q 12 hr for 10–14 days. **PO for prophylaxis of recurrent UTI** 200 mg of SMZ and 40 mg of TMP at bedtime 3 times weekly.[277] **PO for shigellosis** 800 mg of SMZ and 160 mg of TMP q 12 hr for 5 days.[278] **IV for severe UTI or shigellosis** 40–50 mg/kg/day of SMZ and 8–10 mg/kg/day of TMP, in 2–4 equally divided doses, q 6–12 hr for 5 days for shigellosis and up to 14 days for severe UTI. **PO or IV for *Pneumocystis carinii* pneumonia** 100(PO) or 75(IV) mg/kg/day of SMZ and 20(PO) or 15(IV) mg/kg/day of TMP, in 4 equally divided doses, q 6 hr for up to 14 days.[279] **PO for *Pneumocystis carinii* infection prophylaxis** 20 mg/kg/day of SMZ and 4 mg/kg/day of TMP in 2 equally divided doses.[277,279]

Dosage Individualization. Dosage should be reduced in patients with severe renal impairment. No dosage adjustment is necessary for patients with Cl_{cr} greater than 30 ml/min.[277,278,280] For UTI in patients with Cl_{cr} less than 30 ml/min, give normal dosage for 1–6 doses.[277,278] For patients with Cl_{cr} between 10–30 ml/min, follow with ½ usual dose; with Cl_{cr} less than 10 ml/min, follow with ¼–½ usual dose,[277,278] although this probably does not produce effective urinary concentrations, and some authorities advocate full dosage.[281] For systemic infections treated with higher doses, monitor plasma levels.

Pediatric Dose. PO for UTI, shigellosis (over 12 yr) same as adult dose; (2 months–12 yr) 40 mg/kg/day of SMZ and 8 mg/kg/day of TMP (Susp 1 ml/kg/day) in 2 equally divided doses. **PO for otitis media** same as UTI. **IV for severe UTI or shigellosis** (2 months and over) same as adult mg/kg dose. **PO or IV for *Pneumocystis carinii* pneumonia** (2 months and over) same as adult mg/kg dose. **PO for *Pneumocystis carinii* infection prophylaxis** (2 months and over) same as adult mg/kg dose.

Dosage Forms. Susp 40 mg/ml of SMZ and 8 mg/ml of TMP; Tab 400 mg of SMZ and 80 mg of TMP, 800 mg of SMZ and 160 mg of TMP; Inj 80 mg/ml of SMZ and 16 mg/ml of TMP.

Patient Instructions. This medication should be taken with a full 8 ounce glass of water on an empty stomach (1 hr before or 2 hr after meals) for best absorption. Drink several additional glasses of water daily, unless directed otherwise.

Pharmacokinetics and Biopharmaceutics. *Fate.* SMZ and TMP are 90-100% absorbed orally.[282] In normal adults, peak plasma concentrations of 20-50 mcg/ml of SMZ and 0.9-1.9 mcg/ml of TMP occur about 1-4 hr after administration of 800 mg of SMZ and 160 mg of TMP.[282] An additional 10-20 mcg/ml of SMZ exists in the plasma as inactive metabolites.[280] IV infusion over 1 hr of 800 mg of SMZ and 160 mg of TMP in adults produces peak plasma levels of 46.3 mcg/ml of SMZ and 3.4 mcg/ml of TMP.[283] SMZ and TMP are widely distributed in the body, although TMP is much more widely distributed due to its higher lipophilicity; TMP is 45% protein bound and has a V_d of 1-2 L/kg.[282] SMZ has a V_d of 0.36 L/kg and is 60% protein bound.[277,282] TMP concentrations in various tissues and fluids (including the prostate, bile and sputum) are several times greater than concomitant plasma concentrations. CSF concentrations in normal adults are approximately 50% of plasma concentrations. SMZ usually appears in much lower concentrations in body tissues and fluids.[278,282,283] SMZ undergoes extensive liver metabolism, producing N^4-acetylated and N^4-glucuronidated derivatives; 85% is excreted in the urine within 24-72 hr, 10-30% as unchanged drug. Nearly all TMP is excreted in the urine within 24-72 hr, 50-75% as unchanged drug.[280,282] The pharmacokinetics of these drugs are essentially unchanged when given in combination.[280,282] The pH of the urine influences the renal tubular excretion of these compounds, but does not significantly alter overall elimination.[278,280]

$t_{1/2}$. Approximately 8-11 hr (average 9) for SMZ in normal adults;[278,283] 6-15 hr for TMP in normal adults.[277,278,283] Increased in the presence of severe renal failure (20-30 hr or more) for TMP; SMZ unchanged, although data are conflicting due to the measurement of inactive metabolites.[277,278,280,282,284]

Adverse Reactions. Blood dyscrasias (primarily thrombocytopenia, leukopenia and megaloblastic anemia and hemolytic anemia in patients with G6PD deficiency) have been reported in association with SMZ and TMP, although they are probably no more common than with SMZ alone.[277,278] In usual doses, TMP does not affect plasma folate levels as determined by radioisotopic techniques,[285] although effects on folate metabolism may be more significant in patients with pre-existing folate depletion (eg, alcoholics, the elderly, pregnant or malnourished patients).[277] Also, calcium leucovorin reverses antifolate effects without interfering with antimicrobial action.[277,279] SMZ and TMP have been implicated as nephrotoxins, especially in patients with pre-existing renal impairment, but more recent observations have not supported this contention and generally conclude that the combination is safe and effective in these patients.[281,286] It appears that SMZ and TMP compete for tubular excretion with creatinine and reduce the Cl_{cr} in some patients, although glomerular filtration is maintained.[290] May cause jaundice and kernicterus in neonates, and rashes and other hypersensitivity reactions similar to those caused by other sulfonamides.[277,278]

Contraindications. Pregnancy; infants less than 2 months.

Precautions. Lactation; history of hypersensitivity reaction to sulfonamide derivatives; G6PD deficiency; impaired renal or hepatic function. See Drug Interactions chapter.

Parameters to Monitor. Baseline and periodic CBC for patients on long-term or high-dose treatment.

Notes. The efficacy and safety of SMZ and TMP has been demonstrated in numerous other infectious conditions (eg, chronic UTI, chronic bronchitis, sepsis, enteric fever, prostatitis, endocarditis and gonorrhea) and is considered an effective alternative to conventional therapy in most cases.[277,278,284] SMZ is available as a single agent (Gantanol®-Susp 100 mg/ml; Tab 500 mg) and is similar to sulfisoxazole in effectiveness. TMP is available as a single agent (Trimpex®-Tab 100 mg) and has been shown to be effective in acute UTI.[284,287] It does not appear to be as effective in patients with chronic UTI and it has not undergone adequate testing for the treatment of systemic infections.[277,278,284] It has a potential advantage in patients with allergy or toxicity attributed to the sulfonamide;[284,288] however, the relative potential for the single agent to permit the development of resistance is unsettled.[289] In vitro data indicate that SMZ and TMP exhibit maximum synergistic activity at a concentration ratio of 20:1; the 5:1 formulation results in plasma concentrations which approximate this ratio in patients with normal renal function; tissue and body fluid concentration ratios vary widely from the optimum, although adequate synergistic effect occurs at these ratios.[277,278,282] Efficacy of SMZ and TMP in the treatment of *Pneumocystis carinii* pneumonitis is equivalent to pentamidine which makes the combination a valuable alternative, due to its increased safety and availability.[277,279]

Sulfasalazine

Azulfidine®,
Various

Pharmacology. Sulfasalazine (SS) is a conjugate of sulfapyridine (SP) and 5-aminosalicylic acid (5-ASA) which has no antibacterial activity before hydrolysis to its components, and is not used for treating infections. 5-ASA has anti-inflammatory activity which includes potent inhibition of prostaglandin synthesis; this probably accounts for the usefulness of SS in inflammatory bowel disease. SP does not appear to contribute to the anti-inflammatory effect of SS.[291,292]

Administration and Adult Dose. PO for inflammatory bowel disease 1-2 g/day in 4 divided doses initially, increasing (usually by 1 g/day) each week to response and tolerance, to a usual maximum of 3-4 g/day. Doses of 8-12 g/day in 4 divided doses have been used. After optimum response is achieved, doses may be decreased to 500 mg qid for maintenance. Maintenance doses may be discontinued after several years without symptoms.

Pediatric Dose. PO for inflammatory bowel disease 40-60 mg/kg/day in 3-6 divided doses initially, followed after adequate response by maintenance doses of 30 mg/kg/day in 4 divided doses.

Dosage Forms. EC Tab 500 mg; Susp 250 mg/5 ml; Tab 500 mg.

Patient Instructions. Take each dose after meals or with food, and drink at least 1 full glass of water with each dose; drink several additional glasses of water daily. This medication must be taken continually to be effective. Report any nausea, vomiting, excessive change in appetite or abrupt change in character or volume of stools.

Pharmacokinetics and Biopharmaceutics. *Onset and Duration.* Maximum effect in 1-2 weeks; duration 8-12 hr following a dose.

Plasma Levels. SP concentrations of 20-50 mcg/ml have been correlated with optimum response in some studies,[293] but not in others;[291] plasma levels are probably not a reliable index of therapeutic effect. Levels over 50 mcg/ml are associated with increased toxicity and are most likely in slow acetylators.[294-296]

Fate. SS is about 30% absorbed from the small intestine, but is almost completely secreted unchanged in the bile.[297] It is then metabolized in the large bowel, probably by intestinal bacteria, to SP and 5-ASA. Most of SP is absorbed from the colon, metabolized by the liver and excreted in the urine; slow acetylators have higher plasma SP concentrations. 5-ASA is eliminated in the feces. After an oral dose of SS, about 91% is recovered in the urine in 3 days as SP, SP metabolites and small amounts of SS.[297,298]

$t_{1/2}$. (SP) 5–13 hr, depending on acetylator phenotype.[291]

Adverse Reactions. Anorexia, nausea, vomiting, epigastric pain and headache occur frequently, especially with high doses and plasma SP levels;[291,294,295,298] reversible infertility occurs frequently in males.[299] Skin rash is reported occasionally; hemolytic anemia and leukopenia occur rarely. Impairment of dietary folate absorption has been reported.[340]

Contraindications. Intestinal tract obstruction; history of sulfonamide allergy.

Precautions. Pregnancy (despite promising reports of safety).[300] Use with caution in renal impairment, slow acetylators or G6PD deficiency. See Drug Interactions chapter.

Parameters to Monitor. Observe patient for therapeutic response (decrease in crampy diarrhea) and toxicity (headache, anorexia, epigastric pain, nausea). Obtain baseline and periodic WBC and reticulocyte counts. Plasma SP levels may be useful in monitoring for toxicity.[291,294,295,298]

Notes. Primarily useful in maintaining and prolonging periods of remission in ulcerative colitis[295] and in Crohn's disease of the colon,[294] often in combination with oral and/or rectal corticosteroids or oral azathioprine. There are no studies comparing EC and uncoated tablet preparations.

Sulfisoxazole and Salts   Gantrisin®, Various

Pharmacology. A synthetic structural analogue of para-aminobenzoic acid (PABA) which, like other sulfonamides, competitively inhibits the synthesis of dihydropteroic acid (an inactive folic acid precursor) from PABA in bacteria. Bacteriostatically active against many bacteria, although acquired resistance has narrowed the indications primarily to lower UTI. Resistance can occur due to bacterial mutation which reduces the affinity of the folic acid synthesizing enzyme for sulfonamide or which increases bacterial production of PABA. Resistance also results from decreased bacterial permeability, which may be R-factor mediated and transferred among bacterial populations.[18]

Administration and Adult Dose. PO (as sulfisoxazole or sulfisoxazole acetyl) 2–4 g initially, then 4–8 g/day in 4–6 divided doses; PO (as sulfisoxazole acetyl in vegetable oil emulsion) 4–5 g q 12 hr. IM, IV, or SC 50 mg/kg initially, then 100 mg/kg/day in 2–4 equally divided doses. The initial loading dose is probably of no value.[343] Vag 250–500 mg (2.5–5 g of Crm 10%) bid.

Dosage Individualization. Most sources recommend that the dosing interval be extended to 18–24 hr[124,206] or that the drug be avoided[301] in patients with severely impaired renal function. However, the degree of accumulation and risk of toxicity is probably quite small, and full doses may be necessary to achieve therapeutic levels in the urinary tract.[124]

Pediatric Dose. **PO** (over 2 months) (as sulfisoxazole or sulfisoxazole acetyl) 75 mg/kg initially, then 150 mg/kg/day in 4–6 equally divided doses; **PO** (over 2 months) (as sulfisoxazole acetyl in vegetable oil emulsion) 60–75 mg/kg q 12 hr. **PO** do not exceed 6 g/day. **IM, IV, or SC** (over 2 months) same as adult dose in mg/kg.

Dosage Forms. **Susp** (as acetyl) 100 mg/ml, (as acetyl in vegetable oil emulsion) 200 mg/ml; **Syrup** (as acetyl) 100 mg/ml; **Tab** 500 mg; **Inj** (as diolamine) 400 mg/ml; **Ophth Oint** (as diolamine) 4%; **Ophth Sol** (as diolamine) 4%; **Vag Crm** 10%.

Patient Instructions. Oral forms should be taken with a full 8 ounce glass of water on an empty stomach (1 hr before or 2 hr after meals) for best absorption. Drink several additional glasses of water daily, unless directed otherwise.

Pharmacokinetics and Biopharmaceutics. *Fate.* Nearly 100% absorbed orally, with peak plasma concentrations of approximately 10–15 mcg/ml at 2–4 hr after a 2 g dose.[301-303] IM administration produces similar plasma concentrations.[302] Sulfisoxazole acetyl form is deacetylated in the GI tract and absorbed as free sulfisoxazole; it produces a delayed and lower peak plasma concentration.[302] V_d is 0.16 L/kg; about 85–90% protein bound.[303] Distribution is largely restricted to extracellular space, with low concentrations in many tissues and fluid; CSF concentrations equal 10–50% of plasma concentrations; fetal plasma concentrations equal 50% of maternal concentrations.[18,302] Extensive liver metabolism to N^4-acetylated derivative. Approximately 95% of a single dose is excreted in the urine within 24 hr, 40–60% as unchanged active drug.[18,301-303]

$t_{1/2}.$ In normal adults 5–7 hr (average 6); approximately 11 hr with severe renal impairment.[18,124,301] Alkalinization of the urine decreases the half-life to 4.4 hr in normal adults.[301]

Adverse Reactions. Reactions are infrequent, but include blood dyscrasias (primarily thrombocytopenia and leukopenia and hemolytic anemia in patients with G6PD deficiency) and hypersensitivity reactions. Jaundice and kernicterus can occur in neonates due to displacement of bilirubin from albumin binding sites. Nephrotoxicity due to crystalluria is unlikely due to the high solubility of sulfisoxazole, although in patients with renal failure the accumulation of the less soluble acetylated metabolite may increase this risk.[18,301,302]

Contraindications. Pregnancy at term; infants less than 2 months.

Precautions. Pregnancy; history of hypersensitivity reaction to sulfonamide derivatives; G6PD deficiency; impaired renal or hepatic function. See Drug Interactions chapter.

Parameters to Monitor. Baseline and periodic CBC and urinalysis for patients on long-term or high-dose treatment.

Notes. Drug of choice in acute, uncomplicated UTI in females; development of resistance limits its usefulness in the treatment of recurrent or persistent infections.

8:36 URINARY GERMICIDES

Methenamine Hippurate	Hiprex®, Urex®
Methenamine Mandelate	Mandelamine®

Pharmacology.   Methenamine acts as a weak urinary antiseptic via hydrolysis in acidic urine to ammonia and formaldehyde. Mandelic and hippuric acids may exert a mild antiseptic effect.

Administration and Adult Dose.   PO 1 g bid (as hippurate); 1 g qid (as mandelate).

Pediatric Dose.   PO (6–12 yr) 500 mg–1 g bid (as hippurate), 500 mg qid (as mandelate). **PO** (under 6 yr) 20 mg/kg qid (as mandelate).

Dosage Forms.   (As hippurate) **Tab** 1 g. (As mandelate) **Gran** 500 mg, 1 g packets; **Susp** 250, 500 mg/5 ml; **Tab** 250, 500 mg, 1 g.

Patient Instructions.   Take with adequate amounts of fluids to ensure adequate urine flow. Antacids may antagonize the activity of this drug unless measures are taken to ensure an acid urine.

Pharmacokinetics and Biopharmaceutics. *Plasma Levels.* Not for infections outside the urinary tract.
   Fate. Rapidly absorbed and excreted in the urine (90% within 24 hr). Inactive in plasma; in urine it is converted to ammonia and bactericidal formaldehyde if pH is 5.7 or less.[318,319] Mandelic and hippuric acids do not significantly lower urine pH in usual doses.[320]
   $t_{1/2}$. (Methenamine) 2–6 hr.[321]

Adverse Reactions.   Occasional GI distress; urinary tract irritation, albuminuria and hematuria with excessive doses or prolonged therapy.

Contraindications.   Moderate to severe impairment of renal function (ineffective urinary concentrations expected); severe liver disease.

Precautions.   Pregnancy.

Parameters to Monitor.   Urinalysis and/or cultures initially and at completion of treatment or periodically during prolonged treatment. Check urine pH periodically during therapy with a dipstick or nitrazine paper.

Notes.   Acidification of the urine is usually necessary, especially with infection due to urea-splitting organisms (eg, *Proteus mirabilis*). Oral ascorbic acid in doses of 1 g qid or more is usually recommended to acidify the urine; however, acidification may be inconsistent and short-lived.[320,322] Methenamine is probably of little value in preventing or treating infections in patients with indwelling urinary catheters,[320] although it may reduce the occurrence of catheter blockage and resulting infections.[323,324] More effective agents (eg, sulfamethoxazole-trimethoprim) are available for preventing infections in men with urinary tract abnormalities[325] and women experiencing recurrent UTIs.[326]

Nitrofurantoin	Furadantin®, Macrodantin®, Various

Pharmacology.   A nitroheterocyclic compound active against most bacteria which commonly cause urinary tract infections. Most *Proteus* sp.

are moderately resistant and *Pseudomonas aeruginosa* is usually resistant. Mechanism of action is unknown, although reactive metabolites may bind covalently to DNA.[321,327]

Administration and Adult Dose. PO 5-7 mg/kg/day in 4 divided doses (usually 50-100 mg qid); 1-2 mg/kg/day as a single dose for chronic suppression.[328] IV not recommended — see Notes.

Pediatric Dose. PO (over 1 month) 5-7 mg/kg/day in 4 divided doses.

Dosage Forms. Cap (as macrocrystals) 25, 50, 100 mg; **Susp** 5 mg/ml; **Tab** 50, 100 mg; **Inj** (as sodium) 180 mg.

Patient Instructions. This drug should be taken with food, milk or an antacid to minimize stomach upset and increase absorption.

Pharmacokinetics and Biopharmaceutics. *Plasma Levels.* Not sufficient for infections outside the urinary tract.
    Fate.   Usually well-absorbed orally from either the crystalline or macrocrystalline form, although absorption occurs more slowly with the latter.[321,329] Marked bioinequivalence may exist among different products;[330,331] however, only products having grossly deficient bioavailability are likely to be ineffective.[332] V_d is about 0.5-0.7 L/kg; 60-65% plasma protein bound. Rapid metabolism by unknown pathways results in subtherapeutic plasma and tissue concentrations (except renal tissue). Usual doses result in a 50-250 mcg/ml peak concentration in the urine with normal renal function, with 30-50% appearing as unchanged drug within 12 hr.[321]
    $t_{1/2}$. 1 hr in normal adults; probably not significantly longer with renal impairment; no data on the effect of liver impairment.[321]

Adverse Reactions. Nausea and vomiting are frequent and dose-related, probably less frequent with the macrocrystalline form.[333] Occasional rashes and other hypersensitivity reactions occur.[334,335] Ascending polyneuropathy associated with prolonged, high-dose therapy and/or use of the drug in patients with renal failure occurs, and can be fatal or may slowly reverse after drug discontinuation.[336] Severe, acute pneumonitis, usually appearing soon after initiation of therapy and resolving very rapidly with its discontinuation, can occur. Severe, chronic interstitial pulmonary fibrosis occurs which is only partially reversible;[337] recent evidence suggests that pulmonary reactions are not rare.[334] Hemolysis may occur in patients with G6PD deficiency. Rare hepatotoxicity may take the form of chronic active hepatitis.[338]

Contraindications. Moderate to severe impairment of renal function (creatinine clearance less than 40 ml/min) resulting in ineffective urine concentrations and potentially toxic plasma concentrations. Pregnancy at term, and infants less than 1 month of age, due to inadequate metabolic clearance by fetus and neonate.

Precautions. Pregnancy; lactation; G6PD deficiency; pre-existing lung disease or peripheral neuropathy.

Parameters to Monitor. Initial renal function tests. Check for signs of peripheral neuropathy during prolonged therapy.

Notes. Not for infections outside the urinary tract. Macrodantin® is the macrocrystalline form. Has mutagenic activity in mammalian cells;[321,339] however, there is no evidence of carcinogenicity in humans. IV nitrofurantoin (Ivadantin®) is not recommended due to the availability of more systemically effective antimicrobials.

8:40 OTHER ANTI-INFECTIVES

General References: 304, 305, 317

Metronidazole   Flagyl®

Pharmacology.   A nitroimidazole with activity against *T. vaginalis* (trichomoniasis), *E. histolytica* (amebiasis) and *Giardia lamblia* (giardiasis), and is bactericidal against nearly all obligate anaerobic bacteria, including *Bacteroides fragilis*. It is essentially inactive against aerobic and micro-aerophilic bacteria. Reduced by a nitroreductase enzyme within sensitive organisms to highly reactive intermediates which disrupt DNA and inhibit nucleic acid synthesis.

Administration and Adult Dose.   **PO for trichomoniasis** 1–2 g as a single dose, or 500 mg bid for 5 days, or 250 mg tid for 7 days.[306,307] **PO for symptomatic intestinal amebiasis (amebic dysentery)** 750 mg tid for 5–10 days. **PO for extraintestinal amebiasis** 750 mg tid for 5–10 days;[308] some practitioners include a drug effective against the intestinal cyst form, because occasional failures with metronidazole therapy have been reported — see Notes. **PO or IV for anaerobic infections** 15 mg/kg (usually 1 g) initially, followed by 7.5 mg/kg (usually 500 mg) q 6 hr to maximum of 4 g/day. Infuse each IV dose over 1 hr. **PO for giardiasis** 250 mg bid-tid for 7–10 days or 2 g/day as a single dose for 3 days;[304,306] see Notes. **PO for "nonspecific" vaginitis due to *H. vaginalis*** 500 mg bid for 7 days.[304]

Dosage Individualization.   Dose is not altered with impaired renal function.[304,305] Patients with severe hepatic disease metabolize metronidazole slowly, with resultant accumulation of metronidazole and its metabolites in the plasma. For such patients, doses below those usually recommended should be administered cautiously, although specific guidelines are not available; close monitoring of plasma metronidazole levels as well as signs of toxicity is recommended.

Pediatric Dose.   **PO for amebic dysentery or extraintestinal amebiasis** 35–50 mg/kg/day in 3 divided doses for 5–10 days, to maximum of 2.4 g/day. **PO for giardiasis** 25 mg/kg/day in 2–3 divided doses for 7–10 days, to maximum of 750 mg/day.[309] See Notes.

Dosage Forms.   Tab 250, 500 mg; Inj 500 mg

Patient Instructions.   May occasionally cause a harmless dark coloration of the urine and metallic taste in mouth. Nausea, vomiting and faintness may occur if alcohol is taken during therapy with this drug.

Pharmacokinetics and Biopharmaceutics. Fate.   Very well absorbed orally, with 250 and 500 mg producing peak concentrations of 5 and 12 mcg/ml, respectively at 1–2 hr in adults.[307,310] IV infusions over 1 hr produce plasma levels identical to those seen after equivalent PO doses. IV 7.5 mg/kg q 6 hr produces steady-state peak and trough levels of 24 and 19 mcg/ml, respectively.[306] V_d is 0.6–0.8 L/kg (ie, about equal to total body water); 10–20% protein bound;[307] wide distribution with therapeutic levels in many tissues, including abscesses, bile, bone and CSF.[304,311] Extensively metabolized in the liver by hydroxylation. oxidation and glucuronide formation; 44–80% excreted in the urine in 24 hr, about 8–20% as unchanged drug.[307,312]

$t_{1/2}$.   6–8 hr in adults;[307,310,312] not increased with impaired renal function;[304] prolonged variably with severe hepatic impairment.

Adverse Effects. Metallic taste in mouth and GI complaints may be frequent with high doses. Occasional dizziness, vertigo and paresthesias have been reported with very high doses. Reversible mild neutropenia reported occasionally.[304-306,313] Reversible, rare, but severe peripheral neuropathy may occur with high doses given over prolonged periods. Pseudomembranous colitis has been reported with oral metronidazole.[314,315] The IV preparation is associated occasionally with phlebitis at the infusion site. Experimental production of tumors in some rodent species and mutations in bacteria has raised serious concern regarding potential carcinogenicity; to date, mammalian testing and human epidemiologic research have not detected a significant risk, although further data are needed.[304,313]

Contraindications. First trimester of pregnancy, although there is no direct evidence of teratogenicity in humans or animals.[304,306]

Precautions. Pregnancy; patients with active CNS disease or neutropenia. See Drug Interactions chapter.

Parameters to Monitor. Before and after the completion of any lengthy or repeated courses of therapy, monitor WBC count.[304]

Notes. Therapy of amebiasis with metronidazole alone is somewhat controversial. For *asymptomatic* patients passing cyst forms of the parasite, metronidazole is not useful; PO diiodohydroxyquin 650 mg tid for 20 days has been effective in only 60–70% of such cases; and **PO diloxanide furoate** (Furamide®) 500 mg tid for 10 days is 80–85% effective — see Drugs Available from CDC chart. For *symptomatic* patients with amebic dysentery or extra-intestinal amebiasis, **IM emetine hydrochloride** 1 mg/kg/day in 1–2 divided doses for 7 days, to maximum of 60 mg/day has been successful, usually in combination with **PO chloroquine phosphate** 10 mg/kg/day in 2 divided doses for 2–3 weeks, to maximum of 500 mg/day. **IM or SC dehydroemetine** 1–1.5 mg/kg/day for 10 days appears to be as effective as emetine and may have less cardiac toxicity[308] — see Drugs Available from CDC chart.

The treatment of *asymptomatic* trichomoniasis is controversial. Signs of endocervical inflammation or erosion on physical exam are considered an indication for treatment. Also, most practitioners choose to treat asymptomatic male consorts, because lack of such treatment may be a cause of treatment failure or recurrent infection of the female partner.[304,306,313]

For the treatment of giardiasis, metronidazole appears to be about as effective as **PO quinacrine hydrochloride** (Atabrine®) 100 mg tid for 7 days.[304]

Proper reconstitution of the IV preparation is important. IV metronidazole reacts with aluminum; aluminum needles should not be used. First, reconstitute with 4.4 ml of sterile water or saline (preserved or nonpreserved). Then dilute dose in normal saline, D5W or lactated Ringer's to a final concentration of no more than 8 mg/ml. Finally, neutralize with 5 mEq of sodium bicarbonate for each 500 mg of drug. Do not refrigerate neutralized solution. Also available as prepared, stabilized solution (Flagyl I.V. RTU®).

Tinidazole (Investigational - Pfizer)   Fasigyn®

Tinidazole is an investigational nitroimidazole, similar to metronidazole in *in vitro* activity against protozoa and anaerobic bacteria. In clinical trials tinidazole appears to be more effective in the treatment of giardiasis and amebiasis, especially in single-dose regimens. Peak plasma levels of tinidazole are 20% greater than metronidazole and persist longer due to a longer elimination half-life (12.5 hr). Side effects are similar to those observed with metronidazole. In several studies PO 50 mg/kg as a single dose was very effective in the treatment of giardiasis; PO 2 g/day for 2 days for amebic liver abscess and 2 g/day for 3 days for intestinal amebiasis were also very effective.[316,317]

References, 8:00 Anti-Infective Agents

1. Most H. Treatment of common parasitic infections of man encountered in the United States. N Engl J Med 1972;287:495-8, 698-702.

2. Katz M. Anthelmintics. Drugs 1977;13:124-36.

3. Botero D. Chemotherapy of human intestinal parasitic diseases. Annu Rev Pharmacol Toxicol 1978;18:1-15.

4. Miller MH. Protozoan and helminth parasites—a review of current treatment. In: Jucker E, ed. Progress in drug research, vol. 20. Basel: Birkhauser Verlag, 1976:433-62.

5. Brugmans JP, Thienpont DC, van Wijngaarden I et al. Mebendazole in enterobiasis: radiochemical and pilot clinical study in 1,278 subjects. JAMA 1971;217:313-6.

6. Miller MJ, Krupp IM, Little MD et al. Mebendazole: an effective anthelmintic for trichuriasis and enterobiasis. JAMA 1974;230:1412-4.

7. Wolfe MS, Wershing JM. Mebendazole: treatment of trichuriasis and ascariasis in Bahamian children. JAMA 1974;230:1408-11.

8. Chavarria AP, Swartzwelder JC, Villarejos VM et al. Mebendazole, an effective broad-spectrum anthelmintic. Am J Trop Med Hyg 1973;22:592-5.

9. Sargent RG, Savory AM, Mina A et al. A clinical evaluation of mebendazole in the treatment of trichuriasis. Am J Trop Med Hyg 1974;23:375-7.

10. Hanna S, Tang A. Human urinary excretion of piperazine citrate from syrup formulations. J Pharm Sci 1973;62:2024-5.

11. Parsons AC. Piperazine neurotoxicity: "worm wobble." Br Med J 1971;4:792.

12. Goodwin LG, Standen OD. Treatment of ascariasis with various salts of piperazine. Br Med J 1958;1:131-3.

13. Rogers EW. Excretion of piperazine salts in urine. Br Med J 1958;1:136-7.

14. Pitts NE, Migliardi JR. Antiminth (pyrantel pamoate): the clinical evaluation of a new broad-spectrum anthelmintic. Clin Pediatr 1974;13:87-94.

15. Bumbalo TS, Fugazzotto DJ, Wyczalek JV. Treatment of enterobiasis with pyrantel pamoate. Am J Trop Med Hyg 1969;18:50-2.

16. Smith TC, Kinkel AW, Gryczko CM et al. Absorption of pyrvinium pamoate. Clin Pharmacol Ther 1976;19:802-6.

17. Buchanan RA, Barrow WB, Heffelfinger JC et al. Pyrvinium pamoate. Clin Pharmacol Ther 1974;16:716-9.

18. Mandell GL, Douglas RG, Bennett JE, eds. Principles and practice of infectious diseases. New York: John Wiley & Sons, 1979.

19. DeTorres OH. A closer look at aminoglycosides. Clin Ther 1981;3:399-412.

20. Pechere J-O, Dugal R. Clinical pharmacokinetics of aminoglycoside antibiotics. Clin Pharmacokinet 1979;4:170-99.

21. Barza M, Scheife RT. Drug therapy reviews: antimicrobial spectrum, pharmacology and therapeutic use of antibiotics – Part 4: aminoglycosides. Am J Hosp Pharm 1977;34:723-77.

22. Pien FD, Ho PWL. Antimicrobial spectrum, pharmacology, adverse effects, and therapeutic use of amikacin sulfate. Am J Hosp Pharm 1981;38:981-9.

23. Appel GB, Neu HC. Gentamicin in 1978. Ann Intern Med 1978;89:528-38.

24. Leroy A, Humbert G, Oksenhendler G et al. Pharmacokinetics of aminoglycosides in subjects with normal and impaired renal function. Antibiot Chemother 1978;25:163-80.

25. Moellering RC. Microbiological considerations in the use of tobramycin and related aminoglycosidic aminocyclitol antibiotics. Med J Aust (Spec Suppl)1977;2:4-8.

26. Brogden RN, Pinder RM, Sawyer PR et al. Tobramycin: a review of its antibacterial and pharmacokinetic properties and therapeutic use. Drugs 1976;12:166-200.

27. Evans WE, Schentag JJ, Jusko W, eds. Applied pharmacokinetics: principles of therapeutic drug monitoring. San Francisco: Applied Therapeutics, 1980.

28. Casillas E, Kenny MA, Minshew BH et al. Effect of ionized calcium and soluble magnesium on the predictability of the performance of the Mueller-Hinton agar susceptibility testing of *Pseudomonas aeruginosa* with gentamicin. Antimicrob Agents Chemother 1981;19:997-92.

29. Mendelson J, Portnoy J, Dick V et al. Safety of the bolus administration of gentamicin. Antimicrob Agents Chemother 1976;9:633-8.

30. Davey PG, Gonda I, Harpur ES et al. Review of recent studies on control of aminoglycoside antibiotic therapy. J Clin Hosp Pharm 1980;5:175-95.

31. Bauer LA, Blouin RA, Griffen WO et al. Amikacin pharmacokinetics in morbidly obese patients. Am J Hosp Pharm 1980;37:519-22.

32. Zaske DE, Cipolle RJ, Strate RG, Gentamicin dosing requirements: wide interpatient variations in 242 surgery patients with normal renal function. Surgery 1980;87:164-70.

33. Sarubbi FA, Hull JH. Amikacin serum concentrations; prediction of levels and dosage guidelines. Ann Intern Med 1978;89:612-8.

34. Ericsson CD, Duke JH, Pickering LK. Clinical pharmacology of intravenous and intraperitoneal aminoglycoside antibiotics in the prevention of wound infections. Ann Surg 1978;188:66-70.

35. Richey GD, Schleupner CJ. Peritoneal fluid concentrations of gentamicin in patients with spontaneous bacterial peritonitis. Antimicrob Agents Chemother 1981;19:312-5.

36. French MA, Cerra FB, Plaut ME et al. Amikacin and gentamicin accumulation pharmacokinetics and nephrotoxicity in critically ill patients. Antimicrob Agents Chemother 1981;19:147-52.

37. Zaske DE, Cipolle RJ, Strate RG et al. Rapid gentamicin elimination in obstetric patients. Obstet Gynecol 1980;56:559-64.

38. Schentag JJ, Gengo FM, Plaut ME et al. Urinary casts as an indicator of renal tubular damage in patients receiving aminoglycosides. Antimicrob Agents Chemother 1979;16:468-74.

39. Keating MJ, Sethi MR, Bodey GP et al. Hypocalcemia with hypoparathyroidism and renal tubular dysfunction associated with aminoglycoside therapy. Cancer 1977;39:1410-4.

40. Fee WE, Aminoglycoside ototoxicity in the human. Laryngoscope 1980;90 (Suppl 24):1-19.

41. Schentag JJ, Plaut ME, Cerra FB. Comparative nephrotoxicity of gentamicin and tobramycin: pharmacokinetic and clinical studies in 201 patients. Antimicrob Agents Chemother 1981;19:859-66.

42. Frimodt-Moller N, Maigaard S, Madsen PO. Comparative nephrotoxicity among aminoglycosides and beta-lactam antibiotics. Infection 1980;8:283-9.

43. Barza M, Lauermann MW, Tally FP et al. Prospective, randomized trial of netilmicin and amikacin, with emphasis on eighth-nerve toxicity. Antimicrob Agents Chemother 1980;17:707-14.

44. Bock BV, Edelstein PH, Meyer RD. Prospective comparative study of efficacy and toxicity of netilmicin and amikacin. Antimicrob Agents Chemother 1980;17:217-25.

45. Smith CR, Lipsky JJ, Laskin OL et al. Double-blind comparison of the nephrotoxicity and auditory toxicity of gentamicin and tobramycin. N Engl J Med 1980;302:1106-9.

46. Hottendorf GH, Barnett D, Gordon LL et al. Nonparallel nephrotoxicity dose-response curves of aminoglycosides. Antimicrob Agents Chemother 1981;19:1024-8.

47. Medoff G, Kobayashi GS. Strategies in the treatment of systemic fungal infections. N Engl J Med 1980;302:145-55.

48. Kobayashi GS, Medoff G. Antifungal agents: recent developments. Annu Rev Microbiol 1977;31:291-308.

49. Bennett JE. Chemotherapy of systemic mycoses. N Engl J Med 1974;290:30-2,320-3.

50. Newberry WM. Drug treatment of systemic mycoses. Semin Drug Treat 1972;2:313-29.

51. Hoeprich PD. Chemotherapy of systemic fungal diseases. Annu Rev Pharmacol Toxicol 1978;18:205-31.

52. Gotz VP, Mar DD, Roche JJ. Compatibility of amphotericin B with drugs used to reduce adverse reactions. Am J Hosp Pharm 1981;38:378-9.

53. Jurgens RW, DeLuca PP, Papadimitriou D. Compatibility of amphotericin B with certain large-volume parenterals. Am J Hosp Pharm 1981;38:377-8.

54. Alazraki NP, Fierer J, Halpern SE et al. Use of a hyperbaric solution for administration of intrathecal amphotericin B. N Engl J Med 1974;290:641-6.

55. Wise GJ, Wainstein S, Goldberg P et al. Candidal cystitis: management by continuous bladder irrigation with amphotericin B. JAMA 1973;224:1636-7.

56. Block ER, Bennett JE, Livoti LG et al. Flucytosine and amphotericin B: hemodialysis effects on the plasma concentration and clearance. Ann Intern Med 1974;80:613-7.

57. Louria DB. Some aspects of the absorption, distribution, and excretion of amphotericin B in man. Antibiot Med Clin Ther 1958;5:295-301.

58. Bindschadler DD, Bennett JE. A pharmacologic guide to the clinical use of amphotericin B. J Infect Dis 1969;120:427-36.

59. Atkinson AJ, Bennett JE. Amphotericin B pharmacokinetics in humans. Antimicrob Agents Chemother 1978;13:271-6.

60. Maddux MS, Barriere SL. A review of complications of amphotericin-B therapy: recommendations for prevention and management. Drug Intell Clin Pharm 1980;14:177-81.

61. Burks LC, Aisner J, Fortner CL et al. Meperidine for the treatment of shaking chills and fever. Arch Intern Med 1980;140:483-4.

62. Tarala RA, Smith JD. Cryptococcosis treated by rapid infusion of amphotericin B. Br Med J 1980;2:28.

63. Smale LE, Waechter KG. Dissemination of coccidiomycosis in pregnancy. Am J Obstet Gynecol 1970;107:356-61.

64. Miller RP, Bates JH. Amphotericin B toxicity: a follow-up report of 53 patients. Ann Intern Med 1969;71:1089-95.

65. Lufter CH, Ball WD. Activity of amphotericin B after filtration (letter). Drug Intell Clin Pharm 1980;14:719.

66. D'Arcy PF, Scott EM. Antifungal agents. In: Jucker E, ed. Progress in drug research, vol. 22. Basel: Birkhauser Verlag, 1978:94-147.

67. Steer PL, Marks MI, Klite PD et al. 5-fluorocytosine: an oral antifungal compound. Ann Intern Med 1972;76:15-22.

68. Horn JR, Giusti DL. The pharmacokinetics of flucytosine in cryptococcal meningitis. Drug Intell Clin Pharm 1975;9:180-8.

69. Cutler RE, Blair AD, Kelly MR. Flucytosine kinetics in subjects with normal and impaired renal function. Clin Pharmacol Ther 1978;24:333-42.

70. MacLeod SM, Ti TY, Williams RB et al. Parenteral 5-fluorocytosine for candidiasis. Drug Intell Clin Pharm 1979;13:72-5.

71. Goldman L. Griseofulvin. Med Clin North Am 1970;54:1339-45.

72. Epstein WL, Shah V, Riegelman S. Dermatopharmacology of griseofulvin. Cutis 1975;15:271-5.

73. Rowland M, Riegelman S, Epstein WL. Absorption kinetics of grisecfulvin in man. J Pharm Sci 1968;57:984-9.

74. Lin C-C, Magat J, Chang R et al. Absorption, metabolism and excretion of ^{14}C-griseofulvin in man. J Pharmacol Exp Ther 1973;187:415-22.

75. Straughn AB, Meyer MC, Raghow G et al. Bioavailability of microsize and ultra-microsize griseofulvin products in man. J Pharmacokinet Biopharm 1980;8:347-62.

76. Sohn CA. Evaluation of ketoconazole. Clin Pharm 1982;1:217-24.

77. Borgers M. Mechanism of action of antifungal drugs, with special reference to the imidazole derivatives. Rev Infect Dis 1980;2:520-34.

78. Stranz MH. Miconazole. Drug Intell Clin Pharm 1980;14:86-95.

79. Stevens DA, Levine HB, Deresinski SC. Miconazole in coccidioidomycosis: II. therapeutic and pharmacologic studies in man. Am J Med 1976;60:191-202.

80. Lewi PJ, Boelaert J, Daneels R et al. Pharmacokinetic profile of intravenous miconazole in man: comparison of normal subjects and patients with renal insufficiency. Eur J Clin Pharmacol 1976;10:49-54.

81. Stevens DA. Miconazole in the treatment of systemic fungal infections. Am Rev Respir Dis 1977;116:801-6.

82. Nightingale CH, Greene DS, Quintiliani R. Pharmacokinetics and clinical use of cephalosporin antibiotics. J Pharm Sci 1975;64:1899-927.

83. Moellering RC, Swartz MN. The newer cephalosporins. N Engl J Med 1976;294:24-8.

84. Barza M, Miao PVW. Antimicrobial spectrum, pharmacology and therapeutic use of antibiotics, part 3: cephalosporins. Am J Hosp Pharm 1977;34:621-9.

85. Meyers BR. The cephalosporins. NY State J Med 1977;77:1128-32.

86. O'Callaghan CH. Description and classification of the newer cephalosporins and their relationship with the established compounds. J Antimicrob Chemother 1979;5:635-71.

87. Weinstein AJ. The cephalosporins: activity and clinical use. Drugs 1980;19:137-54.

88. Murray BE, Moellering RC. Cephalosporins. Annu Rev Med 1981;32:559-81.

89. Bergman HD. Cefamandole. Drug Intell Clin Pharm 1979;13:144-9.

90. Quintiliani R, Nightingale CH. Cefazolin. Ann Intern Med 1978;89(part 1):650-6.

91. Singhvi SM, Heald AF, Schreiber EC. Pharmacokinetics of cephalosporin antibiotics: protein-binding considerations. Chemotherapy 1978;24:121-33.

92. Neu HC. Comparison of pharmacokinetics of cefamandole and other cephalosporin compounds. J Infect Dis 1978;137(Suppl):S80-7.

93. Andriole VT. Pharmacokinetics of cephalosporins in patients with normal or reduced renal function. J Infect Dis 1978;137(Suppl):S88-97.

94. Schrogie JJ, Rogers JD, Yeh KC et al. Pharmacokinetics and comparative pharmacology of cefoxitin and cephalosporins. Rev Infect Dis 1979;1:90-7.

95. Brogard JM, Comte F, Pinget M. Pharmacokinetics of cephalosporin antibiotics. Antibiot Chemother 1978;25:123-62.

96. Gardner ME, Fritz WL, Hyland RN. Antibiotic-induced seizures: a case attributed to cefazolin and a review of the literature. Drug Intell Clin Pharm 1978;12:268-71.

97. Lerner PI, Lubin A. Coagulopathy with cefazolin in uremia. N Engl J Med 1974;290:1324. Letter.

98. Barza M. The nephrotoxicity of cephalosporins: an overview. J Infect Dis 1978;137(Suppl):S60-73.

99. Petz LD. Immunologic cross-reactivity between penicillins and cephalosporins: a review. J Infect Dis 1978;137(Suppl):S74-9.

100. Mashimo K, Kunii O. Clinical trials of cefoperazone in the field of internal medicine in Japan. Clin Ther 1980;3:159-72.

101. Dudley MN, Barriere SL. Cefotaxime: microbiology, pharmacology, and clinical use. Clin Pharm 1982;1:114-24.

102. Geddes AM, Acar JF, Knothe H (eds.). Cefotaxime: a new cephalosporin antibiotic. J Antimicrob Chemother 1980;6(Suppl A):1-303.

103. Brogden RN, Heel RC, Speight TM et al. Cefoxitin: a review of its antibacterial activity, pharmacological properties and therapeutic use. Drugs 1979;17:1-37.

104. Fernex M, Havas L. Introduction and review – reports on ceftriaxone (Rocephin*). Chemotherapy (Basel) 1981;27(Suppl 1):1-8.

105. Stoeckel K, McNamara PJ, Brandt R et al. Effects of concentration-dependent plasma protein binding on ceftriaxone kinetics. Clin Pharmacol Ther 1981;29:650-7.

106. Norrby R, Foord RD, Hedlund P. Clinical and pharmacokinetic studies on cefuroxime. J Antimicrob Chemother 1977;3:355-62.

107. Polk RE. Moxalactam evaluation. Drug Intell Clin Pharm 1982;16:104-12.

108. Reed MD, Bertino JS, Aronoff SC et al. Evaluation of moxalactam. Clin Pharm 1982;1:124-34.

109. Derry JE. Evaluation of cefaclor. Am J Hosp Pharm 1981;38:54-8.

110. Bergman HD. Cefaclor. Drug Intell Clin Pharm 1980;14:11-6.

111. Chow M, Quintiliani R, Cunha BA et al. Pharmacokinetics of high dose oral cephalosporins. J Clin Pharmacol 1979;19:185-94.

112. Humbert G, Fillastre JP, Leroy A et al. Pharmacokinetics of cefoxitin in normal subjects and in patients with renal insufficiency. Rev Infect Dis 1979;1:118-25.

113. Shimizu K. Cefoperazone: absorption, excretion, distribution, and metabolism. Clin Therapeut 1980;3:60-79.

114. Parsons JN, Romano JM, Levison ME. Pharmacology of a new 1-oxa-β-lactam (LY 127935) in normal volunteers. Antimicrob Agents Chemother 1980;17:226-8.

115. Lam M, Manion CV, Czerwinski AW. Pharmacokinetics of moxalactam in patients with renal insufficiency. Antimicrob Agents Chemother 1981;19:461-4.

116. Srinivasan S, Francke EL, Neu HC. Comparative pharmacokinetics of cefoperazone and cefamandole. Antimicrob Agents Chemother 1981;19:298-301.

117. Patel IH, Miller K, Weinfeld R et al. Multiple intravenous dose pharmacokinetics of ceftriaxone in man. Chemotherapy 1981;27(Suppl 1):47-56.

118. Leroy A, Humbert G, Fillastre JP. Pharmacokinetics of moxalactam in subjects with normal and impaired renal function. Antimicrob Agents Chemother 1981;19:965-71.

119. Wise R, Wright N, Willis PJ. Pharmacology of cefotaxime and its desacetyl metabolite in renal and hepatic disease. Antimicrob Agents Chemother 1981;19:526-31.

120. Bolton WK, Scheld WM, Spyker DA et al. Pharmacokinetics of cefoperazone in normal volunteers and subjects with renal insufficiency. Antimicrob Agents Chemother 1981;19:821-5.

121. Washington JA. The in vitro spectrum of the cephalosporins. Mayo Clin Proc 1976;51:237-50.

122. Meissner HC, Smith AL. The current status of chloramphenicol. Pediatrics 1979;64:348-56.

123. Slaughter RL, Pieper JA, Cerra FB et al. Chloramphenicol sodium succinate kinetics in critically ill patients. Clin Pharmacol Ther 1980;28:69-77.

124. Bennett WM, Muther RS, Parker RA et al. Drug therapy in renal failure: dosing guidelines for adults. part 1: antimicrobial agents, analgesics. Ann Intern Med 1980;93(part 1):62-89.

125. Sack CM, Koup JR, Smith AL. Chloramphenicol pharmacokinetics in infants and young children. Pediatrics 1980;66:579-84.

126. Glazer JP, Danish MA, Plotkin SA et al. Disposition of chloramphenicol in low birth weight infants. Pediatrics 1980;66:573-9.

127. Kauffman RE, Miceli JN, Strebel L et al. Pharmacokinetics of chloramphenicol and chloramphenicol succinate in infants and children. J Pediatr 1981;98:315-20.

128. Pickering LK, Hoecker JL, Kramer WG, et al. Clinical pharmacology of two chloramphenicol preparations in children: sodium succinate (iv) and palmitate (oral) esters. J Pediatrics 1980;96:757-61.

129. Weiss CF, Glazko AJ, Weston JK. Chloramphenicol in the newborn infant: a physiologic explanation of its toxicity when given in excessive doses. N Engl J Med 1960;262:787-94.

130. Koup JR, Lau AH, Brodsky B et al. Chloramphenicol pharmacokinetics in hospitalized patients. Antimicrob Agents Chemother 1979;15:651-7.

131. Lindberg AA, Nilsson LH, Bucht H et al. Concentration of chloramphenicol in the urine and blood in relation to renal function. Br Med J 1966;3:724-8.

132. Suhrland LG, Weisberger AS. Delayed clearance of chloramphenicol from serum in patients with hematologic toxicity. Blood 1969;34:466-71.

133. Scott JL, Finegold SM, Belkin GA et al. A controlled double-blind study of the hematologic toxicity of chloramphenicol. N Engl J Med 1965;272:1138-42.

134. Saidi P, Wallerstein RO, Aggeler PM. Effect of chloramphenicol on erythropoiesis. J Lab Clin Med 1961;57:247-56.

135. Meade RH. Drug therapy reviews: antimicrobial spectrum, pharmacology and therapeutic use of erythromycin and its derivatives. Am J Hosp Pharm 1979;36:1185-9.

136. Fraser DG. Selection of an oral erythromycin product. Am J Hosp Pharm 1980;37:1199-205.

137. Ginsburg CM, Eichenwald HF. Erythromycin: a review of its uses in pediatric practice. J Pediatr 1976;89:872-84.

138. Nicholas P. Erythromycin: clinical review. NY State J Med 1977;77:2088-94, 2243-6.

139. Miller AC. Erythromycin in legionaires' disease: a re-appraisal. J Antimicrob Chemother 1981;7:217-22.

140. Wilson JT, van Boxtel CJ. Pharmacokinetics of erythromycin in man. Antibiot Chemother 1978;25:181-203.

141. van Marion WF, van der Meer JWM, Kalff MW, et al. Ototoxicity of erythromycin. Lancet 1978;2:214-5.

142. Reeves DS, Bullock DW. The aminopenicillins: development and comparative properties. Infection 1979;7(Suppl 5):S425-33.

143. Barza M, Weinstein L. Pharmacokinetics of the penicillins in man. Clin Pharmacokinet 1976;1:297-308.

144. Barza M. Antimicrobial spectrum, pharmacology and therapeutic use of antibiotics. part 2: penicillins. Am J Hosp Pharm 1977;34:57-67.

145. Bergan T. Penicillins. Antibiot Chemother 1978;25:1-122.

146. Neu HC. Amoxicillin. Ann Intern Med 1979;90:356-60.

147. Reeves DS, Bullock DW. The aminopenicillins: development and comparative properties. Infection 1979;7(Suppl 5):S425-33.

148. Jusko WJ, Lewis GP, Schmitt GW. Ampicillin and hetacillin pharmacokinetics in normal and anephric subjects. Clin Pharmacol Ther 1973;14:90-9.

149. Lewis GP, Jusko WJ. Pharmacokinetics of ampicillin in cirrhosis. Clin Pharmacol Ther 1975;18:475-84.

150. Sjovall J, Magni L, Bergan T. Pharmacokinetics of bacampicillin compared with those of ampicillin, pivampicillin and amoxycillin. Antimicrob Agents Chemother 1978;13:90-6.

151. Ehrnebo M, Nilsson S-O, Boreus LO. Pharmacokinetics of ampicillin and its prodrugs bacampicillin and pivampicillin in man. J Pharmacokinet Biopharm 1979;7:429-51.

152. Eshelman FN, Spyker DA. Pharmacokinetics of amoxicillin and ampicillin: crossover study of the effect of food. Antimicrob Agents Chemother 1978;14:539-43.

153. Yoshioka H, Takimoto M, Riley HD. Pharmacokinetics of ampicillin in the newborn infant. J Infect Dis 1974;129:461-4.

154. Kagan BM. Ampicillin rash. West J Med 1977;126:333-5.

155. Gotz V, Romankiewicz JA, Moss J et al. Prophylaxis against ampicillin-associated diarrhea with a lactobacillus preparation. Am J Hosp Pharm 1979;36:754-7.

156. George WL. Antimicrobial agent-associated colitis and diarrhea. West J Med 1980;133:115-23.

157. Appel GB, Neu HC. The nephrotoxicity of antimicrobial agents. N Engl J Med 1977;296:663-70, 722-8, 784-7.

158. Gill MA, DuBe JE, Young WW. Hypokalemic, metabolic alkalosis induced by high-dose ampicillin sodium. Am J Hosp Pharm 1977;34:528-31.

159. Neu HC. The pharmacokinetics of bacampicillin. Rev Infect Dis 1981;3:110-6.

160. Nordbring F. Review of side-effects of aminopenicillins. Infection 1979;7(Suppl 5):S503-6.

161. Latos DL, Bryan CS, Stone WJ. Carbenicillin therapy in patients with normal and impaired renal function. Clin Pharmacol Ther 1975;17:692-700.

162. Hoffman TA, Cestero R, Bullock WE. Pharmacodynamics of carbenicillin in hepatic and renal failure. Ann Intern Med 1970;73:173-8.

163. Knirsch AK, Hobbs DC, Korst JJ. Pharmacokinetics, toleration, and safety of indanyl carbenicillin in man. J Infect Dis 1973;127(Suppl):S105-8.

164. Libke RD, Clarke JT, Ralph ED et al. Ticarcillin vs carbenicillin: clinical pharmacokinetics. Clin Pharmacol Ther 1975;17:441-6.

165. Cox CE. Pharmacology of carbenicillin indanyl sodium in renal insufficiency. J Infect Dis 1973;127(Suppl):S157-62.

166. Tabernero Romo JM, Corbacho L, Sanchez L et al. Effects of carbenicillin on blood coagulation: a study in patients with chronic renal failure. Clin Nephrol 1979;11:31-4.

167. Pickering LK, Gearhart P. Effect of time and concentration upon interaction between gentamicin, tobramycin, netilmicin or amikacin and carbenicillin or ticarcillin. Antimicrob Agents Chemother 1979;15:592-6.

168. Nauta EH, Mattie H. Dicloxacillin and cloxacillin: pharmacokinetics in healthy and hemodialysis subjects. Clin Pharmacol Ther 1976;20:98-108.

169. Russo J, Russo ME. Comparative review of two new wide-spectrum penicillins: mezlocillin and piperacillin. Clin Pharm 1982;1:207-16.

170. Center for Disease Control. Syphilis: recommended treatment schedules, 1976. Recommendations established by the venereal disease control advisory committee. Ann Intern Med 1976;85:94-6.

171. Levit F. Syphilis therapy still imperfect. JAMA 1976;236:2213-4.

172. Barrett-Connor E. Current status of the treatment of syphilis. West J Med 1975;122:7-11.

173. Trentham DE, McCravey JW, Masi AT. Low-dose penicillin for gonococcal arthritis. a comparative therapy trial. JAMA 1976;236:2410-2.

174. Brewin A, Arango L, Hadley K et al. High-dose penicillin therapy and pneumococcal pneumonia. JAMA 1974;230:409-13.

175. Public Health Service recommendations for treatment of gonorrhea. West J Med 1979;130:286-9.

176. Galpin JE, Chow AW, Yoshikawa TT et al. "Pseudoanaphylactic" reactions from inadvertent infusion of procaine penicillin G. Ann Intern Med 1974;81:358-9.

177. Bradberry JC, Owens J. Acute psychotic reaction to procaine penicillin. Am J Hosp Pharm 1975;32:411-3.

178. Bryan CS, Stone WJ. "Comparably massive" penicillin G therapy in renal failure. Ann Intern Med 1975;82:189-95.

179. Myre S, Zaske D. Anaphylactic shock following oral penicillin – report of two cases. Am J Hosp Pharm 1976;33:268-9.

180. Green GR, Rosenblum AH, Sweet LC. Evaluation of penicillin hypersensitivity: value of clinical history and skin testing with penicilloyl-polylysine and penicillin G. J Allergy Clin Immunol 1977;60:339-45.

181. Anon. Penicillin allergy. Med Lett Drugs Ther 1978;20:14-5.

182. Winston DJ, Murphy W, Young LS et al. Piperacillin therapy for serious bacterial infections. Am J Med 1980;69:255-61.

183. Thompson MIB, Russo ME, Matsen JM. Piperacillin pharmacokinetics in subjects with chronic renal failure. Antimicrob Agents Chemother 1981;19:450-3.

184. Simon GL, Snydman DR, Tally FP et al. Clinical trial of piperacillin with acquisition of resistance by Pseudomonas and clinical relapse. Antimicrob Agents Chemother 1980;18:167-70.

185. Brogden RN, Heel RC, Speight TM et al. Ticarcillin: a review of its pharmacological properties and therapeutic efficacy. Drugs 1980;20:325-52.

186. Barza M, Schiefe RT. Antimicrobial spectrum, pharmacology and therapeutic use of antibiotics part 1: tetracyclines. Am J Hosp Pharm 1977;34:49-57.

187. Baptista RJ, Harvie RJ, Guen R. The tetracyclines: an overview. US Pharmacist 1979;4:33-44.

188. Siegel D. Tetracyclines: new look at old antibiotic. NY State J Med 1978;78:950-5, 1115-20.

189. Sack DA, Kaminsky DC, Sack RB et al. Prophylactic doxycycline for travelers' diarrhea: results of a prospective double-blind study of Peace Corps volunteers in Kenya. N Engl J Med 1978;298:758-63.

190. Heaney D, Eknoyan G. Minocycline and doxycycline kinetics in chronic renal failure. Clin Pharmacol Ther 1978;24:233-9.

191. Allen JC. Minocycline. Ann Intern Med 1976;85:482-7.

192. Leigh DA. Antibacterial activity and pharmacokinetics of clindamycin. J Antimicrob Chemother 1981;7(Suppl A):3-9.

193. Roberts AP, Eastwood JB, Gower PE et al. Serum and plasma concentrations of clindamycin following a single intramuscular injection of clindamycin phosphate in maintenance haemodialysis patients and normal subjects. Eur J Clin Pharmacol 1978;14:435-9.

194. Palmer DMD, Sales JEL, Lincomycin and clindamycin. Antibiot Chemother 1978;25:204-16.

195. Avant GR, Schenker S, Alford RH. The effect of cirrhosis on the disposition and elimination of clindamycin. Am J Dig Dis 1975;20:223-30.

196. Hinthorn DR, Baker LH, Romig DA et al. Use of clindamycin in patients with liver disease. Antimicrob Agents Chemother 1976;9:498-501.

197. DeHaan RM, Vanden Bosch WD, Metzler CM. Clindamycin serum concentrations after administration of clindamycin palmitate with food. J Clin Pharmacol 1972;12:205-11.

198. DeHaan RM, Metzler CM, Schellenberg D et al. Pharmacokinetic studies of clindamycin phosphate. J Clin Pharmacol 1973;13:190-209.

199. Brown RB, Martyak SN, Barza M et al. Penetration of clindamycin phosphate into the abnormal human biliary tract. Ann Intern Med 1976;84:168-70.

200. Swartzberg JE, Maresca RM, Remington JS. Gastrointestinal side effects associated with clindamycin. Arch Intern Med 1976;136:876-9.

201. George WL. Antimicrobial agent-associated colitis and diarrhea. West J Med 1980;133:115-23.

202. Milstone EB, McDonald AJ, Scholhamer CF. Pseudomembranous colitis after topical application of clindamycin. Arch Dermatol 1981;117:154-5.

203. Borriello SP, Larson HE. Antibiotic and pseudomembranous colitis. J Antimicrob Chemother 1981;7(Suppl A):53-62.

204. Anon. Antibiotic colitis—new cause, new treatment. Med Lett Drugs Ther 1979;21:97-8.

205. Koch-Weser J, Sidel VW, Federman EB et al. Adverse effects of sodium colistimethate: manifestations and specific reaction rates during 317 courses of therapy. Ann Intern Med 1970;72:857-68.

206. Appel GB, Neu HC. The nephrotoxicity of antimicrobial agents (parts 1, 2, 3). N Engl J Med 1977;296:663-70, 722-8, 784-7.

207. Froman J, Gross L, Curatola S. Serum and urine levels following parenteral administration of sodium colistimethate to normal individuals. J Urol 1970;103:210-4.

208. Feeley TW, du Moulin GC, Hedley-Whyte J et al. Aerosol polymyxin and pneumonia in seriously ill patients. N Engl J Med 1975;293:471-5.

209. Davia JE, Siemsen AW, Anderson RW. Uremia, deafness, and paralysis due to irrigating antibiotic solutions. Arch Intern Med 1970;125:135-9.

210. Garrod LP, Lambert HP, O'Grady F, eds. Antibiotic and Chemotherapy. 4th ed. Edinburgh: Churchill Livingstone, 1973.

211. Jackson EA, McLeod DC. Pharmacokinetics and dosing of antimicrobial agents in renal impairment, part i. Am J Hosp Pharm. 1974;31:36-52.

212. Kunin CM. More on antimicrobials in renal failure. Ann Intern Med 1968;69:397-8.

213. Center for Disease Control. Gonorrhea: CDC recommended treatment schedules, 1979. Morb Mortal Wkly Rep 1979;28:13-21.

214. McCormack WM. Finland M. Spectinomycin. Ann Intern Med 1976;84:712-6.

215. Kusumi R, Metzler C, Fass R. Pharmacokinetics of spectinomycin in volunteers with renal insufficiency. Chemotherapy 1981;27:95-8.

216. Novak E, Gray JE, Pfeifer RT. Animal and human tolerance of high-dose intramuscular therapy with spectinomycin. J Infect Dis 1974;130:50-5.

217. Karney WW, Pedersen AHB, Nelson M et al. Spectinomycin versus tetracycline for the treatment of gonorrhea. N Engl J Med 1977;296:889-94.

218. Thornsberry C, Jaffee H, Brown ST et al. Spectinomycin-resistant Neisseria gonorrhoeae. JAMA 1977;237:2405-6.

219. Keighley MRB, Burdon DW, Arabi Y et al. Randomized controlled trial of vancomycin for pseudomembranous colitis and postoperative diarrhoea. Br Med J 1978;2:1667-9.

220. Bartlett JG, Tedesco FJ, Shull S et al. Symptomatic relapse after oral vancomycin therapy of antibiotic-associated pseudomembranous colitis. Gastroenterology 1980;78:431-4.

221. Lindholm DD, Murray JS. Persistence of vancomycin in the blood during renal failure and its treatment by hemodialysis. N Engl J Med 1966;274:1047-51.

222. Eykyn S, Phillips I, Evans J. Vancomycin for staphylococcal shunt site infections in patients on regular haemodialysis. Br Med J 1970;3:80-2.

223. Morris AJ, Bilinsky RT. Prevention of staphylococcal shunt infections by continuous vancomycin prophylaxis. Am J Med Sci 1971;262:87-92.

224. Moellering RC, Krogstad DJ, Greenblatt DJ. Vancomycin therapy in patients with impaired renal function: a nomogram for dosage. Ann Intern Med 1981;94:343-6.

225. Tedesco F, Markham R, Gurwith M et al. Oral vancomycin for antibiotic-associated pseudomembranous colitis. Lancet 1978;2:226-8.

226. Kirby WMM, Divelbiss CL. Vancomycin: clinical and laboratory studies. Antibiot Ann 1956;57:107-17.

227. Nielsen HE, Hansen HE, Korsager B et al. Renal excretion of vancomycin in kidney disease. Acta Med Scand 1975;197:261-4.

228. Newfield P, Roizen MF. Hazards of rapid administration of vancomycin. Ann Intern Med 1979;91:581.

229. Esposito AL. Gleckman RA. Vancomycin: a second look. JAMA 1977;238:1756-7.

230. Cook FV. Farrar WE. Vancomycin revisited. Ann Intern Med 1978;88:813-8.

231. Geraci JE. Vancomycin. Mayo Clin Proc 1977;52:631-4.

232. Pinsker KL, Koerner SK. Chemotherapy of tuberculosis. Am J Hosp Pharm 1976;33:275-83.

233. Leff AR, Leff DR, Brewin A. Tuberculosis chemotherapy practices in major metropolitan health departments in the United States. Am Rev Respir Dis 1981;123:176-80.

234. Hyslop NE. Drug therapy of tuberculosis. N Engl J Med 1976;295:106-7.

235. Andrew OT. Schoenfeld PY, Hopewell PC et al. Tuberculosis in patients with end-stage renal disease. Am J Med 1980;68:59-65.

236. Lee CS. Gambertoglio JG, Brater DC et al. Kinetics of oral ethambutol in the normal subject. Clin Pharmacol Ther 1977;22:615-21.

237. Lee CS. Brater DC, Gambertoglio JG et al. Disposition kinetics of ethambutol in man. J Pharmacokinet Biopharm 1980;8:335-46.

238. Leibold JC. The ocular toxicity of ethambutol and its relation to dose. Ann NY Acad Sci 1966;135:904-9.

239. American Thoracic Society. Guidelines for short-course tuberculosis chemotherapy. Am Rev Resp Dis 1980;121:429-30.

240. Centers for Disease Control. Follow-up of guidelines for short-course tuberculosis chemotherapy. Morb Mortal Wkly Rep 1980;29:183-9.

241. Gold CH, Buchanan N, Tringham V et al. Isoniazid pharmacokinetics in patients in chronic renal failure. Clin Nephrol 1976;6:365-9.

242. Centers for Disease Control. Adverse drug reactions among children treated for tuberculosis. Morb Mortal Wkly Rep 1980;29:589-91.

243. Chow MSS, Ronfeld RA. Pharmacokinetic data and drug monitoring: I. antibiotics and antiarrhythmics. J Clin Pharmacol 1975;15:405-18.

244. Ellard GA, Gammon PT. Pharmacokinetics of isoniazid metabolism in man. J Pharmacokinet Biopharm 1976;4:83-113.

245. Bowersox DW, Winterbauer RH, Stewart GL et al. Isoniazid dosage in patients with renal failure. N Engl J Med 1973;289:84-7.

246. Acocella G, Bonollo L, Garimoldi M et al. Kinetics of rifampicin and isoniazid administered alone and in combination to normal subjects and patients with liver disease. Gut 1972;13:47-53.

247. Goldman AL, Braman SS. Isoniazid: a review with emphasis on adverse effects. Chest 1972;62:71-7.

248. Gronhagen-Riska C, Hellstrom P-E, Froseth B. Predisposing factors in hepatitis induced by isoniazid-rifampin treatment of tuberculosis. Am Rev Respir Dis 1978;118:461-6.

249. Kopanoff DE, Snider DE, Caras GJ. Isoniazid-related hepatitis: a US Public Health Service cooperative surveillance study. Am Rev Respir Dis 1978;117:991-1001.

250. Bernstein RE. Isoniazid hepatotoxicity and acetylation during tuberculosis chemoprophylaxis. Am Rev Respir Dis 1980;121:429-30.

251. Sievers ML, Herrier RN. Treatment of acute isoniazid toxicity. Am J Hosp Pharm 1975;32:202-6.

252. Glassroth J, Robins AG, Snider DE. Tuberculosis in the 1980s. N Engl J Med 1980;302:1441-50.

253. Byrd RB, Horn BR, Solomon DA et al. Toxic effects of isoniazid in tuberculosis chemoprophylaxis: role of biochemical monitoring in 1,000 patients. JAMA 1979;241:1239-41.

254. Schatz M, Patterson R, Kloner R et al. The prevalence of tuberculosis and positive tuberculin skin tests in a steroid-treated asthmatic population. Ann Intern Med 1976;84:261-5.

255. Dash LA, Comstock GW, Flynn JPG. Isoniazid preventive therapy: retrospect and prospect. Am Rev Respir Dis 1980;121:1039-44.

256. American Thoracic Society. Treatment of mycobacterial disease. Am Rev Respir Dis 1977;115:185-7.

257. Wason S, Lacouture PG, Lovejoy FH. Single high-dose pyridoxine treatment for isoniazid overdose. JAMA 1981;246:1102-4.

258. Jacobson JA, Fraser DW. A simplified approach to meningococcal disease prophylaxis. JAMA 1976;236:1053-4.

259. Anon. Preventing spread of meningococcal disease. Med Lett Drugs Ther 1981;23:37-8.

260. Acocella G. Clinical pharmacokinetics of rifampicin. Clin Pharmacokinet 1978;3:108-27.

261. Siegler DI, Bryant M, Burley DM et al. Effect of meals on rifampicin absorption. Lancet 1974;2:197-8.

262. Sippel JE, Mikhail IA, Girgis NI•et al. Rifampin concentrations in cerebrospinal fluid of patients with tuberculous meningitis. Am Rev Respir Dis 1974;109:579-80.

263. Curci G, Claar E, Bergamini N et al. Studies on blood serum levels of rifampicin in patients with normal and impaired liver function. Chemotherapy 1973;19:197-205.

264. Capelle P, Dhumeaux D, Mora M et al. Effect of rifampicin on liver function in man. Gut 1972;13:366-71.

265. Gupta S, Grieco MH, Siegel I. Suppression of T-lymphocyte rosettes by rifampin: studies in normals and patients with tuberculosis. Ann Intern Med 1975;82:484-8.

266. Black HR, Griffith RS, Peabody AM. Absorption, excretion and metabolism of capreomycin in normal and diseased states. Ann NY Acad Sci 1966;135:974-82.

267. Ellard GA, Mitchison DA, Girling DG et al. The hepatic toxicity of isoniazid among rapid and slow acetylators of the drug. Am Rev Respir Dis 1978;118:628-9.

268. Hirsch MS, Swartz MN. Antiviral agents. N Engl J Med 1980;302:903-7, 949-53.

269. Spector SA, Connor JD, Hintz M et al. Single-dose pharmacokinetics of acyclovir. Antimicrob Agents Chemother 1981;19:608-12.

270. Cupps TR, Strauss SE, Waldmann TA. Successful treatment with acyclovir of an immunodeficient patient infected simultaneously with multiple herpesviruses. Am J Med 1981;70:882-6.

271. Saral R, Burns WH, Laskin OL et al. Acyclovir prophylaxis of herpes-simplex-virus infections: a randomized, double-blind, controlled trial in bone-marrow-transplant recipients. N Engl J Med 1981;305:63-7.

272. Chang T-W, Snydman DR. Antiviral agents: action and clinical use. Drugs 1979;18:354-76.

273. Smith RA, Sidwell RW, Robins RK. Antiviral mechanisms of action. Annu Rev Pharmacol Toxicol 1980;20:259-84.

274. Whitley R, Alford C, Hess F et al. Vidarabine: a preliminary review of its pharmacological properties and therapeutic use. Drugs 1980;20:267-82.

275. Hopefl AW. Treatment of disseminated herpes zoster infections. Drug Intell Clin Pharm 1979;13:255-9.

276. Whitley RJ, Soong S-J, Hirsch MS et al. Herpes simplex encephalitis: vidarabine therapy and diagnostic problems. N Engl J Med 1981;304:313-8.

277. Rubin RH, Swartz MN. Trimethoprim-sulfamethoxazole. N-Engl J Med 1980;303:426-32.

278. Gleckman R, Alvarez S, Joubert DW. Drug therapy reviews: trimethoprim-sulfamethoxazole. Am J Hosp Pharm 1979;36:893-906.

279. Winston DJ, Lau WK, Gale RP et al. Trimethoprim-sulfamethoxazole for the treatment of *Pneumocystis carinii* pneumonia. Ann Intern Med 1980;92:762-9.

280. Bergan T, Brodwall EK, Vik-Mo H et al. Pharmacokinetics of sulfadiazine, sulfamethoxazole and trimethoprim in patients with varying renal function. Infection 1979;7(Suppl 4):S382-6.

281. Bennett WM, Craven R. Urinary tract infections in patients with severe renal disease: treatment with ampicillin and trimethoprim-sulfamethoxazole. JAMA 1976;236:946-8.

282. Reeves DS, Wilkinson PJ. The pharmacokinetics of trimethoprim and trimethoprim/sulfonamide combinations, including penetration into body tissues. Infection 1979;7(Suppl 4):S330-41.

283. Grose WE, Bodey GP, Loo TL. Clinical pharmacology of intravenously administered trimethoprim-sulfamethoxazole. Antimicrob Agents Chemother 1979;15:447-51.

284. Wormser GP, Keusch GT. Trimethoprim-sulfamethoxazole in the United States. Ann Intern Med 1979;91:420-9.

285. Bateson MC, Hayes JPLA, Pendahrker P. Cotrimoxazole and folate metabolism. Lancet 1976;2:339-40.

286. Rosenfeld JB, Najenson T, Grosswater Z. Effect of long-term co-trimoxazole therapy on renal function. Med J Aust 1975;2:546-8.

287. Trimethoprim study group. Comparison of trimethoprim at three dosage levels with co-trimoxazole in the treatment of acute symptomatic urinary tract infection in general practice. J Antimicrob Chemother 1981;7:179-83.

288. Friesen WT, Hekster YA, Vree TB. Trimethoprim: clinical use and pharmacokinetics. Drug Intell Clin Pharm 1981;15:325-30.

289. Guerrant RL, Wood SJ, Krongaard L et al. Resistance among fecal flora of patients taking sulfamethoxazole-trimethoprim or trimethoprim alone. Antimicrob Agents Chemother 1981;19:33-8.

290. Kainer G, Rosenberg AR. Effect of co-trimoxazole on the glomerular filtration rate of healthy adults. Chemotherapy (Basel) 1981;27:229-32.

291. Klotz U, Maier K, Fischer C et al. Therapeutic efficacy of sulfasalazine and its metabolites in patients with ulcerative colitis and Crohn's disease. N Engl J Med 1980;303:1499-1502.

292. van Hees P, Bakker JH, van Tongeren JHM. Effect of sulfapyridine, 5-aminosalicylic acid, and placebo in patients with idiopathic proctitis: a study to determine the active therapeutic moiety of sulphasalazine. Gut 1980;21:632-5.

293. Das KM, Eastwood MA, McManus JPA et al. The metabolism of salicylazosulfapyridine in ulcerative colitis. Gut 1973;14:631-41.

294. Singleton JW, Law DH, Kelley ML et al. National cooperative Crohn's disease study: adverse reactions to study drugs. Gastroenterology 1979;77:870-82.

295. Goldman P, Peppercorn MA. Sulfasalazine. N Engl J Med 1975;293:20-3.

296. Das K, Dubin R. Clinical pharmacokinetics of sulfasalazine Clin Pharmacokinet 1976;1:406-25.

297. Das DM, Chowdhury B, Zapp B et al. Small bowel absorption of sulfasalazine and its hepatic metabolism in human beings, cats, and rats. Gastroenterology 1979;77:280-4.

298. Das KM, Eastwood MA, McManus JPA et al. Adverse reactions during salicylazosulfapyridine therapy and the relation with drug metabolism and acetylator phenotype. N Engl J Med 1973;289:491-5.

299. Birnie GG, McLeod TIF, Watkinson G. Incidence of sulfasalazine-induced male infertility. Gut 1981;22:452-5.

300. Mogadam M, Dobbins WO, Korelitz BI et al. Pregnancy in inflammatory bowel disease: effect of sulfasalazine and corticosteroids on fetal outcome. Gastroenterology 1981;80:72-6.

301. Jackson EA, McLeod DC. Pharmacokinetics and dosing of antimicrobial agents in renal impairment, part ii. Am J Hosp Pharm 1974;31:137-48.

302. Weinstein L, Madoff MA, Samet CM. The sulfonamides. N Engl J Med 1960;263:793-800, 842-9, 900-7.

303. Chow MSS, Ronfeld RA. Pharmacokinetic data and drug monitoring: 1. antibiotics and antiarrhythmics. J Clin Pharmacol 1975;13:405-18.

304. Goldman P. Metronidazole. N Engl J Med 1980;303:1212-8.

305. Brogden RN, Heel RC, Speight TM et al. Metronidazole in anaerobic infections: a review of its activity, pharmacokinetics and therapeutic use. Drugs 1978;16:387-417.

306. Finegold SM. Metronidazole. Ann Intern Med 1980;93:585-7.

307. Amon I, Amon K, Huller H. Pharmacokinetics and therapeutic efficacy of metronidazole at different dosages. Int J Clin Pharmacol 1978;16:384-6.

308. Krogstad DJ, Spencer HC, Healy GR. Current concepts in parasitology: amebiasis. N Engl J Med 1978;298:262-5.

309. Wolfe MS. Giardiasis. JAMA 1975;233:1362-5.

310. Bergan T, Bjerke PEM, Fausa O. Pharmacokinetics of metronidazole in patients with enteric disease compared to normal volunteers. Chemotherapy 1981;27:233-8.

311. Warner JF, Perkins RL, Cordero L. Metronidazole therapy of anaerobic bacteremia, meningitis, and brain abscess. Arch Intern Med 1979;139:167-9.

312. Nilsson-Ehle I, Ursing B, Nilsson-Ehle P. Liquid chromatographic assay for metronidazole and tinidazole: pharmacokinetic and metabolic studies in human subjects. Antimicrob Agents Chemother 1981;19:754-60.

313. Goldman P. Metronidazole: proven benefits and potential risks. Johns Hopkins Med J 1980;147:1-9.

314. Saginur R, Hawley CR, Bartlett JG. Colitis associated with metronidazole therapy. J Infect Dis 1980;141:772-4.

315. Thomson G, Clark AH, Hare K et al. Pseudomembranous colitis after treatment with metronidazole. Br Med J 1981;282:864-5.

316. Noguchi Y, Tanaka T. Aspects of the pharmacology and pharmacokinetics of nitroimidazoles with special reference to tinidazole. Drugs 1978;15(Suppl 1):10-5.

317. Bakshi JS, Ghiara JM, Nanivadekar AS. How does tinidazole compare with metronidazole? A summary report of the Indian trials in amoebiasis and giardiasis. Drugs 1978;15(Suppl 1):33-42.

318. Musher DM, Griffith DP. Generation of formaldehyde from methenamine: effect of pH and concentration, and antibacterial effect. Antimicrob Agents Chemother 1974;6:708-11.

319. Hamilton-Miller JMT, Brumfitt W. Methenamine and its salts as urinary tract antiseptics: variables affecting the antibacterial activity of formaldehyde, mandelic acid and hippuric acid in vitro. Invest Urol 1977;14:287-91.

320. Vainrub B, Musher DM. Lack of effect of methenamine in suppression of, or prophylaxis against, chronic urinary tract infection. Antimicrob Agents Chemother 1977;12:625-9.

321. Hoener B, Patterson SE. Nitrofurantoin disposition. Clin Pharmacol Ther 1981;29:808-16.

322. McLeod DC, Nahata MC. Methenamine therapy and urinary acidification with ascorbic acid and cranberry juice. Amer J Hosp Pharm 1978;35:654 (letter).

323. Wibell L, Scheyius A, Norrman K. Methenamine-hippurate and bacteriuria in the geriatric patient with a catheter. Acta Med Scand 1980;207:469-73.

324. Norberg B, Norberg A, Parkhede U et al. Effect of short-term high-dose treatment with methenamine hippurate on urinary infection in geriatric patients with an indwelling catheter. Eur J Clin Pharmacol 1979;15:357-61.

325. Kalowski S, Nanra RS, Friedman A et al. Controlled trial comparing co-trimoxazole and methenamine hippurate in the prevention of recurrent urinary tract infections. Med J Aust 1975;1:585-7.

326. Freeman RB, McFate Smith W, Richardson JA et al. Long-term therapy for chronic bacteriuria in men, USPHS cooperative Study. Ann Intern Med 1975;83:133-47.

327. Chamberlain RE. Chemotherapeutic properties of prominent nitrofurans. J Antimicrob Chemother 1976;2:325-36.

328. Bailey RR, Grower PE, Roberts AP et al. Prevention of urinary tract infections with low-dose nitrofurantoin. Lancet 1971;2:1112-4.

329. Gleckman R, Alvarez S, Joubert DW. Drug therapy reviews: nitrofurantoin. Am J Hosp Pharm 1979;36:342-51.

330. DiSanto AR, Chodos DJ, Phillips JP et al. Clinical bioavailability of nitrofurantoin — a case of bioinequivalence. Int J Clin Pharmacol 1976;13:220-7.

331. Rosenberg HA, Bates TR. The influence of food on nitrofurantoin bioavailability. Clin Pharmcol Ther 1976;20:227-32.

332. Cadwallader DE, Bates TR, Swarbrick J. Bioavailability monograph: nitrofurantoin. J Amer Pharm Assoc 1975;NS15:409-12.

333. Kalowski S, Radford N, Kincaid-Smith P. Crystalline and macrocrystalline nitrofurantoin in the treatment of urinary tract infection. N Engl J Med 1974;290:385-6.

334. Holmberg L, Boman G, Bottiger LE et al. Adverse reactions to nitrofurantoin. Analysis of 921 reports. Amer J Med 1980;69:733-8.

335. Koch-Weser J, Sidel VW, Dexter M et al. Adverse reactions to sulfisoxazole, sulfamethoxazole, and nitrofurantoin. Arch Intern Med 1971;399-404.

336. Toole JF, Parrish ML. Nitrofurantoin polyneuropathy. Neurology 1973;23:554-9.

337. Isreal KS, Brahear RE, Sharma HM et al. Pulmonary fibrosis and nitrofurantoin. Am Rev Respir Dis 1973;108:353-6.

338. Tolman KG. Nitrofurantoin and chronic active hepatitis. Ann Intern Med 1980;92:119-20.

339. McCalla DR. Biological effects of nitrofurans. J Antimicrob Chemother 1977;3:517-9.

340. Halsted CH, Gandhi G, Tamura T. Sulfasalazine inhibits the absorption of folates in ulcerative colitis. N Engl J Med 1981;305:1513-7.

341. Strauss SE. Acyclovir for chronic mucocutaneous herpes simplex virus infection in immunosuppressed patients. Ann Intern Med 1982;96:270-7.

342. Corey L et al. A trial of topical acyclovir in genital herpes simplex virus infections. N Engl J Med 1982;306:1313-9.

343. Prince RA, Cassel DH, Hepler CD et al. Comparative trial of two sulfisoxazole regimens in acute urinary tract infection. Drug Intell Clin Pharm 1981;15:863-6.

344. Cunha BA. Ed. Antimicrobial therapy. Med Clin North Am 1982;66:1-316.

10:00 ANTINEOPLASTIC AGENTS

General References: 1-4

Introduction

THE AGENTS INCLUDED IN THIS SECTION are those having widespread use in cancer chemotherapy. The list is not exhaustive, however, and many agents with therapeutic importance in small patient populations are not included.

Cancer chemotherapeutic agents as a class are the most toxic drugs in use. Adverse reactions listed represent those most likely to occur with the usual doses and methods of use; infrequent, but serious reactions are also listed. Information on the dosing of these drugs has largely been determined empirically, and clinical investigations are continually being performed to find safer and more effective dosage regimens. Thus, doses in this section should only be considered as guidelines based on the most widely accepted usage at the time of this writing.

Because space does not permit in-depth discussions of the toxicity, dosing and other aspects of these drugs, the reader should become familiar with specific agents before initiating treatment. References are provided in this section for more detailed information concerning the proper and safe use of these agents. If specific investigational protocols are available, these may also provide information that is unavailable in other sources, especially with regard to dosage and dosing regimens.

Class Instructions. This drug is very potent and some side effects can be expected to occur with its use. Be sure that you understand the possible dangers as well as the possible benefits of the drug before you begin to take it.

Because this drug can decrease your body's ability to fight infections, any signs of infection such as fever, shaking chills or sore throat should be reported immediately. Unusual bruising or bleeding, shortness of breath, or painful or burning urination should also be reported. The use of aspirin-containing products should be avoided, and alcohol should be avoided or used in moderation. Nausea, vomiting or hair loss may sometimes occur with this drug. The severity of these effects depends on the individual, the dose and other drugs that may be given at the same time.

This drug may cause temporary or sometimes permanent sterility in men and women. It may also cause birth defects if the father is taking the drug at the time of conception or if the mother is taking it any time during pregnancy. If you are breast feeding, this drug may appear in the milk and cause problems in your baby; therefore, an alternate form of feeding your baby should be used.

Alkylating Agents, Oral

Busulfan	Myleran®
Chlorambucil	Leukeran®
Melphalan	Alkeran®

Pharmacology. Water soluble compounds which alkylate DNA, forming a variety of covalent cross-links. The drugs are polyfunctional and may form more than one covalent bond to susceptible cell constituents (typically the N_7 position of guanine). Cell cycle phase-nonspecific and chemically stable enough for oral absorption before significant alkylator activation occurs.

Administration, Dose and Dosage Forms.

	BUSULFAN	CHLORAMBUCIL	MELPHALAN
Administration	PO	PO	PO; IV (investigational)
Adult Dose	Up to 8 mg/day (usually 1–3 mg/day)	0.1–0.2 mg/kg/day for 1 day; or 6–12 mg/day maintenance; or 0.4 mg/kg q 2–4 weeks[5]	0.25 mg/kg/day for 4 days; or 2–4 mg/day maintenance
Pediatric Dose	—	—	—
Dosage Forms	Tab 2 mg	Tab 2 mg	Tab 2 mg Inj 100 mg (investigational)

Dosage Individualization. Studies in nephrectomized animals demonstrate markedly increased myelotoxicity with standard melphalan doses. Thus, one group currently recommends a 50% decrease in the melphalan dose for BUN > 30 mg/dl or Cr_s > 1.5 mg/dl.

Patient Instructions. See Class Instructions.

Pharmacokinetics and Biopharmaceutics.

	BUSULFAN	CHLORAMBUCIL	MELPHALAN[6,7]
Fate.			
Absorption	Reported by manufacturer to be well absorbed orally	Reported by manufacturer to be well absorbed orally	Oral absorption erratic and incomplete; some patients show no levels after standard doses
Distribution	Homogeneous; good ascites penetration; exact V_d not known; binds extensively to proteins	—	V_d 0.5–0.6 L/kg
Metabolism	Extensively metabolized, major fraction as methanesulfonic acid	Rapid metabolism to a number of uncharacterized metabolites	Spontaneous degradation to mono- and dihydroxy products
Excretion	No intact drug found in urine; however, metabolites are renally excreted	< 1% unchanged drug in urine over 24 hr	24-hr urinary excretion only 10–15% of a dose
$t_{1/2}$.	Rapid plasma clearance—90% of dose after 3 min	2 hr (intact drug); 2.5 hr (major metabolite, aminophenylacetic acid)	IV administration: $t_{1/2\alpha}$ 8 min $t_{1/2\beta}$ 108 min; Oral administration: terminal $t_{1/2}$ 90 min

Adverse Reactions. Dose-limiting toxicity for this group is typically myelosuppression, with somewhat delayed nadirs of 14–21 days for leukopenia and thrombocytopenia after pulse dosing; daily administration results in chronic low indices with cumulative effects. Not uncommonly, blood counts continue to drop after drug discontinuation; fatal pancytopenias are reported. Therefore, routine hematologic assessments are important with chronic daily dosing regimens. There may be some selectivity for different normal cell lines by these drugs; busulfan and perhaps chlorambucil are thought to selectively depress granulocytes, relatively sparing platelets and lymphoid elements. The nadir for busulfan can be prolonged (4–6 weeks); continuous administration frequently leads to severe myelosuppression (especially platelets) continuing after the drug is discontinued. Nausea and vomiting are rare with chronic dosing, although large single doses can be strongly emetic. Pulmonary fibrosis can occur with all these drugs, especially busulfan; symptoms include cough, dyspnea and fever, while histopathologic changes include bilateral fibrosis. High-dose corticosteroids may help early evolving pulmonary disease due to melphalan and chlorambucil, but "busulfan lung" is usually fatal within 6 months of diagnosis.[8-10] Busulfan frequently causes hyperpigmentation (especially of intertriginous areas) and broad suppression of testicular, ovarian and adrenal function (occasionally leading to Addisonian crisis). Chronic daily administration of these drugs predisposes patients to drug-induced carcinogenesis, often heralded by preleukemic pancytopenias culminating in acute myelocytic leukemias. Allergic hypersensitivity reported, especially with melphalan. With prolonged use, sterility occurs with all alkylators; females appear more sensitive than males.

Contraindications. Documented hypersensitivity; inadequate marrow reserve.

Precautions. See Dosage Individualization for melphalan use in renal failure.

Parameters to Monitor. Routine (at least monthly) WBC and platelet counts; reduce dosage at first sign of significant myelosuppression (ie, WBC < 2,500-3,500/cu mm or platelets < 60,000-100,000/cu mm). Conversely, patients receiving oral melphalan should be assessed for evidence of mild to moderate myelotoxicity to ensure that some absorption is occurring.

Amsacrine (Investigational - Bristol)

Amsacrine is an intercalator-like antineoplastic derived from an acridine dye. It has some activity against nonlymphocytic leukemia at doses of 75-90 mg/M^2/day for 5-7 days and solid tumors at 120 mg/M^2 once q 3-4 weeks. Each dose is diluted in 500 ml of D5W (only) to minimize phlebitis. Caution should be used in preparing solutions to avoid inhalation of the powder or contact with skin; wear mask and rubber gloves during preparation. Use only a glass syringe to prepare, because of possible inactivation by plastic. Preliminary studies indicate primary hepatic metabolism with a half-life of 2.5 hr. Major toxicities are dose-related leukopenia and thrombocytopenia; rarely, cardiac arrest occurs if hypokalemia is present.[11]

Anthracycline Agents

Daunorubicin   Cerubidine®
Doxorubicin   Adriamycin®

Pharmacology. Tetracyclic amino sugar-linked antibiotics which are actively taken up by cells and concentrated in the nucleus; intercalation or fitting between DNA base pairs occurs (which slightly uncoils the DNA helix). Other biochemical lesions produced include quinone moiety-generated production of free oxygen and hydroxyl radicals with lipid peroxidation of mitochondrial membranes and direct free radical DNA denaturation. Both agents are primarily cell cycle phase-nonspecific, although daunorubicin is late S or G$_2$ phase-specific in intermediate doses.

Administration, Dose and Dosage Forms.

	DAUNORUBICIN	DOXORUBICIN
Administration	IV push, infusion	IV push, infusion
	Both compounds are extremely toxic if inadvertently extravasated; very careful IV technique is mandatory.	
Adult Dose	30-60 mg/M^2/day for 1-3 days; generally not repeated more often than q 3 weeks	60-90 mg/M^2 for 1 dose or 20-30 mg/M^2/day for 3 days; generally not repeated more often than q 3 weeks[a]
Pediatric Dose	Same as adult dose	Same as adult dose
Cumulative Dose Limits[b]	550 mg/M^2, up to 850 mg/M^2	550 mg/M^2 400 mg/M^2 with prior chest irradiation
Dosage Forms	Inj 20 mg	Inj 10, 50 mg

Continued

a. Low weekly doses appear to be less toxic and may allow attainment of greater cumulative doses (> 550 mg/M^2).[13]

b. Attainment of maximal cumulative dose generally precludes continued use, despite evidence of continuing drug response; however, some patients may continue to respond without development of cardiomyopathy.[12]

Patient Instructions.   Immediately report any change in sensation (eg, stinging) at injection site during infusion; this may be an early sign of infiltration. See also Class Instructions.

Pharmacokinetics and Biopharmaceutics.

Fate.

Absorption	Extensively degraded to inactive aglycone in GI tract
Distribution	Both drugs actively enter cells rapidly, with subsequent concentration in the nucleus. Tissue concentrations are highest in lung, kidney, spleen, small intestine and liver; insignificant amounts are found in the CNS. Avid tissue binding probably responsible for prolonged terminal half-lives and V_d of drugs 500–600 L/M^2
Metabolism	Both drugs extensively metabolized, primarily to active alcohol metabolites; further metabolized by liver microsomes to inactive aglycones and demethylated glucuronide and sulfate conjugates[14]

	DAUNORUBICIN	DOXORUBICIN
Excretion		
Biliary	20–30% of a dose	40–60% of a dose
Urinary	14–23% as unchanged drug and metabolites (primarily daunorubicinol)	5–10% as metabolites over 5 days[16]
$t_{1/2}$.	α 45 min β 18.5 hr (daunorubicinol $t_{1/2}$ 27 hr)[15]	α 30 min β 3 hr γ 17 hr (32 hr for metabolites)[16]

Dosage Individualization.   Cumulative doses of both agents must be reduced in patients with prior irradiation of the cardiac chest region or in patients over 70 yr. Doxorubicin requires no dose adjustment for severe renal impairment, while with daunorubicin theoretically 75% of the dose would be recommended in severe renal impairment. Doxorubicin doses, however, *must* be substantially reduced with severe hepatic dysfunction:[16]

SERUM BILIRUBIN (MG/DL)	% OF DOXORUBICIN DOSE RECOMMENDED
≤ 1.2	100 (no reduction)
1.2–3	50
> 3	25 (75% reduction)

Adverse Reactions.   Myelosuppression, affecting both platelets and WBCs constitutes the major acute dose-limiting side effect. Typical nadirs range from 9–14 days, with recovery nearly complete within 3 weeks of administration. Stomatitis, nausea and vomiting are dose-dependent and frequent; prophylactic antiemetics are often helpful. Alopecia usually occurs; during low-dose adjuvant chemotherapy administration regional scalp hypothermia may decrease hair loss. Severe, protracted ulceration and necrosis can occur with inadvertent perivenous infiltration of either drug; partially effective local antidotes include subcutaneous injection of low-dose corticosteroids (50–100 mg hydrocortisone) and icepacking. Large evolving lesions necessitate early plastic surgery consultation. Chronic anthracycline use can lead to severe and often fatal cardiomyopathy — see Cumulative Dose Limits; symptoms are nonspecific and indicative of advanced CHF such as shortness of breath, edema and fatigue. The frequency is low (overall 2.2%),[17] when total dose limits are observed and may be lower when monthly doses are given over several days or by continuous infusion. During drug infusion, various nonspecific ECG changes may occur; these do *not* imply an increased risk of cardiotoxicity. Graded endomyocardial biopsy and graded radionuclide angiography have proved most effective for assessment of the emergence of severe cardiomyopathy. Other reactions include transient allergic phlebitis during administration and a radiation-synergy phenomenon involving heightened tissue reactions in concurrently or previously irradiated tissues, especially the esophagus (avoid by spacing weeks apart).

Contraindications. Pre-existing bone marrow suppression (WBCs < 3,000/cu mm; platelets < 120,000/cu mm); myocardial infarction in previous 6 months; history of CHF.

Precautions. Careful administration technique is mandatory to avoid extravasation and tissue necrosis. A number of conditions or other drugs may interact with the anthracyclines: vinca alkaloids (cross-resistance); amphotericin B (increased drug uptake); phenobarbital (increased rate of aglycone production); hepatocellular disease or cirrhosis (slowed production of alcohol metabolites). Most of these drug interactions have only been studied in vitro and require substantial clinical confirmation.

Parameters to Monitor. Pretreatment and at least monthly WBC and platelet counts. General cardiac status and serial radionuclide scans of the heart in high-risk patients.

Notes. Both drugs compatible with usual IV solutions; incompatible with $NaHCO_3$ and fluorouracil. IV push doses are best reconstituted with NS or D5W; avoid sterile water. Such reconstitutions are stable for prolonged periods and can withstand freezing and thawing. Doxorubicin is widely effective in numerous solid tumors, such as ovarian, thyroid and gastric carcinomas, sarcomas and cancer of the breast as well as hematologic malignancies, such as the lymphomas and leukemias.[18] Daunorubicin's activity is limited primarily to acute myelogenous leukemia (AML). Other anthracyclines include **carminomycin, carubicin,** and **zorubicin.**[19]

Asparaginase   Elspar®

Pharmacology. Macromolecular protein isolated from *E. coli* and other bacteria, which hydrolyzes the essential amino acid asparagine in the serum, thus depriving susceptible lymphocyte-derived malignancies of a necessary element for protein synthesis. Cell cycle G_1 phase-specific.

Administration and Adult Dose. IV or preferably IM for combination therapy of acute leukemia 200 IU/day for 28 days;[20] or 1,000–6,000 IU/M^2/day for 5 days;[21] or 20,000 IU/M^2/week.[22] Very recent investigational protocols have successfully used twice weekly doses up to 100,000 IU.

Pediatric Dose. IV or preferably IM 1,000–6,000 IU/M^2/day for 5 days,[21,23] up to 20,000 IU/M^2/week.

Dosage Forms. Inj 10,000 IU vial. A 10,000 IU/2 ml vial of *Erwinia* asparaginase (investigational) is available from National Cancer Institute (NSC 106977) for use in patients allergic to *E. coli* preparation.

Patient Instructions. Asparaginase often causes allergic reactions which can occasionally be life-threatening. This drug may also alter blood sugar and might aggravate diabetes. Report any abdominal pain immediately. See also Class Instructions.

Pharmacokinetics and Biopharmaceutics. *Fate.* IV and IM produce equivalent plasma levels. Negligible distribution out of vascular compartment with minimal urinary and biliary excretion. Clearance is probably immune-mediated. Asparaginase is still detectable in plasma 13–22 days after administration.

$t_{1/2}$. α phase 4–9 hr; β phase 1.4–1.8 days.

Adverse Reactions. Moderate to severe nondose-related hypersensitivity reactions occur in about 20–35% of patients (IM use may reduce allergic complications); prophylactic antihistamines may sometimes be helpful. Usually not emetic or myelotoxic, but can transiently lower blood sugar followed by a pancreatitis-induced hyperglycemia. Elevated serum cholesterol, severely elevated hepatic enzymes and depressed clotting factors (especially profound for fibrinogen) and decreased albumin synthesis may occur. Lethargy and somnolence occur, which may be more frequent in adults.[24] Fatal hyperthermia has been reported.

Contraindications. Anaphylaxis to commercial *E. coli* preparation (use *Erwinia* preparation); severe pancreatitis or history of pancreatitis.

Precautions. Onset of abdominal pain (amylase elevation), any changes in mental status or severe elevation of prothrombin time require drug discontinuation. Some elevations of liver function tests should be anticipated. Anaphylaxis can occur with any dose and facilities for treatment should be at hand. Intradermal scratch tests and desensitization procedures are only sometimes predictive or preventive for anaphylaxis.[20,25]

Parameters to Monitor. Hepatic enzymes, amylase and prothrombin time routinely and all vital signs upon administration.

Notes. Reconstitute with normal saline or D5W (2 ml maximum for IM use); stable at least 24 hr; do not filter.

Azacitidine (Investigational - NCI)   Mylosar®

Azacitidine is a pyrimidine antimetabolite used in refractory acute myelocytic leukemia. It is given IV in doses of 150–400 mg/M^2/day for 5–10 days as a continuous infusion, or by SC injections. Ringer's lactate (RL) is the only diluent recommended (stable only 8–10 hr in RL). Most of a dose is eliminated in the urine as metabolites. The short terminal half-life (3.5–4.2 hr) and the cell cycle S phase-specific action each mandate continuous drug infusion or multiple SC doses for maximal efficacy. Primary toxicities are myelosuppression, primarily leukopenia (10-day nadir) and moderate to severe nausea and vomiting. Rarer toxicities include neurologic muscle pain and weakness, transient fever, rhabdomyolysis and renal tubular damage with occasionally profound hypophosphatemia. Severe hepatic failure and coma have occurred in patients with metastatic liver involvement.[26]

Bleomycin Sulfate   Blenoxane®

Pharmacology. A mixture of 13 glycopeptide fractions produced by *Streptomyces verticillus.* Antineoplastic effects include single and double strand DNA scission, producing excission of thymine bases, possibly mediated through binding with ferric iron and subsequent production of highly reactive hydroxyl and $\cdot O_2$ radicals. Cell cycle phase-specific with maximal activity occurring in the G_2 (premitotic) phase of cell division.[27]

Administration and Adult Dose. IM test dose 1-2 U may be useful in malignant lymphoma patients to assess exaggerated hyperpyrexic response. If no reaction occurs in 2-4 hr, give regular dose. **SC, IM or IV** 10-20 U/M² 1-2 times/week.[27] **IV continuous infusion** 15-20 U/day for 4-5 days.[28] Experimental evidence in animals favors continuous administration as lessening pulmonary toxicity and maximizing cell kill. A total lifetime dose limit of 400 U is recommended to avoid pulmonary fibrosis. **Intracavitary for pleural effusion** 15-240 U.[29]

Dosage Individualization. Significant dose reduction has been recommended in renal impairment:[30]

SERUM CREATININE (MG/DL)	% OF DOSE RECOMMENDED
2.5-4.0	25 (75% reduction)
4.0-6.0	20
6.0-10.0	5-10 (90-95% reduction)

Pediatric Dose. SC, IM or IV 10-20 U/M² 1-2 times/week in combination regimens. **IV continuous infusion** 15-20 U/M²/day for 4-5 days, usually as a single agent.

Dosage Forms. Inj 15 U ampule.

Patient Instructions. Report any coughing, shortness of breath or wheezing. Skin rashes, shaking chills or transient high fever may occur following administration. Hyperpigmentation of skin fold areas, scars, pressure areas or sites of trauma may occur. See also Class Instructions.

Pharmacokinetics and Biopharmaceutics. *Fate.* Poorly absorbed topically; roughly half of intracavitary-administered drug may be systemically available. Following an IV dose of about 15 U/M², levels of 10-1,000 micro-units/ml are obtained.[28] Steady-state levels during continuous infusion of 20 U/day are 50-200 micro-units/ml.[31] 50-60% of dose recovered in the urine (20-40% as active drug). Tissue inactivation is mediated by specific bleomycin-hydrolase, an enzyme observed to be low in skin and lung, the two main toxicity targets of the drug.

$t_{1/2}$. α phase 24 min; β phase 2-4 hr; possibility of a third elimination phase exists.

Adverse Reactions. Acute fever and a cutaneous, generalized erythema with edema, eventually leading to hyperpigmentation and skin thickening are frequent. Chronically, the most serious toxicity is pulmonary fibrosis manifested by dry cough, rales, dyspnea and bilateral infiltrates. Pulmonary function studies show hypoxemia and reduced CO diffusing capacity. Pulmonary toxicity is usually not noted below 150 mg/M^2, increasing to 55% at doses above 283 mg/M^2 and 66% at 360 mg/M^2;[32] life-threatening pulmonary fibrosis is rare if dosage limits are observed. Prior chest radiotherapy and age over 70 yr predispose patients to toxicity. Low-dose hypersensitivity pneumonitis which may be responsive to corticosteroids also occurs.[33]

Precautions.   Use with extreme caution in patients with renal or pulmonary disease, in those with lymphoma and in those over 70 yr.

Parameters to Monitor.   Calculate cumulative dose at each treatment. Monitor temperature initially, especially in lymphoma patients. Assess renal function prior to dosing. Pulmonary damage is best monitored with CO diffusing capacity and forced vital capacity; specific serial pulmonary function studies have been suggested during therapy. Characteristic x-ray findings include changes suggestive of progressive bilateral fibrosis.

Notes.   1 mg of bleomycin equals 1 unit of activity. Reconstituted solution is stable for 1 month under refrigeration and 2 weeks at room temperature. Incompatible with divalent cations (especially copper), ascorbic acid and compounds with sulfhydryl groups. Vincristine, which is known to arrest cells at the G$_2$-M junction, experimentally enhances bleomycin cell kill (bleomycin following vincristine by 6–24 hr).

Cisplatin   Platinol®

Pharmacology.   A planar coordinate dichlorodiammino compound of platinum. Aquated in vivo to a positively charged species that can attack nucleophilic sites in DNA such as purine and pyrimidine bases. Action is cell cycle phase-nonspecific.

Administration and Adult Dose.   IV bolus or continuous infusion (usually with aggressive hydration) single doses up to 120 mg/M^2 have been used.[34] Einhorn testicular cancer regimen calls for 20 mg/M^2/day for 5 days.[35] See Notes.

Dosage Individualization.   Reduce dosage in renal impairment; specific dose reduction guidelines have not been established.

Pediatric Dose.   IV maximum single dose 100 mg/M^2 q 2–3 weeks; IV 10–20 mg/M^2/day for 4–5 days, repeat q 3–4 weeks.

Dosage Forms.   Inj 10, 50 mg vials.

Patient Instructions.   Maintain adequate hydration; be prepared for severe nausea and vomiting following drug administration. See also Class Instructions.

Pharmacokinetics and Biopharmaceutics. *Plasma Levels.*   In vitro cell culture data suggest cytotoxicity at levels of 50 mcg/ml for 1 hr or 5 mcg/ml for 8 hr.
   Fate.   Peak plasma levels of free platinum following a 100 mg/M^2 bolus are about 3.4 mcg/ml when given with mannitol (12.5 g) and 2.7 mcg/ml without mannitol.[36] Over 90% of platinum is protein bound to RBCs, albumin and pre-albumin. Freely distributed to most organs including kidneys, liver, skin and lungs; minimal accumulation in CSF only after repeated doses. Cumulative 24-hr urinary excretion of platinum is 60% with mannitol, 40% without.

$t_{1/2}$. Free platinum 48 min (without mannitol); 59 min (with mannitol). Terminal $t_{1/2}$ 58–73 hr, probably reflecting release of protein-bound drug.[37]

Adverse Reactions. Primary toxicity is weakly dose-related nephrotoxicity. Major acute toxicity is severe and often prolonged (days) nausea and vomiting, which may be managed with aggressive prophylaxis using butyrophenones, such as droperidol, metoclopramide or (investigationally) high-dose corticosteroids. Ototoxicity, frequent hypomagnesemia and occasional "stocking-glove" peripheral neuropathy are reported. Slight leukopenia, thrombocytopenia and frequent anemia occur. Very rare toxicities include transient cortical dysfunction (blindness) and hypersensitivity (including anaphylaxis).

Contraindications. Marked renal insufficiency (Cr_s over 1.5–2 mg/dl). Anaphylaxis; however, some patients experiencing prior anaphylaxis have been successfully retreated with cisplatin and concomitant antihistamines, epinephrine and corticosteroids.

Precautions. Use cautiously in renal impairment and with other nephrotoxic drugs, especially aminoglycosides.[38] Assure adequate hydration prior to administration. Both furosemide and mannitol are used to decrease platinum nephrotoxicity, although each apparently retards free platinum elimination.

Parameters to Monitor. Assess renal function prior to each dose (eg, serial BUN and/or Cr_s) and serum magnesium levels periodically.

Notes. Reconstitute with sterile water; may then be mixed in saline-containing solutions; stable for 24 hr in mannitol. Do not expose solution to metals (eg, metal drippers or cannulae) because platinum may rapidly plate onto these surfaces.

Cyclophosphamide   Cytoxan®

Pharmacology. Inactive in vitro and must be enzymatically activated in the liver to yield both active alkylating compounds and toxic metabolites.[39] Cell cycle phase-nonspecific.

Administration and Adult Dose. IV (usually) or PO in high-dose intermittent regimens maximum of 40–50 mg/kg given once or over 2–5 days, repeat q 2–4 weeks — these doses are not well tolerated orally. IV 10–15 mg/kg q 7–10 days or 3–5 mg/kg twice weekly. IV doses may be given in any convenient volume of all common IV solutions. **Continuous daily dosing PO** 1–5 mg/kg/day. Continuous doses must be individualized to patient reponse.

Dosage Individualization. No dosage alteration appears necessary in renal impairment, because differences in toxicity between normals and patients with renal failure have not been seen.[40]

Pediatric Dose. Same as adult dose.

Dosage Forms. Tab 25, 50 mg; Inj 100, 200, 500 mg.

Patient Instructions. Drink 2–3 quarts of fluids daily (1–2 quarts in smaller children) and urinate frequently; oral doses should *not* be taken at bedtime. Report any blood in the urine. See also Class Instructions.

Pharmacokinetics and Biopharmaceutics. *Fate.* Oral absorption averages 97%. Metabolized to active compounds (including the highly toxic nonalkylating aldehyde, acrolein, and the principle alkylator, phosphoramide mustard) primarily by hepatic microsomal mixed-function oxidase. Alkylating metabolites are 50% protein bound; V_d is about 0.7 L/kg.[41] Renal elimination accounts for 22% of drug and 60% of metabolites,[41,42] with a mean renal clearance of 11 ml/min of unchanged drug.[43] Elimination is linear over a wide range of doses.[39]

$t_{1/2}$. (Plasma alkylating activity) 6.5–8 + hours; slightly longer in patients on allopurinol or those previously exposed to cyclophosphamide.[41,44]

Adverse Reactions.   Nausea and vomiting are frequent. Dose-limiting toxicity is myelosuppression with a WBC nadir of about 10 days; platelets are also suppressed, perhaps to a lesser extent. The drug is locally nonirritating. Renally eliminated active metabolites occasionally cause sterile hemorrhagic cystitis which may resolve slowly, often leading to a fibrotic, contracted bladder. Bladder epithelial changes range from minimal to frank neoplasia. An early sign of cystitis is microscopic hematuria which can lead to frank hemorrhage. Prophylactic hydration is recommended; N-acetylcysteine (Mucomyst®) bladder irrigations may have antidotal activity. Rarely, bladder dysplasia can lead to bladder cancer after very high doses or with concurrent or prior bladder radiation. Cross-allergenicity with other alkylators, such as mechlorethamine, may occur. Ovarian and testicular function may be permanently lost following high-dose, long-term therapy. Rare reactions include a high-dose fatal cardiomyopathy, "allergic" interstitial pneumonitis and a transient condition similar to SIADH which is preventable with vigorous isotonic hydration.

Contraindications.   Previous life-threatening hypersensitivity to cyclophosphamide; significant leukopenia and thrombocytopenia; hemorrhagic cystitis; pulmonary toxicity due to prior alkylator therapy.

Precautions.   Pregnancy. Consider dosage reduction or discontinuation of drug in patients who develop infections; use with caution in impaired renal or hepatic function.

Parameters to Monitor.   Prior to induction therapy dosing, the patient should be assessed for adequate numbers of WBCs (generally > 3,500/cu mm and platelets > 120,000/cu mm). With chronic dosing, these counts should be assessed at least monthly. Hematuria should be closely followed, especially if a patient has received a large cumulative dose.

Notes.   Do not dilute with benzyl alcohol-preserved solutions. Dissolution of powder is quite slow; vigorous shaking and/or slight warming may hasten dissolution. Diluted solution is stable for 24 hr at room temperature and 6 days under refrigeration. Widely used in both hematologic and solid malignances and as an immunosuppressant in a variety of autoimmune disorders.

Cytarabine   Cytosar®

Pharmacology.   Arabinoside sugar analogue of the natural pyrimidine nucleoside cytidine. Cytarabine is cell cycle S phase-specific with activity markedly enhanced by continuous administration over several days.

Administration and Adult Dose. IV for remission induction 100–150 mg/M^2/day as a continuous infusion for 5–10 days.[45] Recent experimental therapy has successfully used induction doses of up to 3 g/M^2 q 12 hr as a 2-hr infusion for 4–12 doses in refractory AML.[46] **SC for remission induction** 100 mg/M^2 q 12 hr for 5–10 days. **SC for remission maintenance** 70–100 mg/M^2/day for 5 days in 4 divided doses. **Intrathecal** (IT) 70 mg/M^2 (usually 100 mg) 1–2 times weekly, diluted with nonpreserved isotonic solutions only (eg, normal saline, D5W, Ringer's lactate).[47] See Notes.

Pediatric Dose. IV or SC same as adult dose. **Intrathecal** (3 yr or older) 70 mg/M^2, diluted as above, repeated no more often than q 3–5 days; (2–3 yr) reduce dose by 1/6; (1–2 yr) reduce dose by 1/3; (< 1 yr) reduce dose by 1/2.

Dosage Forms. Inj 100, 500 mg.

Patient Instructions. See Class Instructions.

Pharmacokinetics and Biopharmaceutics. *Plasma Levels.* 0.05–0.1 mcg/ml necessary for cytotoxic effects;[48] this is similar to reported "therapeutic" levels of 0.1–0.4 mcg/ml produced by 60-min continuous infusion of 17–80 mg.[49]
   Fate. Not systemically bioavailable following oral absorption. After injection, there is a large interpatient variation in levels attained as measured by various assay techniques.[50] It is widely distributed and deactivated by cytidine deaminase, primarily in the liver. The deamination product, uracil arabinoside (ARA-U), is inactive and rapidly excreted in the urine; 24 hr after injection, 72% of the dose is recovered in the urine as ARA-U, only 8% as unchanged drug.[51] The CSF to plasma ratio is 0.4 with slow elimination from the CSF due to low CNS deaminating activity; however, to attain therapeutic CSF concentrations following standard IV doses, additional IT injections are required. About 13% is bound to plasma proteins; reported V_ds are quite variable: 20–270 L[49] and 70–760 L.[50]
   $t_{1/2}$. α phase 1.6–12 min; β phase 9–111 min.[49,51] Following intrathecal administration CNS half-life of 2–11 hr has been reported.[52]

Adverse Reactions. Principle side effect is dose-related myelosuppression with a leukopenic nadir of 3–11 days and a thrombocytopenic nadir of 12–14 days; megaloblastosis is typically noted in the recovering bone marrow and in the rare cases in which anemia develops. Mild to moderate nausea and vomiting are frequent; prophylactic anti-emetics are often suppressive. Mild oral ulceration occurs occasionally. A flu-like syndrome is occasionally produced, manifested by arthralgias, fever and sometimes rash. Hepatic enzyme elevation is rare, even with 3 g/M^2 doses; one instance of SIADH reported with this large dose.[46]
   Intrathecal toxicities are dose-related and include transient headaches and vomiting.[47] Seizures and paraplegia are very rare and involve high-dose, closely spaced treatments.

Precautions. Significant myelosuppression is *not* a contraindication, because marrow hypoplasia with complete suppression of the leukemic clone is the desired clinical endpoint; however, extensive supportive facilities must be available during therapy, including WBC and platelet transfusion capability.

Parameters to Monitor. Routine WBC and platelet counts; RBC indices.

Notes. Physically incompatible with sodium methotrexate and fluorouracil; avoid direct admixture. Chemically stable in solution for up to 7 days at room temperature. IT doses should *not* be diluted with bacteriostatic diluents. Patients may be taught sterile technique for self-dosing of SC drug for remission maintenance. The use of small reconstitution volumes (1 ml/100 mg) and rotation of injection sites should be observed. Clinical activity is limited primarily to selected hematologic malignancies (eg, AML, ALL, DHL).

Fluorouracil

Fluorouracil®,
Adrucil®,
Efudex®

Pharmacology. 5-fluorinated antimetabolite of the DNA pyrimidine precursor uracil. Inhibits thymidine formation, thereby blocking DNA synthesis. Some fluorouracil may be incorporated into RNA, inhibiting subsequent protein synthesis. Cell cycle S phase-specific.

Administration and Adult Dose. Rapid IV 15 mg/kg/week for 4 weeks, followed by 20 mg/kg/week until severe toxicity develops. Drug is stopped until resolution is complete, then resumed at 5 mg/kg/week.[53] **IV "loading course"** 12 mg/kg (800 mg maximum) as a single dose daily for 4 days, then 12–15 mg/kg/week is recommended by manufacturer; however, it has been associated with severe, life-threatening bone marrow toxicity.[54] **IV continuous infusion** 1–2 g/day for up to 5 days has been used by special treatment centers; continuous infusion does not consistently increase antitumor efficacy, but does appear to lessen hematologic toxicity.[55] Equivalent **PO** doses are used, but are associated with very slight clinical response. **Intra-arterial, intraperitoneal and intracavitary** administration have also been used. **Top for neoplastic keratoses** 5% cream daily for 1–2 weeks, applied as a thin layer with gloved hand or nonmetal applicator. Skin response progresses sequentially through erythema, vesiculation, erosion, ulceration necrosis and finally regranulation. Treatment is usually stopped once erosion is evident to allow healing to occur over the next 1–2 months.

Pediatric Dose. Generally indicated for adult malignancies, although theoretically, equivalent mg/kg doses could be used in children.

Dosage Forms. Inj 500 mg/10 ml; **Top Crm** 5%; **Top Soln** 2, 5%.

Patient Instructions. Avoid prolonged exposure to strong sunlight; report any severe sores in the mouth immediately. See also Class Instructions.

Pharmacokinetics and Biopharmaceutics. *Fate.* Oral doses are erratically and incompletely absorbed with bioavailability of 50–80%, lessened by mixing with acidic fruit juices.[56] V_d is about 25–35 L/kg with drug diffusing to effusions and CSF (peak CSF levels of $6–8 \times 10^{-8}$ mol/L after a 15 mg/kg IV bolus). Extensively and rapidly metabolized, primarily in the liver, to a variety of inactive metabolites which are renally excreted. Up to 15% of unchanged drug is renally excreted, 90% within 6 hr of administration. Fluoroacetate and citrate metabolites found in the CSF are believed to mediate rare CNS toxicities.

$t_{1/2}$. α phase about 8 min; β phase 12–37 min.[57]

Adverse Reactions. Dose-limiting toxicity is myelosuppression (when given by bolus injection) with leukopenic and thrombocytopenic nadirs at 7–14 days. Severe stomatitis 5–8 days after therapy can herald severe impending myelosuppression; this is unpredictably seen with large bolus doses (> 12 mg/kg). Oral dosing increases severity of the frequent mild diarrhea. GI ulceration is occasionally severe, although acute nausea and vomiting are usually mild. Cutaneous toxicities include mild to moderate alopecia, hyperpigmentation of skin and veins and rashes which are often worsened by sunlight. Rare toxicities involve CNS dysfunction manifested by ataxia, confusion, visual disturbances and headaches. Very rarely, cardiotoxicity has been reported.

Contraindications. Pre-existing severe myelosuppression (WBC < 2,000/cu mm, platelet count < 100,000/cu mm).

Precautions. Concurrent allopurinol appears to block one activation pathway, possibly reducing fluorouracil hematologic toxicity. Fluorouracil can inhibit the antipurine effects of methotrexate. The clinical significance of these two interactions is unclear.

Parameters to Monitor. Pretreatment and monthly assessment of bone marrow function, particularly WBC and platelet counts. In the weeks following dosing, observe for severe stomatitis which may herald life-threatening myelosuppression.

Notes. If precipitate is noted in ampule, gently warm in a water bath and/or vigorously shake to redissolve. Fluorouracil is physically incompatible with diazepam, doxorubicin, cytarabine and methotrexate injections. Mild to moderate activity in GI tract tumors and in breast cancer; topical application is often curative in superficial skin cancers.

Hexamethylmelamine (Investigational - NCI)

Hexamethylmelamine may act as an antimetabolite to inhibit DNA and RNA synthesis; metabolites may also have alkylating activity. It is used in combination chemotherapy of ovarian, cervical and lung cancers, taken orally in doses ranging from 4–12 mg/kg/day in 4 divided doses for periods up to 3–6 weeks. Use of a single dose at night may lessen acute toxicity. Hexamethylmelamine is N-demethylated to pentamethylmelamine by hepatic microsomal enzymes. Over half a dose is renally excreted in 24 hr. Oral absorption is incomplete and erratic, and may be dose-dependent. Nausea, vomiting and abdominal cramps may be dose-limiting in some patients. Neurotoxic effects are frequent, including agitation, hallucinations and confusion; these are reversible and amenable to dose reduction. Leukopenia and thrombocytopenia are typically mild. **Pentamethylmelamine** is a water-soluble (injectable) derivative now also in clinical trials.[58]

Immunotherapeutic Agents
BCG
Levamisole   Tramisol®
(Investigational - Janssen)

BCG or Bacillus Calmette-Guerin is an attenuated bovine strain of *M. tuberculosis;* it is a nonspecific immunostimulant used in a variety of malignant diseases such as acute leukemia (by systemic "scarification"), malignant melanoma (by intralesional injection) and lung cancer (by intrapleural instillation). Available products include investigational high-viability Pasteur fresh frozen vaccine, and lyophilized lower-viability strains such as the

Glaxo strain of Eli Lilly and the Connaught strain of Canada. Toxicities include local reactions at the scarification site (erythema, pruritus and eventual crusting) and systemic responses of fever, chills, myalgias and arthralgias. PPD conversion is also expected. Rare adverse reactions include local draining lymphadenopathy, anaphylaxis, pulmonary and hepatic granulomas and occasional disseminated "BCG-osis". Thrombocytopenia is frequent with intralesional therapy in melanoma.[59]

Levamisole is the l-isomer of the imidazole anthelmintic agent tetramisole; it is orally administered and thought to modulate immunity by restoring depressed T-lymphocyte function and phagocytic macrophage activity. In high or continuous daily dosing, levamisole can act as an immunosuppressant. The drug is currently undergoing investigation as an immunomodulator for use in various disseminated cancers and in rheumatoid arthritis. Adverse reactions are infrequent; they include agranulocytosis, skin rash and rare febrile responses, predominantly seen in continuously dosed arthritics. Vasculitis has also been seen. Renal and hepatic toxicity is not reported and the drug is typically well tolerated in 80–95% of patients treated.[60]

Mechlorethamine Hydrochloride   Mustargen®

Pharmacology. This prototype bischloroethylamine is a polyfunctional alkylating agent. In solution, the compound readily ionizes to an active form which can alkylate at a number of nucleophilic protein sites, principally the N_7 position of guanine in both DNA and RNA. This action is cell cycle phase-nonspecific.

Administration and Adult Dose. **IV for Hodgkin's disease** (in the classical "MOPP" regimen) 6 mg/M^2 by careful push on days 1 and 8 of a monthly treatment cycle.[61] Vein irritation and sclerosis occur in exposed veins; therefore, it is common to begin venipunctures low on the limb and move up serially, and to administer mechlorethamine last in a combination drug sequence. **IV as a single agent** up to 0.4 mg/kg as a single monthly dose. **Top for mycosis fungoides and psoriasis** 10 mg/60 ml of water, applied to the affected body areas 1–2 times/day.[62]

Pediatric Dose. **IV** same as adult dose.

Dosage Forms. **Inj** 10 mg.

Patient Instructions. See Class Instructions.

Pharmacokinetics and Biopharmaceutics. *Fate.* Chemical cyclization occurs in vivo to form positively charged carbonium ions which rapidly react with various cellular components; unchanged drug cannot be detected in the blood within minutes of administration. Less than 0.01% of unchanged drug is recovered in the urine; however, up to 50% of labeled products may be found in urine within 24 hr.[63]

Adverse Reactions. The major dose-limiting toxicity is myelosuppression: leukopenic nadir 6–8 days, thrombocytopenic nadir 10–16 days. Extravasation causes delayed and protracted (months) ulceration and necrosis; a 1/6 molar sodium thiosulfate solution (4 ml of 10% sodium thiosulfate plus 6 ml sterile water) and copious flushing with water may be used as topical antidotes to lessen serious tissue damage. Nausea and vomiting within the first 3 hr are severe, and, rarely, may last over 1 day. Primary reproductive failure and alopecia are frequent in both males and females. IV or topical use can cause maculopapular rashes and sometimes severe sensitivity reactions (anaphylaxis and occasional cross-reactivity with other alkylating agents).

Contraindications. Prior severe hypersensitivity reactions; pre-existing profound myelosuppression.

Precautions. Patients with lymphomas (especially "bulky" lymphomas) should receive prophylactic allopurinol 2–3 days prior to therapy to prevent hyperuricemia and urate nephropathy following massive tumor lysis. Every effort should be made to avoid topical contact with this highly vesicant drug (except during topical therapy).

Parameters to Monitor. Pretreatment and at least monthly assessment of bone marrow function, particularly WBC and platelet counts.

Notes. Mechlorethamine is a powerful vesicant and should be prepared with great caution. Use mask and rubber gloves during preparation and avoid inhalation of dust and vapors, or contact with skin and mucous membranes, especially the eyes. Injection should be used within 1 hr of preparation; topical solution and ointment are stable for 1 month under refrigeration.[64] Because of its extreme acute toxicity, use is limited primarily to malignant lymphomas[61] and topically in mycosis fungoides, a cutaneous non-Hodgkin's lymphoma.[65]

Methotrexate

Mexate®,
Various

Pharmacology. Folic acid analogue which binds to dihydrofolate reductase, blocking formation of the DNA nucleotide thymidine; purine synthesis is also inhibited. Most active in S phase.

Administration and Adult Dose. *Single Agent Therapy:* for **choriocarcinoma IM, IV, PO** 15–30 mg/day for 5 days, repeated q 1–2 weeks for 3–5 courses; **mycosis fungoides IM** 50 mg once weekly or 25 mg twice weekly; **head and neck cancer IM, IV, PO** 25–50 mg/M^2 once weekly (watch for cumulative myelosuppression with continued dosing on this regimen); **meningeal leukemia Intrathecal (IT)** 12 mg/M^2 in a preservative-free, isotonic diluent (eg, Elliott's B solution, patient's own CSF or D5LR); **high-dose therapy IV** (50–100 mg/M^2) with leucovorin rescue should be used only by experts in major research centers; **psoriasis IM, or PO** maintenance 5–10 mg initially then **PO, IM or IV** 10–25 mg/week, to maximum of 50 mg/week, depending on clinical response; chronic daily dosing results in increased hepatotoxicity compared to weekly oral or parenteral doses.

Combined Modality Therapy: for **acute lymphocytic leukemia** various schedules are reported for remission-maintenance therapy **IM, IV** 30 mg/M^2 twice weekly, or 7.5 mg/kg/day for 5 days, or **PO** 2.5 mg/kg/day for 2 weeks; repeat at monthly intervals; **Burkitt's lymphoma PO, IV, IM** 0.625–2.5 mg/kg/day for 1–2 weeks, then off drug for 7–10 days; **breast cancer IV, IM** (combined with cyclophosphamide and fluorouracil) 40 mg/M^2 days 1 and 8, repeat monthly.[66]

Dosage Individualization. Patients with any "third space" fluids (eg, ascites, pleural effusions) should receive reduced doses due to retention and slow release of drug from these compartments.[67]

Pediatric Dose. **IM, IV for remission maintenance** same as adult dose for acute lymphoblastic leukemia. **Intrathecally for meningeal cancer,** use age-adjusted dosing rather than mg/M^2 dose.[68] See the following page.

AGE (YR)	IT DOSE (MG)
> 3	12
2–3	10
1–2	8
< 1	6

Dosage Forms. Tab 2.5 mg; Inj (as sodium) 50 mg/2 ml (preserved solution); 20, 50, 100 mg (nonpreserved powder).

Patient Instructions. See Class Instructions.

Pharmacokinetics and Biopharmaceutics. *Plasma Levels.* Following high-dose therapy, a threshold for bone marrow and mucosal toxicity approximates 1.0×10^{-6} mol/L 48 hr after dosing. To prevent toxicity, plasma levels should be kept below 10^{-5} mol/L at 24 hr, 5×10^{-7} mol/L at 48 hr and 5×10^{-8} mol/L at 72 hr.[69]

Fate. PO and IM absorption are rapid, peaking at 1–2 and 0.1–1 hr, respectively. Following IT dosing there is slow diffusion of drug into the bloodstream. PO and IM doses less than 30 mg/M^2 are completely absorbed; larger doses are only about 50–70% absorbed. About 60–70% is bound to plasma proteins; V_d is 0.5–1.0 L/kg. Over 90% of a dose is excreted in the urine, 90% unchanged after IV and 60–70% unchanged after PO; methotrexate solubility is markedly decreased in acid urine.

$t_{1/2}$. Elimination from the plasma can be described by 2 or 3 phases. α phase 0.75 min, β phase 2–4 hr, γ phase 10–26 hr;[70] the biological significance of the final phase (if real) is unclear.

Adverse Reactions. Nearly all reactions are dose and duration related. The primary toxicity is hematologic suppression, principally leukopenia with the nadir at 7–14 days depending upon the administration schedule (more prolonged with daily dosing). Thrombocytopenia and macrocytic anemia occur also. Mucosal ulcerations of the mouth and tongue, and diarrhea may occasionally become severe within 1–3 weeks after administration, sometimes heralding severe myelotoxicity. Mild to moderate nausea and vomiting just after dosing occur occasionally and erythematous rashes have been reported. Leukoencephalopathy occurs rarely with either IV or IT use. Other toxicities following IT use include nausea and vomiting, meningismus, paresthesias and, rarely, convulsions. Chronic daily dosing in psoriasis has led to hepatocellular damage including fibrocongestive liver changes and atrophy of the liver.

Contraindications. Pregnancy; severe renal or hepatic dysfunction; psoriasis patients with pre-existing bone marrow depression.

Precautions. Renal function must be adequate prior to administration of this drug. Concomitant vinca alkaloids (vincristine or vinblastine) can impair methotrexate elimination from the CSF; similarly, probenecid diminishes renal elimination. Both interactions augment the biological effects of a given dose of methotrexate. Asparaginase given 1 week prior to or 24 hr after methotrexate appears to reduce methotrexate hematologic toxicities.

Parameters to Monitor. Monitoring should include assessment of pretreatment hepatic, renal and bone marrow function (including WBCs, platelets and RBCs). High doses should be followed with 24 hr and/or 48 hr plasma levels and institution of appropriate leucovorin rescue. The urine should also be alkalinized prior to high doses to enhance methotrexate solubility.

Notes. If overdosage occurs, the antidote is calcium leucovorin (citrovorum factor) which can be given IV or IM in methotrexate-equivalent doses up to 75 mg q 6 hr for 4 doses. A delay of greater than 36 hr lessens the chance of rescue. Reconstitute lyophilized forms with normal saline, D5W or Elliott's B solution (for IT use). Reconstituted solutions are chemically stable for 7 days at room temperature. Physically incompatible with fluorouracil, prednisolone sodium phosphate and cytarabine. Clinically useful in a variety of hematologic and solid tumors as well as nonmalignant hyperplastic conditions such as psoriasis.

Nitrosoureas

Carmustine
Lomustine

BiCNU®
CeeNU®

Pharmacology. Highly lipid soluble drugs which are metabolized to active alkylating and carbamoylating moieties. Several key cellular enzymatic steps are inhibited, including those involving DNA polymerase and RNA protein synthesis. There is typically only partial cross-resistance to classical alkylators. The nitrosoureas are cell cycle phase-nonspecific and even have significant activity on G_0 (resting phase) cells.

Administration, Dose and Dosage Forms.

	CARMUSTINE	LOMUSTINE
Administration	IV in 100–200 ml D5W over 15–45 min	PO only
Adult Dose	75–100 mg/M²/day for 1–2 days or 200 mg/M² as single dose, or 80 mg/M²/day for 3 days,[71] repeat at 6–8 week intervals	100–130 mg/M² as single dose, repeat at 6–8 week intervals
Pediatric Dose	Same as adult dose	
Dosage Forms	Inj 100 mg (with alcohol diluent)	Cap 100 mg (2)* + 40 mg (2) + 10 mg (2)

*commercial packet totals 300 mg.

Dosage Individualization. Elderly patients or those with heavily pretreated bone marrows should receive 50–75% of the recommended dose and/or expanded treatment intervals (8 weeks minimum). Lomustine absorption is rapid; thus, vomiting 45 or more minutes after ingestion does not require redosing.

Patient Instructions. Lomustine should be taken on an empty stomach. See also Class Instructions.

Pharmacokinetics and Biopharmaceutics.

	CARMUSTINE	LOMUSTINE
Fate.		
Absorption	—	Complete after 30 min[72]
Distribution	Both drugs are diffusely distributed with decreasing relative concentrations in spleen, liver and ovaries; both achieve substantial penetration into CNS with simultaneous CSF levels of $> 50\%$ of plasma for intact carmustine and metabolites[73] and $> 30\%$ for intact lomustine and metabolites;[72] enterohepatic cycling of active metabolites is possible and may explain subsequent peaks in nitrosourea plasma levels at 1 and 4 hr	
Metabolism	Both drugs are rapidly and extensively metabolized (partially by liver microsomal enzymes) to a number of active products which have long plasma half-lives compared to the parent compounds	
Excretion	30% urinary drug recovery as metabolites after 24 hr, 65% after 96 hr[73]	50% urinary drug recovery as metabolites after 12 hr, 60% after 48 hr; $< 5\%$ fecal excretion
$t_{1/2}$.	Intact drug 5 min; biological effect 15–30 min; metabolites slow decay over 3–4 days	Intact drug 15 min; cyclohexyl and carbonyl metabolites: α phase 4–5 hr, β phase 30–50 hr; chloroethyl metabolite 72 hr

Adverse Reactions. Major dose-limiting toxicity is delayed and potentially cumulative myelosuppression; nadirs are unusually prolonged with leukopenic at approximately 35 days and thrombocytopenic at about 30 days. Thus, doses are not repeated more often than q 6 weeks.[74] Nausea and vomiting are frequent; prophylactic phenothiazine antiemetics are moderately effective. Carmustine frequently causes severe pain at injection site and venospasm which may be reduced by slow, dilute infusions. Both drugs may transiently raise liver enzymes; nephrotoxicity is consistently reported following cumulative doses $\geq 1,500$ mg/M^2. Pulmonary fibrosis also reported, usually following cumulative doses $> 1,000$ mg/M^2;[75] variant carmustine-induced pulmonary fibrosis, highly responsive to early drug discontinuation and corticosteroids, has been reported.[76] Other rare toxicities include CNS effects (eg, confusion, lethargy, ataxia), stomatitis and alopecia. In animal models the nitrosoureas are highly carcinogenic and several cases of leukemia after nitrosourea therapy have been reported.

Contraindications.   Demonstrated hypersensitivity; significant pre-existing myelosuppression.

Precautions. Pregnancy. Clinical resistance to carmustine and perhaps other nitrosoureas is significantly reduced by concomitant amphotericin B administration. Experimentally in rats, carmustine, lomustine and the investigational drug semustine are cleared much more rapidly (with reduced antitumor activity) by pretreatment with phenobarbital, which stimulates microsomal enzymes.

Notes. Carmustine should be stored under refrigeration; appearance of an oily film in the vial is evidence of decomposition, and such vials should be discarded. Carmustine is incompatible with sodium bicarbonate. Semustine is an oral investigational methyl derivative of lomustine with no outstanding advantages over presently available agents; it is available from NCI.

Podophylotoxins
Etoposide
Teniposide (Investigational - Bristol)

VePesid®
Vumon®

Etoposide and teniposide are podophyllum derivatives which possess cell cycle S and G_2 phase-specific cytotoxic activities and irreversibly inhibit cell progression into mitosis. Etoposide (diluted in saline only) has clinical activity in small cell lung cancer with IV doses up to 140 mg/M^2 or 50 mg/M^2/day for 5 days. Teniposide has clinical activity primarily in lymphomas and in pediatric acute leukemias in IV doses of 100 mg/M^2/week or 50 mg/M^2/day for 5 days, up to 165 mg/M^2 twice weekly. The half-life of etoposide is 3–15 hr (average 11); it is highly protein bound and eliminated largely as metabolites in the feces. Teniposide is > 90% protein bound and is eliminated much more slowly than etoposide. Teniposide half-lives are α phase 45 min, β phase 4 hr, and γ phase 11–39 hr (average 20); 40% of a dose is eliminated in the feces and CSF drug levels are high (27% of plasma levels). The dose-limiting side effect of both drugs is myelosuppression with the leukopenic nadir at 10–14 days. Nausea and vomiting are typically mild (more severe after oral etoposide). Hypotension is reported with rapid drug infusions. Rarely, severe hypersensitivity reactions (including anaphylaxis), alopecia and chemical phlebitis during infusion occur.[77,78] Etoposide is available as Inj 100 mg.

Purine Analogues
Azathioprine
Mercaptopurine
Thioguanine

Imuran®
Purinethol®
Thioguanine

Pharmacology. The thiolated purines act as antimetabolites following metabolic activation to the nucleotide forms (phosphorylated ribose sugar attachment). Subsequently, purine biosynthesis is interrupted at a number of enzymatic sites, including the conversion of inosinic acid to adenine- or xanthine-based ribosides. DNA and RNA synthesis is halted in a cell cycle S phase-specific fashion.

Administration, Dose and Dosage Forms.

	AZATHIOPRINE	MERCAPTOPURINE	THIOGUANINE
Administration	PO, IV	PO, IV (investigational)	PO, IV (investigational)
Adult Dose Initial:	3–5 mg/kg/day	500–700 mg/M^2/day for 5 days	—
Maintenance	1–2 mg/kg/day	80–100 mg/M^2/day	2–3 mg/kg/day
Pediatric Dose Initial:	3–5 mg/kg for 1 dose	500–700 mg/M^2/day for 5 days	—
Maintenance:	1–2 mg/kg/day	80–100 mg/M^2/day	2–3 mg/kg/day
Dosage Forms	Tab 25, 50 mg Inj 100 mg	Tab 50 mg Inj 500 mg (investigational)	Tab 40 mg Inj 75 mg (investigational)

Dosage Individualization. Purine antimetabolite toxicities are not consistently increased in patients with renal failure.[79,80] See Precautions.

Patient Instructions. To maximize absorption, these drugs should not be taken with meals. Nausea and vomiting are rare with usual doses. See also Class Instructions.

Pharmacokinetics and Biopharmaceutics.

	AZATHIOPRINE	MERCAPTOPURINE	THIOGUANINE
Fate.			
Absorption	Reportedly well absorbed; however, no published studies are available; may have significant first-pass hepatic extraction		
Distribution	Approximately 30% protein bound; freely distributed throughout the body including placental transfer; CSF/plasma ratios: 0.19 for mercaptopurine, 0.16 for thioguanine		
Metabolism	Rapid conversion to mercaptopurine; this is not altered in renal failure	Metabolized extensively by xanthine oxidase, also methylated to active metabolite and sulfurated to inactive thiouric acid	Predominantly eliminated by methylation to inactive metabolites
$t_{1/2}$.	IV azathioprine: 12.5 min; mercaptopurine after PO azathioprine: ½–4 hr (1 hr onset)	36–90 min	α phase 15 min β phase 11 hr

Adverse Reactions. The dose-limiting toxicity is myelosuppression (leukopenia and thrombocytopenia). Mild to moderate mucositis occurs with large doses, but nausea and vomiting are rare with low daily maintenance doses. Predominantly cholestatic liver toxicities are reported rarely with long-term therapy. Significant crystalluria with hematuria reported with large IV mercaptopurine doses.[81] Restrictive lung disease is also described with azathioprine, which reverses upon drug discontinuation. A single case of azathioprine-induced acute renal insufficiency has been reported; allergic hypersensitivity was suspected.[82] A variety of rashes have also been described with this class of agents. Chronic immunosuppressive therapy with any of these agents exposes patients to a significant risk of carcinogenesis; CNS lymphomas and acute myeloid leukemia are the tumors most frequent.[83]

Contraindications. Significant or impending severe bone marrow depression.

Precautions. Patients on allopurinol *must* receive substantially reduced doses of mercaptopurine or azathioprine (1/3–1/4 the normal dose), to avoid life-threatening myelosuppression. Thioguanine is primarily methylated as the eliminating step; thus, no dose reduction is necessary with concomitant allopurinol.

Parameters to Monitor. WBC and platelet counts and total bilirubin at least monthly.

Notes. Azathioprine is also used for severe rheumatoid arthritis.

Streptozocin   Zanosar®

Streptozocin is a glucose-containing nitrosourea. It has some selective cytotoxic activity in insulinomas and malignant carcinoid and is active to a lesser extent in other adenocarcinomas of the GI tract. The drug inhibits DNA synthesis via inhibition of pyrimidine biosynthesis and blockade of key enzymatic sites in gluconeogenesis pathways. It is cell cycle phase-nonspecific. The drug is administered IV 1–1.5 g/M^2/week or 500 mg/M^2/day for 5 days, repeated every 6 weeks. The drug is rapidly and extensively metabolized (unchanged drug half-life = 35 min) and only 10–20% is renally excreted unchanged. It is highly lipophilic, achieving good CNS penetration. Streptozocin and metabolites have a short distribution phase ($t_{1/2}$ 6 min) followed by possibly two elimination phases representing active metabolites ($t_{1/2\ \beta}$ 3.5 hr, $t_{1/2\ \gamma}$ 40 hr). Common acute toxicities include nausea, vomiting and phlebitis; carefully avoid extravasation. The drug is only mildly myelotoxic, but is extremely nephrotoxic. Signs of streptozocin nephrotoxicity include various renal tubular defects as well as proteinuria; adequate hydration may offer some protection. It also selectively destroys pancreatic beta cells.[84] Available as Inj 1 g.

Tamoxifen Citrate   Nolvadex®

Pharmacology. Synthetic nonsteroidal anti-estrogen which binds to cytosol estrogen receptor (ER) proteins in hormonally sensitive organs including the breast, prostate, uterus and ovary.[85] Subsequently, the tamoxifen-receptor complex is translocated to the cell nucleus wherein estrogen-dependent growth-stimulatory mRNA synthesis is halted.

Administration and Adult Dose. PO 10–20 mg/M^2/day in 2 divided doses (usually 20 mg bid in premenopausal patients and 10 mg bid in postmenopausal patients). To rapidly achieve steady-state levels, an initial 2-week course of 40 mg/M^2 bid, followed by the standard maintenance dose has been recommended.[86]

Dosage Forms. Tab 10 mg.

Patient Instructions. Lactation may occur while on tamoxifen. In premenopausal patients the chance of becoming pregnant is increased and mechanical contraceptive use should be instituted. See also Class Instructions.

Pharmacokinetics and Biopharmaceutics. *Onset and Duration.* Therapeutic levels attained with 10–20 mg/M^2/day in ≥ 7 days, versus 3 hr after the loading dose regimen of ≥ 40 mg/M^2 bid.[86] There is no long-term antitumor effect after drug discontinuation.

Plasma Levels. There does not appear to be a direct relationship between levels and response or time to response, but all responders have tamoxifen levels > 180 mg/ml at the time of remission.

Fate. Well absorbed orally with a peak level of 42 ng/ml (12 ng/ml of N-desmethyl metabolite) achieved 3–4 hr after a 20 mg dose.[87] Initially, the N-desmethyl concentration is only 50% of the tamoxifen level, but by 21 days the 2 fractions are roughly equal. With low-dose continuous therapy, mean steady-state tamoxifen levels of ≥ 260 ng/ml are achieved after 16 weeks. Following absorption, tamoxifen is slowly, but extensively metabolized, mainly to N-desmethyl tamoxifen which is equally anti-estrogenic to tamoxifen. Neither is readily conjugated and both undergo hepatic hydroxylation and conjugation followed by elimination into the bile and feces; levels are measurable for up to 6 weeks after drug discontinuation.[86]

$t_{1/2}$. (Tamoxifen) 4 days; (N-desmethyl tamoxifen) 9 days.[87] With chronic dosing, these half-lives increase slightly.[86]

Adverse Reactions. Well tolerated, producing rare myelosuppression (usually in heavily pretreated patients). Menopausal symptomatology, including hot flashes, nausea and rarely vomiting, is produced in a third of patients. Menstrual difficulties include irregularity, vaginal bleeding and pruritus vulvae. A serious disease "flare" is infrequently seen during initial therapy involving hypercalcemia and an increase in bone or soft tissue pain;[88] this often subsides even with continued therapy and may indicate early tumor response. Retinopathy has occurred only after very large doses (> 120 mg/day for 1 yr).[89]

Precautions. Pregnancy. Use with caution in patients with pre-existing leukopenia and thrombocytopenia.

Notes. The response rate in breast cancer is about 50–70% in ER positive patients, whereas the rate in ER negative patients is only about 5–10%.[90]

Vinca Alkaloids

Vinblastine
Vincristine
Vindesine

Velban®
Oncovin®
Eldisine®

Pharmacology. Periwinkle plant derived antimitotic agents; cytotoxic activity is related to specific binding to microtubule protein, blocking formation of the mitotic spindle apparatus necessary for cell division. The vincas are lethal at high concentrations and at lower concentrations dividing cells are arrested in metaphase. Occasionally, vincas may be used to synchronize tumor cell populations for subsequent treatment by G_2-M phase-specific agents such as bleomycin.

Administration, Dose and Dosage Forms.

	VINBLASTINE	VINCRISTINE	VINDESINE
Administration	IV push, infusion	IV push	IV push, infusion
Adult Dose	IV push 4–12 mg/M^2 as a single agent, repeat up to once weekly; or 1.5–1.7 mg/M^2/day for 5 days as a continuous infusion[91]	0.4–1.4 mg/M^2/week (2 mg typical single dose limit)	IV push 3 mg/M^2 q 1–2 weeks; or 1.5 mg/M^2/day for 5–7 days as a continuous infusion[92]
Pediatric Dose	IV push 4–10 mg/M^2, repeat up to once weekly	1.4–2 mg/M^2/week (2 mg typical single dose limit)	IV push 4 mg/M^2 q 1–2 weeks
Dosage Forms	Inj 10 mg	Inj 1, 5 mg	Inj 5 mg

Dosage Individualization. Vinblastine and vindesine may require substantial (75%) dose reduction in heavily pretreated patients (drugs, radiation therapy). All the vinca alkaloids are extensively (50%) eliminated in the bile and doses must be reduced by approximately 50–75% in the presence of severe hepatobiliary dysfunction.

Patient Instructions. See Class Instructions.

Pharmacokinetics and Biopharmaceutics.

Fate.

Distribution	Pharmacokinetic patterns can be described by a three compartment open model: an initial short phase with rapid tissue uptake (V_d approximating total body water) and a long terminal phase of about 1 day with a large V_d reflecting slow drug release from tissue binding sites. Vincas do not effectively penetrate the CNS or other fatty tissues and achieve highest levels in liver, gallbladder and spleen. See also $t_{1/2}$ on page 368
Metabolism	Approximately 50% of renally and fecally excreted products are closely related metabolites. An example is the formation of desacetyl vinblastine (which is more active on a weight basis than vinblastine) following either vindesine or vinblastine
Excretion	The vinca alkaloids appear to be eliminated primarily in the bile and feces, some in the urine

	VINBLASTINE	VINCRISTINE	VINDESINE
Urine (cumulative)	–	10% (24 hr)	13% (24 hr)
	33% (72 hr)	13% (72 hr)	19% (72 hr)
Feces (cumulative)	–	33% (24 hr)	–
	21% (72 hr)	67% (72 hr)	–

Continued

	VINBLASTINE	VINCRISTINE	VINDESINE
Pharmacokinetic Parameters[93,94]			
V_d central (L/kg)	0.7	0.33	0.054
$V_d \gamma$ (L/kg)	27.3	8.4	8.8
$t_{1/2}$·			
$t_{1/2} \alpha$ (hr)	0.062	0.077	0.037
$t_{1/2} \beta$ (hr)	0.164	2.3	0.9
$t_{1/2} \gamma$ (hr)	25	85	24

Adverse Reactions. Myelosuppression is the dose-limiting toxicity for vinblastine and vindesine with the leukopenic nadir at 4–10 days; unless patients have been heavily pretreated (ie, with drugs or radiation), recovery from leukopenia is rather prompt, sometimes facilitating weekly or semi-monthly dosing. Significant thrombocytopenia is rare and with vindesine the platelet count may actually increase; defective erythropoiesis is also reported for vindesine. The major toxicity of vincristine is peripheral neuropathy manifested by paresthesias, constipation, jaw pain, diminished deep tendon reflexes, and rarely, bladder atony or paralytic ileus. These slowly resolve over a month and necessitate substantial dose reduction if present at the time of dosing. Seizures have been reported very rarely. Mild laxatives may be useful for constipation. The vincas are extremely toxic if inadvertently extravasated; hyaluronidase (150 U/3 ml) may be effective as a local antidote. Infrequently, nausea and vomiting can occur, along with transiently severe pain in tumor masses (with vinblastine, vindesine). Alopecia is common with all agents.

Contraindications. (Vinblastine and vindesine) severe bone marrow compromise from prior therapy; (all vincas) severe peripheral nervous system effects from prior doses, particularly paralytic ileus.

Precautions. Use with caution in patients with neurologic deficiencies or hepatic disease. Vinca administration (especially vincristine) has been associated with increased cellular retention of methotrexate (increased even in CNS tissues).

Parameters to Monitor. (Vinblastine and vindesine) pretreatment and at least monthly WBC and hemoglobin/hematocrit assessments; (vincristine) serial peripheral neurologic assessments; (all vincas) biliary function prior to dosing and making dosage adjustments for impaired hepatobiliary status.

Notes. Protect these drugs from light and store under refrigeration. Useful in hematologic neoplasms (primarily nonmyelotoxic vincristine) and in solid tumors (primarily vinblastine).

Miscellaneous Agents

Dacarbazine	DTIC®
Dactinomycin	Cosmegen®
Mithramycin	Mithracin®
Mitomycin	Mutamycin®
Procarbazine	Matulane®

Pharmacology.

DRUG	CHEMICAL CLASS	MECHANISM OF ACTION	MAJOR CLINICAL APPLICATION
Dacarbazine	Imidazole analog of a purine precursor	Alkylation of DNA via several azo-metabolites; primarily phase-nonspecific	Malignant melanoma (10–20% objective response rates)[95]
Dactinomycin	Tricyclic, peptide-containing antibiotic	Intercalation of DNA, results in decreased mRNA synthesis; phase-nonspecific	Sarcomas; choriocarcinomas[96]
Mithramycin	Complex polycyclic, sugar-linked antibiotic	DNA intercalation; phase-nonspecific; separate calcium lowering effect	Control of hypercalcemia due to malignancy;[97] testicular cancer
Mitomycin	Antibiotic with quinone, urethane and aziridine groups	Activation chemically and metabolically to a variety of alkylator moieties; phase-nonspecific, but maximum efficacy in G_1 and S phase	GI tract tumors; bladder cancers (topical and systemic)[98]
Procarbazine	N-methyl hydrazine	Auto-oxidation and microsomal activation to several alkylating species; S phase-specific	Hodgkin's and non-Hodgkin's lymphomas; brain tumors

Administration, Dose and Dosage Forms.

DRUG	ADMINISTRATION/DOSE	DOSAGE INDIVIDUALIZATION	DOSE FORMS
Dacarbazine	IV up to 850 mg/M^2 as single dose, repeat in 3–4 weeks; or up to 250 mg/M^2/day for 5 days, repeat in 3–4 weeks	Reduce dose for decreased renal and/or hepatic function	Inj 100, 200 mg

Continued

DRUG	ADMINISTRATION/DOSE	DOSAGE INDIVIDUALIZATION	DOSE FORMS
Dactinomycin	Adult: IV 2 mg/week, for 3 weeks or 500 mcg/day for up to 5 days Pediatric: IV 450 mcg/M^2/day (up to 500 mcg) for up to 5 days, repeat in 3–4 weeks	Reduce dose for decreased hepato-biliary function	Inj 0.5 mg
Mithramycin	Hypercalcemia: IV 25 mcg/kg/day for 3–4 days Testicular tumors: IV 25–30 mcg/kg/day for up to 5 days	Reduce dose 25–50% for moderate to severe renal failure	Inj 2.5 mg
Mitomycin	Single agent: IV 20 mg/M^2 as a single dose Combination therapy: IV 5–10 mg/M^2, repeat in 4–6 weeks (up to 60 mg/week intravesical bladder therapy)	Watch for delayed and prolonged myelosuppression	Inj 5 mg
Procarbazine	PO 50–200 mg/M^2/day for 10–20 days, repeat in 3–4 weeks[99]	Base dosage on ideal body weight, Reduce dose for BUN > 40 mg/dl, Cr_s > 2.0 mg/dl or serum bilirubin > 3.0 mg/dl	Caps 50 mg

Patient Instructions. See Class Instructions.
Dacarbazine: Major nausea and vomiting should be anticipated; thought to be lessened with successive courses. Pain on injection and a flu-like syndrome may also occur. **Procarbazine:** Due to MAO inhibition, patients should avoid concurrent ingestion of alcoholic beverages, sympathomimetics, tricyclic or MAO-inhibiting antidepressants, and tyramine-rich foods.

Pharmacokinetics and Biopharmaceutics.

DRUG	FATE	$t_{1/2}$
Dacarbazine	Extensively metabolized, some microsomally mediated (50% N-demethylation); 5% protein bound; 30–45% urinary excretion (maximal at 6 hr)	α 35 min β 5 hr (approx); 7.2 hr with renal and hepatic dysfunction in one patient[100]
Dactinomycin	30% drug recovery in urine and feces after 1 week; no CNS penetration; probably concentrated in the bile	Terminal $t_{1/2}$ > 36 hr[101]
Mithramycin	40% urinary elimination; good penetration of CNS; metabolism unknown	Unknown

Continued

DRUG	FATE	$t_{1/2}$
Mitomycin	10–30% urinary recovery; rapidly eliminated, primarily by hepatic metabolism	Dose-dependent ($t_{1/2}$ increases with dose): α 5–10 min β 1 hr (approx)[102]
Procarbazine	Rapid, complete PO absorption; CNS levels equal to plasma by 0.5–1.5 hr; extensively metabolized by hepatic microsomes and by auto-oxidation; some reactive oxidation products include H_2O_2, $\cdot OH$ and $\cdot O_2$ (superoxide) free radicals; 70% recovered in urine as acid metabolite, < 5% as unchanged drug	7–10 min (unchanged drug)

Adverse Reactions.

DRUG	DOSE-LIMITING TOXICITY	FREQUENT SIDE EFFECTS[a]	RARE TOXICITIES
Dacarbazine	Myelosuppression (leukopenic nadir 21–25 days)	Nausea and vomiting (occasionally severe)	Flu-like syndrome within 1 week (myalgia, fever, malaise)
Dactinomycin	Myelosuppression (nadir 7–10 days)	Nausea and vomiting, mucositis, diarrhea, reversible alopecia	Radiation "recall" toxicity, severe ulceration if extravasated
Mithramycin	Hemorrhagic tendency (decreased platelet number and responsiveness, depressed clotting factor synthesis)[103]	Mild to moderate myelosuppression, nausea and vomiting, nephrotoxicity (proteinuria, increased creatinine) and hepatotoxicity (increased LDH, SGOT)	Stomatitis, progressive skin thickening, hyperpigmentation
Mitomycin	Myelosuppression (long leukopenic nadir 3–4 weeks) thrombocytopenia *and* anemia; all may be cumulative	Nausea, vomiting, diarrhea, alopecia, nephrotoxicity	Interstitial pneumonia (corticosteroids helpful); severe ulceration if extravasated
Procarbazine	Pancytopenic myelosuppression (nadir 2–3 weeks)	CNS effects: paresthesias, dizziness, headache, ataxia, nightmares, depression, hallucinations (up to 30% of patients); also mild to moderate nausea and vomiting (rapid tolerance usually develops)	Flu-like syndrome, allergic pneumonitis and rash

Continued

a. All agents in this group are mutagenic and teratogenic, and also cause sterility in most patients. These effects are both dose- and duration-dependent and are especially common with procarbazine.

Contraindications and Precautions.

DRUG	CONTRAINDICATIONS	PRECAUTIONS
Dacarbazine	Pre-existing severe bone marrow aplasia	Microsomal enzyme inhibition might alter drug toxicity
Dactinomycin	Pre-existing severe bone marrow aplasia	Avoid concomitant radiation therapy; avoid extravasation
Mithramycin	Thrombocytopenia or pre-existing bleeding diathesis; hypocalcemia; severe renal or hepatic dysfunction	Combine cautiously (if at all) with other drugs affecting platelet function (eg, aspirin)
Mitomycin	Pre-existing myelosuppression and anemia	May act synergistically with doxorubicin to increase cardiotoxicity (CHF)
Procarbazine	Severe hypersensitivity; unstable mental status; pre-existing severe bone marrow aplasia	Avoid concomitant MAO inhibitors, alcohol, tricyclic antidepressants, sympathomimetics, tyramine-containing foods; microsomal enzyme-inducing drugs may augment procarbazine cytotoxicity; procarbazine potentiates barbiturates, narcotics and other drugs primarily metabolized in the liver

Parameters to Monitor. Mithramycin. Evaluate serum calcium and hepatic function routinely; patients developing a progressive facial blush should be closely followed for subsequent development of life-threatening bleeding. **Mitomycin.** Pretreatment and monthly bone marrow function, hemoglobin and hematocrit. **Procarbazine.** Periodic neurologic and monthly bone marrow function may be useful.

Notes. Dacarbazine. Very light sensitive; avoid all light during storage and minimize light exposure after reconstitution. Acute toxicity may be worsened by exposure to light. Reconstituted solution is clear to pale yellow and is stable for 8 hr at room temperature. Pink coloration denotes drug decomposition. **Dactinomycin.** Reconstitute with preservative-free diluents. Significantly adsorbed to cellulose filters; avoid in-line filtration. **Mithramycin.** Unstable in acidic solutions (eg, D5W); physically incompatible with divalent cations. Reconstituted solution is stable for 48 hr under refrigeration (24 hr if further diluted in 1 L D5W). **Mitomycin.** Protect reconstituted solution from light.

References, 10:00 Antineoplastic Agents

1. Dorr RT, Fritz WL, comps. Cancer chemotherapy handbook. New York: Elsevier, 1980.
2. See-Lasley K, Ignoffo RJ, comps. Manual of oncology therapeutics. St. Louis: CV Mosby, 1981.
3. Pratt WB, Rudden RW, comps. The anticancer drugs. New York: Oxford University Press, 1979.
4. Haskell CM, ed. Cancer treatment. Philadelphia: WB Saunders, 1980.

5. Sawitsky A, Rai KR, Glidewell O et al. Comparison of daily versus intermittent chlorambucil and prednisone therapy in the treatment of patients with chronic lymphocytic leukemia. Blood 1977;50:1049-59.

6. Alberts DS, Chang SY, Chen H-SG et al. Oral melphalan kinetics. Clin Pharmacol Ther 1979;26:737-45.

7. Alberts DS, Chang SY, Chen H-SG et al. Kinetics of intravenous melphalan. Clin Pharmacol Ther 1979;26:73-80.

8. Taetle R, Dickman PS, Feldman PS. Pulmonary histopathologic changes associated with melphalan therapy. Cancer 1978;42:1239-45.

9. Heard BE, Cooke RA, Busulfan lung. Thorax 1968;23:187-93.

10. Lane SD, Besa EC, Justh G et al. Fatal interstitial pneumonitis following high-dose intermittent chlorambucil therapy for chronic lymphocytic leukemia. Cancer 1981;47:32-6.

11. Issell BF. Amsacrine (AMSA). Cancer Treat Rev 1980;7:73-83.

12. Von Hoff DD, Rozencweig M, Layard M et al. Daunomycin-induced cardiotoxicity in children and adults: a review of 110 cases. Am J Med 1977;62:200-8.

13. Weiss AJ, Metter GE, Fletcher WS et al. Studies on adriamycin using a weekly regimen demonstrating its clinical effectiveness and lack of cardiac toxicity. Cancer Treat Rep 1976;60:813-22.

14. Bachur NR. Adriamycin (NSC-123127) pharmacology. Cancer Chemother Rep (part 3)1975;6:153-8.

15. Huffman DH, Benjamin RS, Bachur NR. Daunorubicin metabolism in acute nonlymphocytic leukemia. Clin Pharmacol Ther 1972;13:895-905.

16. Benjamin RS, Wiernik PH, Bachur NR. Adriamycin chemotherapy — efficacy, safety, and pharmacologic basis of an intermittent single high-dosage schedule. Cancer 1974;33:19-27.

17. Von Hoff DD, Layard MW, Basa P et al. Risk factors for doxorubicin-induced congestive heart failure. Ann Intern Med 1979;91:710-7.

18. Blum RH, Carter SK. Adriamycin: a new anticancer drug with significant clinical activity. Ann Intern Med 1974;80:249-59.

19. Young RC, Ozols RF, Meyers CE. The anthracycline antineoplastic drugs. N Engl J Med 1981;305:139-53.

20. Clarkson B, Krakoff I, Burchenal J et al. Clinical results of treatment with E. coli l-asparaginase in adults with leukemia, lymphoma, and solid tumors. Cancer 1970;25:279-305.

21. Sutow WW, George S, Lowman JT et al. Evaluation of dose and schedule of l-asparaginase in multidrug therapy of childhood leukemia. Med Pediatr Oncol 1976;2:387-95.

22. Pratt CB, Simone JV, Zee P et al. Comparison of daily versus weekly l-asparaginase for the treatment of childhood acute leukemia. J Pediatr 1970;77:474-83.

23. Nesbit M, Chard R, Evans A et al. Evaluation of intramuscular versus intravenous administration of l-asparaginase in childhood leukemia. Am J Pediatr Hematol Oncol 1979;1:9-13.

24. Haskell CM, Canellos GP, Leventhal BG et al. L-asparaginase: therapeutic and toxic effects in patients with neoplastic disease. N Engl J Med 1969;281:1028-35.

25. Ohnuma T, Holland JF, Freeman A et al. Biochemical and pharmacological studies with asparaginase in man. Cancer Res 1970;30:2297-305.

26. Von Hoff DD, Slavik M, Muggia FM, 5-Azacytidine: a new anticancer drug with effectiveness in acute myelogenous leukemia. Ann Intern Med 1976;85:237-45.

27. Bennett JM, Reich SD. Bleomycin. Ann Intern Med 1979;90:945-8.

28. Alberts DS, Chen H-SG, Liu R et al. Bleomycin pharmacokinetics in man. Cancer Chemother Pharmacol 1978;1:177-81.

29. Paladine W, Cunningham TJ, Sponzo R et al. Intracavitary bleomycin in the management of malignant effusions. Cancer 1976;38:1903-8.

30. Crooke ST, Comis RL, Einhorn LH et al. Effects of variations in renal function on the clinical pharmacology of bleomycin administered as an IV bolus. Cancer Treat Rep 1977;61:1631-36.

31. Kramer WG, Feldman S, Broughton A et al. The pharmacokinetics of bleomycin in man. J Clin Pharmacol 1978;18:346-52.

32. Sostman HD, Matthay RA, Putnam CE. Cytotoxic drug-induced lung disease. Am J Med 1977;62:608-15.

33. Yagoda A, Mukherji B,Young C et al. Bleomycin, an antitumor antibiotic: clinical experience in 274 patients. Ann Intern Med 1972;77:861-70.

34. Prestayko AW, D'Aoust JC, Issell BF et al. Cisplatin (cis-diamminedichloroplatinum II). Cancer Treat Rev 1979;6:17-39.

35. Einhorn LH, Donohue J. Cis-diamminedichloroplatinum, vinblastine, and bleomycin combination chemotherapy in disseminated testicular cancer. Ann Intern Med 1977;87:293-8.

36. Belt RJ, Himmelstein KJ, Patton TF et al. Pharmacokinetics of non-protein-bound platinum species following administration of cis-dichlorodiammineplatinum (II). Cancer Treat Rep 1979;63:1515-21.

37. DeConti RC, Toftness BR, Lange RC et al. Clinical and pharmacological studies with cis-diamminedichloroplatinum (II). Cancer Res 1973;33:1310-5.

38. Gonzalez-Vitale JC, Hayes DM, Cvitkovic E et al. Acute renal failure after cis-dichlorodiammineplatinum (II) and gentamicin-cephalothin therapies. Cancer Treat Rep 1978;62:693-8.

39. Brock N, Gross R, Hohorst H-J et al. Activation of cyclophosphamide in man and animals. Cancer 1971;6:1512-29.

40. Grochow LB, Colvin M. Clinical pharmacokinetics of cyclophosphamide. Clin Pharmacokinet 1979;4:380-94.

41. Bagley CM, Bostick FW, DeVita VT. Clinical pharmacology of cyclophosphamide. Cancer Res 1973;33:226-33.

42. Mouridsen HT, Jacobsen E. Pharmacokinetics of cyclophosphamide in renal failure. Acta Pharmacol Toxicol 1975;36:409-14.

43. Cohen JL, Jao JY, Jusko WJ. Pharmacokinetics of cyclophosphamide in man. Br J Clin Pharmacol 1971;43:667-80.

44. Juma FD, Rogers HJ, Trounce JR. Pharmacokinetics of cyclophosphamide and alkylating activity in man after intravenous and oral administration. Br J Clin Pharmacol 1979;8:209-17.

45. Southwest Oncology Group. Cytarabine for acute leukemia in adults. Arch Intern Med 1974;133:251-9.

46. Rudnick SA, Cadman EC, Capizzi RL et al. High dose cytosine arabinoside (HDARAC) in refractory acute leukemia. Cancer 1979;44:1189-93.

47. Band PR, Holland JF, Bernard J et al. Treatment of central nervous system leukemia with intrathecal cytosine arabinoside. Cancer 1973;32:744-58.

48. Wan SH, Huffman DH, Azarnoff DL et al. Pharmacokinetics of 1-β-D-arabinofuranosylcytosine in humans. Cancer 1974;34:392-7.

49. van Prooijen R, van der Kleijn E, Haanen C. Pharmacokinetics of cytosine arabinoside in acute myeloid leukemia. Clin Pharmacol Ther 1977;21:744-50.

50. Harris AL, Potter C, Bunch C et al. Pharmacokinetics of cytosine arabinoside in patients with acute myeloid leukaemia. Br J Clin Pharmacol 1979;8:219-27.

51. Ho DHW, Frei E. Clinical pharmacology of 1-β-D-arabinofuranosylcytosine. Clin Pharmacol Ther 1971;12:944-54.

52. Chabner BA, Myers CE, Oliverio VT. Clinical pharmacology of anticancer drugs. Semin Oncol 1977;4:165-91.

53. Jacobs EM, Reeves WJ, Wood DA et al. Treatment of cancer with weekly 5-fluorouracil; study by the Western cooperative Cancer Chemotherapy Group (WCCCG). Cancer 1971;27:1302-5.

54. Horton J, Olson KB, Sullivan J et al. 5-Fluorouracil in cancer: an improved regimen. Ann Intern Med 1970;73:897-900.

55. Seifert P, Baker LH, Reed ML et al. Comparison of continuously infused 5-fluorouracil with bolus injection in treatment of patients with colorectal adenocarcinoma. Cancer 1975;36:123-8.

56. Cohen JL, Irwin LE, Marshall GJ et al. Clinical pharmacology of oral and intravenous 5-fluorouracil (NSC-19893). Cancer Chemother Rep 1974;58 (part 1):723-31.

57. Kirkwood JM, Ensminger W, Rosowsky A et al. Comparison of pharmacokinetics of 5-fluorouracil and 5-fluorouracil with concurrent thymidine infusions in a phase I trial. Cancer Res 1980;40:107-13.

58. Legha SS, Slavik M, Carter SK. Hexamethylmelamine: an evaluation of its role in the therapy of cancer. Cancer 1976;38:27-35.

59. Hortobagyi GN, Richman SP, Dandridge K et al. Immunotherapy with BCG administered by scarification. Cancer 1978;42:2293-303.

60. Symoens J, Veys E, Mielants M et al. Adverse reactions to levamisole. Cancer Treatment Rep 1978;62:1721-30.

61. DeVita VT, Serpick AA, Carbone PP. Combination chemotherapy in the treatment of advanced Hodgkin's disease. Ann Intern Med 1970;73:881-95.

62. Taylor JR, Halprin KM. Topical use of mechlorethamine in the treatment of psoriasis. Arch Dermatol 1972;106:362-64.

63. Gilman AG, Goodman LS, Gilman A, eds. Goodman and Gilman's the pharmacological basis of therapeutics. 6th ed. New York: Macmillan, 1980.

64. Taylor JR, Halprin KM, Levine V et al. Mechlorethamine hydrochloride solutions and ointment. Arch Dermatol 1980;116:783-5.

65. Van Scott EJ, Kalmanson JD. Complete remissions of mycosis fungoides lymphoma induced by topical nitrogen mustard (HN2). Cancer 1973;32:18-30.

66. Bonadonna G, Brusamolino E, Valagussa P et al. Combination chemotherapy as an adjuvant treatment in operable breast cancer. N Engl J Med 1976;294:405-10.

67. Evans WE, Pratt CB. Effect of pleural effusion on high-dose methotrexate kinetics. Clin Pharmacol Ther 1978;24:68-72.

68. Bleyer WA. Clinical pharmacology of intrathecal methotrexate II. An improved dosage regimen derived from age-related pharmacokinetics. Cancer Treat Rep 1977;61:1419-25.

69. Isacoff WH, Morrison PF, Aroesty J et al. Pharmacokinetics of high-dose methotrexate with citrovorum factor rescue. Cancer Treat Rep 1977;61:1665-74.

70. Shen DD, Azarnoff DL. Clinical pharmacokinetics of methotrexate. Clin Pharmacokinet 1978;3:1-13.

71. Fewer D, Wilson CB, Boldrey EB et al. The chemotherapy of brain tumors. JAMA 1972;222:549-52.

72. Sponzo RW, De Vita VT, Oliverio VT. Physiologic disposition of 1-(2-chloroethyl)-3-cyclohexyl-1-nitrosourea (CCNU) and 1-(2-chloroethyl)-3-(4-methyl cyclohexyl)-1-nitrosourea (MeCCNU) in man. Cancer 1973;31:1154-9.

73. De Vita VT, Carbone PP, Owens A et al. Clinical trials with 1,3-bis(2-chloroethyl)-1-nitrosourea, NSC-409962. Cancer Res 1965;25:1876-81.

74. Oliverio VT. Toxicology and pharmacology of the nitrosoureas. Cancer Chemother Rep 1973;4(part 3):13-20.

75. Aronin PA, Mahaley MS, Rudnick SA et al. Prediction of BCNU pulmonary toxicity in patients with malignant gliomas. N Engl J Med 1980;303:183-8.

76. Durant JR, Norgard MJ, Murad TM et al. Pulmonary toxicity associated with bischloroethylnitrosourea (BCNU). Ann Intern Med 1979;90:191-4.

77. Allen LM, Creaven PJ. Comparison of the human pharmacokinetics of VM-26 and VP-16, two antineoplastic epipodophyllotoxin glucopyranoside derivatives. Eur J Cancer 1975;11:697-707.

78. Rozencweig M, VonHoff DD, Henney JE et al. VM-26 and VP 16-213: a comparative analysis. Cancer 1977;40:334-42.

79. Lin S-N, Jessup K, Floyd M et al. Quantitation of plasma azathioprine and 6-mercaptopurine levels in renal transplant patients. Transplantation 1980;29:290-4.

80. Bach JF, Dardenne M. The metabolism of azathioprine in renal failure. Transplantation 1971;12:253-9.

81. Duttera MJ, Carolla RL, Gallelli JF et al. Hematuria and crystalluria after high-dose 6-mercaptopurine administration. N Engl J Med 1972;287:292-4.

82. Sloth K, Thomsen AC. Acute renal insufficiency during treatment with azathioprine. Acta Med Scand 1971;189:145-8.

83. Penn I, Starzl TE. A summary of the status of de novo cancer in transplant recipients. Transplant Proc 1972;4:719-32.

84. Schein PS, O'Connell MJ, Blom J et al. Clinical antitumor activity and toxicity of streptozotocin (NSC-85998). Cancer 1974;34:993-1000.

85. Patterson JS, Battersby LA. Tamoxifen: an overview of recent studies in the field of oncology. Cancer Treat Rep 1980;64:775-8.

86. Fabian C, Sternson L, Barnett M. Clinical pharmacology of tamoxifen in patients with breast cancer: comparison of traditional and loading dose schedules. Cancer Treat Rep 1980;64:765-73.

87. Adam HK, Patterson JS, Kemp JV. Studies on the metabolism and pharmacokinetics of tamoxifen in normal volunteers. Cancer Treat Rep 1980;64:761-4.

88. Plotkin D, Lechner JJ, Jung WE et al. Tamoxifen flare in advanced breast cancer. JAMA 1978;240:2644-6.

89. Beck M, Mills PV. Ocular assessment of patients treated with tamoxifen. Cancer Treat Rep 1979;63:1833-4.

90. Lippman ME, Allegra JC. Receptors in breast cancer: estrogen receptor and endocrine therapy of breast cancer. N Engl J Med 1978;299:930-3.

91. Yap H-Y, Blumenschein GR, Keating MJ et al. Vinblastine given as a continuous 5-day infusion in the treatment of refractory advanced breast cancer. Cancer Treat Rep 1980;64:279-83.

92. Bodey GP, Yap H-Y, Yap B-S et al. Continuous infusion vindesine in solid tumors. Cancer Treat Rev 1980;7(Suppl):39-45.

93. Owellen RJ, Root MA, Hains FO. Pharmacokinetics of videsine and vincristine in humans. Cancer Res 1977;37:2603-7.

94. Nelson RL, Dyke RW, Root MA. Comparative pharmacokinetics of vindesine, vincristine and vinblastine in patients with cancer. Cancer Treat Rev 1980;7(Suppl):17-24.

95. Carter SK, Friedman MA. 5-(3,3-dimethyl-l-triazeno)-imidazole-4-carboxamide(DTIC, DIC, NSC-45388)—a new antitumor agent with activity against malignant melanoma. Eur J Cancer 1972;8:85-92.

96. Frei E. The clinical use of actinomycin. Cancer Chemother Rep 1974;58:49-54.

97. Slayton RE, Schnider BI, Elias E et al. New approach to the treatment of hypercalcemia: the effect of short-term treatment with mithramycin. Clin Pharmacol Ther 1971;12:833-7.

98. DeFuria MD, Bracken RB, Johnson DE et al. Phase I-II study of mitomycin C topical therapy for low-grade, low-stage transitional cell carcinoma of the bladder; an interim report. Cancer Treat Rep 1980;64:225-230.

99. Spivack SD. Procarbazine. Ann Intern Med 1974;81:795-800.

100. Loo TL, Housholder GE, Gerulath AH et al. Mechanism of action and pharmacology studies with DTIC (NSC-45388). Cancer Treat Rep 1976;60:149-52.

101. Tattersall MHN, Sodergren JE, Sengupta SK et al. Pharmacokinetics of actinomycin D in patients with malignant melanoma. Clin Pharmacol Ther 1975;17:701-8.

102. Crooke ST, Bradner WT. Mitomycin C: a review. Cancer Treat Rev 1976;3:121-39.

103. Kennedy BJ. Metabolic and toxic effects of mithramycin during tumor therapy. Am J Med 1970;49:494-503.

12:00 AUTONOMIC DRUGS

12:04 PARASYMPATHOMIMETIC (CHOLINERGIC) AGENTS

Physostigmine Salicylate   Antilirium®

Pharmacology. A centrally active reversible cholinesterase inhibitor most commonly used in the management of severe overdoses of drugs with anticholinergic properties, particularly tricyclic antidepressants.

Administration and Adult Dose. IV as a therapeutic trial 1–2 mg (no faster than 1 mg/min), may repeat in 10–15 min to a maximum total of 4 mg; lowest effective dose may be repeated q 30–60 min as needed.[1]

Pediatric Dose. IV as a therapeutic trial 0.5 mg slowly, may repeat q 10 min to a total of 2 mg; lowest effective dose may be repeated q 30–60 min as needed.[1]

Dosage Forms. Inj 1 mg/ml.

Pharmacokinetics and Biopharmaceutics. *Onset and Duration.* Onset rapid; peak 5–10 min;[2] duration variable from 30–60 min[3,4] to several hr.[5]

   Fate. Rapidly hydrolyzed by cholinesterase.[6]

Adverse Reactions. Dose-related salivation, urination, emesis, defecation, bronchospasm, increased respiratory secretions, muscle weakness, bradycardia and hypotension may occur.[1-3] Onset of these symptoms requires drug discontinuation. Convulsions have been reported.[2]

Contraindications. Asthma; gangrene; diabetes; cardiovascular disease; intestinal or urinary obstruction.

Precautions. Rapid IV injection should be avoided to reduce the possibility of bradycardia, hypersalivation and convulsions.

Parameters to Monitor. Anticholinergic signs; symptoms of cholinergic excess; level of patient consciousness.

Notes. Physostigmine need not be given in all tricyclic antidepressant overdoses, only those with severe or life-threatening signs such as hallucinations, coma with respiratory depression, uncontrollable seizures or severe hypertension.[1] Physostigmine excess can be countered with 0.5 mg atropine per 1 mg of physostigmine administered.[3]

12:08 PARASYMPATHOLYTIC (CHOLINERGIC BLOCKING) AGENTS

General References: 7-9

Class Instructions. These drugs may cause dry mouth, constipation, blurring of vision, or drowsiness. Until the extent of these latter effects is known, caution should be used when driving, operating machinery, or performing other tasks requiring mental alertness. Avoid excessive concurrent use of alcohol and other drugs which cause drowsiness.

Atropine Sulfate

Various

Pharmacology. A competitive antagonist of acetylcholine at peripheral muscarinic and central receptors, causing an increase in heart rate and decreased salivary secretion, GI motility, sweating and urinary bladder contractability.

Administration and Adult Dose. **PO, SC, IM or IV for GI anticholinergic effect** 400–600 mcg qid (with meals and at bedtime); **SC, IM or IV for preanesthetic medication** 300–600 mcg about one hr before induction.

Pediatric Dose. **PO or SC for general use** 10 mcg/kg q 4–6 hr.

Dosage Forms. **Tab** 0.4 mg; **Hyp Tab** 0.3, 0.4, 0.6 mg; **Inj** 0.3, 0.4, 0.5, 0.6, 1, 1.3 mg/ml.

Patient Instructions. See Class Instructions.

Pharmacokinetics and Biopharmaceutics. *Fate.* Rapidly and well absorbed from GI tract; up to 93% of an injected dose is excreted into the urine within 24 hr, of which 30–50% is unchanged drug.[10,11]
   $t_{1/2}$. 12.5–38 hr.[10]

Adverse Reactions. Toxic effects are dose-related and frequent, especially in children. The following may occur in adults: at 0.5 mg—slight dryness of nose and mouth, bradycardia, inhibition of sweating (may lead to fever); at 1 mg—definite dryness of nose and mouth, thirst, acceleration of heart (possibly preceded by slowing), slight mydriasis; 2 mg—marked dry mouth, tachycardia, palpitation, mydriasis, slight blurring of near vision, flushed and dry skin; 5 mg—increase in above symptoms, plus speech disturbance, swallowing difficulty, headache, hot and dry skin, restlessness with asthenia; greater than 10 mg—above symptoms in the extreme, ataxia, excitement, disorientation, hallucinations, delirium and coma.

Contraindications. Acute angle glaucoma; adhesions (synechiae) between the iris and lens of the eye; asthma; obstructive disease of GI tract; obstructive uropathy; intestinal atony of elderly or debilitated patients; megacolon complicating ulcerative colitis; hiatal hernia with reflux esophagitis; unstable cardiovascular status in acute hemorrhage.

Precautions. Pregnancy. Patients over 40 yr, particularly those with any severe heart disease, hypertension, ulcerative colitis, ileus, chronic lung disease, hyperthyroidism, autonomic neuropathy, hepatic or renal disease, or prostatic hypertrophy (these latter patients may experience urinary hesitancy, and should micturate at time of administration). Overdosage may cause a curare-like action. See Drug Interactions chapter.

Notes. Used principally as a spasmolytic and as a preoperative drying agent; anticholinergics have only a limited role in peptic ulcer disease, but may be useful for persistent pain or lack of ulcer healing under routine management, or for patients with a high ulcer recurrence rate.[7] Generally, anticholinergics with no central activity (eg, propantheline) are preferred in ulcer regimens.

Benztropine Mesylate   Cogentin®

Pharmacology. A competitive antagonist of acetylcholine at peripheral muscarinic and central receptors; also possesses antihistaminic properties. Primarily used to treat both idiopathic and drug-induced parkinsonism.

Administration and Adult Dose. **PO, IM or IV for parkinsonism** 1–2 mg/day, to maximum of 6 mg/day in two divided doses; initiate at a low dose, then increase in 0.5 mg increments at 5–6 day intervals; reduce dosage or terminate other concomitant antiparkinson drugs gradually. **PO, IM or IV for drug-induced extrapyramidal symptoms** 1–4 mg once or twice daily.

Pediatric Dose. Contraindicated in children under 3 yr.

Dosage Forms. **Tab** 0.5, 1, 2 mg; **Inj** 1 mg/ml.

Patient Instructions. See Class Instructions.

Adverse Reactions. The most frequent adverse effects are dose-related and include dry mouth, blurred vision, nervousness, tachycardia, nausea, constipation, drowsiness, decreased sweating, urinary retention and other signs of cholinergic blockade—see Atropine.

Contraindications. Children under 3 yr; narrow angle glaucoma.

Precautions. Pregnancy. Use cautiously in children, in the elderly and in those with cardiac, hepatic or renal disorders (eg, cardiac arrhythmias, urinary retention), hypertension, glaucoma, obstructive diseases of the GI or genitourinary tracts, and prostatic hypertrophy (see Atropine). Use with caution in hot weather or in patients with a tendency to anhidrosis, and in the treatment of CNS drug-induced extrapyramidal disorders, due to the possibility of intensifying mental symptoms to the point of toxic psychosis. See Drug Interactions chapter.

Notes. May aggravate, rather than lessen, phenothiazine-induced tardive dyskinesia.[12] Long-term prophylactic use in patients receiving antipsychotic drugs is probably not warranted when based on the prevalence of extrapyramidal symptoms.[18] See also Antiparkinson Agents 92:00.

Propantheline Bromide   Pro-Banthine®, Various

Pharmacology. A competitive antagonist of acetycholine at peripheral muscarinic receptors, but not centrally. Used primarily as adjunctive therapy in duodenal ulcer treatment and other hypersecretory states where it has an additive effect with cimetidine in reducing acid secretion.

Administration and Adult Dose. **PO for GI conditions** 15 mg tid 1 hr ac and 30 mg hs. **IM, IV** 30 mg or more q 6 hr initially; maintenance dose is 1/2 of full therapeutic dose.

Dosage Individualization. Use one-half of the usual adult dose in geriatric patients.

Pediatric Dose. **PO** 1.5 mg/kg/day in divided doses.

Dosage Forms. **Tab** 7.5, 15 mg; **Inj** 30 mg; **SR Tab** 30 mg—not recommended—see Notes.

Patient Instructions. Take with a full glass of water on an empty stomach, 1 hr before meals. See also Class Instructions.

Pharmacokinetics and Biopharmaceutics. *Onset and Duration.* PO onset 1-1.5 hr, duration 3-6 hr; IM, IV onset 30 min, duration 3-4 hr.
   Fate. Incomplete oral absorption;[13] absorption may be enhanced by antacids and decreased by food.[14,15]

Adverse Reactions. See Atropine (note that atropine doses do not apply to propantheline); CNS effects are less than with atropine.

Contraindications. Gastric ulceration as well as those for atropine—see Atropine.

Precautions. See Atropine.

Notes. The ratio between equally effective oral and parenteral doses may be as great as 30 to 1; the SR dosage form appears to be ineffective.

Trihexyphenidyl Hydrochloride

Artane®,
Various

Pharmacology. A competitive antagonist of acetylcholine at peripheral muscarinic and central receptors. Primarily used to treat both idiopathic and drug-induced parkinsonism.

Administration and Adult Dose. **PO for parkinsonism** 1-2 mg first day, then increase by 2 mg increments at 3-5 day intervals to total of 6-10 mg/day in 3 to 4 divided doses (some patients, especially postencephalitic, may require 12-15 mg/day); **PO** 1-2 mg tid is usually adequate for concomitant use with levodopa.

Dosage Forms. **Elxr** 2 mg/5 ml; **SR Cap** 5 mg; **Tab** 2, 5 mg.

Patient Instructions. See Class Instructions.

Adverse Reactions. See Benztropine.

Contraindications. Narrow angle glaucoma is a relative contraindication.

Precautions. See Benztropine.

Parameters to Monitor. Periodic gonioscopic evaluations and monitoring of intraocular pressures.

Notes. See Benztropine.

12:12 SYMPATHOMIMETIC (ADRENERGIC) AGENTS

General References, Antiasthmatic: 16, 17
Shock: 18, 19

Class Instructions.   **Anti-asthmatic inhalers.** Extend length of mouthpiece (to slow rate of inhalation and thereby increase penetration into airways) by rolling a 6-inch length of paper into a tube and inserting into mouthpiece. To use inhaler, tilt head up and place mouthpiece extension into mouth. While breathing normally, release one dose of aerosolized medication, inhale, remove inhaler from mouth and hold breath for 5 seconds. Do not exceed prescribed dose. Report if symptoms do not completely clear or the inhaler is required more than three times in 24 hours. Clean mouthpiece weekly with hot water and soap. Store away from heat and direct sunlight. Bronchodilators may cause nervousness, tremors (especially with terbutaline or albuterol) or rapid heart rate. Report if these effects continue after dosage reduction, or if chest pain, dizziness or headache occur, or if asthmatic symptoms are not relieved.

Dobutamine Hydrochloride   Dobutrex®

Pharmacology. A sympathomimetic amine which acts directly on cardiac β_1-adrenergic receptors and, at low doses, has only a slight agonist effect on β_2- and α-adrenergic receptors; this specificity is dose-dependent and is lost at high doses. At low doses, it increases myocardial contractility without significantly increasing heart rate. Unlike dopamine, dobutamine does not release stored catecholamines, nor does it have any effect on dopaminergic receptors.[20,21]

Administration and Adult Dose. IV for inotropic support, by infusion only (in any nonalkaline IV fluid), 2.5 mcg/kg/min initially, increasing gradually in increments of 2.5 mcg/kg/min up to 20 mcg/kg/min, titrating to desired response in each patient. Most patients can be maintained on 10 mcg/kg/min or less. Although infusions up to 40 mcg/kg/min have been used, doses over 20 mcg/kg/min should be used with caution because of increased risks of tachycardia and tachydysrhythmias.[22]

Pediatric Dose. Safety and efficacy not established; however, limited experience with IV infusions of 2 and 7.7 mcg/kg/min indicates that the drug may be safe.[23]

Dosage Forms. Inj 250 mg.

Pharmacokinetics and Biopharmaceutics. *Onset and Duration.* Onset 1–2 min; peak within 10 min; duration less than 10 min.
    Fate. Eliminated primarily in the liver to inactive glucuronide conjugates and 3-O-methyldobutamine.[22]
    $t_{1/2}$. About 2 min.[22]

Adverse Reactions. Ventricular dysrhythmias may occur (although less likely than with other catecholamines). Occasionally marked increases in heart rate or systolic blood pressure occur; reduction of dosage usually reverses these effects rapidly. Patients with atrial fibrillation may be at risk of developing rapid ventricular responses, because dobutamine facilitates A-V conduction. Nausea, headache, angina and shortness of breath are occasionally noted.

Contraindications. Idiopathic hypertrophic subaortic stenosis.

Precautions. Correct hypovolemia before using in patients who are hypotensive. Use with caution in patients receiving cyclopropane or halogenated hydrocarbon anesthesia. Although most cases of extravasation cause no signs of tissue damage, at least one case of dermal necrosis following a 2.5 mcg/kg/min infusion has been reported.

Parameters to Monitor. Heart rate, arterial blood pressure, urine output, pulmonary artery wedge pressure, cardiac index, ECG for ectopic activity and infusion rate of solution.

Notes. Physically incompatible with sodium bicarbonate and other alkaline solutions.

Dobutamine Dilution Guide

AMOUNT ADDED		VOLUME OF DILUENT	FINAL CONCENTRATION
MG	VOLUME (RECONSTITUTED)		
250	1 vial (10 ml)	1000 ml	250 mcg/ml*
250	1 vial (10 ml)	500 ml	500 mcg/ml*
250	1 vial (10 ml)	250 ml	1000 mcg/ml*

*Recommended concentrations, but concentrations up to 5 mg/ml have been used.

Dopamine Hydrochloride   Intropin®

Pharmacology. A catecholamine which acts directly on peripheral dopaminergic receptors to produce renal and mesenteric vasodilation as well as β_1- and α-adrenergic receptors. Additionally, it acts indirectly by releasing norepinephrine from sympathetic nerve storage sites. Ranges are approximately as follows: dopaminergic 0.5–2 mcg/kg/min, β_1 1–10 mcg/kg/min, α 10+ mcg/kg/min.[24]

Administration and Adult Dose. **IV for shock, by infusion only** (in any nonalkaline IV fluid) 2–5 mcg/kg/min initially, increasing gradually in increments of 5–10 mcg/kg/min up to 20–50 mcg/kg/min, titrating dosage to desired response in each patient. Most patients can be maintained on 20 mcg/kg/min or less. Doses over 50 mcg/kg/min should be used only with careful monitoring of urinary output. **IV for chronic refractory congestive heart failure** 0.5–1 mcg/kg/min initially, increasing gradually until increases in urine flow, diastolic blood pressure or heart rate are observed. Most patients respond to 1–3 mcg/kg/min.[24,25]

Pediatric Dose. Safety and efficacy not established; however, limited experience with IV infusions of 0.3–25 mcg/kg/min indicates that the drug may be efficacious and safe.[26]

Dosage Forms. Inj 40, 80 mg/ml.

Pharmacokinetics and Biopharmaceutics. *Onset and Duration.* Onset 2–4 min;[27] duration less than 10 min.
  Fate. 75% metabolized to homovanillic acid (HVA) and other metabolites; 25% metabolized to norepinephrine and excreted in urine as HVA and metabolites of HVA and norepinephrine; very little is excreted as unchanged dopamine.[28]

Adverse Reactions. Ventricular arrhythmias may occur (although less likely than with other catecholamines); reduce dose if increased number of ventricular ectopic beats occurs. Hypotension at low infusion rates indicates that rate should be rapidly increased; hypertension may occur at high infusion rates. Nausea, vomiting and angina pectoris are occasionally seen. Gangrene of the extremities has occurred in patients with profound shock given large doses of dopamine for long periods of time.

Contraindications.   Pheochromocytoma; presence of uncorrected tachyarrhythmias or ventricular fibrillation.

Precautions. Correct hypovolemia before using in patients with shock. If increased diastolic pressure, decreased pulse pressure or decreased urine flow occurs, decrease infusion rate and observe patient for signs of excessive vasoconstriction. Use with caution in patients with occlusive vascular disease, and extreme caution in patients receiving cyclopropane or halogenated hydrocarbon anesthesia. Avoid extravasation of solution; however, if it occurs, the area may be infiltrated with 5–10 mg of phentolamine diluted in 10 ml normal saline.

Parameters to Monitor. In shock, closely monitor heart rate, pulmonary artery wedge pressure, cardiac index, arterial blood pressure, arterial blood gases, acid-base balance, toe temperature, urine output, infusion rate of solution and for signs of vasoconstriction or extravasation (eg, blanching).[29]

Notes. Physically incompatible with sodium bicarbonate or other alkaline solutions.

Dopamine Dilution Guide

AMOUNT ADDED		VOLUME	FINAL
MG	VOLUME	OF DILUENT	CONCENTRATION
200	5 ml (1 amp-40 mg/ml)	250 ml	800 mcg/ml*
200	5 ml (1 amp-40 mg/ml)	500 ml	400 mcg/ml*
400	5 ml (1 amp-80 mg/ml)	500 ml	800 mcg/ml*
800	10 ml (2 amps-80 mg/ml)	500 ml	1600 mcg/ml

*Recommended concentrations, but concentrations up to 3.2 mg/ml have been used.

Epinephrine and Salts

Adrenalin®, Medihaler-Epi®,
Sus-Phrine®, Various

Pharmacology. Stimulates α- (vasoconstriction, pressor effects), β_1- (increased myocardial contractility and conduction), and β_2-adrenergic (bronchodilation and vasodilation) receptors. Used for reversible bronchospasm and hypersensitivity reactions.

Administration and Adult Dose. SC for anaphylaxis 0.3–0.5 mg (0.3–0.5 ml of 1:1000 aqueous solution), may repeat q 10–15 min,[30] to maximum of 1 mg/dose and 5 mg/day; SC for asthma, same dose as above, may repeat q 20 min for 3 doses, then q 4 hr prn. SC aqueous suspension (free base) for asthma 0.5–1.5 mg (0.1–0.3 ml of 1:200 or 0.2–0.6 ml of 1:400), may repeat with 0.5–1.5 mg no sooner than q 6 hr. Inhal (metered dose) not recommended because of low efficacy and ultra-short duration of action; β_2 selective agonists (eg, terbutaline, albuterol) are preferred. See also Medical Emergencies chapter.

Pediatric Dose. SC 0.01 mg/kg/dose, to maximum of 0.5 mg/dose of 1:1000 aqueous solution, may repeat q 15 min for 3 doses, then q 4 hr prn. SC aqueous suspension (1 month to 12 yr) 0.005 ml/kg/dose of 1:200, to maximum of 0.15 ml/dose for children 30 kg or less, may repeat q 6 hr. For 1:400 aqueous suspension, double the dose.

Dosage Forms. **Inhal** (bitartrate/HCl) 0.16, 0.2, 0.27 mg free base/spray; **Soln** 1, 2.25%; **Inj** (aqueous solution as HCl) 1 mg/ml (1:1000); **Inj** (aqueous suspension as free base) 2.5 mg/ml (1:400), 5 mg/ml (1:200).

Patient Instructions.   See Class Instructions.

Pharmacokinetics and Biopharmaceutics. *Onset and Duration.*
Onset SC (aqueous solution or suspension) 3–10 min; Inhal peak 3–5 min; duration SC (aqueous suspension) up to several hr;[31] Inhal 15–30 min.
   Fate.   Oral drug rapidly inactivated in GI tract. Parenteral action terminated by uptake into adrenergic neurons. Metabolism is by MAO and COMT.[31,32]

Adverse Reactions.   Dose-related restlessness, anxiety, tremor, weakness, dizziness, headache, palpitations and hypertension. Anginal pain may occur when coronary insufficiency is present. Cardiac arrhythmias, cerebral hemorrhage from a sharp rise in blood pressure from overdose, and elevation of blood glucose.[32] Local necrosis from repeated injections and tolerance with prolonged use may occur.

Contraindications.   Intra-arterial administration is not recommended due to marked vasoconstriction; use with local anesthetics in fingers or toes; during general anesthesia with halogenated hydrocarbons or cyclopropane;[32] α-adrenergic blocker-induced (including phenothiazines) hypotension; cerebral arteriosclerosis; organic heart disease.

Precautions.   Allow sufficient time to elapse before changing to another systemic sympathomimetic agent. Use with caution in the elderly and in patients with cardiovascular disease, hypertension, diabetes or hyperthyroidism; in psychoneurotic patients and in pregnancy. Avoid use with drugs that sensitize heart to arrhythmias.

Parameters to Monitor.   Blood pressure, heart rate, relief of asthmatic or allergic symptoms.

Notes.   Do not use solution if it is brown in color or contains a precipitate. Protect solution from light. Suspension provides a sustained effect; shake suspension well prior to use. Nonprescription inhalers have only a transient effect because of their low dose.[16] They should be used only by patients who have infrequent symptoms (less than once/week) and obtain total relief of symptoms from administration of two inhalations.

Isoproterenol Salts — Anti-Asthmatic Uses

Isuprel®, Medihaler-Iso®, Various

Pharmacology.   A nonspecific β-adrenergic agonist used as a bronchodilator. β-agonist effect may result from increased cyclic AMP by activation of adenyl cyclase.

Administration and Adult Dose.   **Inhal** (metered dose—both HCl and sulfate forms) 1–2 inhalations with 1–5 min between inhalations, may repeat up to 3 times daily. **Inhal in pulmonary function testing only** (compressed air-driven nebulizer) 0.5 ml of 0.5% soln in 2 ml normal saline, repeated in 1–2 hr prn, under medical supervision. **IV, PO, SL not recommended.**[16]

Pediatric Dose.   **Inhal** same as adult dose; smaller lung volumes automatically result in smaller amount administered.

Dosage Forms.   **Inhal** (metered dose) 0.08, 0.120, 0.131 mg/spray; **Inhal**

Soln 0.25, 0.5, 1%; **Inj** 0.2 mg/ml. **SL Tab** not recommended.[16] Isoproterenol is formulated as the hydrochloride or sulfate salt.

Patient Instructions. See Class Instructions.

Pharmacokinetics and Biopharmaceutics. *Onset and Duration.*
Onset Inhal within 2 min; peak effect 3-5 min.[33] Duration—see Sympathomimetic Bronchodilators Comparison Chart.
   Fate. Poorly and irregularly absorbed after PO or SL administration.[34] After aerosol use, 80% excreted in urine as sulfate conjugate, because most of the dose is deposited in the oropharynx, swallowed and metabolized in the gut. Less than 4% of the overall dose is metabolized by COMT to 3-O-methyl isoproterenol, but a large portion of the dose reaching the lung is metabolized to this substance, which is a weak β-adrenergic blocker.[35]

Adverse Reactions. Dose-related tachycardia, palpitation, nervousness, nausea and vomiting may occur.

Contraindications.   Pre-existing cardiac arrhythmias associated with tachycardia; more than 4 doses/day (except under medical supervision).

Precautions. Use with caution in patients with coronary insufficiency. Excessive use of aerosol may cause a refractory state to develop; deaths have been reported after overuse of aerosol.

Parameters to Monitor. Question patient concerning number of inhalations per day, relief of symptoms and duration of benefit.

Notes. No longer recommended for use in the relief of acute asthmatic symptoms, but remains useful for pulmonary function testing because of rapid onset. Isuprel® Compound Elixir is an irrational formulation; the drug is degraded in the gut.

Isoproterenol Hydrochloride—   Isuprel®,
Cardiac Uses   Various

Pharmacology. A direct acting, nonspecific β-adrenergic agonist whose primary cardiovascular actions are on the heart (inotropic and chronotropic) and skeletal muscle vasculature (vasodilation).

Administration and Adult Dose. **IV for shock by infusion in 5% dextrose only** titrate dosage to desired response in each patient or to heart rate of no more than 130 beats/min.[18] Usual dosage range is 0.05-0.2 mcg/kg/min (usually 1-4 mcg/min).[18,19] Rates of over 30 mcg/min have been used in advanced states of shock. See also Medical Emergencies chapter.

Pediatric Dose. **IV for shock by infusion in 5% dextrose only** begin at 0.1 mcg/kg/min, titrating to response. Infusions of up to 2.7 mcg/kg/min have been used in status asthmaticus without significant toxicity.[36]

Dosage Forms. **Inj** 200 mcg/ml (1:5000).

Pharmacokinetics and Biopharmaceutics. *Onset and Duration.*
SL onset variable, up to 30 min; duration 1-2 hr.[31,34] IV onset immediate; duration 8 min with low dose, up to 50 min with large doses.[37]
   Fate.   After oral administration, drug is rapidly and extensively metabolized to inactive sulfate conjugate, probably in the intestine. After IV administration, 50% is excreted unchanged in the urine, 25-35% metabolized by COMT to 3-O-methyl metabolite which is then excreted unchanged or as sulfate conjugate. The 3-O-methyl metabolite is a weak β-blocker, but

has a short half-life. Termination of drug activity appears to be by uptake into adrenergic neurons rather than metabolism.[37]

Adverse Reactions.   Flushing of face, sweating, mild tremors, nervousness, headache, tachycardia with palpitation can occur. Anginal pain in patients with angina pectoris has been reported.

Contraindications.   Tachycardia caused by digitalis intoxication; patients with pre-existing arrhythmias associated with tachycardia (except ventricular tachycardias and arrhythmias that require isoproterenol's inotropic effect for therapy).

Precautions.   Correct hypovolemia before use in patients with shock. Do not administer simultaneously with epinephrine. Use with caution, and in carefully adjusted doses, in patients with coronary insufficiency, hyperthyroidism or sensitivity to sympathomimetics. Doses sufficient to raise the heart rate above 130 beats/min may induce ventricular arrhythmias.

Parameters to Monitor.   When used in situations other than resuscitation from cardiac arrest, closely monitor ECG, heart rate, pulmonary artery wedge pressure, cardiac index, arterial blood pressure, arterial blood gases, acid-base balance, urine output and infusion rate of solution; may be advisable to slow, or temporarily stop infusion if heart rate exceeds 100 beats/min.

Notes.   Physically incompatible with sodium bicarbonate or other alkaline solutions.

Isoproterenol Dilution Guide

AMOUNT ADDED		VOLUME OF	
MG	VOLUME	5% DEXTROSE	FINAL CONCENTRATION
1	5 ml (1:5000)	500 ml	2 mcg/ml (1:500,000)*
2	10 ml (1:5000)	500 ml	4 mcg/ml (1:250,000)

*Recommended concentration, but concentrations of 10 times this have been used.

Metaproterenol Sulfate   Alupent®, Metaprel®

Pharmacology.   A predominantly β_2-adrenergic agonist (bronchodilator); not as selective or long-acting as terbutaline or albuterol.[16]

Administration and Adult Dose.   PO 20 mg 4–6 times/day. Inhal (metered dose) 1.3–1.95 mg (2–3 inhalations), repeated not more often than q 3–4 hr, to maximum of 7.8 mg (12 inhalations)/day. Inhal (compressed air-driven nebulizer) 0.2–0.3 ml in 2.5 ml normal saline under medical supervision, not more often than q 4 hr.

Pediatric Dose.   PO (under 6 yr) 5 mg 4–6 times/day; (6–9 yr or under 27 kg) 10 mg 4–6 times/day; (over 9 yr or 27 kg) 20 mg 4–6 times/day. Inhal (metered dose) same as adult dose.

Dosage Forms.   Syrup 10 mg/5 ml; Tab 10, 20 mg; Inhal 0.65 mg/metered dose (300 doses/inhaler); Inhal Soln 5%.

Patient Instructions.   See Class Instructions.

Pharmacokinetics and Biopharmaceutics.   *Onset and Duration.*
Onset Inhal 5–30 min; PO peak 1–2 hr. Duration—see Sympathomimetic Bronchodilators Comparison Chart.

Fate. Only 40% of oral drug is absorbed due to first-pass metabolism in liver; excreted primarily as glucuronic acid conjugates.[31]

Adverse Reactions. Sympathomimetic effects, such as tachycardia, nervousness, tremor and nausea may occur and are usually dose-related. Occasional reactions are palpitations, vomiting and bad taste.

Contraindications. Cardiac arrhythmias.

Precautions. Pregnancy. Use with caution in patients with coronary artery disease or CHF.

Parameters to Monitor. See Isoproterenol.

Notes. As effective as isoproterenol by inhalation, but has longer duration of action and fewer cardiac side effects.[33,38] Oral use adds therapeutic benefit to theophylline for only 1 hr after each dose. Store inhalant solution at room temperature and protect from light.

Norepinephrine Bitartrate   Levophed®

Pharmacology. A catecholamine which directly stimulates β_1- and α-adrenergic receptors. It has little action on β_2-receptors.

Administration and Adult Dose. IV for shock, by infusion only (in any nonalkaline IV fluid) 8–12 mcg of base/min initially, adjusting rate to maintain a systolic blood pressure of about 80–100 mm Hg (but no more than 40 mm Hg below pre-existing systolic pressure); average maintenance dosage ranges from 2–4 mcg of base/min.

Pediatric Dose. IV for shock by infusion only 2 mcg/M^2/min initially, titrating to desired blood pressure, to maximum of 6 mcg/M^2/min.

Dosage Forms. Inj 1 mg (of levarterenol base)/ml.

Pharmacokinetics and Biopharmaceutics. *Onset and Duration.* Onset rapid; duration 1–2 min after discontinuing infusion.[31]
   Fate. After oral administration, drug is rapidly inactivated in GI tract. IV action is terminated by uptake into adrenergic neurons; drug is metabolized primarily by COMT, and to a lesser extent by MAO, to inactive metabolites and their conjugates.[31,34]

Adverse Reactions. Dose-related hypertension (sometimes indicated by headache), reflex bradycardia, increased peripheral vascular resistance and decreased cardiac output. Volume depletion may occur if fluid is not replaced.

Contraindications. Hypotension secondary to uncorrected blood volume deficit; mesenteric or peripheral vascular thrombosis, unless drug is lifesaving; cyclopropane or halogenated hydrocarbon anesthesia.

Precautions. Use with caution in patients receiving MAO inhibitors or tricyclic antidepressants (may cause profound hypertension). Administer into a large vein (antecubetal or femoral preferred) to avoid necrosis secondary to vasoconstriction; avoid the leg veins in elderly patients or in those with occlusive vascular diseases. Avoid extravasation of solution; however, if it occurs, the area may be infiltrated with 5–10 mg of phentolamine diluted in 10 ml normal saline.

Parameters to Monitor. In shock, closely monitor heart rate, pulmonary artery wedge pressure, cardiac index, arterial blood pressure, arterial blood gases, acid-base balance, urine output, infusion rate of solution and for signs of vasoconstriction or extravasation (eg, blanching).

Notes. Do not use solution if it has a brown color or precipitate. 2 mg of norepinephrine bitartrate = 1 mg norepinephrine base.

Norepinephrine Dilution Guide

AMOUNT ADDED		VOLUME OF	FINAL
MG (BASE)	VOLUME	5% DEXTROSE	CONCENTRATION
2 mg	2 ml	500 ml	4 mcg/ml*
4 mg	4 ml	500 ml	8 mcg/ml*
8 mg	8 ml	500 ml	16 mcg/ml†

*Recommended pediatric concentration.
†Recommended adult concentration.

Pseudoephedrine Hydrochloride Sudafed®, Novafed®, Various

Pharmacology. An indirect acting agent that stimulates α, β_1 and β_2-adrenergic receptors via release of endogenous adrenergic amines.

Administration and Adult Dose. PO 60–120 mg qid prn;[39] PO SR Cap/Tab 120 mg q 8–12 hr.

Pediatric Dose. PO 120–240 mg/day divided into 4 doses for rapid release products and into 2–3 doses for slow release. Do not give SR 120 mg to patients under 12 yr.

Dosage Forms. SR Cap 60, 120 mg; Syrup 30 mg/5 ml; Tab 30, 60 mg; SR Tab (as sulfate) 120 mg.

Patient Instructions. Take last dose a few hours before bedtime if insomnia occurs with bedtime administration.

Pharmacokinetics and Biopharmaceutics. *Onset and Duration.* Onset 15–30 min; duration 3 hr,[40] 8–12 hr for SR dosage form.[31]
   Fate. SR formulations (Novafed®, Sudafed® S.A.) are the only two formulations with documented bioavailability. Partly metabolized to inactive metabolite(s) and 6% metabolized to active metabolite, norpseudoephedrine.[41] 55–75% excreted unchanged in urine.[31]
   $t_{1/2}$. Average 7 hr; urinary flow and pH dependent: 9–16 hr at pH 8; 5–8 hr at pH 5.5–6; 3–6 hr at pH 5.[41,42]

Adverse Reactions. Mild transient nervousness, insomnia, irritability or headache.

Contraindications. Severe hypertension; coronary artery disease; MAO inhibitor therapy.

Precautions. Use with caution in patients with hypertension, diabetes mellitus, ischemic heart disease, increased intraocular pressure or prostatic hypertrophy. Elderly patients may be particularly sensitive to CNS effects. If use is necessary in infants with phenylketonuria, reduce dose to avoid possible increased agitation.[43]

Parameters to Monitor. Nasal stuffiness, blood pressure, CNS stimulation.

Notes. Used primarily for decongestion of nasal mucosa and eustachian tubes.[44,45] Combination with an antihistamine may provide additive benefit in seasonal allergic rhinitis, because antihistamines do not relieve nasal stuffiness.[46]

Ritodrine Hydrochloride   Yutopar®

Pharmacology. A selective β_2-adrenergic agonist, with actions similar to terbutaline, used to inhibit contractions of uterine smooth muscle.

Administration and Adult Dose. **IV for premature labor** 100 mcg/min as a continuous infusion, increased, if needed, in 50 mcg/min increments at 10 min intervals to desired effect, side effects or a maximum of 350 mcg/min. Continue infusion for 12 hr after cessation of contractions. An infusion control device should be used. **IM**, although not FDA approved, has been used with doses comparable to IV, given at 4 hr intervals.[34,47] **PO** 10 mg q 2 hr for 24 hr, starting 30 min before cessation of IV infusion, then 10–20 mg q 4–6 hr, to maximum of 120 mg/day.[48]

Dosage Forms. **Tab** 10 mg; **Inj** 50 mg/5 ml.

Patient Instructions. This drug may cause nervousness, trembling or an unusually fast or pounding heartbeat; report any other adverse effects. Do not double up on missed doses.

Pharmacokinetics and Biopharmaceutics. *Onset and Duration.* Onset IV within minutes; PO 30–60 min.[49]
  Fate. Oral bioavailability is about 30%.[49] Infusions of 150 mcg/min yield plasma levels of 32–52 ng/ml. A 10 mg oral dose results in peak levels of 5–15 ng/ml.[47] Cord blood levels approach maternal plasma levels. V_d is 0.71 L/kg; 32% plasma protein bound. Excretion as unchanged drug and inactive conjugates is 90% complete in 24 hr.[49]
  $t_{1/2}$. α phase (IV only) 6–9 min; β phase 1.3–2.6 hr; γ phase 10 hr or more.[49]

Adverse Reactions. Dose-related β-adrenergic effects on the cardiovascular system include elevated maternal and fetal heart rates and widening of the maternal pulse pressure. Oral use results in lesser or delayed cardiovascular effects. Other frequent effects are palpitations, trembling, nausea, vomiting and headache. Rare cardiac effects include chest pain or tightness and arrhythmias, adult respiratory distress syndrome, angina, pulmonary edema and death. Rare fetal effects include hypoglycemia, ileus, hypocalcemia and hypotension.[50,69]

Contraindications. Eclampsia and severe pre-eclampsia; hemorrhage; intra-uterine fetal death; chorio-amnioitis; maternal cardiac disease; hypertension; pulmonary hypertension; hyperthyroidism; uncontrolled diabetes mellitus; bronchial asthma under treatment with β-adrenergic agents or corticosteroids; pregnancy before the 20th week.[50]

Precautions. Maternal pulmonary edema and death has been reported usually in patients treated concomitantly with ritodrine and corticosteroids. When used with ritodrine, sympathomimetic drugs exert additive effects; β-blockers exert inhibitory effects. Hypotensive effects may be potentiated by anesthetic agents. Use with caution in pre-eclampsia, hypertension or diabetes.[69]

Parameters to Monitor. Fetal and maternal heart rates, maternal blood pressure, serum potassium and glucose levels during IV infusion, signs and symptoms of pulmonary edema and adult respiratory distress syndrome.

Notes. Other β-adrenergic agonists, such as terbutaline, isoxsuprine and fenoterol have been used in a fashion similar to ritodrine for premature labor.[50]

Sympathomimetic Agents for Hemodynamic Support[a]

DRUG	INJECTABLE DOSAGE FORMS	ADRENERGIC RECEPTOR SELECTIVITY				TOTAL PERIPHERAL RESISTANCE	CARDIAC OUTPUT
		INOTROPIC ACTIVITY (β_1)	CHRONOTROPIC ACTIVITY (β_1)	VASODILATION (β_2)	VASOCONSTRICTION (α)		
Phenylephrine[b] Neo-Synephrine®	10 mg/ml (1%)	0	0[c]	0	+++++	↑	↓
Norepinephrine[d] Levophed®	1 mg/ml (of base)	++	++[c]	0	++++	↑	0/↓
Epinephrine Adrenalin® Various	1 mg/ml (1:1000) 0.1 mg/ml (1:10,000)	+++	+++	++	++++	↓	↑
Dopamine Intropin®	40, 80 mg/ml	++	+/++[e]	++	+/++	↓/↑[e]	↑
Dobutamine Dobutrex®	250 mg/vial	++	0/+[e]	+	0/+[e]	↓	↑
Isoproterenol Isuprel® Various	200 mcg/ml (1:5000)	++++	++++	+++++	0	↓	↑

Continued

Sympathomimetic Agents for Hemodynamic Support[a]

DRUG	INJECTABLE DOSAGE FORMS	ADRENERGIC RECEPTOR SELECTIVITY					TOTAL PERIPHERAL RESISTANCE	CARDIAC OUTPUT
		INOTROPIC ACTIVITY (β_1)	CHRONO-TROPIC ACTIVITY (β_1)	VASO-DILATION (β_2)	VASO-CONSTRICTION (α)			
Phentolamine[f] Regitine®	5 mg/ml	—	g	—	—	—	↓	↑

Key. +++++ = Pronounced effect; + = Minimal effect; 0 = No effect; ↓ = Decreased; ↑ = Increased

a. This table compares only a few of the many factors important in the treatment of shock. Consult references 18, 19, 25 for a complete guide. Cross-table comparisons of the adrenergic selectivity properties between this table and the Sympathomimetic Bronchodilators Comparison Chart cannot be made for the following reasons: (1) the rating scale of this table reflects a finer degree of differentiation of effects (hence 0-5+ vs. 0-4+); (2) the routes of administration are different; and (3) vascular β_2 receptors appear to respond slightly differently from bronchiolar β_2 receptors.

b. Used to ↑ BP to reflexly ↑ vagal tone in paroxysmal supraventricular tachycardias.

c. Decrease in heart rate may result from reflex mechanisms.

d. Primarily used to increase peripheral vascular resistance in volume-repleted hypotensive patients.

e. Dose-dependent.

f. α-adrenergic blocking agent; useful in severe vasoconstriction (ie, extravasation of norepinephrine or dopamine).

g. Increase in heart rate may result from reflex and direct mechanisms.

Sympathomimetic Bronchodilators Comparison Chart[a,b]

DRUG	ADULT DOSAGE RANGE	DOSAGE FORMS	β-ADRENERGIC RECEPTOR SELECTIVITY		DURATION[c]	COMMENTS
			CARDIAC β_1	BRON-CHIOLAR β_2		
Epinephrine Adrenalin® Various	SC 0.3–0.5 mg Inhal not recommended	Inj 1 mg/ml Inhal not recommended	+ + +	+ +	Short; may repeat SC in 15–30 min	Massage of SC injection site may hasten onset
Epinephrine Aq Susp Sus-Phrine®	SC 0.5 mg, then 0.5–1.5 mg q 6 hr prn	Inj 2.5, 5 mg/ml	+ + +	+ +	Up to several hr	Massage of SC injection site may hasten onset
Isoproterenol Isuprel®	Inhal 1–2 sprays; IV, PO, SL Tab not recommended	Inhal 0.25, 0.5, 1% Inj, PO, SL Tab not recommended	+ + +	+ + +	Inhal 30–60 min	See monograph
Isoetharine Bronkometer® Bronkosol®	Inhal 1–2 sprays q 4 hr	Inhal (soln) 0.1, 0.125, 0.2, 0.25, 0.5, 1%; (metered dose) 0.34 mg/spray	+ +	+ +	1 hr	Short duration is a disadvantage

Continued

Sympathomimetic Bronchodilators Comparison Chart[a,b]

DRUG	ADULT DOSAGE RANGE	DOSAGE FORMS	β-ADRENERGIC RECEPTOR SELECTIVITY CARDIAC β_1	β-ADRENERGIC RECEPTOR SELECTIVITY BRON-CHIOLAR β_2	DURATION[c]	COMMENTS
Metaproterenol Alupent® Metaprel®	PO 20 mg 4-6 times/day Inhal 2-3 sprays q 3-4 hr; or (diluted soln) 0.2-0.3 mg q 4 hr (q 1-2 hr under medical supervision)	Syrup 10 mg/5 ml Tab 10, 20 mg Inhal (soln) 5%; (metered dose) 0.65 mg/spray	++	+++	PO 4 hr Inhal (metered) dose) 1-3 hr Inhal (soln) 3 hr	See monograph
Terbutaline Brethine® Bricanyl®	PO 5 mg 4-6 times/day SC 0.25 mg 1-2 times in any 4 hr Inhal 1-2 mg diluted with 2 ml normal saline q 3-4 hr (q 1 hr under medical supervision)	Tab 2.5, 5 mg Inj 1 mg/ml	+	++++	PO 4-8 hr SC 1.5-4 hr Inhal 5 hr	Muscle tremors with PO and SC dosing initially and in high doses; ↓PO dose to 2.5 mg tid if side effects present.[d]

Continued

Sympathomimetic Bronchodilators Comparison Chart[a,b]

DRUG	ADULT DOSAGE RANGE	DOSAGE FORMS	β-ADRENERGIC RECEPTOR SELECTIVITY		DURATION[c]	COMMENTS
			CARDIAC β_1	BRON-CHIOLAR β_2		
Albuterol Proventil® Ventolin®	PO 2-8 mg tid-qid Inhal 1-2 sprays q 4-6 hr	Tab 2, 4 mg Inhal (metered dose) 0.09 mg/spray	±	+ + + +	PO 4-8 hr Inhal 4-6 hr	Drug of choice if patient can be taught use of metered dose inhaler[d]
Fenoterol Berotec®- Boehringer-Ingelheim	PO 5-10 mg 3-4 times/day Inhal 1-2 sprays 3-4 times/day	—	±	+ + + +	PO 6-8 hr Inhal 8 hr	May have more β-agonist activity than albuterol; skeletal muscle tremors with PO and SC dosing[d] Investigational

a. From references 16, 17, 31, 32, 34, 38, 51-57.
b. See footnote "a", in Sympathomimetic Agents For Hemodynamic Support Comparison Chart.
c. The duration of β-receptor agonists varies among studies. The values listed are approximate for single-dose use. The duration of action and intensity of effect of β-agonists appears to decrease by about one-half with continuous use.[16,55]
d. It is unclear whether the increase in heart rate seen with selective β_2-agonists represents residual β_1 effects, reflex tachycardia secondary to peripheral vasodilation or both. Muscle tremor is a direct β_2 effect on skeletal muscle.[31]

12:16 SYMPATHOLYTIC (ADRENERGIC BLOCKING) AGENTS

General References: 58

Ergotamine Tartrate   Ergomar®, Ergostat®, Gynergen®

Pharmacology. An ergot alkaloid with peripheral α-adrenergic blocking properties. Mechanism in migraine is thought to be vasoconstriction of cranial blood vessels, with concomitant decrease in the amplitude of pulsations.

Administration and Adult Dose. PO for migraine 1–2 mg initially, or **SL** 2 mg initially, then PO 1 mg or SL 2 mg each half hr prn, to maximum of 6 mg/day or 10 mg/week; **Inhal** one inhalation (0.36 mg) initially, then q 5+ min, to maximum of 6 inhalations/day or 15 inhalations/week; **SC or IM** 0.25–0.5 mg, then 0.25 mg in 40 min if needed, to maximum of 1 mg/week.

Pediatric Dose. Safety and efficacy not established.

Dosage Forms. Inhal 9 mg/ml; SL Tab 2 mg; Tab 1 mg; Inj 0.5 mg/ml.

Patient Instructions. Initiate therapy at first signs of attack. Take only as directed and do not exceed specified dosages.

Pharmacokinetics and Biopharmaceutics. *Onset and Duration.* Onset PO averages up to 5 hr, SC or IM 15 min to 2 hr.[59]
Plasma Levels. A high frequency of adverse reactions has been associated with plasma levels above 1.8 ng/ml.[60]
Fate. Absorption from GI tract is irregular, whereas there is better absorption from parenteral sites; SL is considered least well absorbed. Average peak plasma levels are variously reported as 0.6 ng/ml attained in 1 hr[60] and 0.36 ng/ml attained in 1–2 hr[61] following a single 2 mg oral dose; and 1.5 ng/ml 15 min after a 0.25 mg IM dose[60] and 1.94 ± 0.34 ng/ml 30 min following a 0.5 mg IM dose.[61] Rectal administration of a 2 mg dose produces plasma levels slightly higher than oral use.[60,61] There is great variation in plasma levels, and in most subjects plasma levels showed a second increase in 24–48 hr.[61] Metabolized by the liver, with 90% of metabolites excreted in bile.[59]
$t_{1/2}$. α phase 1.8–3.6 hr; β phase 17–25 hr after a 1 mg oral dose.[62]

Adverse Reactions. Frequently nausea, vomiting, weakness in legs, muscle pains in extremities and numbness or tingling of fingers and toes occur; occasional headache, precordial distress and pain and transient tachycardia or bradycardia occur; rarely, gangrene or serious cardiovascular effects have been reported.

Contraindications. Pregnancy; occlusive or peripheral vascular disease; coronary heart disease; hypertension; hepatic or renal impairment; sepsis; severe pruritus.

Precautions. Avoid overdosing or prolonged administration due to the potential for ergotism and gangrene.

Notes. Evidence indicates that caffeine facilitates the absorption of oral ergotamine,[63] but the stimulant action of preparations containing caffeine (eg, Cafergot®) may keep patients from the beneficial effect of sleep.[64] Propranolol may prove useful in migraine prevention for some patients.[58,65,66]

Methysergide Maleate   Sansert®

Pharmacology.   Mechanism of clinical action is unknown; it is a peripheral competitive antagonist of serotonin, blocking increased blood vessel permeability and affecting the pain threshold; inhibits histamine release from mast cells and stabilizes platelets against release of serotonin.

Administration and Adult Dose.   **PO prophylaxis** of frequent and/or severe vascular headaches 2 mg/day initially, then adjust by 2 mg q 3–4 days, to maximum of 8 mg/day in divided doses. Three weeks are required for a therapeutic trial; if efficacy is not demonstrated, further administration is unlikely to be of benefit. Drug must be discontinued (by decreasing dosage over 2–3 weeks) for one month q 6 months, in order to avoid serious fibrotic changes.

Pediatric Dose.   Not recommended.

Dosage Forms.   **Tab** 2 mg.

Patient Instructions.   Take with meals or food when possible. Immediately report cold, numb and painful hands and feet; leg cramps on walking; dysuria; any type of girdle, flank or chest pain, or any associated symptomatology.

Pharmacokinetics and Biopharmaceutics.   *Onset and Duration.* Onset 1–2 days; duration 1–2 days following discontinuation.[59]
  Fate.   Rapidly absorbed from GI tract. Following a 2 mg tid regimen, a simulated mean steady-state plasma level (drug and metabolites) of 40 ng/ml is attained. Metabolized by the liver, with 56% excreted in the urine as unchanged drug and metabolites.[67]
  $t_{1/2}$.   10 hr.[67]

Adverse Reactions.   About one-third of patients develop some type of adverse effect.[66,68] Usually, these include nausea, vomiting and GI pain, drowsiness or insomnia, ataxia, muscle pains, dizziness, edema, weight gain, hyperesthesia; occasionally, psychic disturbances (eg, feelings of dissociation or unreality), alopecia and rash. Rare, but potentially life-threatening, are fibrotic and cardiovascular changes including retroperitoneal or pleuropulmonary fibrosis and fibrosis of cardiac valves; the fibrotic process may result in vascular insufficiency.

Contraindications.   Pregnancy; peripheral or coronary vascular disease; severe arteriosclerosis or hypertension; phlebitis or cellulitis of the lower limbs; pulmonary disease; collagen diseases or fibrotic processes; impaired liver or renal function; valvular heart disease; debilitated states and serious infections.

Precautions.   Methysergide has no place in the management of an acute attack. All patients using methysergide should be under close medical supervision.

Parameters to Monitor.   Patients should be monitored for symptoms of fibrotic or vascular change and examined regularly. Each patient should have an annual intravenous pyelogram.[58]

Notes.   Fibrotic manifestations often regress when the drug is withdrawn. Propranolol may prove useful in migraine prevention for some patients;[58,65] in a comparative study, propranolol was as effective as methysergide with fewer severe side effects.[66]

References, 12:00 Autonomic Drugs

1. Anon. Physostigmine for tricyclic antidepressant overdosage. Med Lett Drugs Ther 1980;22:55.
2. Newton RW. Physostigmine salicylate in the treatment of tricyclic antidepressant overdosage. JAMA 1975;231:941-3.
3. Rumack BH. Anticholinergic poisoning: treatment with physostigmine. Pediatrics 1973;52:449-51.
4. Burks JS, Walker JE, Rumack BH et al. Tricyclic antidepressant poisoning: reversal of coma, choreoathetosis and myoclonus by physostigmine. JAMA 1974;230:1405-7.
5. Snyder BD, Blonde L, McWhirter WR. Reversal of amitriptyline intoxication by physostigmine. JAMA 1974;230:1433-4.
6. Taylor P. Anticholinesterase agents. In: Gilman AG, Goodman LS, Gilman A, eds. Goodman and Gilman's the pharmacological basis of therapeutics. 6th ed. New York: Macmillan, 1980;100-19.
7. Ivey KJ. Anticholinergics: do they work in peptic ulcer? Gastroenterology 1975;68:154-66.
8. Klett CJ, Caffey E. Evaluating the long-term need for antiparkinson drugs by chronic schizophrenics. Arch Gen Psychiatry 1972;26:374-9.
9. Bohman T, Myren J, Flaten O. The effect of trimipramine, cimetidine, and atropine on gastric secretion. Scand J Gastroenterol 1980;15:177-82.
10. Kalser SC, McClain PC. Atropine metabolism in man. Clin Pharmacol Ther 1970;11:214-27.
11. Kalser SC. The fate of atropine in man. Ann NY Acad Sci 1971;179:667-83.
12. Kiloh LG, Smith JS, Williams SE. Antiparkinson drugs as causal agents in tardive dyskinesia. Med J Aust 1973;2:591-3.
13. Beermann B et al. On the metabolism of propantheline in man. Clin Pharmacol Ther 1972;13:212-20.
14. de Saintonge, Herxheimer A. Sodium bicarbonate enhances the absorption of propantheline in man. Eur J Clin Pharmacol 1973;5:239-42.
15. Gibaldi M, Grundhofer B. Biopharmaceutic influences on the anticholinergic effects of propantheline. Clin Pharmacol Ther 1975;18:457-61.
16. Weinberger M, Hendeles L. Pharmacotherapy of asthma. Am J Hosp Pharm 1976;33:1071-80.
17. Ahrens RC, Hendeles L, Weinberger M. The clinical pharmacology of drugs used in the treatment of asthma. In Yaffe SJ, ed. Pediatric pharmacology: therapeutic principles in practice. New York: Grune & Stratton, 1980;233-80.
18. Tarazi RC. Sympathomimetic agents in the treatment of shock. Ann Intern Med 1974;81:364-71.
19. Weil MH, Shubin H, Carlson R. Treatment of circulatory shock: use of sympathomimetic and related vasoactive agents. JAMA 1975;231:1280-6.
20. Leier CV, Heban PT, Huss P et al. Comparative systemic and regional hemodynamic effects of dopamine and dobutamine in patients with cardiomyopathic heart failure. Circulation 1978;58:466-75.
21. Anon. Dobutamine (Dobutrex). Med Lett Drugs Ther 1979;21:15-6.
22. Sonnenblick EH, Frishman WH, LeJemtel TH. Dobutamine: A new synthetic cardioactive sympathetic amine. N Engl J Med 1979;300:17-22.
23. Driscoll DJ, Gillette DC, Duff DF et al. Hemodynamic effects of dobutamine in children. Am J Cardiol 1979;43:581-5.
24. Goldberg LI. Dopamine—clinical uses of an endogenous catecholamine. N Engl J Med 1974;291:707-10.
25. Rosenblum R. Physiologic basis for the therapeutic use of catecholamines. Am Heart J 1974;87:527-30.
26. Driscoll DJ, Gillette PC, McNamara DG. The use of dopamine in children. J Pediatr 1978;92:309-14.
27. Allwood MJ et al. Peripheral vascular effects of noradrenaline, isopropylnoradrenaline and dopamine. Br Med Bull 1963;19:132-6.
28. Goodall McC, Alton H. Metabolism of 3-hydroxytyramine (dopamine) in human subjects. Biochem Pharmacol 1968;17:905-14.
29. Ruiz CE, Weil MH, Carlson RW. Treatment of circulatory shock with dopamine. JAMA 1979;242:165-8.
30. Kelly JF, Patterson R. The treatment of anaphylaxis. Ration Drug Ther 1973;7(11):1-5.
31. Kepler JA, ed. American hospital formulary service. Washington, DC: American Society of Hospital Pharmacists, 1959-1982.
32. Weiner N. Norepinephrine, epinephrine, and the sympathomimetic amines. In: Gilman AG, Goodman LS, Gilman A, eds. Goodman and Gilman's the pharmacological basis of therapeutics. 6th ed. New York: Macmillan, 1980;138-75.
33. Holmes TH, Morgan B. A comparative clinical trial of metaproterenol and isoproterenol as bronchodilator aerosols. Clin Pharmacol Ther 1968;9:615-24.
34. Wade A, ed. Martindale, the extra pharmacopoeia. 27th edition. London: The Pharmaceutical Press, 1977.
35. Blackwell EW, Briant RH, Conolly ME et al. Metabolism of isoprenaline after aerosol and direct intrabronchial administration in man and dog. Br J Pharmacol 1974;50:587-91.
36. Wood DW, Downes JJ, Scheinkopf H et al. Intravenous isoproterenol in the management of respiratory failure in childhood status asthmaticus. J Allergy Clin Immunol 1972;50:75-81.
37. Conolly ME. Davies DS, Dollery CT et al. Metabolism of isoprenaline in dog and man. Br J Pharmacol 1972;46:458-72.
38. Chervinsky P, Belinkoff S. Comparison of metaproterenol and isoproterenol aerosols: spirometric evaluation after two months' therapy. Ann Allergy 1969;27:611-6.
39. Hendeles L, Weinberger M, Wong L. Medical management of noninfectious rhinitis. Am J Hosp Pharm 1980;37:1496-1504.
40. Bickerman HA. Physiologic and pharmacologic studies on nasal airway resistance (RN). Proceedings of conference on current research methodology in the evaluation of proprietary medicines. Washington, DC: The Proprietary Association 1971; Dec 8.
41. Brater DC, Kaojarern S, Benet LZ et al. Renal excretion of pseudoephedrine. Clin Pharmacol Ther 1980;28:690-4.
42. Kuntzman RG, Tsai I, Brant L et al. The influence of urinary pH on the plasma half-life of pseudoephedrine in man and dog and a sensitive assay for its determination in human plasma. Clin Pharmacol Ther 1971;12:62-67.

43. Spielberg SP, Schulman JD. A possible reaction to pseudoephedrine in a patient with phenylketonuria. J Pediatr 1977;90:1026.

44. Anon. Establishment of a monograph for OTC cold, cough, allergy, bronchodilator and antiasthmatic products. Fed Regist 1976;41:38312-424.

45. Roth RP, Cantekin EI, Bluestone CD et al. Nasal decongestant activity of pseudoephedrine. Ann Otol Rhinol Laryngol 1977;86:235-42.

46. Empey DW, Bye C, Hodder M et al. A double-blind crossover trial of pseudoephedrine and triprolidine, alone and in combination, for the treatment of allergic rhinitis. Ann Allergy 1975;34:41-6.

47. Spellacy WN, Cruz AC, Birk SA et al. Treatment of premature labor with ritodrine: a randomized controlled study. Obstet Gynecol 1979;54:220-3.

48. Creasy RK, Golbus MS, Laros RK et al. Oral ritodrine maintenance in the treatment of preterm labor. Am J Obstet Gynecol 1980;137:212-6.

49. Gandar R, deZoeten LW, van der Schoot JB. Serum level of ritodrine in man. Eur J Clin Pharmacol 1980;17:117-22.

50. Anon. Adverse reactions from treating premature labor with beta agonists. FDA Drug Bull 1981;11:13-4.

51. Dulfano MJ, Glass P. The bronchodilator effects of terbutaline: route of administration and patterns of response. Ann Allergy 1976;37:357-66.

52. Anon. Metaproterenol. Med Lett Drugs Ther 1974;16:45-6.

53. Avery GS. Salbutamol: a review. Drugs 1971;1:274-302.

54. O'Donnell SR, Wanstall JC. Evidence that the efficacy (intrinsic activity) of fenoterol is higher than that of salbutamol on β-adrenoceptors in guinea-pig trachea. Eur J Pharmacol 1978;47:333-40.

55. Plummer AL. The development of drug tolerance to beta$_2$ adrenergic agents. Chest 1978;73:949-57.

56. Steen SN, Smith R, Kuo J et al. Comparison of the bronchodilator effects of oral therapy with fenoterol hydrobromide and ephedrine. Chest 1977;72:291-5.

57. Pennock BE, Rogers RM, Ryan BR et al. Aerosol administration of fenoterol hydrobromide (Th 1165A) in subjects with reversible obstructive airway disease. Chest 1977;72:731-6.

58. Scheife RT, Hills JR. Migraine headache: signs and symptoms, biochemistry, and current therapy. Am J Hosp Pharm 1980;37:365-74.

59. Gilman AG, Goodman LS, Gilman A, eds. Goodman and Gilman's the pharmacological basis of therapeutics. 6th ed. New York: Macmillan, 1980.

60. Orton DA, Richardson RJ. Ergotamine absorption and toxicity. Postgrad Med J 1982;58:6-11.

61. Ala-Hurula V, Myllyla VV, Arvela P et al. Systemic availability of ergotamine tartrate after oral, rectal and intramuscular administration. Eur J Clin Pharmacol 1979;15:51-5.

62. Aellig WH, Nuesch E. Comparative pharmacokinetic investigations with tritium-labeled ergot alkaloids after oral and intravenous administration in man. Int J Clin Pharmacol 1977;15:106-12.

63. Schmidt R, Fanchamps A. Effect of caffeine on intestinal absorption of ergotamine in man. Eur J Clin Pharmacol 1974;7:213-6.

64. Wilkinson M. Migraine—treatment of acute attack. Br Med J 1971;2:754-5.

65. Anon. Propranolol for prevention of migraine headaches. Med Lett Drugs Ther 1979;21:77-8.

66. Behan PO, Reid M. Propranolol in the treatment of migraine. Practitioner 1980;224:201-4.

67. Meier J, Schreier E. Human plasma levels of some anti-migraine drugs. Headache 1976;16:96-104.

68. Anon. Drugs for migraine. Med Lett Drugs Ther 1976;18:55-6.

69. Anon. Ritodrine update. FDA Drug Bull 1982;12:4.

20:00 BLOOD FORMATION AND COAGULATION

20:04 ANTIANEMIA DRUGS

20:04.04 IRON PREPARATIONS

General References: 1, 2

Ferrous Salts   Various

Pharmacology. Ferrous salts are soluble forms of iron, an essential nutrient which functions primarily as the oxygen-binding core of heme in red blood cells (as hemoglobin), muscles (as myoglobin) and the respiratory enzyme, cytochrome C.

Administration and Adult Dose. PO 2-3 mg/kg/day of elemental iron in divided doses.[3] Consult Ferrous Salts Comparison Chart for usual dosage ranges for individual salts. Dose-related adverse effects may be decreased by using suboptimal dosages, by increasing the daily dose gradually, or by administering with a small amount of food (although this latter method reduces absorption). After hemoglobin is normalized, oral therapy should continue for approximately 3 months to replenish iron stores.

Dosage Individualization. Iron requirement during pregnancy is approximately twice that of the normal, nonpregnant woman due to an expanding blood volume and the demands of the fetus and placenta. A prophylactic dose of 30–60 mg/day elemental iron during the second and third trimesters has been recommended to prevent depletion of maternal iron stores. Iron deficient patients may need higher doses.[4,5]

Pediatric Dose. PO for prophylaxis 1 mg/kg/day of elemental iron in single or divided doses. **PO for treatment** 6 mg/kg/day of elemental iron in 3 divided doses.

Dosage Forms. See Ferrous Salts Comparison Chart.

Patient Instructions. This drug should be taken with a full glass of water on an empty stomach (1 hr before to 2 hr after meals) for best absorption. If gastric distress or nausea occurs, a small quantity of food may be taken with the drug, but do not take with antacids as absorption will be significantly impaired. Stools will probably become black. Keep out of the reach of children.

Pharmacokinetics and Biopharmaceutics. *Onset and Duration.* Response to equivalent amounts of oral or parenteral therapy is essentially the same. Reticulocytes increase within 3–7 days and reach a peak of 5–15% about the tenth day, and an initially rapid increase in hemoglobin occurs in 2 weeks.[6] Three to six months of therapy are generally required for restoration of iron stores.[1]

Plasma Levels. 50–150 mcg/dl. A decrease in the transferrin saturation (serum iron ÷ total iron binding capacity x 100) is an indication of pre-anemic iron deficiency. A transferrin saturation less than 16% confirms iron deficiency.[1] See Laboratory Indices chapter. In overdosage, toxicity may occur at levels greater than 350 mcg/dl. Chelation therapy is indicated at levels greater than 500 mcg/dl and possibly with levels over 350 mcg/dl if the patient is symptomatic.

Fate. Iron is absorbed primarily from the duodenum at a rate dependent on the amount of iron in storage sites. About 10% of dietary iron is absorbed in normal subjects, 20% in iron deficient patients and as much as 70% of medicinal iron during marked iron deficiency or increased erythropoiesis. In the plasma, iron is oxidized to the ferric state, combined with transferrin, and either utilized or stored as ferritin (mostly in the reticuloendothelial system and hepatocytes). The average loss in the healthy adult male is about 1 mg/day. Gastrointestinal loss of extravasated red cells, iron in bile and exfoliated mucosal cells accounts for two-thirds of this iron. The other third is lost in the skin and urine. Menstruating women have an additional loss of about 0.5 mg/day.

Adverse Reactions. Occasional GI irritation, constipation, diarrhea, and stained teeth (liquid preparations only — dilute and use a drinking straw).

Contraindications. Hemochromatosis, hemosiderosis and hemolytic anemias in which no true iron deficiency exists.

Precautions. Use with caution in patients with peptic ulcer, regional enteritis and ulcerative colitis. Serious acute poisoning (which can be fatal) occurs frequently in children: in a 15 kg child as little as 1 g of ferrous sulfate may cause toxic symptoms.[7] Food and antacids significantly impair the absorption of iron —see Drug Interactions chapter.

Parameters to Monitor. Periodic reticulocyte count, hemoglobin and hematocrit—see Onset and Duration.

Notes. Ferrous salts are used in prevention and treatment of iron deficiency anemias. Such anemias occur most frequently with exceptional blood losses (eg, pathological bleeding, menstruation) and during periods of rapid growth (eg, infancy, adolescence, pregnancy). Iron is ineffective in hemoglobin disturbances not caused by iron deficiency. Concurrent administration of high doses of ascorbic acid may enhance absorption (particularly when given with sustained-release formulations), but cost/benefit does not warrant its use. Wide variation in dissolution and absorption exists among sustained-release and enteric-coated products, and the frequency of adverse effects, while negligible, probably reflects the small amount of ionic iron available for absorption due to transport of the iron past the duodenum and proximal jejunum.[8]

Ferrous Salts Comparison Chart

DRUG	ADULT DOSE (CAP OR TAB/DAY)	SOLID DOSAGE FORMS[a]	ELEMENTAL IRON/CAP OR TAB (PERCENT)	(MG FE)	OTHER DOSAGE FORMS[a]
Ferrous Fumarate	1–2	SR Cap 350 mg	33	115	Drp 45 mg/0.6 ml
		SR Tab 300 mg	33	100	Susp 100 mg/5 ml
	1–4	Tab (Chewable) 100 mg	33	33	
	1–4	Tab 195, 200 mg	33	64,66	
	1–2	Tab (Chewable) 100, 200, 225 mg	33	33,66,74	
	1–2	Tab 325 mg	33	108	
Ferrous Gluconate	3–6	Cap 325 mg	12	38	Elxr 300, 325 mg/5 ml
	1	SR Cap 435 mg	12	50	
	3–6	Tab 320, 325 mg	12	37,38	
Ferrous Sulfate Exsiccated	3	Cap 190 mg	30	57	
	1–2	SR Cap 167 mg	30	50	
	3–4	Tab 200 mg	30	60	

Continued

Ferrous Salts Comparison Chart

DRUG	ADULT DOSE (CAP OR TAB/DAY)	SOLID DOSAGE FORMS[a]	ELEMENTAL IRON/CAP OR TAB (PERCENT)	ELEMENTAL IRON/CAP OR TAB (MG FE)	OTHER DOSAGE FORMS[a]
Ferrous Sulfate					
Hydrous	—	SR Cap/Tab Various	20	—	Drp 75 mg/0.6 ml
	3–6	Tab 195 mg	20	39	Elxr 195 mg/4 ml
	3	Tab 300, 325 mg	20	60,65	Elxr 162.5, 220 mg/5 ml
					Syrup 90 mg/5 ml

a. Doses listed represent total iron salt, not elemental iron.

Iron Dextran Injection   Imferon®, Various

Pharmacology. See Ferrous Salts. The overall response to parenteral iron is not significantly different from orally administered iron, and therefore, iron dextran is indicated *only* when oral iron therapy is determined to be ineffective or impossible.

Administration and Adult Dose. The total cumulative amount required for restoration of hemoglobin and body stores of iron can be approximated from the formula:

0.66 × body weight in kg

$$\times \left(100 - \frac{\text{patient's hemoglobin in g/dl}}{14.8} \times 100 \right)$$

$$= \text{total mg iron to be injected.}$$

To calculate dose in ml, divide the result by 50. The requirements for infants weighing 13.6 kg (30 lb) or less are 80% of the amount calculated from the formula. **Deep IM** (in upper outer quadrant of buttock using Z-track technique) 25 mg (0.5 ml) test dose the first day, then, if no adverse reaction, proceed to administer (until the total calculated amount is reached) a daily dose not to exceed 25 mg (0.5 ml) for infants under 4–5 kg, 50 mg (1 ml) for children under 9 kg, 100 mg (2 ml) for patients under 50 kg, and 100–250 mg (2–5 ml) for others. **Slow IV** test dose of 25 mg (0.5 ml) the first day, then, if no adverse reaction, proceed (until the total calculated amount is reached) by daily increments over 2–3 days, to maximum daily dose of 100 mg. Although FDA approval is for administration by small daily IV injections, this method offers no greater efficacy or patient safety than **total dose IV infusion**, in which the total calculated dose of iron dextran is diluted in 200–250 ml of normal saline (dextrose solutions cause increased local phlebitis) and infused (after a 25 mg test dose is delivered over 5 minutes) over a period of 1–2 hr.[9]

Pediatric Dose. See Administration and Adult Dose.

Dosage Forms. 50 mg elemental iron/ml. **Inj for IM or IV use** (contains no preservative) 2, 5 ml ampule. **Inj for IM use only** (contains 0.5% phenol as preservative) 10 ml vial.

Pharmacokinetics and Biopharmaceutics. *Onset and Duration.* Hematological response is equivalent to oral therapy, although total body stores of iron are replaced when the above dosage regimens are used.

Fate. Following IV administration, the inert complex is gradually cleared from the plasma by the reticuloendothelial cells of the liver, spleen and bone marrow; in doses greater than 500 mg the clearance rate is 10–20 mg/hr. The iron dextran is then dissociated and released as free ferric iron (at a rate controlled by the serum iron level), which combines with transferrin and is incorporated into hemoglobin within the bone marrow.[9,10]

$t_{1/2}$. 6 hr with doses less than 500 mg;[10] 2.3–3 days with greater doses.[11]

Adverse Reactions. Immediate anaphylactoid reactions, which may be life threatening, occur rarely. Delayed systemic reactions resembling serum sickness and starting within 4–48 hr after injection are characterized by lymphadenopathy, myalgia, arthralgia, fever and headache. IM injections are associated with variable degrees of soreness and inflammation at the injection site and with brown skin discoloration at the injection site. Hypotension and peripheral vascular "flushing" are seen with too rapid IV administration.

Contraindications.   Anemias other than iron deficiency anemia; hemochromatosis; hemosiderosis; subcutaneous administration.

Precautions.   Pregnancy. Use with extreme caution in the presence of serious liver impairment. Patients with rheumatoid arthritis may have an acute exacerbation or reactivation of joint pain and swelling following IV administration. History of allergies and/or asthma. Epinephrine should be immediately available.

Parameters to Monitor.   See Ferrous Salts.

20:12 COAGULANTS AND ANTICOAGULANTS

20:12.04 ANTICOAGULANTS

General References: 46-48

Class Instructions.   These drugs are potentially harmful when taken with nonprescription or prescription drugs. Consult the physician or pharmacist when considering the use of other medications, particularly aspirin-containing products.

Heparin Calcium
Heparin Sodium

Calciparine®

Various

Pharmacology.   A heterogeneous group of mucopolysaccharides derived from the mast cells of animal tissues. It binds with antithrombin III, accelerating the rate at which antithrombin III neutralizes *activated forms* of factors XII, XI, IX, X, VII, and II. Its action is immediate and occurs in vitro and in vivo.

Administration and Adult Dose.   Express dose in units only; dose must be individually titrated to desired effect (usually 1.5-2.5 times control clotting test used).[14-16] **IV for thrombophlebitis** (continuous infusion) 70-100 U/kg initially, then 10-15 U/kg/hr; (intermittent) 75-125 U/kg q 4 hr. **IV for pulmonary embolus** (continuous infusion) 70-100 U/kg initially, then 25 U/kg/hr; alternatively, 5000 U initially, then 1000 U/hr; (intermittent) 75-125 U/kg q 4 hr.[12-14] Duration of therapy for thrombophlebitis or pulmonary embolus is 7-10 days, followed by oral anticoagulation (usually initiated during the first few days of heparin therapy).[15] **SC for prophylaxis of deep vein thrombosis** 5000 U 2 hr before surgery, repeated q 8-12 hr until patient is ambulatory.[17,18]

Dosage Individualization.   Patients with pulmonary embolus seem to require larger heparin doses than patients with thrombophlebitis.[13,16] There is no good evidence that renal or liver disease significantly affect dosage considerations.[20]

Pediatric Dose.   Same as adult dose in U/kg.

Dosage Forms.   **Inj** 1000, 5000, 10,000, 20,000, 40,000 U/ml (sodium); **Inj** 5000 U/0.2 ml (calcium).

Patient Instructions.   See Class Instructions.

Pharmacokinetics and Biopharmaceutics. *Onset and Duration.*
Onset immediate after IV administration.

Fate. No biotransformation in plasma or liver, nor any renal excretory mechanism has been identified as primarily responsible for heparin elimination; transfer and storage in reticuloendothelial cells has been suggested.[16,20] V_d is 70 ml/kg (approximates plasma volume).

$t_{1/2}$. (Pharmacologic) 93 min (deep venous thrombosis); 52 min (pulmonary embolus).[19] Half-life appears to be dose-related; higher doses lead to increased half-life and decreased clearance.[13,20]

Adverse Reactions. Hemorrhage; thrombocytopenia (more common with bovine-lung than porcine-intestinal mucosa heparin),[21] osteoporosis with prolonged use of large doses.[16,20]

Contraindications. Active bleeding or bleeding tendencies (eg, hemophilia, purpura, increased capillary permeability); threatened abortion; subacute bacterial endocarditis, suspected intracranial hemorrhage; inaccessible ulcerative lesions (especially of the GI tract); visceral carcinoma; regional or lumbar block anesthesia; severe hypertension; shock; and after eye, brain, or spinal cord surgery.

Precautions. Avoid IM injections due to risk of hematoma formation. See Antiplatelet Drugs Comparison Chart and Drug Interactions chapter.

Parameters to Monitor. APTT or ACT for therapeutic effects; hematocrit, stool guaiac, urinalysis (for hematuria) for toxicity.

Notes. Women over 60 yr may have a higher risk of bleeding complications.[16] Continuous IV infusion may be less hazardous than intermittent IV administration.[22] Questionable efficacy in acute MI; current treatment practices (eg, coronary care units, early ambulation) may themselves have reduced any need for or benefit from anticoagulants.[23,24] Biological source of heparin (porcine mucosa vs beef lung) apparently has no effect on anticoagulant potency.[25]

Warfarin Sodium   Coumadin®, Panwarfin®

Pharmacology. Prevents the conversion of vitamin K back to its active form from the vitamin K epoxide. This impairs formation of the vitamin K-dependent clotting factors VII, IX, X and II (prothrombin).

Administration and Adult Dose. PO or IV maintain at 2–10 mg/day, titrating dose to 1½–2½ times control prothrombin time (PT).

Dosage Individualization. Large variability in response requires that dosage be carefully individualized in all patients. Patients with liver disease, CHF, hyperthyroidism, or fever and the elderly may be particularly sensitive to warfarin. Renal failure does not enhance the hypoprothombinemic response to warfarin; however, these patients may have compromised hemostatic mechanisms which predispose to bleeding.[26]

Dosage Forms. Tab 2, 2.5, 5, 7.5, 10 mg; Inj 50 mg.

Patient Instructions. See Class Instructions.

Pharmacokinetics and Biopharmaceutics. *Onset and Duration.*
Peak PT effect 36–72 hr;[27] at least 5–7 days of warfarin therapy are required before full therapeutic effect is achieved.[28] Duration after discontinuation is dependent on resynthesis of vitamin K-dependent clotting factors II, VII, IX and X (about 4–5 days).

Fate. Completely absorbed orally; greater than 97% bound to plasma proteins.[29,30] Undergoes oxidative biotransformation in the liver, producing warfarin alcohols which have some minor anticoagulant activity.[31,32] The warfarin enantiomers are metabolized by different routes. Less than 1% excreted unchanged in the urine.[29]

$t_{1/2}$. Average 42 hr,[33] unchanged in acute hepatic disease.[34] Enantiomer half-lives: R warfarin 20–70 hr; S warfarin 18–34 hr.[35]

Adverse Reactions. Hemorrhage; rarely necrosis of the skin, purple-toe syndrome.

Contraindications. Pregnancy; hemorrhagic tendencies; blood dyscrasias; surgery or trauma; severe hepatic or renal disease; disturbances of intestinal flora; severe hypertension.

Precautions. Many drug interactions—see Drug Interactions chapter. Avoid IM injections due to risk of hematoma formation. Several other factors may influence response: diet, travel and environment. Monitor patients with liver disease, CHF, hyperthyroidism or fever especially carefully.

Parameters to Monitor. PT daily until stabilized, then weekly to monthly to monitor therapeutic effect; hematocrit, stool guaiac, urinalysis (for hematuria) for toxicity. Also monitor for ecchymosis, hemoptysis and epistaxis.

Notes. Loading dose has no therapeutic advantage and may be unsafe due to excessive depression of factor VII.[36] Phytonadione (vitamin K_1) begins to restore the PT toward normal within 4–8 hr, although large doses may subsequently induce a resistance to anticoagulant effect lasting one or more weeks.[37] S warfarin enantiomer appears to be a more potent anticoagulant than R warfarin.[35]

Antiplatelet Drugs

THE USE OF ANTICOAGULANTS has been found useful in preventing venous thrombosis. They are, however, less effective in preventing arterial thrombosis, possibly because of differences in factors leading to the formation of venous and arterial thrombi. Venous thrombi contain primarily fibrin in combination with some platelet aggregates. Also, the amount of platelets adhering to venous walls is limited. On the other hand, a platelet nidus plays the major role in the formation of arterial thrombi and thrombi which form on prosthetic surfaces. These considerations have led to the investigation of drugs affecting platelet function as a new approach to the prevention of thrombosis.

Despite the large number of clinical trials that have been performed, very few recommendations can presently be made concerning the usefulness of antiplatelet drugs in preventing thrombus formation. Agents offering the most promise are reviewed in the following table. These agents probably act by different mechanisms to inhibit platelet function. The use of combination antiplatelet drug therapy may prove the best approach. The table follows on the next page.

Antiplatelet Drugs Comparison Chart

CLINICAL USE	DRUGS AND DOSES USED				COMMENTS
	ASPIRIN	SULFINPYRAZONE	DIPYRIDAMOLE		
Transient Ischemic Attacks	A 1,300 mg/day	B 600–800 mg/day	C 400–800 mg/day		Aspirin reduced the prevalence of stroke and death in men only. Patients with previous MI or hypertension responded poorly [38]
Acute Myocardial Infarction	B 300–975 mg/day	B 800 mg/day	B 400 mg/day		Aspirin (975 mg/day) with dipyridamole (225 mg/day) showed a greater influence on mortality than aspirin alone or placebo, especially when initiated early after MI. [39] The trial claiming effectiveness of sulfinpyrazone in preventing sudden death has been criticized for inconsistent classification and exclusion of data. [40,41] There is evidence that sulfinpyrazone (400 mg bid) significantly reduces reinfarctions and thromboembolic events. [59] No difference in cardiac deaths was observed
AV Shunts	B 160 mg/day	A 600 mg/day	D		Low dose aspirin (≤ 160 mg/day) may be more effective than higher doses in preventing thrombosis because of its potential to block thromboxane synthesis without affecting vascular prostacyclin (see Aspirin) [42] Continued

Antiplatelet Drugs Comparison Chart

CLINICAL USE	DRUGS AND DOSES USED				COMMENTS
	ASPIRIN	SULFINPYRAZONE	DIPYRIDAMOLE		
Heart Valves	(see Comments)	D 800 mg/day	C 150 mg/day		Studies suggest that dipyridamole (400 mg/day) or aspirin (1,000 mg/day) added to conventional oral anticoagulant therapy is more effective than oral anticoagulants alone. Aspirin (1,000 mg/day) in combination with dipyridamole (100 mg/day) appears to be better than placebo, but not as effective as oral anticoagulants alone [43]
Venous Thrombosis	B 600–1,500 mg/day	B 800 mg/day	C 400 mg/day		
Coronary Artery Bypass Operation	A (see Comments)	D	A (see Comments)		Dipyridamole in combination with aspirin appears to reduce early vein graft occlusion. Dosages were as follows: dipyridamole 100 mg qid for 2 days prior to operation, 100 mg on the day of operation at 6 AM and 1 hr after surgery, then 75 mg plus aspirin 325 mg 7 hr post-op and tid thereafter [60]

Key: A = Proven clinical efficacy; B = Promising, but inconclusive clinical efficacy; C = Little or no clinical efficacy; D = Little or no information on clinical efficacy. Adapted from references 38–45.

20:40 THROMBOLYTIC AGENTS

General References: 49-52

Streptokinase   Kabikinase®, Streptase®

Pharmacology.   A bacterial protein derived from group C β-hemolytic streptococci. Acts indirectly, forming a streptokinase-plasminogen activator complex which activates other plasminogen converting it to the proteolytic enzyme plasmin. Plasmin then hydrolyzes fibrin, factors V, VIII, II, complement and kallikreinogen.

Administration and Adult Dose.   IV loading dose 250,000 IU over 30 min, followed by infusion of 100,000 IU/hr for 12-72 hr. Institute heparin therapy—see Parameters to Monitor. **Selective intra-arterial infusion** (investigational) 5,000 IU/hr for 5-16 hr.[53] **Selective intracoronary artery infusion** 20,000 IU (average) bolus, then 2,000 IU/min for about 1 hr.[54] See Notes.

Dosage Individualization.   The recommended fixed dosage schedule results in sufficient activation of plasminogen in 95% of patients.[49] An increase in dosage is sometimes necessary in patients with high titer antistreptokinase antibodies (eg, recent streptococcal infection or recent treatment with streptokinase).

Pediatric Dose.   Safety and efficacy not established.

Dosage Forms.   Inj 100,000, 250,000, 600,000, 750,000 IU.

Pharmacokinetics and Biopharmaceutics. *Onset and Duration.* Onset of effect on coagulation (fibrinolytic activity) is immediate following IV loading dose. Peak fibrinolytic effect 6-8 hr into the infusion. Duration of fibrinolytic effect 8-24 hr following discontinuation of the infusion.[55]

Fate.   Plasma clearance results, in part, from formation of an antigen-antibody complex which remains soluble and is rapidly removed. It is postulated that the reticuloendothelial system also contributes to clearance.[56]

$t_{1/2}$.   Demonstrates biphasic elimination characteristics; the initial half-life α phase averages 18 min and is related to antigen-antibody formation, β phase averages 83 min and appears to be related to clearance by the reticuloendothelial system.[56]

Adverse Reactions.   Surface bleeding complications occur frequently and are primarily related to invasive procedures (eg, venous cutdowns, arterial punctures and sites of surgical intervention). Severe internal bleeding reported occasionally; however, its prevalence is no greater than with standard anticoagulant therapy. Rarely, cerebral hemorrhage occurs. Occasional allergic reactions include fever, urticaria, itching, flushing and musculoskeletal pain. Anaphylactoid reactions occur rarely with the preparation now in use.[50]

Contraindications.   Active internal bleeding or cerebrovascular accident within the last 2 months. Major relative contraindications include major surgery within the last 10 days, recent serious GI bleeding, recent trauma and severe hypertension. Minor relative contraindications are bacterial endocarditis, severe hepatic or renal disease, pregnancy, diabetic hemorrhagic retinopathy, likelihood of a left heart thrombus and age greater than 75 yr.[50]

Precautions.   Avoid IM injections and drugs that affect clotting and platelet function.

Parameters to Monitor. Monitor thrombin time, activated partial thromboplastin time or prothrombin time to detect activation of the fibrinolytic system, performed 3-4 hr after initiating therapy and q 12 hr throughout treatment.[50,51] No correlation has been made between clotting test results and likelihood of hemorrhage or efficacy,[57] however, prolongation of the thrombin time to 2-5 times normal control value has been recommended.[51] Institute anticoagulant therapy with heparin after completion of the thrombolytic infusion. When the coagulation test being used no longer exceeds twice normal control (usually 3-4 hr after discontinuation of the thrombolytic agent) heparin therapy is initiated without a loading dose.[50]

Notes. Recommended only for treatment of thrombosis involving the popliteal vein or deep veins of the thigh and pelvis, and for patients in whom pulmonary emboli has caused obstruction of blood flow to one or more lung segments or when clinical shock is present.[50] The effectiveness of thrombolytic therapy is markedly diminished in patients with thrombosis of more than 5 days duration.[49] Thrombolytic therapy may help prevent venous valvular damage and the development of venous hypertension.[50,58] Streptokinase costs about $200 for 24 hr of therapy versus about $2,000 for 12 hr of urokinase therapy. Low-dose streptokinase by selective intra-arterial infusion has been used successfully to treat arterial occlusion, while minimizing hemorrhagic complications.[53] Streptokinase by selective intracoronary artery infusion has been used for short periods of time in the management of acute transmural myocardial infarction in patients with coronary artery occlusion.[54]

Urokinase   Abbokinase®

Pharmacology. An enzymatic protein produced by human renal-parenchymal cells. Acts directly to activate plasminogen, converting it to the proteolytic enzyme plasmin. Plasmin then hydrolyzes fibrin, factors V, VIII, II, complement and kallikreinogen.

Administration and Adult Dose. IV loading dose 4,400 IU/kg over 10 min, followed by continuous infusion of 4,400 IU/kg/hr for 12 hr.

Dosage Individualization. No special guidelines established.

Pediatric Dose. Safety and efficacy not established.

Dosage Forms. Inj 250,000 IU.

Pharmacokinetics and Biopharmaceutics. *Onset and Duration.* Onset of fibrinolytic activity immediate following IV loading dose; duration of fibrinolytic effect up to 12 hr after discontinuation.
  Fate. Not known.
  $t_{1/2}$. About 16 min (estimated).

Adverse Reactions. See Streptokinase. Allergic reactions occur much less frequently than with streptokinase.

Contraindications. See Streptokinase.

Precautions. See Streptokinase.

Parameters to Monitor. See Streptokinase.

Notes. Approved only for treatment of massive pulmonary embolus where significant filling defects involving 2 or more lobar pulmonary arteries are present, or for pulmonary emboli accompanied by unstable hemodynamics. See Streptokinase.

References, 20:00 Blood Formation and Coagulation

1. Dallman PR. Iron deficiency: diagnosis and treatment. West J Med 1981;134:496-505.

2. Hamstra RD, Block MH, Schocket AL. Intravenous iron dextran in clinical medicine. JAMA 1980;243:1726-31.

3. Camitta BM, Nathan DG. Anemia in adolescence: 1. disturbances of iron balance. Postgrad Med 1975;57:143-6.

4. Trace elements—Iron. In: Committee on Dietary Allowances. National Research Council. Recommended dietary allowances. 9th ed. Washington, DC: National Academy of Sciences, 1980:137-43.

5. Berkowitz RL, Coustan DR. Mochizuki TK, eds. Handbook for prescribing medications during pregnancy. Boston: Little, Brown, 1981:240-42.

6. Gilman AG, Goodman LS, Gilman A, eds. Goodman and Gilman's the pharmacological basis of therapeutics. 6th ed. New York: Macmillan, 1980.

7. Stein M, et al. Acute iron poisoning in children. West J Med 1976;125:289-97.

8. Middleton EJ, et al. Studies on the absorption of orally administered iron from sustained-release preparations. N Engl J Med 1966;274:136-39.

9. Hanson DB, Hendeles L. Guide to total dose intravenous iron dextran therapy. Am J Hosp Pharm 1974;31:592-5.

10. Kepler JA, ed. American hospital formulary service. Washington, DC: American Society of Hospital Pharmacists, 1959-82.

11. Wood JK, Milner PFA, Pathak UN. The metabolism of iron-dextran given as a total-dose infusion to iron deficient Jamaican subjects. Br J Haematol 1968;14:119-29.

12. Salzman EW, Deykin D, Shapiro RM et al. Management of heparin therapy: controlled prospective trial. N Engl J Med 1975;292:1046-50.

13. Simon TL, Hyers TM, Gaston JP et al. Heparin pharmacokinetics: increased requirements in pulmonary embolism. Br J Haematol 1978;39:111-20.

14. Basu D, Gallus A, Hirsh J et al. A prospective study of the value of monitoring heparin treatment with the activated partial thromboplastin time. N Engl J Med 1972;287:324-7.

15. Genton E. Guidelines for heparin therapy. Ann Intern Med 1974;80:77-82.

16. Coon WW. Some recent developments in the pharmacology of heparin. J Clin Pharmacol 1979;19:337-49.

17. Gallus AS, Hirsh J, Tuttle RJ et al. Small subcutaneous doses of heparin in prevention of venous thrombosis. N Engl J Med 1973;288:545-51.

18. Gallus AS, Hirsh J, O'Brien SE et al. Prevention of venous thrombosis with small, subcutaneous doses of heparin. JAMA 1976;235:1980-2.

19. Hirsh J, van Aken WG, Gallus AS et al. Heparin kinetics in venous thrombosis and pulmonary embolism. Circulation 1976;53:691-5.

20. Estes JW. Clinical pharmacokinetics of heparin. Clin Pharmacokinet 1980;5:204-20.

21. Bell WR, Royall RM. Heparin-associated thrombocytopenia: a comparison of three heparin preparations. N Engl J Med 1980;303:902-7.

22. Glazier RL, Crowell EB. Randomized prospective trial of continuous vs intermittent heparin therapy. JAMA 1976;236:1365-7.

23. Goldman L, Feinstein AR. Anticoagulants and myocardial infarction. Ann Intern Med 1979;90:92-4.

24. Selzer A, Use of anticoagulant agents in acute myocardial infarction: statistics or clinical judgment? Am J Cardiol 1978;41:1315-7.

25. McMahon FG, Jain AK, Ryan JR et al. Anticoagulant potency of mucosal and lung heparin. Clin Pharmacol Ther 1975;17:79-82.

26. O'Reilly RA, Aggeler PM. Determinants of the response to oral anticoagulant drugs in man. Pharmacol Rev 1970;22:35-96.

27. Nagashima R, O'Reilly RA, Levy G. Kinetics of pharmacologic effects in man: the anticoagulant action of warfarin. Clin Pharmacol Ther 1969;10:22-35.

28. Kazmier FJ, Spittell JA, Thompson JJ et al. Effect of oral anticoagulants on factors VII, IX, X, and II. Arch Intern Med 1965;115:667-73.

29. O'Reilly RA, Aggeler PM, Leong LS. Studies on the coumarin anticoagulant drugs: a comparison of the pharmacodynamics of dicumarol and warfarin in man. Thrombosis and Diathesis Haemorrhagica 1964;11:1-22.

30. Bachmann K, Shapiro R. Protein binding of coumarin anticoagulants in disease states. Clin Pharmacokinet 1977;2:110-26.

31. Yacobi A, Udall JA, Levy G. Serum protein binding as a determinant of warfarin body clearance and anticoagulant effect. Clin Pharmacol Ther 1976;19:552-8.

32. Lewis RJ, Trager WF, Robinson A et al. Warfarin metabolites: the anticoagulant activity and pharmacology of warfarin alcohols. J Lab Clin Med 1973;81:925-31.

33. O'Reilly RA, Aggeler PM, Leong LS. Studies on the coumarin anticoagulant drugs: the pharmacodynamics of warfarin in man. J Clin Invest 1963;42:1542-51.

34. Williams RL. Schary WL, Blaschke TF et al. Influence of acute viral hepatitis on disposition and pharmacologic effect of warfarin. Clin Pharmacol Ther 1976;20:90-7.

35. Breckenridge A, Orme M, Wesseling H et al. Pharmacokinetics and pharmacodynamics of the enantiomers of warfarin in man. Clin Pharmacol Ther 1974;15:424-30.

36. O'Reilly RA, Aggeler PM. Studies on coumarin anticoagulant drugs. Initiation of warfarin therapy without a loading dose. Circulation 1968;38:169-77.

37. Deykin D. Warfarin therapy (second of two parts). N Engl J Med 1970;283:801-3.

38. The Canadian Cooperative Study Group. A randomized trial of aspirin and sulfinpyrazone in threatened stroke. N Engl J Med 1978;299:53-9.

39. The Persantine-Aspirin Reinfarction Study Research Group. Persantine and aspirin in coronary heart disease. Circulation 1980;62:449-61.

40. The Anturane Reinfarction Trial Research Group. Sulfinpyrazone in the prevention of cardiac death after myocardial infarction. N Engl J Med 1978;298:289-95.

41. The FDA'S Critique of the Anturane Reinfarction Trial. N Engl J Med 1980;303:1488-92.

42. Harter HR, Burch JW, Majerus PW et al. Prevention of thrombosis in patients on hemodialysis by low-dose aspirin. N Engl J Med 1979;301:577-9.

43. Weiss HJ. Antiplatelet therapy (2 parts). N Engl J Med 1978;298:1344-7;1403-6.

44. Genton E, Gent M, Hirsh J et al. Platelet-inhibiting drugs in the prevention of clinical thrombotic disease (3 parts). N Engl J Med 1975;293:1174-78;1236-40;1296-1300.

45. Hirsh J. Antiplatelet drugs in thromboembolism. Postgrad Med 1979;66:119-27.

46. Thomas DP. Heparin in the prophylaxis and treatment of venous thromboembolism. Semin Hematol 1978;15:1-17.

47. Wessler S, Gitel SN. Heparin: new concepts relevant to clinical use. Blood 1979;53:525-44.

48. Fenech A, Douglas AS. Individualization of oral anticoagulant therapy. Drugs 1979;18:48-57.

49. Marder VJ. The use of thrombolytic agents: choice of patient, drug administration, laboratory monitoring. Ann Intern Med 1979;90:802-8.

50. Sherry S, Bell WR, Duckert H et al. Thrombolytic therapy in thrombosis: a National Institutes of Health consensus development conference. Ann Intern Med 1980;93:141-4.

51. Bell WR, Meek AG. Guidelines for the use of thrombolytic agents. N Engl J Med 1979;301:1266-70.

52. Verstraete M. Biochemical and clinical aspects of thrombolysis. Semin Hematol 1978;15:35-54.

53. Katzen BT, van Breda A. Low dose streptokinase in the treatment of arterial occlusions. AJR 1981;136:1171-8.

54. Mathey DG, Kuck K-H, Tilsner V et al. Nonsurgical coronary artery recanalization in acute transumural myocardial infarction. Circulation 1981;63:489-99.

55. Fletcher AP, Alkjaersig N, Sherry S. The maintenance of a sustained thrombolytic state in man. I. Induction and effects. J Clin Invest 1959;38:1096-110.

56. Fletcher AP, Alkjaersig N, Sherry S. The clearance of heterologous protein from the circulation of normal and immunized man. J Clin Invest 1958;37:1306-15.

57. Marder VJ, Soulen RL, Atichartakarn V et al. Quantitative venographic assessment of deep vein thrombosis in the evaluation of streptokinase and heparin therapy. J Lab Clin Med 1977;89:1018-29.

58. Arnesen H, Hoiseth A, Ly B. Streptokinase or heparin in the treatment of deep vein thrombosis. Acta Med Scand 1982;211:65-8.

59. Anturan Reinfarction Italian Study. Sulphinpyrazone in post-myocardial infarction. Lancet 1982;1:237-42.

60. Chesebro JH, Clements IP, Fuster V et al. A platelet-inhibitor-drug trial in coronary-artery bypass operations. N Engl J Med 1982;307:73-8.

24:00 CARDIOVASCULAR DRUGS

24:04 CARDIAC DRUGS

General References: 1-4

Amiodarone (Investigational - Labaz)   Cordarone®

Amiodarone is a class III antiarrhythmic agent which prolongs effective refractory period markedly without altering conduction velocity or automaticity. It has a broad spectrum of activity against re-entrant tachycardias such as those associated with Wolf-Parkinson-White syndrome and recurrent ventricular tachycardia. Amiodarone is also a peripheral vasodilator and slows resting heart rate without a decrease in contractility. The drug is variably absorbed (about 50%) and widely distributed. Although the elimination half-life has yet to be determined, it is estimated to be 30 days or greater. Side effects include a slate-grey skin discoloration and yellow-brown corneal microdeposits. The significance of the corneal deposits is unknown; however, it seemingly does not impair vision. Amiodarone may cause a "low T_3 syndrome" due to inhibition of peripheral conversion of T_4 to T_3. Pulmonary fibrosis and neurotoxicity attributed to this agent have also been reported. IV dose is 5–10 mg/kg slowly. PO maintenance doses range from 200–800 mg/day.[5,6]

Amrinone (Investigational - Winthrop)   Inocor®

Amrinone is an inotropic agent that acts to increase contractility by a mechanism different from digitalis glycosides or adrenergic agents. The exact mode of action has not been determined. Heart rate and blood pressure remain unchanged, although vascular resistance drops, due to direct relaxant effects or indirect sympathetic withdrawal. The drug is apparently well absorbed orally with a duration of action of 4-7 hr. Adverse reactions include thrombocytopenia, nephrogenic diabetes insipidus and fever. No arrhythmogenic action has been demonstrated. Amrinone has been administered at doses of 2-4 mg/kg orally bid-tid.[7,8]

Aprindine (Investigational - Lilly)   Fibocil®

Aprindine is a potent class I antiarrhythmic effective in a wide variety of supraventricular and ventricular tachyarrhythmias. This agent generally causes minimal adverse hemodynamic effects, although the significance of its negative inotropic actions remains uncertain. Aprindine is absorbed orally and a significant amount of drug is found in the urine unchanged. At least one metabolite, N-desethylaprindine, possesses antiarrhythmic activity. Distribution half-life is about 1.7 hr and elimination half-life averaged 30 hr in one study. Elimination is quite variable, however, with myocardial infarction patients clearing the drug considerably slower ($t_{1/2}$ 60 hr). Neurologic toxicity is most bothersome and includes tremor, dizziness, ataxia, psychosis and hallucinations. Other serious reactions include agranulocytosis and cholestatic jaundice. A PO or IV loading dose of 200-300 mg may be given with a maintenance dose of 100-150 mg/day in 2 divided doses. Desired therapeutic levels are 1-3 mcg/ml. Toxicity is more prevalent at plasma levels greater than 2 mcg/ml.[5,9]

Bretylium Tosylate   Bretylol®

Pharmacology. An antiarrhythmic with actions thought to be due to an initial catecholamine release and subsequent catecholamine depletion and/or direct effect independent of the adrenergic nervous system.[10] It causes an initial increase in blood pressure, heart rate and myocardial contractility (catecholamine release) followed by hypotension (neuronal blockade).[11] Its greatest usefulness is in severe ventricular tachyarrhythmias resistant to other antiarrhythmics.

Administration and Adult Dose. IM or IV 5 mg/kg, over 5-10 min with additional doses of 10 mg/kg repeated as necessary, to maximum of 40 mg/kg total if no response. Maintenance can be given as IM or IV 5-10 mg/kg q 6 hr or an IV infusion of 1-2 mg/min.

Dosage Individualization. In renal impairment, lower doses may be required.[12]

Dosage Forms. Inj 50 mg/ml.

Pharmacokinetics and Biopharmaceutics. *Onset and Duration.* IV onset may be delayed by 20-60 min of administration; duration is usually 6-12 hr after a single dose.[13] Due to persistent myocardial levels, duration after multiple doses may be much longer.[14]

Fate. A quaternary ammonium compound absorbed only 15-20% after oral administration.[13] After IV dosing, bretylium is primarily cleared renally, with about 70-85% excreted in the urine unchanged.[15,16] One study estimated V_d to be 8.2 L/kg;[16] not bound to plasma proteins.[17]

$t_{1/2}$. α phase about 25 min; β phase 5.5-7.8 hr.[15-17] In a patient with severe renal dysfunction, $t_{1/2}$ reported to be 31.4 hr.[12]

Adverse Reactions. Hypotension (usually orthostatic) via adrenergic blockade is most common. The drop in mean arterial pressure is usually not more than 20 mm Hg; however, sometimes it can be severe, necessitating drug discontinuation.[18] Nausea and vomiting may occur after fast IV administration.[18]

Contraindications. Suspected digitalis-induced ventricular tachycardia (may increase the rate of ventricular tachycardia or the likelihood of ventricular fibrillation).[19]

Precautions. Bretylium should be used with caution if hypotension exists prior to its administration.[11] Keep patients supine until tolerance to hypotension develops. Prolonged effects may occur and dosage reduction in patients with impaired renal function may be required.

Parameters to Monitor. Close monitoring of blood pressure and constant ECG monitoring is required.

Digitoxin
Crystodigin®, Various

Pharmacology. See Digoxin.

Administration and Adult Dose. PO or IV loading dose 0.8–1.4 mg in divided doses over 12–24 hr at intervals of 6–8 hr;[20] alternatively, 10–15 mcg/kg loading dose. **Daily maintenance dose** 10% of total digitalizing dose.

Dosage Individualization. Unlike digoxin, no significant maintenance dosage changes are needed in patients with impaired renal function.[21]

Pediatric Dose. PO or IV digitalizing dose 25–35 mcg/kg in divided doses over 12–24 hr at intervals of 6–8 hr. **Daily maintenance dose** 10–20% of total digitalizing dose.[22]

Dosage Forms. Elxr 50 mcg/ml; Soln 20 mcg/drop; Tab 0.05, 0.1, 0.15, 0.2 mg; Inj 0.2, 0.25 mg/ml.

Patient Instructions. See Digoxin.

Pharmacokinetics and Biopharmaceutics. *Onset and Duration.* IV onset 25–120 min; IV peak 4–12 hr;[23] somewhat slower with PO dosing.
   Plasma Levels. Therapeutic 15–30 ng/ml; toxic, greater than 35 ng/ml. Considerable overlap exists between toxic and therapeutic ranges.
   Fate. Definitive data unavailable, but probably well absorbed with approximately 70% absorbed from the small bowel and 15% from the stomach.[24,25] Eliminated primarily by hepatic metabolism; 30–50% of the drug is excreted in urine and feces as unchanged drug.[24] About 8% of daily losses of digitoxin are due to metabolic conversion to digoxin; however, even in severe renal dysfunction, accumulation of digoxin is not significant.[20] About 14% of the absorbed drug is enterohepatically recycled.[25] Because greater than 90% is plasma protein bound, V_d is less than that of digoxin, being approximately 0.6 L/kg.[25]
   $t_{1/2}$. α phase 1–2 hr; β phase 2.4–16.4 days (average 7.6)[25]

Adverse Reactions. See Digoxin.

Precautions. See Digoxin.

Parameters to Monitor. See Digoxin.

Digoxin
Lanoxin®, Various

Pharmacology. Digitalis glycosides exert positive inotropic effects through improvement of availability of calcium to myocardial contractile elements, thereby increasing cardiac output in heart failure. Antiarrhythmic actions of digitalis glycosides are primarily due to an increase in AV nodal refractory period via increased vagal tone, sympathetic withdrawal and direct mechanisms.[26] Additionally, digitalis exerts a moderate direct vasoconstrictor action on arterial and venous smooth muscle.[27]

Administration and Adult Dose. IV loading dose 10 mcg/kg for patients in sinus rhythm; 13-15 mcg/kg for negative chronotropic action (ie, atrial fibrillation) in divided doses over 12-24 hr at intervals of 6-8 hr.[28] PO dose should be adjusted for percent oral absorption (see Fate). Usually, 0.5 mg is given initially, then 0.25 mg q 6 hr until desired effect or total digitalizing dose is achieved. **Maintenance dose** = (total body stores) × (% lost/day), where total body stores is the original calculated loading dose and % lost/day is 14 + (Cl_{cr} ÷ 5). Usual maintenance doses range from 0.125 to 0.5 mg/day.[28] A dosing nomogram has also been described.[29] **IM not recommended.**[30]

Dosage Individualization. Decrease loading and maintenance dose in renal impairment. Base dose on ideal body weight in obese individuals.

Pediatric Dose. PO total digitalizing dose (TDD) (premature newborn) 20-30 mcg/kg; (full-term newborn) 25-35 mcg/kg; (1-24 months) 35-60 mcg/kg; (2-5 yr) 30-40 mcg/kg; (5-10 yr) 20-35 mcg/kg; (over 10 yr) 10-15 mcg/kg. IV total digitalizing dose 80% of oral TDD. In all ages, give 1/2 TDD first, then 1/4 TDD every 6-8 hr for 2 doses. PO, IV maintenance dose (premature newborn) 20-30% of oral TDD; (all other ages) 25-35% of oral TDD. Maintenance doses are given in 2 divided doses in children under 10 yr. All doses are based on ideal body weight.

Dosage Forms. Elxr 50 mcg/ml; Tab 0.125, 0.25, 0.375, 0.5 mg; Inj 0.25 mg/ml; Caps 0.05, 0.1, 0.2 mg — see Notes.

Patient Instructions. Report feelings of fatigue, anorexia, nausea, abdominal discomfort or visual disturbances such as hazy vision, photophobia, spots or halos and red-green blindness.[31]

Pharmacokinetics and Biopharmaceutics. *Onset and Duration.* IV onset 14-30 min; peak 1.5-5 hr;[23] somewhat slower with PO dosing.
   Plasma Levels. Therapeutic 0.5-2 ng/ml; toxic, greater than 3 ng/ml. Considerable overlap exists between therapeutic and toxic ranges.[32] Signs or symptoms of digitalis toxicity may be evident below 3 ng/ml, especially if other risk factors are present.[32]
   Fate. Oral absorption is 60-75% from tablets; 85% from elixir.[33] Differences in tablet dissolution rates and altered bioavailability for various brands has been reported.[34] Excreted 60-80% unchanged in the urine in normal patients.[33] Active metabolites include digitoxigenin, bis-digitoxoside, digoxigenin monodigitoxoside and dihydrodigoxin.[33] Enterohepatic recycling of digoxin may be as high as 30%.[35] V_d is 7-8 L/kg; protein binding to albumin is 20-30%.[33]
   $t_{1/2}$. α phase 0.5-1 hr; β phase 1.6 days;[33] β phase 3.5-4.5 days in anephric patients.[28]

Adverse Reactions. Arrhythmias, listed in decreasing prevalence, are premature ventricular beats, second and third degree heart block, AV junctional tachycardia, atrial tachycardia with block, ventricular tachycardia and SA nodal block.[36,37] GI symptoms include abdominal discomfort, anorexia, nausea and vomiting. CNS side effects occur frequently, yet are nonspecific, such as weakness, lethargy, disorientation, agitation and nervousness. Visual disturbances are common, and include blurred vision, yellow or green tinting, flickering lights or halos or red-green color blindness. Hallucinations and psychosis have been reported. Rare reactions include gynecomastia, hypersensitivity and thrombocytopenia.[31]

Contraindications. Hypertrophic obstructive cardiomyopathy, except for supraventricular arrhythmias;[38] suspected digitalis intoxication; second or third degree heart block in the absence of mechanical pacing.

Precautions. Electrolyte abnormalities predisposing to digitalis toxicity include hypokalemia, hypomagnesemia and hypercalcemia. Hypothyroidism may reduce digoxin requirements due to lower V_d and clearance.[33] Cardioversion in patients receiving digitalis glycosides may result in refractory ventricular tachycardia or fibrillation.[39] If electrical cardioversion is necessary, initial treatment should be at low energy levels or with prophylactic antiarrhythmics (phenytoin or lidocaine) given prior to the shock.[39] Use with caution in patients with pulmonary disease, because hypoxia may sensitize the myocardium to arrhythmias and increase the risk of toxicity.[40] Serious bradyarrhythmias may occur with sick sinus syndrome, but controversy exists concerning the significance of its effects on the SA node.[41] Digitalis glycosides may increase infarct size in the nonfailing heart.[42] Quinidine may cause an increase in both digitoxin[43] and digoxin[44] levels — see Drug Interactions chapter.

Parameters to Monitor. Digitalis plasma levels need only be obtained when compliance, effectiveness or systemic availability is questioned or toxicity is suspected.[45,46] Heart rate, ECG for digitalis-induced arrhythmias, subjective complaints of toxicity, renal function (BUN, creatinine), serum electrolytes (especially potassium) frequently initially, then monthly to bimonthly when stabilized.

Notes. Obtain blood samples for digoxin levels at least 6-8 hr after a dose to allow central and tissue compartment equilibration. Lanoxicaps® are more bioavailable than Lanoxin®; 0.1 mg capsule is equivalent to 0.125 mg tablet.

Diltiazem   Cardizem®

Diltiazem is a calcium antagonist that is useful in the treatment of coronary artery spasm. More work must be done to establish its role in angina pectoris, hypertension and supraventricular arrhythmias. Diltiazem is well absorbed after oral administration and extensively metabolized in the liver; β half-life is 4.1-5.6 hr. Diltiazem is 80% protein bound. Side effects include AV nodal block, hypotension, headache and GI upset. The safety of concurrent administration of beta-blockers with diltiazem needs to be determined. Dosage is 30 mg qid initially, increasing at 1-2 day intervals, to maximum of 240 mg/day in 3 or 4 doses.[47,48] Available as tab 30, 60 mg.

Disopyramide   Norpace®

Pharmacology. Qualitatively has the same electrophysiological actions as procainamide and quinidine.[49] It causes an increase in systemic vascular resistance through a vasoconstrictor action;[50] additionally, may exert a profound negative inotropic effect[51] and has significant anticholinergic properties systemically and on the heart.

Administration and Adult Dose. PO loading dose 300-400 mg. Maintenance dose 100-400 mg q 6 hr. Large maintenance doses such as 300-400 mg q 6 hr should be reserved for patients with resistant arrhythmias such as recurrent ventricular tachycardia.

Dosage Individualization. In patients less than 50 kg, or with heart failure, hepatic disease or moderate renal insufficiency (creatinine clearance greater than 40 ml/min), load with 200 mg, then give 100 mg q 6 hr. In patients with severe renal insufficiency, give normal loading dose, then usual maintenance doses at prolonged intervals as follows:

CREATININE CLEARANCE	MAINTENANCE INTERVAL
15–40 ml/min	10 hr
5–15 ml/min	20 hr
1–5 ml/min	30 hr

Dosage Forms. Cap 100, 150 mg.

Patient Instructions. Report any symptoms such as difficulty in urinating, constipation, blurred vision or dry mouth to the physician or pharmacist. Shortness of breath, weight gain or edema should also be reported.

Pharmacokinetics and Biopharmaceutics. *Onset and Duration.* PO onset within 1 hr. Duration varies with individual differences in drug disposition, but is usually 6–12 hr.

Plasma Levels. Usual range is 2–4 mcg/ml[52] with toxicity more likely over 4 mcg/ml. However, levels of 7 mcg/ml or greater may be required occasionally in some resistant ventricular dysrhythmias.[53]

Fate. Oral absorption is rapid; systemic availability is 50–80%.[54] About 50% excreted unchanged in the urine.[55] The major metabolite is an N-monodealkylated form that possesses weak antiarrhythmic activity and appears in the urine.[56,57] V_d is about 0.8 L/kg in normal subjects.[55] The percent of unbound drug in plasma varies from 19–46% over a plasma concentration range of 2–8 mcg/ml.[57,58]

$t_{1/2}$. α phase 2–4 min (IV);[57] β phase is concentration dependent. The variability in protein binding may be responsible for dose-dependent kinetics.[58] $t_{1/2}$ β ranges from 4.4–8.2 hr in normals;[55] prolonged with renal dysfunction, averaging 12.7 hr in one study[59] and 18.6 hr (mean) reported in 8 patients with ventricular dysrhythmias.[60]

Adverse Reactions. The most significant adverse reactions include dry mouth, urinary retention, blurred vision and constipation, and often require dosage reduction or drug discontinuation. Occasionally causes hypotension, probably by its negative inotropic action.[56] Ability to exacerbate CHF is most prevalent in patients with left ventricular dysfunction.[51] Through its vagolytic action, it may cause sinus tachycardia. Severe bradycardia, AV nodal block, or asystole may occur, especially in patients with SA or AV nodal disease.[61] A syndrome with ventricular tachycardia or fibrillation, similar to quinidine syncope, has been reported.[62] May occasionally cause nausea, vomiting or rash; rarely, hepatic cholestasis, psychosis, peripheral neuropathy or hypoglycemia occur.[54]

Contraindications. History of disopyramide-induced heart block or serious ventricular arrhythmias; second or third degree heart block or bifasicular bundle branch block; long QT syndrome; severe CHF or cardiogenic shock.

Precautions. In atrial fibrillation or flutter, digitalis or propranolol should be given prior to disopyramide to block the AV node. QRS or QT prolongation greater than 35% of baseline measurement is an indication for disopyramide discontinuation. Use very cautiously in patients with CHF, because of negative inotropic and vasoconstrictive actions.[50,51] If possible, other antiarrhythmics should be used in patients with prostatic hypertrophy or pre-existing urinary retention. Disopyramide may exacerbate glaucoma or myasthenia gravis.

Parameters to Monitor. Because of concentration-dependent protein binding, total drug levels unreliably reflect active drug concentration. Plasma levels and symptoms or signs of toxicity should be closely monitored in patients with altered states of drug disposition such as renal dysfunction. Daily ECG should be observed for QT, QRS or PR prolongation. Obtain frequent vital signs initially for evidence of adverse hemodynamic effects (ie, CHF), and less frequently when a maintenance dose is attained. Question the patient about anticholinergic manifestations, such as urinary and visual abnormalities.

Lidocaine   Xylocaine®, Various

Pharmacology. Electrophysiological actions differ in healthy and diseased cardiac tissues—see Electrophysiologic Actions of Antiarrhythmics Comparison Chart.[63,64] Most antiarrhythmic activity may be due to blockade of the fast sodium channel in Purkinje fibers.[64] Used in the acute treatment of ventricular arrhythmias associated with myocardial infarction or digitalis intoxication. Effectiveness in the treatment of atrial arrhythmias (except PSVT associated with extranodal AV pathways) is limited.

Administration and Adult Dose. IV loading dose for ventricular tachycardia or fibrillation 100 mg (1-1.5 mg/kg) over 1 min; if ineffective, may repeat with 50-100 mg q 5-10 min, to maximum of 300 mg.[65] IV maintenance 2-4 mg/min infusion.[65] IV for post-MI prophylaxis of primary ventricular fibrillation 100 mg followed by infusion of 3 mg/min.[66] IM for prehospital, post-MI, arrhythmia prophylaxis 200-300 mg. PO not recommended.

Dosage Individualization. In CHF, use one-half of IV loading doses.[65] In liver disease or CHF, initial maintenance infusion is 1 mg/min with maximum of 2-3 mg/min.[65] In myocardial infarction without CHF, maintenance infusion rate may have to be decreased by 30-50% in 24 hr.[65]

Pediatric Dose. IV loading dose 0.5-1.5 mg/kg, may repeat q 10 min, to maximum of 200-300 mg. IV maintenance 20-50 mcg/kg/min infusion.[22]

Dosage Forms. Inj 10, 20, 40, 100 mg/ml.

Patient Instructions. Report minor toxicities such as drowsiness, perioral numbness or tingling, dizziness or nausea, during maintenance infusion.

Pharmacokinetics and Biopharmaceutics. *Onset and Duration.* IV onset immediate; duration after initial IV bolus is 10-20 min.[67] IM onset 10 min; duration 3 hr.[67]

Plasma Levels. Therapeutic 1.5-6.4 mcg/ml.[66] Toxic reactions are more likely at concentrations over 5 mcg/ml.[65] See Adverse Reactions.

Fate. Lidocaine is absorbed orally; however, a large hepatic first-pass effect limits systemic availability to about 35%.[68] Primarily metabolized in the liver with less than 10% excreted unchanged in the urine.[69] Major metabolites, monoethylglycinexylidide (MEGX) and glycinexylidide (GX) both possess neurotoxic[70] and antiarrhythmic[71] actions. Accumulation of these metabolites in renal impairment or prolonged infusions may contribute to lidocaine toxicity. About 70% bound to plasma proteins;[65] V_d is about 1.3 L/kg in normals, 0.9 L/kg in CHF.[69] Clearance is decreased in both CHF and liver disease.[65,69]

$t_{1/2}$. α phase about 8 min;[67,69] β phase 80-108 min.[65,69] IM absorption $t_{1/2}$ 12-28 min.[65] β phase in CHF or liver disease may be prolonged (about 5.5 hr and 6.6 hr respectively).[65,69] Elimination half-life increases to an average of 3.2 hr 24 hr after MI without CHF.[72]

Adverse Reactions. Dose-related neurologic side effects include dizziness, nausea, drowsiness, speech disturbances, perioral numbness, muscle twitching, confusion, vertigo or tinnitus and usually occur at plasma levels greater than 5 mcg/ml;[65,73] serious toxicities occurring at plasma levels greater than 9 mcg/ml include psychosis, seizures and respiratory depression.[65,73] Sinus arrest or severe bradycardia is associated with sinus node disease, toxic drug levels or concomitant therapy with other antiarrhythmics.[73] Complete AV block may occur, especially in patients with pre-existing bifasicular bundle branch block, AV nodal block or inferior wall MI.[73,74]

Contraindications. History of hypersensitivity to amide-type local anesthetic (rare); second or third degree heart block unless the site of block can be localized to the AV node itself[73] or ventricular pacemaker is functional; severe sinus node dysfunction.

Precautions. Propranolol may decrease lidocaine clearance so that close monitoring is necessary with concomitant administration of these two agents.

Parameters to Monitor. Plasma levels and signs or symptoms of toxicity should be closely monitored in patients with altered drug disposition such as heart failure, hepatic disease, acute MI or prolonged IV infusion (greater than 24 hr). Minor subjective and objective toxicities are extremely important because they are often subtle and may forecast more serious toxicities (ie, seizures). Continuously observe ECG for therapeutic and/or toxic actions. Monitor vital signs such as blood pressure, heart rate and respirations frequently.

Notes. Ethmozin is an investigational antiarrhythmic agent with electrophysiologic actions similar to lidocaine.[75]

Mexiletine   Mexitil®
(Investigational - Boehringer-Ingelheim)

Mexiletine is a local anesthetic class I antiarrhythmic resembling lidocaine in electrophysiological actions and structure. This agent has little or no effect on blood pressure or heart rate, but may depress cardiac output in patients with pre-existing left ventricular dysfunction. Mexiletine has been used primarily for serious ventricular dysrhythmias. Unlike lidocaine, this agent can be used orally. Most of the drug is metabolized, with about 8% excreted unchanged in the urine. Elimination half-life is about 10-12 hr. V_d is large, often 500 L or greater. The most bothersome adverse reactions are neurological and include tremor, dizziness, blurred vision, nystagmus, confusion and seizures. Cardiac toxicities are hypotension, sinus bradycardia, AV dissociation, widening of QRS complexes and exacerbation of sinus node disease. Additionally, nausea and vomiting may occur. An IV loading dose may be given as 1-1.25 g over 8 hr with a maintenance infusion of 0.5-1 g over 24 hr. Oral doses range from 0.6-1 g/day in 3-4 divided doses. With these doses, the desired therapeutic range is 0.75-2 mcg/ml with toxicity occurring frequently with plasma concentrations greater than 2 mcg/ml.[5]

Nifedipine   Procardia®

Nifedipine is a calcium antagonist (class IV antiarrhythmic) used for its vasodilating properties. It has not proved as useful for supraventricular tachycardias. It is used to treat coronary artery spasm, and preliminary studies have shown success in heart failure, hypertension and angina pectoris. The drug is well absorbed and extensively metabolized to inactive compounds. Nifedipine has a duration of action of 6–12 hr and an elimination half-life of about 4 hr. It is 90% protein bound. Most side effects, such as headache, hypotension, flushing and dizziness result from its vasodilatory action. Exacerbation of heart failure, precipitation of anginal pain and constipation have been reported. Although theoretically possible, combination therapy with beta blockers does not seem to result in severe hemodynamic decompensation as does verapamil. Oral doses range from a starting dose of 10 mg tid, to maximum of 120 mg/day in 3–4 divided doses. Nifedipine has also been given by intravenous and sublingual routes. [47,76,77]

Procainamide   Procan®, Procan-SR®, Pronestyl®

Pharmacology. Class I antiarrhythmic that alters normal and ischemic Purkinje action potential in a similar fashion to quinidine.[78] It may decrease systemic blood pressure by causing peripheral ganglionic blockade;[78] it also possesses weak anticholinergic action.

Administration and Adult Dose. PO loading dose 1 g over 2 hr in 2 divided doses. **PO maintenance dose** 1–9 g/day in 4–6 divided doses.[79] **SR** may be given q 8 hr. **IV loading dose** 1–2.5 g at a rate no greater than 20 mg/min.[80,81] **IV maintenance dose** 1.5–5 mg/min (20–80 mcg/kg/min) infusion.[81] **Intermittent IV or IM** 1–9 g/day in 4–6 divided doses.

Dosage Individualization. Decrease loading dose in patients with CHF. Maintenance dose should be reduced in liver disease, the aged and possibly CHF or MI. In renal insufficiency, procainamide and its active metabolite accumulate, necessitating lower maintenance doses.[82]

Pediatric Dose. PO 50 mg/kg/day in 4–6 divided doses. **IV loading dose** 100 mg over 5 min, to maximum of 1 g.[22]

Dosage Forms. Cap, Tab 250, 375, 500 mg; **SR Tab** 250, 500, 750 mg; **Inj** 100, 500 mg/ml.

Patient Instructions. Report any symptoms such as nausea, vomiting, fever, sore throat, arthralgia, rash, chest or abdominal pain or shortness of breath.

Pharmacokinetics and Biopharmaceutics. *Onset and Duration.* PO onset within 1 hr; SR preparation is somewhat slower. IM onset within 1 hr; IV immediate. Duration is usually 3–6 hr.

Plasma Levels. Therapeutic range is 4–10 mcg/ml;[80] toxicity more likely at plasma levels greater than 12 mcg/ml.[83] In some arrhythmias (eg, recurrent ventricular tachycardia), levels of 20 mcg/ml or greater may be required for prevention of arrhythmias.[79] Effective plasma levels of NAPA are 15–25 mcg/ml, with the toxic range overlapping with the therapeutic range.[84]

Fate. Oral absorption is 75–95%;[85] about 50% excreted in the urine as unchanged drug.[86] The remainder is metabolized, mostly to active N-acetylprocainamide (NAPA) by the liver, with smaller amounts excreted as p-aminobenzoic acid.[86] The total quantity of NAPA produced is dependent on liver function and acetylator phenotype.[86] V_d is about 2 L/kg in normals[85] and 1.5 L/kg in CHF;[86] approximately 15% bound to plasma proteins.[85] Total body clearance may be lower in MI.[87]

$t_{1/2}$. α phase about 6 min;[88] β phase in normals 2.5–4.7 hr (average 3.5).[88] $t_{1/2}$ in renal dysfunction 5.3–20.7 hr with anephric patients averaging 10.1

hr.[89] NAPA $t_{1/2}$ 4.3–15.1 hr (average 7).[84] In renal failure, NAPA $t_{1/2}$ may be as long as several days.[82,84]

Adverse Reactions. Hypotension may occur, especially after rapid IV administration. Severe bradycardia, AV nodal block or asystole and ventricular tachyarrhythmias have been reported, but much less so than the syndrome of quinidine syncope.[90,91] GI symptoms occur frequently and include nausea and vomiting; drug fever and dermatological reactions may also occur.[91] Agranulocytosis is rare, but potentially fatal.[92] About 50–80% of patients develop a positive antinuclear antibody (ANA) with 30% developing SLE symptoms; genetically slow acetylators more rapidly develop positive ANA and SLE symptoms.[93] Common symptoms or signs are rash, arthralgias, fever, pericarditis and pleuritis. Although drug cessation usually reverses these symptoms in about 2 weeks, some patients have prolonged manifestations and for others the SLE syndrome may be initially life-threatening.[93] It is possible that NAPA does not carry the risk of SLE.

Contraindications. History of procainamide-induced SLE; second or third degree heart block or bifasicular bundle branch block; long QT syndrome or severe sinus node dysfunction.

Precautions. In atrial fibrillation or flutter, procainamide may paradoxically increase ventricular rate; digitalis or propranolol should be given before procainamide in these situations to block the AV node. QRS or QT prolongation greater than 35% of a baseline measurement should be an indication to withhold further procainamide. Procainamide may exacerbate myasthenia gravis.

Parameters to Monitor. Plasma levels and symptoms or signs of toxicity should be monitored in patients with suspected altered drug disposition such as heart failure, hepatic disease or renal dysfunction. Continuous (with IV) or daily (with PO) ECG should be monitored for QRS, QT or PR prolongation. Blood pressure should be monitored frequently when therapy is initiated (especially with IV), and less frequently when a maintenance dose is determined. Periodically monitor WBC counts and signs of infection for the development of drug-induced agranulocytosis. Observe closely for symptoms of drug-induced SLE.

Notes. Procan-SR® is a wax matrix formulation; the matrix may appear in the stool, but this does not imply a lack of bioavailability.

Propranolol   Inderal®

Pharmacology. A nonselective β-adrenergic blocker used in arrhythmias, hypertension and angina pectoris. Antiarrhythmic mechanism is due to decreased AV nodal conduction in supraventricular tachycardias and blockade of catecholamine-induced dysrhythmias.[94] Antihypertensive mechanism is unknown, but contributing factors are a CNS mechanism, renin blockade and a decrease in myocardial contractility and cardiac output.[95] Propranolol also lowers myocardial oxygen demand by decreasing contractility and heart rate, which symptomatically alleviates anginal pain and increases exercise tolerance in coronary artery disease.[96] See Beta-Adrenergic Blocking Agents Comparison Chart.

Administration and Adult Dose. PO 10–20 mg q 6 hr initially, increasing gradually to desired effects. In hypertension, over 1 g/day has been used; however, consider adding another agent if 480 mg/day is ineffective.[97] In angina pectoris, dose is titrated to pain relief and exercise evidence of β-blockade (bradycardia). The endpoint for dosing in acute arrhythmias is return to sinus rhythm or ventricular rate less than 100 beats/min and hemodynamic stability (in atrial fibrillation or flutter). Twice daily dosing has been shown effective in angina pectoris[99] and hypertension.[97] **PO for post-MI prophylaxis** 180-240 mg/day in 2-3 divided doses. **IV** 1 mg q 5 min to maximum of 0.15 mg/kg; some authors recommend that the first dose be given over 2-10 min.[98,229]

Dosage Individualization. Therapeutic endpoints may be achieved with lower doses in hypothyroidism or liver disease; patients with thyrotoxicosis require higher doses to achieve desired effect.[100]

Pediatric Dose. PO 0.5-1 mg/kg/day in 3-4 divided doses, to maximum of 60 mg/day. **IV** 0.1-0.15 mg/kg, to maximum 10 mg, at a rate of 1 mg q 5 min.[22]

Dosage Forms. Tab 10, 20, 40, 60, 80, 90 mg; **Inj** 1 mg/ml; **SR Caps** 80, 120, 160 mg.

Patient Instructions. Report any symptoms such as shortness of breath, edema, wheezing, fatigue, depression, nightmares or inability to concentrate.

Pharmacokinetics and Biopharmaceutics. *Onset and Duration.*
PO onset variable; duration varies from 6 to at least 12 hr.[97,99,100]

Plasma Levels. No definite relationship between plasma concentrations and therapeutic effect in the treatment of arrhythmias, angina pectoris or hypertension. β-blockade is associated with plasma concentrations greater than 100 ng/ml.[101]

Fate. Rapidly and completely absorbed after oral administration; however, a large hepatic first-pass effect occurs, limiting systemic availability.[100,101] First-pass elimination is saturable with an oral dose greater than about 30 mg.[101] Only 1-4% of a dose is excreted in the urine as unchanged drug.[100] An active metabolite, 4-hydroxypropranolol is formed after oral, but not IV administration.[100] V_d is approximately 200-250 L;[101] about 90% bound to albumin and other plasma proteins.[100] Unlike most other drugs, displacement from plasma proteins increases elimination half-life and V_d due to high tissue affinity (termed nonrestrictive elimination).[102]

$t_{1/2}$. α phase about 10 min;[103] β phase after a single PO dose is approximately 3 hr. With chronic oral therapy, β phase is 4-6 hr; however, it may be as long as 10-20 hr in patients with liver disease.[103]

Adverse Reactions. Adverse effects are usually not dose-related.[104] May cause occasional life-threatening reactions with initial (especially IV) dosing; acute heart failure with pulmonary edema and hypotension, or symptomatic bradycardia and heart block may occur.[104] Acute drug cessation in patients with coronary artery disease may precipitate unstable angina pectoris or MI.[105] May precipitate hypoglycemia, but probably more important in diabetics is its ability to mask hypoglycemic symptoms.[106] May exacerbate symptoms of peripheral vascular disease or Raynaud's disease. β-blockers may exacerbate previously stable asthma or chronic airway obstruction by causing bronchospasm,[104] or renal dysfunction by further depressing GFR.[107] Depression or, less often, psychotic changes may occur.[104]

Contraindications. Severe obstructive pulmonary disease, asthma or active allergic rhinitis; cardiogenic shock or severe heart failure; second or third degree heart block; brittle diabetes; history of hypoglycemic episodes; severe sinus node disease; concomitant MAO inhibitor therapy.

Precautions. In coronary artery disease, discontinue drug by tapering the dose over 4-7 days. Use cautiously in patients with Prinzmetal's vasospastic angina to prevent worsening of chest pain.[108] Caution should be used with peripheral vascular disease or heart failure. Concurrent digitalis therapy may lessen the β-blocker exacerbation of heart failure. See Drug Interactions chapter.

Parameters to Monitor. During IV administration, blood pressure and pulse must be taken q 5 min with constant ECG monitoring for signs of AV nodal block (lengthened PR interval) or bradycardia. Vital signs should be evaluated routinely for hemodynamic endpoints (eg, blood pressure in hypertension and heart rate or pressure-rate quotient in angina pectoris). Question the patient about subjective complaints such as nightmares or fatigue. When a patient at risk for adverse reactions is first given propranolol, signs and symptoms of toxicity must be searched out (eg, heart failure—shortness of breath or edema; bronchospasm—wheezing or shortness of breath; diabetes—blood glucose; peripheral vascular disease—painful or cold extremities).

Notes. Propranolol may be beneficial for treatment of symptomatic hypertrophic obstructive cardiomyopathy by increasing end-diastolic volume and relieving ventricular outflow obstruction.[38] If a β-blocker must be used in lung disease, metoprolol causes alterations in pulmonary function that are more easily reversed by bronchodilators, and is probably a better choice than propranolol.[109]

Quinidine Sulfate
Quinidine Gluconate

Various
Duraquin®, Quinaglute®

Pharmacology. A class I antiarrhythmic which slows conduction velocity, prolongs effective refractory period and decreases automaticity of normal and diseased fibers (see Electrophysiologic Actions of Antiarrhythmics Comparison Chart).[78] Cellular mechanism appears to be blockade of the fast sodium channel.[110] AV nodal conduction may be increased reflexly through vasodilation, attributed to peripheral α-adrenergic blockade or vagolytic action.

Administration and Adult Dose. PO **loading dose** (sulfate salt) 200 mg q 2 hr for 5–6 doses; **maintenance dose** 200–600 mg q 6–8 hr. **SR** products may be given q 12 hr.[111] **IV** (as gluconate) 5–8 mg/kg (3.75–6 mg/kg in CHF) at a rate of 0.3 mg/kg/min.[234] **IM not recommended.** See Notes.

Dosage Individualization. The elderly (over 60 yr) and patients with liver disease or heart failure are likely to have slower clearance and lower initial doses are recommended.[112] After an initial dosage regimen is selected, maintenance doses should be adjusted based on side effects, therapeutic response and plasma levels.

Pediatric Dose. PO **loading dose** (sulfate salt) 3–6 mg/kg, may repeat q 2–3 hr for 5 doses. **PO maintenance** (gluconate salt) 2–10 mg/kg q 3–6 hr; (sulfate salt) 3–6 mg/kg q 3–6 hr.[22]

Dosage Forms. **Tab** (sulfate salt) 100, 200, 300 mg; (polygalacturonate salt) 275 mg; **SR Tab** (gluconate salt) 324, 330 mg; (sulfate salt) 300 mg; **Inj** (sulfate salt) 200 mg/ml; (gluconate salt) 80 mg/ml. See Notes.

Patient Instructions. Report any symptoms such as blurred vision, dizziness, tinnitus, diarrhea, abnormal bleeding or bruising, rash or fainting episodes.

Pharmacokinetics and Biopharmaceutics. *Onset and Duration.* PO onset of sulfate within 1 hr and SR gluconate product somewhat later; IM onset within 1 hr; IV is immediate. Duration 6–8 hr.[113]

Plasma Levels. Therapeutic range about 1–6 mcg/ml depending on assay. Toxicity is more likely with plasma levels greater than 6 mcg/ml.[114]

Fate. Oral sulfate and gluconate are about 70% bioavailable[111,115] with significant first-pass elimination;[112] IM absorption is incomplete.[113] Primarily metabolized in the liver to two active metabolites: 3-hydroxyquinidine and 2'-oxoquinidinone.[116] 10–20% of the dose is excreted unchanged in the urine.[117] V_d is 2–3 L/kg,[115,117] lower in patients with CHF (1.3–2.3 L/kg);[118] 70–95% bound to plasma proteins (primarily albumin).[112,113]

$t_{1/2}$. α phase about 7 min;[117] β phase in normals 6–8 hr.[113,117] In heart failure, clearance is slower and V_d smaller than normal, such that elimination half-life remains about the same.[118] Half-life in alcoholic cirrhosis is prolonged to 8–10 hr.[119]

Adverse Reactions. Cinchonism may occur at high quinidine levels; symptom complex includes tinnitus, blurred vision, headache and nausea; may progress in severe cases to delirium and psychosis. Hypotension may occur, especially after IV administration. Non-dose-related syncope, attributed to the occurrence of drug-induced ventricular tachycardia, fibrillation or torsade de pointes may occur.[120] Asystole or AV nodal block has been reported. Nausea or vomiting may occur. Diarrhea, which may occur in as many as 30% of patients receiving quinidine, may be treated with aluminum hydroxide gel or by using the polygalacturonate salt.[121,122] Idiosyncratic reactions include hepatitis, drug fever, rare anaphylactoid reactions, thrombocytopenia and hemolytic anemia. IM use may cause pain and muscle damage.[113]

Contraindications. History of past immunological reaction to quinidine or quinine; previous occurrence of quinidine-syncope; second or third degree heart block or bifasicular bundle branch block; severe sinus node dysfunction or long QT syndromes.

Precautions. In atrial fibrillation or flutter, quinidine may increase AV nodal conduction and ventricular rate so that digitalis or propranolol should be given first, in an attempt to block AV nodal conduction. QRS or QT prolongation is a therapeutic effect; however, prolongation greater than 35% of baseline measurements may reflect impending drug-induced arrhythmia.[78] Quinidine may exacerbate myasthenia gravis. Care should be taken with concurrent digitalis and quinidine therapy as quinidine increases digoxin or digitoxin plasma levels—see Drug Interactions chapter.

Parameters to Monitor. Plasma levels and signs or symptoms of toxicity should be monitored in patients with altered drug disposition such as CHF or liver disease. ECG, observing for QT, QRS or PR prolongation; blood pressure (especially with IV) should be monitored daily when therapy is initiated. These may be done less frequently when a maintenance dose is determined. Other parameters, such as platelet count, liver enzymes and hematocrit should be routinely monitored only if idiosyncratic reactions are suspected.

Notes. Dosage adjustment should be made when switching from one salt form to another; sulfate salt contains 83% quinidine, gluconate salt 62% and polygalacturonate 60%. Encainide[123] and flecainide[124] are investigational antiarrhythmics with electrophysiologic actions similar to quinidine, procainamide and disopyramide.

Tocainide (Investigational - Astra)   Tonocard®

Tocainide is a class I antiarrhythmic agent similar in structure and electrophysiologic actions to lidocaine. Other than causing a small increase in peripheral vascular resistance, this agent has minimal hemodynamic effects. Tocainide has been used in ventricular dysrhythmias. Unlike lidocaine, the drug is absorbed after oral administration; it escapes first-pass metabolism with about 40% excreted in the urine unchanged. Elimination half-life ranges from 11–15 hr. GI complaints are most frequent and include anorexia, nausea and vomiting. Neurologic disturbances are dose-related and include tremor, paresthesias, blurred vision and dizziness. Tocainide is administered orally at doses of 400–600 mg q 8 hr. Desired therapeutic levels are 6–12 mcg/ml.[5,125]

Verapamil   Calan®, Isoptin®

Pharmacology. A slow channel (calcium-dependent) blocking agent that prolongs AV nodal conduction.[126] It is used to convert re-entrant supraventricular tachycardias and to slow ventricular rate in atrial fibrillation or flutter.[127] Because it decreases contractility and arteriolar resistance, it is used in angina caused by coronary obstruction or vasospasm and may find eventual use in the treatment of hypertension and hypertrophic obstructive cardiomyopathy.

Administration and Adult Dose. **IV for supraventricular arrhythmias** 5–10 mg (0.075–0.15 mg/kg) over at least 2 min (3 min in elderly), may repeat with 10 mg (0.15 mg/kg) in 30 min if arrhythmia is not terminated or desired endpoint is not achieved. **IV constant infusion** 5 mcg/kg/min. **PO for angina** 80 mg tid-qid initially, increasing at daily (for unstable angina) or weekly intervals to usual maintenance dose of 320–480 mg/day.

Pediatric Dose. **IV** (under 1 yr) 0.1–0.2 mg/kg (usually 0.75–2 mg) over 2 min initially, may repeat with same dose in 30 min if initial response inadequate; (1–15 yr) 0.1–0.3 mg/kg to maximum of 5 mg (usually 2–5 mg) over 2 min initially, may repeat with same dose to maximum of 10 mg in 30 min if initial response inadequate.

Dosage Forms. **Inj** 2.5 mg/ml; **Tab** 80, 120 mg.

Pharmacokinetics and Biopharmaceutics. *Onset and Duration.* IV onset immediate; hemodynamic duration 20 min.[128] PO electrophysiologic effect lasts for up to 6 hr,[129] while maximum effects in angina are apparent during the first 24–48 hr of therapy.
Plasma Levels. Effective plasma levels are not well established.
Fate. Although seemingly well absorbed PO, only 10–22% of an oral dose is bioavailable, indicating a significant hepatic first-pass effect.[130] N-demethylated and N-dealkylated metabolites may possess pharmacologic activity.[5] Although the quantity of drug excreted unchanged in the urine is unknown, about 70% of a dose (drug and metabolites) is excreted renally.[5,130]
$t_{1/2}$. α phase 5–30 min; β phase 3.2–7.3 hr in one study.[130]

Adverse Reactions. Major hemodynamic side effects (eg, severe hypotension) and conduction abnormalities (eg, symptomatic bradycardia or asystole) have been reported; these reactions usually occur when the patient is concurrently receiving β-blockers.[5] IV calcium administration (10–20 ml of a 10% solution) may, in part, reverse these adverse effects.[5] Occasionally, dizziness, headache and GI complaints may occur.

Contraindications. Concomitant IV β-blocker administration; shock or severely hypotensive states; second or third degree AV nodal block; sick sinus syndrome, unless functioning ventricular pacemaker is in place; hypotension or heart failure unless due to supraventricular tachyarrhythmias amenable to verapamil therapy.

Precautions. Use with caution in patients receiving digitalis glycosides; although the significance of this interaction is controversial, potential for conduction defects exist.[94] Additionally, verapamil may attenuate digitalis' positive inotropic actions.[5] Use with caution in patients receiving disopyramide.

Parameters to Monitor. Blood pressure readings and constant ECG monitoring should be observed during IV administration. Particular attention should be paid to signs and symptoms of heart failure and hypotension. The ECG should also be monitored for PR prolongation and bradycardia.

Beta-Adrenergic Blocking Agents Comparison Chart[a]

DRUG	DOSAGE FORMS	CARDIO-SELECTIVITY	BETA HALF-LIFE (HOURS)	EXCRETED UNCHANGED IN URINE	PROTEIN BINDING	APPROVED USES	STARTING DOSE	MAXIMUM DOSE
Propranolol Inderal®	Tab 10, 20, 40, 80 mg Inj 1 mg/ml	0	3–6	1%	90%	Hypertension, Angina pectoris, Arrhythmias. Post-MI prophylaxis	40–80 mg/day	480 mg/day
Metoprolol Lopressor®	Tab 50, 100 mg	+ (up to 100 mg)	3–7	39%	10%	Hypertension	100 mg/day	450 mg/day
Nadolol Corgard®	Tab 40, 80, 120 mg	0	17–24	70%	25%	Hypertension, Angina pectoris	40 mg/day	320 mg/day
Atenolol Tenormin®	Tab 50, 100 mg	+ (up to 100 mg)	6–7	85%	10%	Hypertension	50 mg/day	100 mg/day
Timolol[b] Blocadren®	Tab 10, 20 mg	0	4–5	20%	<10%	Hypertension. Post-MI prophylaxis	20 mg/day 20 mg/day	60 mg/day 20 mg/day
Pindolol[c] Visken®	Tab 5, 10 mg	0	3–4	40%	57%	Hypertension	20 mg/day	60 mg/day

a. From references 131-135.
b. Timolol is also available as Timoptic® ophthalmic drops 0.25 and 0.5% for treatment of glaucoma.
c. Pindolol has potent intrinsic agonist activity.

Electrophysiologic Actions of Antiarrhythmics Comparison Chart

CLASS[a]	DRUG	CONDUCTION VELOCITY	REFRACTORY PERIOD	AUTOMATICITY	AV NODAL CONDUCTION	REFERENCES
(Fast Channel Blockers)	**Quinidine**	↓↓	↑↑	↓↓	↑/↓	78,81
	Procainamide	↓↓	↑↑	↓↓	↑/↓	78,81
	Disopyramide	↓↓	↑↑	↓↓	↑	49
	Lidocaine Normal Tissue	o	→	→	o	63,136
	Ischemic Tissue	↓↓	↑	↓↓	o	
	Phenytoin Normal Tissue	o	→	→	↑	137,138
	Ischemic Tissue	↓↓	↑	↓↓	↑	
II (Beta Blockers)	**Propranolol**	→	→	→	↓↓	94
III	**Bretylium**	o	↑↑	↑/o	↑/o	10
IV (Slow Channel Blockers)	**Verapamil**	o	o	o	↓↓	126
	Diltiazem	o	o	o	→	48

Key: ↑ = increase, ↓ = decrease, o = minimal or no effect, ↑/↓ = variable

a. Classification system from reference 5.

24:06 ANTILIPEMIC AGENTS

General References: 139-142

Cholestyramine Resin

Questran®

Pharmacology. An anion exchange resin which binds with bile acids in the intestine to form an insoluble complex that is excreted in the feces. The loss of bile acids leads to an increased catabolism of cholesterol to form new bile acids, resulting in decreased plasma LDL and cholesterol levels.

Administration and Adult Dose. PO for hypercholesterolemia 12-16 g/day initially, adjust incrementally to maximum of 16-32 g/day, in 2 divided doses, preferably just before meals.[140,143] **PO for pruritus of cholestasis** 4 g tid-qid.

Dosage Individualization. Decrease dose in patients with constipation, because impaction may occur.

Pediatric Dose. PO (over 6 yr) 80 mg/kg/tid.

Dosage Forms. Pwdr 4 g resin/9 g packets; 378 g cans.

Patient Instructions. Do not take this drug in dry form; mix with moisturized pulpy fruit (applesauce, crushed pineapple), highly fluid soups or at least 120 ml of liquid—allow to stand for 1-2 min before stirring. Take thyroid preparations 4-6 hr before or after cholestyramine; take other oral medications at least 1 hr before or 4-6 hr after cholestyramine.

Pharmacokinetics and Biopharmaceutics. *Onset and Duration.* 1-3 weeks for the majority of lipid lowering effect to occur; lipids return to pretreatment levels 2-4 weeks after drug discontinuation.[144]
   Fate. Not absorbed from GI tract.

Adverse Reactions. Constipation occurs frequently, especially in the elderly; occasionally nausea, vomiting, flatulence, diarrhea, steatorrhea (at high doses), abdominal distension and cramps occur. Bleeding tendency due to hypoprothrombinemia may occur, as can hyperchloremic acidosis in children.

Contraindications. Complete biliary obstruction.

Precautions. Pregnancy. Discontinue if significant elevation in plasma triglycerides occurs. Interferes with GI absorption of some drugs (especially acidic drugs) and fat-soluble vitamins—see Drug Interactions chapter.

Parameters to Monitor. Plasma lipids every 2 weeks initially, then every month; children should have periodic hemoglobin and plasma folic acid determinations.

Notes. Decreases LDL (reduces plasma cholesterol 20-30%), may increase VLDL. Effectiveness may be enhanced in certain patients by concurrent use with niacin, clofibrate or neomycin.[139,145] Cholestyramine has no efficacy in hyperlipoproteinemias types III, IV or V and should not be used in these conditions.[146] May be useful in treating diarrhea associated with ileal resection,[147] for treating refractory diarrhea associated with pseudomembranous colitis,[148] and as adjunctive treatment for digitoxin intoxication.[149] There appears to be sustained cholesterol reduction in children on long-term treatment.[150]

Clofibrate
Atromid-S®

Pharmacology. Presumably interrupts cholesterol biosynthesis prior to mevalonate formation, increases triglyceride and VLDL clearance and increases biliary excretion of neutral sterols.

Administration and Adult Dose. PO 1.5-2 g/day in 2-4 divided doses.

Dosage Individualization. Reduce dose in renal impairment.[151]

Pediatric Dose. Safety and efficacy not established.

Dosage Forms. Cap 500 mg.

Patient Instructions. This drug may be taken with food or milk to minimize stomach upset.

Pharmacokinetics and Biopharmaceutics. *Onset and Duration.* Triglycerides decrease within 2-5 days; lipids return to pretreatment levels 2-3 weeks after drug discontinuation.[144]

Fate. Well absorbed orally and rapidly metabolized to active metabolite, chlorophenoxyisobutyric acid (CPIB), which attains peak plasma concentrations in 3-6 hr. CPIB is 92-97% bound to plasma proteins, and is eliminated in the urine, 40-70% as glucuronide.[152]

$t_{1/2}$. (CPIB) a phase 6-25 hr (average 15); b phase 54 hr; increased 2- to 6-fold in renal impairment.[151,152]

Adverse Reactions. Nausea, diarrhea and GI distress occur occasionally. Infrequently, headache, drowsiness, dizziness, weakness, weight gain, skin reactions, alopecia, cardiac arrhythmias, leukopenia, anemia, elevated SGOT and SGPT and decreased libido in men occur. Acute myositis with flu-like symptoms may occur, especially with coexisting renal disease. An increased prevalence of cholelithiasis and cholecystitis has been reported,[153,154] as has an increased rate of noncardiovascular deaths.[154]

Contraindications. Pregnancy; lactation; clinically significant hepatic or renal dysfunction; primary biliary cirrhosis. Manufacturer states renal dysfunction to be a contraindication, but the drug may be safe in reduced doses.[151]

Precautions. Peptic ulcer reactivation reported. Manufacturer recommends drug discontinuation several months prior to planned pregnancy. Concurrent oral anticoagulant therapy—see Drug Interactions chapter.

Parameters to Monitor. Plasma lipids every 2 weeks initially, then every month. Periodic liver function tests; periodic CBC because leukopenia and anemia have been reported.

Notes. Decreases VLDL, variable effects on LDL; there is a marked reduction of both cholesterol and triglycerides when Type III hyperlipidemia is treated. Has platelet inhibiting effect. No evidence of long-term decrease in fatal myocardial infarction (MI), but there is a decrease in nonfatal MI.[154]

Colestipol
Colestid®

Pharmacology. An anion exchange resin with a mechanism of action similar to cholestyramine.[155,248]

Administration and Adult Dose. PO for hypercholesterolemia 15–30 g/day, in 2–4 divided doses, preferably just before meals.

Dosage Individualization. Decrease dose in patients with constipation, because impaction may occur.

Dosage Forms. **Granules** 5 g packets, 500 g bottles.

Patient Instructions. Do not take this drug in dry form; mix with moisturized pulpy fruit (applesauce, crushed pineapple), highly fluid soups or at least 120 ml of liquid—stir until completely mixed (will not dissolve). Take thyroid preparations 4–6 hr before or after colestipol; take other oral medications at least 1 hr before or 4–6 hr after colestipol.

Pharmacokinetics and Biopharmaceutics. See Cholestyramine.

Adverse Reactions. See Cholestyramine.

Contraindications. See Cholestyramine.

Precautions. See Cholestyramine.

Parameters to Monitor. See Cholestyramine.

Notes. Decreases LDL (reduces plasma cholesterol 20–30%), may increase VLDL. Effectiveness may be enhanced in certain patients by concurrent use with niacin, clofibrate or neomycin.[145,156,157,248] Unlike cholestyramine, colestipol is tasteless and odorless.

Niacin   Various

Pharmacology. A B-vitamin which, in pharmacologic doses, may reduce the release of free fatty acids to the liver, leading to decreased triglyceride and VLDL synthesis and subsequent formation of LDL.

Administration and Adult Dose. **PO for hyperlipoproteinemia** 100 mg tid initially, increasing by 300 mg/day every 4–7 days to maintenance dose of 1–3 g tid.[158,159]

Pediatric Dose. Safety and efficacy not established.

Patient Instructions. This drug may be taken with food or milk to minimize stomach upset. Transient flushing, itching or headache may occur.

Dosage Forms. **Tab** 25, 50, 100, 500 mg; **Inj** 50, 100 mg/ml. **SR** products not recommended.

Pharmacokinetics and Biopharmaceutics. *Onset and Duration.* (Decrease in plasma triglycerides and cholesterol) onset 1–4 days and 5–7 days, respectively.[160]
   Plasma Levels. Measurable pharmacologic effects occur at 0.1–0.2 mcg/ml; a therapeutic range of 0.5–1 mcg/ml has been suggested.[161]
   Fate. Rapidly absorbed from GI tract, with peak plasma concentrations attained in 20–70 min (average 45). One-third of drug is excreted unchanged in urine.[161]
   $t_{1/2}$. About 45 min.[161]

Adverse Reactions. Frequent dose-related cutaneous flushing and pruritus occurs initially, with tolerance developing in 1–2 weeks. Occasionally, transient headache, nausea, vomiting and diarrhea occur. Carbohydrate intolerance, hyperuricemia, gouty attacks and abnormal liver function tests, each reversible with discontinuation of the drug, occur occasionally.[162-164] An increased frequency of atrial fibrillation and other arrhythmias has been reported.[164] Hepatotoxicity more likely with SR forms.

Contraindications. Active peptic ulcer; hepatic dysfunction.

Precautions. Pregnancy. Use with caution, if at all, in patients with gall bladder disease, or prior history of liver disease, diabetes, hyperuricemia or peptic ulcer. May potentiate hypotensive effect of ganglionic blocking antihypertensive agents.

Parameters to Monitor. Plasma lipids every 2 weeks initially, then every month. Signs of the development of arrhythmias, liver function tests, blood glucose, serum uric acid.

Notes. Decreases VLDL and LDL (triglycerides 26%, cholesterol 10%).[164] In coronary heart disease patients, there is no evidence of a long-term decrease in mortality, but there is a decrease in nonfatal myocardial infarctions.[164] Niacinamide (nicotinamide) is a closely related vitamin, but it has no hypolipoproteinemic effect.

Probucol
Lorelco®

Probucol is a cholesterol lowering agent that is thought to inhibit earlier stages of cholesterol synthesis and increase fecal bile acids. It is moderately effective, reducing plasma cholesterol 10–15% within 1–3 months, with one study reporting an average decrease of 17% at 6 months and 25% after 2 or more years. It also decreases HDL cholesterol and apoprotein A-I. The significance of these changes is not known and the place of probucol in therapy is not well defined. Adverse effects are minimal, with occasional diarrhea and other GI disturbances predominating; transient eosinophilia and a fall in serum aldolase have been reported. Although less than 10% is absorbed, the drug accumulates in adipose tissue and may persist in the blood for over six months after being discontinued. Safety of use for children or during pregnancy has not been established. Dosage is 500 mg bid, taken with morning and evening meals. It is available as 250 mg tablets.[165,248,275]

Gemfibrozil
Lopid®

Gemfibrozil is a hypolipoproteinemic agent structurally related to clofibrate. It lowers LDL and VLDL and elevates HDL cholesterol; total cholesterol is usually unaffected. The drug is well absorbed orally, undergoes enterohepatic circulation and hepatic glucuronidation; the glucuronide is excreted in the urine. The drug's half-life is about 90 minutes. Gemfibrozil is indicated in type IV hyperlipoproteinemia, but neither its place in therapy nor its long-term efficacy in reducing morbidity and mortality are established. Occasional GI side effects include abdominal and epigastric pain, diarrhea, nausea, vomiting and flatulence. Also, rashes, headache, blurred vision, dizziness, leukopenia, muscle pains and liver function test abnormalities have been reported. Its potential to cause gallstones approaches that of clofibrate. The dose of oral anticoagulants may have to be reduced and the doses of insulin and oral hypoglycemics may have to be increased during gemfibrozil therapy. Dosage is 900–1500 mg/day (usually 1200 mg) in 2 equally divided doses given 30 minutes before the morning and evening meals. Available as 300 mg capsules.[277]

Hyperlipoproteinemias: Classification and Treatment[a,b]

TYPE:	I	IIa	IIb	III	IV	V
PREVALENCE:	RARE	COMMON	COMMON	UNCOMMON	COMMON	UNCOMMON
Plasma Lipoprotein Pattern[c]	↑Chylomicrons	↑LDL (β)	↑LDL (β) ↑VLDL (pre-β)	↑Abnormal ILDL	↑VLDL (pre-β)	↑Chylomicrons ↑VLDL (pre-β)
Plasma Lipids	→SL↑Cholesterol ↑Triglycerides	↑Cholesterol	↑Cholesterol SL↑Triglycerides	↑Cholesterol ↑Triglycerides	→SL↑Cholesterol ↑Triglycerides	SL↑Cholesterol ↑Triglycerides
Diet	Low fat	Low cholesterol; ↑polyunsaturates	Low cholesterol; ↑polyunsaturates; restricted calorie & carbohydrate	Low cholesterol; ↑polyunsaturates; restricted calorie	Controlled calorie & carbohydrate; moderately restricted cholesterol	Restricted fat; controlled carbohydrate; moderately restricted cholesterol
Drugs	None	**Cholestyramine or Colestipol and/or Niacin or Probucol**	**Cholestyramine or Colestipol and/or Niacin or Probucol**	**Clofibrate or Niacin**	**Clofibrate or Niacin**	**Niacin or Clofibrate; Norethindrone[d]**

Key: LDL = low-density lipoproteins; VLDL = very low-density lipoproteins; ILDL = intermediate low-density lipoproteins; →SL↑ = normal or slightly elevated

a. Dietary treatment is the basic treatment for all types of hyperlipoproteinemia. In secondary hyperlipoproteinemias, the primary cause should be treated specifically. Drugs are a supplement to dietary control and have additive effects with diet in types II and III.
b. Information in table derived from references 141, 142, 146, 166 and also Drug Ther Bull 1982;20:41-3.
c. Classified by density. Letters in parentheses refer to corresponding lipoprotein pattern in electrophoretic mobility classification system.
d. Norethindrone is a progestational agent that is occasionally used in treating type V hyperlipoproteinemia in female patients.

24:08 HYPOTENSIVE AGENTS

(SEE ALSO BETA-ADRENERGIC BLOCKING AGENTS 24:04)

General References: 246, 274

Class Instructions. This medication can control hypertension, but it will not cure the disease. Long-term compliance is necessary to control hypertension and prevent damage to several body systems. Because hypertension is a disease that does not have characteristic symptoms, only your physician can determine if your blood pressure is being adequately controlled by these medications. Do not start or stop taking medications or adjust the dose without medical supervision, and avoid running out of your medications. Some prescription and over-the-counter medications may interact with your medications for hypertension; make sure that your physician and pharmacist know the names of any other medications you are taking regularly.

This drug may cause drowsiness. Until the extent of this effect is known, caution should be used when driving, operating machinery or performing other tasks requiring mental alertness. Avoid excessive concurrent use of alcohol and other drugs which cause drowsiness. This drug may also cause faintness or dizziness, especially on rising suddenly, standing for prolonged periods or after exertion or alcohol intake.

Captopril

Capoten®

Pharmacology. A competitive inhibitor of angiotensin-converting enzyme, which is responsible for converting angiotensin I to angiotensin II in lung tissue. Angiotensin II is a potent endogenous vasopressor and stimulator of aldosterone release. Reduction in plasma angiotensin II appears to be the mechanism for short-term blood pressure reduction. Other factors, such as increased levels of plasma kinins and prostaglandin E_2 have been postulated to play a role in the long-term antihypertensive effect of captopril. The hypotensive action of captopril results from dilatation of both arteriolar (resistance) and venous (capacitance) vessels.[167]

Administration and Adult Dose. PO 25 mg tid initially, increased to 50 mg tid after 1–2 weeks if control of hypertension is inadequate. If control continues to be inadequate after an additional 1–2 weeks, add a thiazide diuretic (eg, hydrochlorothiazide 25 mg/day) and titrate its dose upward every few weeks as needed until the maximum antihypertensive dose is achieved (eg, hydrochlorothiazide 100–150 mg/day). If control remains inadequate, increase captopril dose to 100 mg tid, then if control is not achieved the maximum dose of 150 mg/tid may be tried.

Dosage Individualization. The initial dose in renal failure should be reduced and dosage increases should be in smaller increments to avoid enhanced hypotensive responses. If a diuretic is required in renal failure, a loop diuretic, such as furosemide, should be used.

Pediatric Dose. Safety and efficacy not established.

Dosage Forms. Tab 25, 50, 100 mg.

Patient Instructions. Do not use potassium supplements while taking this drug. Report the appearance of skin rash, impairment of taste, fever, sore throat or edema. See also Class Instructions.

Pharmacokinetics and Biopharmaceutics. *Onset and Duration.* Onset within 15 minutes; peak 70 min; duration dose-dependent, with a 10 mm Hg or greater decline in supine blood pressure lasting 103 ± 5 min with a 6.25 mg dose; 175 ± 15 min with a 12.5 mg dose; and 287 ± 10 min with a 25 mg dose.[168]

Fate. Bioavailability from radiolabeled doses is about 75%. Peak plasma levels occur about 0.72-0.77 hr following an oral dose.[169] Plasma protein binding is about 30%.[170] During the first 24 hr 38.4% unchanged captopril, 1.48% captopril disulfide and 26.2% polar metabolites are excreted in the urine.[171] Activity of metabolites is unknown.

Adverse Reactions. Frequently skin rashes are reported, with maculopapular and morbilliform eruptions being most common and a few reports of urticaria. Pruritus may be present with any rash; rashes appear to be dose-related and may resolve with dosage reduction, discontinuation, or with continued treatment.[172] Frequently, dysgeusia, characterized by loss or diminution of taste and complaints of bitter or salty taste sensations occurs. It is potentially reversible with continued treatment[173] or may require drug discontinuation.[174] Occasionally proteinuria, nephrotic syndrome, angioedema, neutropenia, agranulocytosis, pancytopenia or hypotension on initiation of therapy occur.[175] Rarely angina, myocardial infarction, tachycardia or hyperkalemia occur; renal dysfunction reported which is reversible on discontinuation of drug.[176-179]

Precautions. Patients on dietary salt restriction, diuretic therapy, or dialysis (salt/volume depletion) should be monitored for hypotensive episodes following the initial dose. If possible, patients should discontinue salt restricted diets and diuretics one week prior to treatment. Use with caution in patients having an increased risk of developing neutropenia or agranulocytosis due to the presence of severe hypertension, impaired renal function, autoimmune or collagen vascular disorders (especially systemic lupus erythematosus), or drugs altering WBC or immune function. Elevation in serum creatinine and BUN may occur in patients with renal artery stenosis, necessitating a reduction in dose or discontinuation of diuretic therapy. Hypotension may occur during surgical procedures, especially if the anesthetic agents produce hypotension; hypotension is responsive to volume expansion. Use with caution with diuretics, sympatholytic agents, agents stimulating renin secretion, potassium supplements and potassium sparing diuretics.

Parameters to Monitor. CBC and differential counts should be performed q 2 weeks for the first 3 months of therapy and periodically thereafter. If the neutrophil count drops below 1,000/cu mm, discontinue therapy; neutrophil count should normalize in 2 weeks. Urinary proteins should be monitored monthly for the first 9 months and periodically thereafter. Periodically monitor serum potassium. Monitor blood pressure response regularly.

Clonidine Hydrochloride   Catapres®

Pharmacology. A central α-adrenergic receptor stimulant in the nucleus tractus solitarius causing a response similar to the baroreceptor reflex, resulting in a decrease in the sympathetic cardioaccelerator and vasoconstrictor outflow from the CNS. This reflex also results in the stimulation of the vagal nucleus, leading to a reduction in heart rate.

Administration and Adult Dose. PO 0.1 mg bid initially, increased by 0.1-0.2 mg/day until control is achieved. The usual dosage range is 0.2-0.8 mg/day, to maximum of 2.4 mg/day.

Dosage Individualization. Renal impairment may require dosage adjustments. At creatinine clearances of 10 ml/min or less, one group recommends that 50-75% of the usual dose be administered.[180]

Dosage Forms. **Tab** 0.1, 0.2, 0.3 mg.

Patient Instructions. Do not abruptly discontinue this drug because this may result in a rapid increase in blood pressure. See also Class Instructions.

Pharmacokinetics and Biopharmaceutics. *Onset and Duration.*
Onset 30-60 min; peak at 2-4 hr;[181] manufacturer lists the duration of action as 6-8 hr; however, several studies show that bid dosing is usually effective.[181-183]

Plasma Levels. Maximal antihypertensive effect seems to be associated with plasma levels of 1.5-2.0 ng/ml;[184-186] levels above this range may result in a reversal of antihypertensive effects.[185]

Fate. About 75% of dose absorbed orally;[185] V_{dss} ranges from 2.1-3.9 L/kg.[185,187] Metabolized in liver with drug and metabolites excreted in the urine; 38% of absorbed drug is excreted unchanged within 24 hr.

$t_{1/2}$. α phase 2.2-28.7 min (average 10.8);[185] β phase 7.4-12.7 hr in single-dose studies[184,186-188] up to 16.4 ± 4.8 hr after multiple doses.[184]

Adverse Reactions. Dry mouth, drowsiness, constipation, dizziness, fatigue and headache occur frequently; anorexia, parotid pain, Raynaud's phenomenon, impotence, vivid dreams or nightmares, insomnia and anxiety are occasional.

Precautions. Use with caution in cerebrovascular disease, coronary insufficiency, recent myocardial infarction or chronic renal dysfunction. See Drug Interactions chapter.

Parameters to Monitor. Blood pressure; patient compliance.

Diazoxide   Hyperstat®, Proglycem®

Pharmacology. A nondiuretic thiazide that reduces total peripheral resistance via direct relaxation of arteriolar smooth muscle. It also increases blood glucose by inhibiting insulin release and by other mechanisms.

Administration and Adult Dose. **IV for hypertension** 300 mg (or 5 mg/kg) administered over 30 seconds or less, may repeat after 30 min if the initial response is inadequate; maintenance injections are repeated q 4-24 hr based on duration of effect. Individuals sensitive to diazoxide may develop hypotension from the standard dose; an alternative dose would be 150 mg IV initially, repeated q 5 min until diastolic pressure is 110 mm Hg or less, to maximum cumulative dose of 600 mg.[190] With maintenance dosing, a diuretic should be given concurrently to prevent the development of tolerance or CHF secondary to sodium and water retention.[191] **PO for hypoglycemia** 1 mg/kg q 8 hr initially, then titrate to response. Usual maintenance dose is 3-8 mg/kg/day in 2-3 doses.

Dosage Individualization. Pregnant women and patients with renal dysfunction may require much lower initial doses and careful titration of maintenance doses to avoid hypotension.[192,193,198]

Pediatric Dose. **IV for hypertension** 5 mg/kg (or 175 mg/M²). **PO for hypoglycemia** (infants and neonates) 3.3 mg/kg q 8 hr initially, then titrate to response. Usual maintenance dose is 8-15 mg/kg/day in 2-3 doses.

Dosage Forms. (Hyperstat®) **Inj** 15 mg/ml; (Proglycem®) **Cap** 50, 100 mg; **Susp** 50 mg/ml.

Patient Instructions. See Class Instructions.

Pharmacokinetics and Biopharmaceutics. *Onset and Duration.* (Hypertension) onset 1–2 min; peak effect 2–3 min; duration 4–12 hr.[194] (Hypoglycemia) onset 1 hr; duration 8 hr.

Plasma Levels. No correlation between elimination phase plasma levels and hypotensive effect.[195]

Fate. Absorbed orally; V_d is 210 ml/kg with normal renal function and 200–290 ml/kg in renal failure;[196] 94% protein bound (84% in renal failure)[192] with binding inversely related to plasma concentration.[195] Metabolized by oxidation and conjugation with sulfate, with 19–22% excreted unchanged in urine.[196]

$t_{1/2}$. β phase 10–72 hr; 20–53 hr in renal failure.[196]

Adverse Reactions. Sodium and water retention and hyperglycemia are frequent with repeated use. Hyperuricemia occurs; however, reports of gout are lacking. Occasionally hypotension, possibly leading to symptoms of myocardial or cerebral ischemia, occurs.

Contraindications. Allergy to thiazides; hypertension secondary to arteriovenous shunt or coarctation of the aorta.

Precautions. Extravasation should be avoided due to the alkalinity of the solution. Drug-induced hyperglycemia may occasionally require treatment in diabetic patients. Renal failure may enhance the hyperglycemic effects.[197] Antihypertensive effects may be enhanced by recent use of methyldopa or reserpine or by the use of other direct-acting vasodilators such as hydralazine, minoxidil, nitroprusside, nitrates or papaverine.

Parameters to Monitor. Periodic serum uric acid level with prolonged use. **Hypertension.** Frequent measurements of blood pressure until stable, then hourly; blood glucose levels with repeated doses, especially in patients with diabetes mellitus and/or renal failure. **Hypoglycemia.** Frequent blood glucose levels initially and periodically after stabilization occurs in several days. Observe for signs of edema.

Guanabenz Acetate   Wytensin®

Guanabenz is a centrally acting alpha-adrenergic agonist that is structurally and pharmacologically similar to clonidine. It has been found to be approximately equivalent to clonidine in efficacy and more effective when given with a thiazide diuretic than when given alone. The most frequent side effects reported include drowsiness, dry mouth, dizziness and weakness; postural hypotension is rare. Abrupt discontinuation of the drug may cause a withdrawal syndrome of sympathetic overactivity (eg, anxiety, insomnia, palpitations) within 16–48 hours; however, unlike clonidine, rebound hypertension is not prevalent. Dosage is initiated at 4 mg bid and increased incrementally to an average of 30–40 mg/day in 2 divided doses to a maximum of 32 mg bid.[189,276] Available as tab 4, 8 mg.

Guanethidine Sulfate   Ismelin®

Pharmacology. A ganglionic blocking agent whose long-term antihypertensive action is due to a reduction in total peripheral resistance produced by norepinephrine depletion from presynaptic storage granules and an inhibition of action potential-induced release of norepinephrine.

Administration and Adult Dose. **PO in ambulatory patients** 10 mg/day initially, increasing daily dose by 10–25 mg/day at 5–7 day intervals, based on patient response. **PO in hospitalized patients** 25–50 mg/day initially, increasing daily dose by 25–50 mg/day or every other day as indicated. Doses may be given once daily.

Pediatric Dose. **PO** 0.2 mg/kg/day or 6 mg/M^2/day initially as a single oral dose, increasing q 7–10 days by the same amount as the initial dose. Final dose may be 5–8 times the starting dose.

Dosage Forms. **Tab** 10, 25 mg.

Patient Instructions. Patients should be cautioned about the use of OTC products containing ephedrine or phenylephrine. See also Class Instructions (the cautions regarding orthostatic hypotension and its precipitating factors should be emphasized).

Pharmacokinetics and Biopharmaceutics. *Onset and Duration.* Maximum hypotensive response may not occur for up to 14 days after initiating or changing dose.
  Plasma Levels. Adrenergic blockade at 8 ng/ml or greater.[199]
  Fate. Bioavailability 3–27% in one study[200] and 43% in another (although this may include metabolites formed before entry into systemic circulation).[201] Metabolized to inactive metabolites and excreted in urine as unchanged drug and metabolites.
  $t_{1/2}$. α phase 1.5 days; β phase 4.1–7.7 days.[202]

Adverse Reactions. Frequently postural or exertional hypotension (producing symptoms of dizziness, weakness, lassitude or syncope), bradycardia and diarrhea occur. Occasionally fluid retention and edema (possibly progressing to CHF), inhibition of ejaculation occur.

Contraindications. Known or suspected pheochromocytoma; frank CHF not due to hypertension; use with MAO inhibitors.

Precautions. Potential aggravation of asthma. Drugs used in surgical anesthesia may enhance the hypotensive action of guanethidine, possibly leading to cardiovascular collapse. The addition of minoxidil to guanethidine therapy may result in a marked decrease in blood pressure. See Drug Interactions chapter.

Parameters to Monitor. Blood pressure routinely.

Notes. Guanadrel is an agent pharmacologically similar to guanethidine, but having a more rapid onset and shorter duration of action.[203] It is available as Hylorel® as Tab 10, 25 mg.

Hydralazine Hydrochloride   Apresoline®, Various

Pharmacology. A vasodilator that reduces total peripheral resistance through a direct relaxation of arterial smooth muscle. A reflex increase in heart rate, cardiac output, plasma renin activity, and sodium and water retention can attenuate its antihypertensive action; therefore, long-term regimens using hydralazine should include a diuretic and a sympatholytic agent.

Administration and Adult Dose. PO 10 mg qid initially, increasing dose during the first week to 25 mg qid; in the second and subsequent weeks the dose may be increased to 50 mg qid, to maximum of 200–300 mg/day. In slow acetylators, the risk of drug-induced systemic lupus erythematosus may be reduced by limiting the total daily dose to 200 mg. Several studies indicate that bid dosing is as effective as qid.[204] **IM or IV** 20–40 mg prn.

Pediatric Dose. PO 0.75 mg/kg/day or 25 mg/M^2/day initially, in 4 divided doses; the dose may be titrated to 10 times the initial dose over a period of 3–4 weeks. **IM or IV** 1.7–3.5 mg/kg/day or 50–100 mg/M^2/day in 4–6 divided doses as needed for continued control of blood pressure.

Dosage Forms. **Tab** 10, 25, 50, 100 mg; **Inj** 20 mg/ml.

Patient Instructions. This drug may cause headache, dizziness or palpitations; report if these symptoms are persistent. Report symptoms (of drug-induced systemic lupus erythematosus) such as fever, arthralgia and generalized malaise. See also Class Instructions.

Pharmacokinetics and Biopharmaceutics. *Onset and Duration.* PO onset 1 hr; duration (following 300 mg/day) a minimum of 30 hr was required for mean arterial pressure to return to 50% of baseline value.[204] IV onset 10–20 min, IM onset 20–40 min; duration for both 3–8 hr.[205]

Plasma Levels. The hypotensive effect is directly related to the plasma concentration of hydralazine; however, no therapeutic or toxic ranges are established.[206]

Fate. Bioavailability depends on acetylator phenotype and is only 6.6% in fast acetylators and 39.3% in slow acetylators, probably due to extensive first-pass acetylation.[207] V_d ranges from 4.2–8.2 L/kg in fast acetylators and 4.2–7.3 L/kg in slow acetylators.[208-210] The drug is extensively metabolized in the liver by acetylation; the acetylation rate is genetically determined. About 11–14% excreted unchanged in the urine after IV and 2–4% after PO dosing;[211] metabolites are excreted in urine.

$t_{1/2}$. β phase 0.34–2.3 hr (independent of acetylator phenotype); renal impairment may increase half-life to 3.8–15.8 hr.[212]

Adverse Reactions. Headache, tachycardia, palpitations, anorexia, nausea and vomiting, diarrhea and angina pectoris occur frequently. Occasionally peripheral neuropathy, dizziness, blood dyscrasias, depression, nasal congestion and flushing occur. SLE occurs, especially in slow acetylators;[213] in these patients, limiting daily dose to 200 mg or less can minimize the risk of SLE.

Contraindications. Coronary artery disease; mitral valvular rheumatic disease.

Precautions. Hypotensive effects may be additive when combined with other parenteral antihypertensive agents such as diazoxide.

Parameters to Monitor. Blood pressure. Baseline and periodic CBC and ANA titers, especially if the patient relates symptoms of drug-induced SLE.

Methyldopa   Aldomet®
Methyldopate Hydrochloride

Pharmacology. The antihypertensive action of methyldopa is thought to be mediated by the metabolite *a*-methylnorepinephrine which interacts with alpha receptors in the brainstem, causing a reflex depression of sympathetic control of arterial blood pressure.

Administration and Adult Dose. PO 250 mg bid-tid initially, increased every few days to maximum of 2-3 g/day in 2-4 divided doses. There is some evidence that a single daily dose at bedtime is effective in some patients.[214] IV usual dose is 250-500 mg q 6 hr to maximum of 1 g q 6 hr.

Dosage Individualization. The dosing interval may have to be extended to 12-24 hr when Cl_{cr} is less than 10 ml/min.[215]

Pediatric Dose. PO 10 mg/kg/day in 2-4 doses initially, to maximum of 65 mg/kg/day or 3 g/day, whichever is less. IV 20-40 mg/kg/day divided into 4 doses q 6 hr, to maximum of 65 mg/kg/day or 3 g/day, whichever is less.

Dosage Forms. Susp 250 mg/5 ml; Tab 125, 250, 500 mg; Inj 250 mg/5 ml.

Patient Instructions. Report changes in mood (depression), loss of appetite, jaundice, abdominal pain or unexplained fevers and arthralgias. See also Class Instructions.

Pharmacokinetics and Biopharmaceutics. *Onset and Duration.* PO gradual onset occurring within 6 hr.[216] IV onset 2-3 hr, maximum 3-5 hr; duration 6-12 hr.[217]

Fate. Oral bioavailability is low and variable, 7.9-61.5% (average 25) in one study[218] and average 32% in another,[219] probably due to extensive first-pass metabolism to 3-O-methyldopa. IV bioavailability is similar to oral, apparently because a significant portion of the methyldopate ester is not hydrolyzed to methyldopa.[220] V_d is 0.28-1.4 L/kg (average 0.69). The drug is excreted in the urine as metabolites, sulfate conjugate and as unchanged drug, with 64% excreted unchanged after IV and 18% after PO dose.[218]

$t_{1/2}$. α phase 0.53 hr;[219] β phase 90-130 min (average 106).[218]

Adverse Reactions. Somewhat dose-related reactions include weight gain, drowsiness, nasal congestion and dizziness frequently. Positive Coombs' test occurs in 10-20%; however, less than 1% develop hemolytic anemia. Occasionally indigestion, depression, diarrhea, nightmares, impotence and orthostatic hypotension occur.[221] Rarely hemolytic anemia, hepatitis and lupus-like syndrome occur.

Contraindications. Active hepatic disease, such as acute hepatitis or active cirrhosis; liver dysfunction associated with previous methyldopa therapy.

Precautions. Use with caution in any patient with a history of prior hepatic disease.

Parameters to Monitor. Pretreatment—CBC, direct Coombs' test and liver function tests to establish baseline values. Maintenance—periodic CBC to monitor for hemolytic anemia and blood dyscrasias and liver function tests.

Minoxidil   Loniten®

Pharmacology. A potent vasodilator that acts by direct relaxation of arteriolar smooth muscle, resulting in a reduction of total peripheral resistance. The subsequent decrease in blood pressure leads to a reflex sympathetic activation, producing an increase in heart rate, cardiac output and renin secretion. A redistribution of renal blood flow also leads to sodium and water retention. Because these factors may attenuate the antihypertensive response, minoxidil should be administered with a sympatholytic agent and a diuretic (often, a loop diuretic is required).

Administration and Adult Dose. PO 5 mg/day initially, increase in 5-10 mg increments q 3 days; usual dosage range 10-40 mg/day, to maximum of 100 mg/day. If a single dose reduces supine blood pressure by more than 30 mm Hg, the total daily dose should be divided into 2 equal doses.

Pediatric Dose. PO 0.2 mg/kg initially as a single daily dose, increased by 50-100% increments q 3 days; usual dosage range is 0.25-1 mg/kg/day, to maximum of 50 mg/day.

Dosage Forms. Tab 2.5, 10 mg.

Patient Instructions. Report any of the following side effects: 20 beat/min increase in resting heart rate; rapid weight gain of more than 5 lbs or the development of edema; respiratory difficulty; development or worsening of chest pain (that may indicate myocardial ischemia); dizziness; lightheadedness; or fainting. See also Class Instructions.

Pharmacokinetics and Biopharmaceutics. *Onset and Duration.* PO onset 30 min; peak 4-8 hr in one study and 7-11 hr in another; duration 2-5 days.[222,223]

  Fate. About 97% of a C^{14}-labeled dose is recovered from the urine over a 4-day period;[224] however, this may not reflect the amount of unchanged drug reaching the systemic circulation. Protein binding is negligible; V_d values reported in the literature vary widely and range from 99-826 L (average 200) in one study, to 542 ± 186 L in another.[222,224] The drug is extensively metabolized to glucuronic acid conjugates and more polar metabolites. In the first 24 hr, $9.8 \pm 7\%$ of the dose is excreted unchanged in the urine.[224]

  $t_{1/2}$. 2.8-4.2 hr.[222,224]

Adverse Reactions. Frequently sodium and water retention, hypertrichosis and reversible ECG T wave changes.[225] Occasionally angina pectoris, CHF and pericardial effusion, sometimes leading to tamponade, occur.[226]

Contraindications. Pheochromocytoma.

Precautions. Degenerative myocardial lesions reported in dogs, but have not been demonstrated in man.[227] The addition of minoxidil to pre-existing guanethidine therapy may result in significant orthostatic hypotension; if possible, discontinue guanethidine 5 days prior to starting minoxidil.

Parameters to Monitor. Blood pressure, pulse rate, body weight, cardiac and pulmonary function regularly.

Nitroprusside Sodium   Nipride®

Pharmacology. A vasodilator that reduces peripheral vascular resistance (afterload) via a direct relaxation of arteriolar smooth muscle and by reducing venous return (preload) by dilation of the venous system.

Administration and Adult Dose. IV by constant infusion average rate 3 mcg/kg/min with a range of 0.5-10 mcg/kg/min. Patients receiving other antihypertensive agents can usually be controlled with a smaller dose. Administration rates should be carefully controlled through the use of microdrip regulators or infusion pumps. See Notes.

Dosage Individualization. Start with low infusion rates and carefully titrate upwards in elderly patients.

Pediatric Dose. **IV by constant infusion**—a report of 20 cases indicates that an average dose of 1.4 mcg/kg/min (0.5–3.5 mcg/kg/min) is required for adequate blood pressure control.[228]

Dosage Forms. Inj 50 mg.

Patient Instructions. See Class Instructions.

Pharmacokinetics and Biopharmaceutics. *Onset and Duration.* Onset 30–60 seconds; peak effect 1–2 min; duration 3–5 min.[217]

Plasma Levels. Therapeutic and toxic levels of parent compound not established. Thiocyanate levels over 10–12 mg/dl are associated with toxicity.[230]

Fate. Cyanide is released from nitroprusside following the interaction of the iron in nitroprusside with RBC sulfhydryl groups. Cyanide is then converted to thiocyanate by the liver enzyme rhodanase; thiocyanate and an insignificant amount of unchanged nitroprusside are eliminated in the urine.

$t_{1/2}$. (Thiocyanate) 1 week, prolonged in renal impairment.

Adverse Reactions. Rapid infusion may lead to nausea, retching, diaphoresis, apprehension, headache, restlessness, muscle twitching, retrosternal discomfort, palpitations, dizziness and abdominal pain, which are relieved by decreasing the infusion rate. Thiocyanate is not particularly toxic and accumulates to toxic levels only following long-term treatment with nitroprusside. Accumulation may be potentiated by renal dysfunction. Toxicity may present as fatigue, anorexia, nausea, headaches, disorientation, psychotic behavior or muscle spasms. Cyanide toxicity can develop quickly if large doses are administered rapidly; this seems to occur only in individuals who appear resistant to nitroprusside and subsequently receive high doses in attempts to reduce blood pressure. Toxicity may present as tachypnea, tachycardia, altered consciousness, convulsions or coma.

Contraindications. Increased intracranial pressure;[231] hypertension secondary to arteriovenous shunts or coarctation of the aorta; use as an agent to produce intraoperative controlled hypotension in patients with inadequate cerebral circulation; Leber's optic atrophy; tobacco amblyopia; vitamin B_{12} deficiency.

Precautions. If an adequate hypotensive response is not achieved after 10 min of infusing a dose of 10 mcg/kg/min the infusion should be stopped, because larger doses increase the risk of cyanide toxicity.[232] Use with caution in renal or hepatic disease.

Parameters to Monitor. Blood pressure should be monitored frequently due to the rapid onset and dissipation of clinical effect. Plasma cyanide and thiocyanate levels should be monitored daily in patients with renal or hepatic dysfunction. Cyanide toxicity is most easily detected by monitoring for metabolic acidosis.

Notes. Reconstitute with 5% dextrose only; protect from light and discard solution 24 hr after preparation.

Prazosin Hydrochloride   Minipress®

Pharmacology. Prazosin causes a postsynaptic α-adrenergic receptor blockade which produces a decrease in total peripheral resistance. Reflex tachycardia usually observed with traditional α-blockers (eg, phentolamine) is infrequent, because of the absence of presynaptic α-receptor blockade. Thus, norepinephrine in the synapse exerts a negative feedback inhibition of further norepinephrine release.[233]

Administration and Adult Dose.   **PO** 1 mg bid-tid initially, increasing slowly based on response. Usual dosage range is 6–15 mg/day, to maximum of 20 mg/day. Doses up to 40 mg/day may produce a response in a few individuals not responding to a lower dose.

Dosage Individualization.   Carefully titrate dose in chronic renal failure.[217]

Pediatric Dose.   Safety and efficacy not established.

Dosage Forms.   **Cap** 1, 2, 5 mg.

Patient Instructions.   To minimize the potential danger from first dose syncope, the initial dose should be taken at bedtime and the patient warned against arising suddenly. See also Class Instructions.

Pharmacokinetics and Biopharmaceutics. *Onset and Duration.*
Onset 1.5 hr after 1.5 mg PO dose.[235] Full antihypertensive response may not be achieved for 2–9 weeks (average 4).[236]
   Plasma Levels.   No studies indicate a reliable association between plasma levels and antihypertensive response following an oral dose. One study with IV administration found an association between plasma levels and response.[237] The relationship of first-dose syncope or faintness to the time of peak plasma concentration remains controversial.
   Fate.   About 55–57% oral bioavailability.[237,238] 92–97% protein bound; V_d 0.45–0.57 L/kg (average 0.51).[239] Metabolized in the liver by demethylation and conjugation; excreted renally as metabolites and 3.4% as unchanged drug.
   $t_{1/2}$. α phase 3 min; β phase 0.65 ± 0.08 hr; γ phase 2.6–3 hr, prolonged in CHF to 6.47 ± 4.6 hr.[237-240]

Adverse Reactions.   Dizziness, headache, drowsiness, weakness, palpitations and nausea occur frequently. Occasionally syncope, tachycardia and abdominal discomfort occur.

Precautions.   First-dose syncope usually occurs within 30–90 min of initial dose. With a 1 mg initial dose, the frequency of syncopal episodes is less than 1%.[241] Syncope seems to be more common in patients on low sodium diets and those on diuretics.

Parameters to Monitor.   Blood pressure routinely.

Notes.   Trimazosin is an investigational agent pharmacologically similar to prazosin which has similarly been used in both hypertension and CHF.[242]

Reserpine   Various

Pharmacology.   Most of reserpine's antihypertensive effect is due to depletion of norepinephrine from postganglionic adrenergic neurons; depletion of monoamines from neurons in the CNS may also contribute to its effect. It depletes neurons by interfering with the storage of neurotransmitters through a blockade of the uptake mechanism.

Administration and Adult Dose.   **PO** 0.5 mg/day for 1–2 weeks, then reduce to a maintenance dose of 0.1–0.25 mg/day. **IM** 0.5–1 mg initially; if additional control is needed, 2 mg may be given after 3 hr; if the response continues to be inadequate after an additional 3 hr, a 4 mg dose may be given; failure to respond to the 4 mg dose is an indication for switching to another antihypertensive. Parenteral resperine should only be used by individuals familiar with its effects when given by this route.

Pediatric Dose. PO 0.07 mg/kg/dose or 2 mg/M^2/dose.

Dosage Forms. Tab 0.1, 0.25, 0.5, 1 mg; Inj 2.5 mg.

Patient Instructions. Report any symptoms of depression (despondency, self-deprecation, early morning insomnia, loss of appetite). See also Class Instructions.

Pharmacokinetics and Biopharmaceutics. *Onset and Duration.*
Onset slow with PO dosing; peak in 3 weeks. Parenteral onset 1½–3 hr, peak 3–4 hr; duration 6–24 + hr.[243]

Fate. Reserpine appears to undergo extensive metabolism in the intestinal mucosa, serum and liver.[244] Less than 1% excreted unchanged in the urine over 7 days.[245]

Adverse Reactions. Mental depression is a dose-related phenomenon, occurring in about 10% of patients treated with reserpine in usual antihypertensive doses.[246] Drowsiness, weakness, GI disturbances (abdominal pain, activation of peptic ulcer disease, diarrhea, epigastric distress), nasal congestion and bradycardia occur occasionally.

Contraindications. Mental depression with suicidal tendencies; electroconvulsive therapy; active peptic ulcer disease; ulcerative colitis.

Precautions. Use with extreme caution in patients with a history of mental depression.

Parameters to Monitor. Blood pressure; signs and symptoms of depression.

Notes. Reserpine is a very weak antihypertensive used alone, but is effective in mild to moderate hypertension in combination with a diuretic and vasodilator.[247]

Drugs For Hypertensive Emergencies Comparison Chart[a]

DRUG	DOSAGE RANGE	ONSET	DURATION	COMMENTS[b,c]
Methyldopa Aldomet®	IV only, 250 mg–1 g q 4–8 hr	2–3 hr	6–12 hr	Hypotensive response is highly variable; does not affect cardiac output or renal blood flow; slow onset
Hydralazine Apresoline®	IM or IV 5–50 mg q 3–6 hr	10–40 min	3–8 hr	Not predictably effective; increases cardiac output; many patients may be sensitive to parenteral doses, resulting in excessive hypotension
Diazoxide Hyperstat® I.V.	IV push 300 mg (or 5 mg/kg) q 4–24 hr[d]	1–2 min	4–12 hr	Acts rapidly and for a long period; increases cardiac output; requires blood pressure monitoring at hourly intervals
Nitroprusside Sodium Nipride®	IV infusion 100 mg/L at a rate of 0.5–10 mcg/kg/min by continuous infusion using microdrip regulator or infusion pump. Average dose is 3 mcg/kg/min	½–1 min	3–5 min	Hypotensive action is predictable and effective; must be given by IV infusion with continuous monitoring of the patient; arterial pressure response adjusted by changing infusion rate, decreases cardiac output; hypotensive effect is enhanced by elevating head of the patient's bed

a. Adapted from references 217 and 249.
b. Reduction of arterial pressure may lead to sodium and fluid retention, thus reducing the antihypertensive effectiveness of these drugs; diuretic drugs should therefore be administered concomitantly during therapy.
c. Consult the monograph of each drug for additional information.
d. Reduced initial doses may avoid occasional hypotensive episodes.

24:12 VASODILATING AGENTS

General References: 250, 257, 258

Class Instructions. This drug may cause headache, dizziness and/or flushing; alcohol may potentiate these side effects. During an acute angina attack, cease activity, assume a sitting position and dissolve 1 tablet under the tongue. Keep this drug in the original container, tightly closed. Patients on chronic therapy should not discontinue these medications abruptly.

Isosorbide Dinitrate   Isordil®, Sorbitrate®, Various

Pharmacology. See Nitroglycerin.

Administration and Adult Dose. SL or Chew Tab for acute anginal attack 2.5–10 mg q 2–4 hr or prn; PO for prophylaxis of angina and for CHF 10–60 mg q 4–6 hr.[250] Dosage must be started low and titrated slowly upward over a period of several days to weeks to patient tolerance or to the desired therapeutic effect. Because of the possibility of tolerance and dependence, patients on long-acting nitrate regimens should be maintained on the lowest effective dosage. The dose should be slowly tapered if nitrates are discontinued.[251] See Notes.

Dosage Forms. Chew Tab 5, 10 mg; SL Tab 2.5, 5, 10 mg; SR Cap 40 mg; SR Tab 40 mg; Tab 5, 10, 20 mg.

Patient Instructions. See Class Instructions.

Pharmacokinetics and Biopharmaceutics. *Onset and Duration.* Onset 5–15 min after SL and Chew Tab administration, 15 min–4 hr after PO administration; duration is 1–4 hr after SL and Chew Tab administration, 4–6 hr after PO administration.[252]

   Fate. Extensive first-pass metabolism by liver after oral administration to less active mononitrate metabolites (2–ISMN, 5–ISMN). Larger doses and chronic administration overcome degradation processes with significant increases in plasma concentration of the parent compound and metabolites.[253]

   $t_{1/2}$. 29 min; metabolites: 2–ISMN, 105 min and 5–ISMN, 7.5 hr.[253]

Adverse Reactions. See Nitroglycerin.

Contraindications. See Nitroglycerin.

Precautions. See Nitroglycerin.

Parameters to Monitor. Observe for headache and other side effects. In angina, monitor frequency of angina. In CHF, monitor hemodynamic and functional measurements.

Notes. Oral nitrates, sometimes in doses greater than recommended by the manufacturer, have been shown to be effective in the prophylaxis of angina pectoris and in the treatment of CHF.[250,253-256] See Vasodilators in Heart Failure Comparison Chart.

Nitroglycerin   Various

Pharmacology. An organic nitrate that specifically relaxes vascular smooth muscle. The venous (capacitance) system is affected to a greater degree than the arterial (resistance) system. Venous pooling, decreased venous return to the heart (preload) and decreased arterial resistance (afterload) reduce intracardiac pressures and left ventricular size, thereby decreasing myocardial oxygen consumption and ischemia. In myocardial ischemia, nitrates may improve regional myocardial blood supply, although total coronary flow decreases or remains the same. The various nitrate preparations have the same pharmacological effects and differ only in dose, onset and duration.[250,252]

Administration and Adult Dose. SL for acute anginal attack 150–600 mcg prn; **PO for prophylaxis of angina and in CHF** 6.5–19.5 mg q 4–6 hr; **Top for prophylaxis and treatment of angina pectoris and CHF** 2.5–5 cm, to maximum of 10–12.5 cm q 3–6 hr.[250,252] Dosage must be started low and titrated slowly upward over a period of several days to weeks to patient tolerance or to the desired therapeutic effect. **Top for prophylaxis and treatment of angina pectoris (SR Patch)** 2.5–15 mg/day, titrated to patient response. **IV for CHF post-MI, angina pectoris, peri-operative blood pressure control or hypotensive anesthesia** 5 mcg/min initially by constant infusion using an infusion pump. Dosage must be titrated to the individual patient's response. Initially increase dose in 5 mcg/min increments q 3–5 min until response noted. If no response occurs at 20 mcg/min, increments of 10 mcg/min and later 20 mcg/min can be used. Once partial blood pressure response occurs, incremental increases should be decreased and intervals increased.[257,258] See Notes.

Dosage Forms. SL Tab 150, 300, 400, 600 mcg; **SR Cap** 2.5, 6.5, 9 mg; **SR Tab** 1.3, 2.6, 6.5 mg; **Inj** 8, 50 mg/10 ml; **Oint** 2%. **SR Patch** (Nitro-Dur®) 2.5, 5, 7.5, 10, 15 mg/24 hr; (Nitrodisc®) 5, 10 mg/24 hr; (Transderm-Nitro®) 2.5, 5, 10, 15 mg/24 hr.

Patient Instructions. See Class Instructions.

Pharmacokinetics and Biopharmaceutics. *Onset and Duration.* Onset immediate after SL and IV administration, 15–30 min after topical administration and very delayed (hours) after SR Tab and Caps; duration is 30–60 min after SL and IV, 3–6 hr after topical and oral administration.[250,252]

   Fate. Well absorbed sublingually and transcutaneously. Metabolized in the liver to less active dinitro and inactive mononitro metabolites; extensive first-pass metabolism occurs after oral administration. Larger doses and chronic administration may saturate metabolism and result in increased plasma concentrations of drug and metabolites.[259] V_d is about 200 L; plasma protein binding is 60% for drug and 30–60% for dinitro metabolites.

   $t_{1/2}$. 1–4.4 min (estimated).[263]

Adverse Reactions. Headache occurs most frequently; occasionally flushing, dizziness, weakness, nausea, vomiting, palpitations, tachycardia and postural hypotension occur. Many of these effects may be minimized by slow upward titration of the dose. Tolerance and dependence may occur with prolonged use. Rashes and exfoliative dermatitis have been reported rarely.

Contraindications. Severe anemia; severe postural hypotension; increased intracranial pressure. Glaucoma has been stated to be a contraindication, but nitrates can probably be used safely in these patients.[250,259]

Precautions. Some tolerance and cross-tolerance with other nitrates may occur with long-term or excessive use. Use with caution in patients with severe renal or hepatic disease, those with low or normal pulmonary capillary wedge pressure and in those receiving drugs that lower blood pressure; see Drug Interactions chapter.

Parameters to Monitor. Observe for headache and other side effects. In angina, monitor frequency of angina. In CHF, obtain hemodynamic and functional measurements. During IV use, blood pressure and heart rate should be constantly monitored in all patients; pulmonary capillary wedge pressure may also be useful in some patients.

Notes. A burning sensation and localized erythema under the tongue is an indication of potency of SL tablets.[260] Large and unpredictable amounts of nitroglycerin are lost through polyvinyl chloride containers, most IV administration sets and tubing, as well as in certain IV filters.[261,262] The injection should always be diluted in glass containers and administered with the special administration sets provided by the manufacturer; in-line filters should be avoided. Stored in glass containers, the diluted injection is stable for 48 hr at room temperature and 7 days under refrigeration. The special administration set (eg, Tridilset®) has a rather large dead-space and the line should be flushed whenever the concentration of solution is changed. See Vasodilators in Heart Failure Comparison Chart.

Nitroglycerin Dilution Guide

AMOUNT ADDED		VOLUME OF DILUENT	FINAL CONCENTRATION
MG	VOLUME		
8	1 amp (8 mg/ml)	250 ml	32 mcg/ml
16	2 amps (8 mg/ml)	250 ml	64 mcg/ml
32	4 amps (8 mg/ml)	250 ml	128 mcg/ml
50	1 amp (50 mg/ml)	250 ml	200 mcg/ml
50	1 amp (50 mg/ml)	500 ml	100 mcg/ml*
100	2 amps (50 mg/ml)	250 ml	400 mcg/ml†
100	2 amps (50 mg/ml)	500 ml	200 mcg/ml
200	4 amps (50 mg/ml)	500 ml	400 mcg/ml†

*Recommended *initial* concentration.
†Recommended *maximum* concentration.

Vasodilators in Heart Failure Comparison Chart[a,b]

DRUG	DOSAGE[c]	DURATION	SITE OF ACTION[d]	HR	MAP	PCWP	CI	SVR
Sodium Nitroprusside Nipride®	IV 15–400 mcg/min	minutes	A,V	0	sl↓	↓	↑	↓
Phentolamine Regitine®	IV 0.1–2.0 mg/min	minutes	A	sl↑	↓	↓	↑	↓
Hydralazine Apresoline® Various	PO 50–100 mg q 6–8 hr	hours	A	0	sl↓	sl↓	↑	↓
Nitroglycerin Various	IV 5–100 mcg/min	minutes	V, (A)	sl↑/↓	↓	↓	↑/↓	sl↓
	TOP 2% 2.5–12.5 cm q 4–6 hr	hours	V, (A)	sl↑/↓	↓	↓	↑/↓	sl↓
Isosorbide Dinitrate Isordil®	PO 10–60 mg q 4–6 hr	hours	V, (A)	sl↑/↓	↓	↓	↑/↓	sl↓
Sorbitrate® Various	Chew Tab 10–40 mg q 4–6 hr	hours	V, (A)	sl↑/↓	↓	↓	↑/↓	sl↓
Prazosin Minipress®	PO 2–7 mg q 6–8 hr	hours	A, V	0	sl↓	↓	↑	↓

Continued

Vasodilators in Heart Failure Comparison Chart[a,b]

DRUG	DOSAGE[c]	DURATION	SITE OF ACTION[d]	HR	MAP	PCWP	CI	SVR
Captopril Capoten®	PO 25–100 mg q 8–12 hr	hours	A, V	↓	↓	↓	↑	↓
Trimazosin Investigational-Pfizer	PO 50–300 mg q 6–8 hr	hours	A, V	o	↓	↓	↑	↓

Key: A = arterial; V = venous; HR = heart rate; MAP = mean arterial pressure; PCWP = pulmonary capillary wedge pressure; CI = cardiac index; SVR = systemic vascular resistance; ↑ = increase; ↓ = decrease; sl = slight; o = no change

a. From references 250, 257, 258, 264-273.

b. These agents have been shown to be effective in the acute treatment of congestive heart failure. Long-term therapy with some of these agents is presently being evaluated and should be assessed in individual patients by measurements of functional and hemodynamic performance.

c. Dosages of these agents should be started low and increased gradually with continuous hemodynamic monitoring. To avoid adverse rebound effects, carefully taper the dosages of these drugs if they are to be discontinued. See Nitroglycerin Notes.

d. Predominant site of action. Parentheses denote lesser activity.

References, 24:00 Cardiovascular Drugs

1. Singh BN. Rational basis of antiarrhythmic therapy: clinical pharmacology of commonly used antiarrhythmic drugs. Angiology 1978;29:206-42.
2. Federman J. Vliestra RE. Antiarrhythmic drug therapy. Mayo Clin Proc 1979;54:531-42.
3. Harrison DC, Meffin PJ, Winkle RA. Clinical pharmacokinetics of antiarrhythmic drugs. Prog Cardiovasc Dis 1977;20:217-42.
4. Mason DT. Digitalis pharmacology and therapeutics: recent advances. Ann Intern Med 1974;80:520-30.
5. Singh BN, Collett JT, Chew CYC. New perspectives in the pharmacologic therapy of cardiac arrhythmias. Prog Cardiovasc Dis 1980;22:243-301.
6. Zipes DP, Troup PJ. New antiarrhythmic agents. Am J Cardiol 1978;41:1005-22.
7. Wynne J, Malacoff RF, Benotti JR et al. Oral amrinone in refractory congestive heart failure. Am J Cardiol 1980;45:1245-9.
8. LeJemtel TH, Keung E, Ribner HS et al. Sustained beneficial effects of oral amrinone on cardiac and renal function in patients with severe congestive heart failure. Am J Cardiol 1980;45:123-9.
9. Danilo P. Aprindine. Am Heart J 1979;97:119-23.
10. Heissenbuttel RH, Bigger JT. Bretylium tosylate: a newly available antiarrhythmic drug for ventricular arrhythmias. Ann Intern Med 1979;91:229-38.
11. Chatterjee K, Mandel WJ, Vyden JK et al. Cardiovascular effects of bretylium tosylate in acute myocardial infarction. JAMA 1973;223:757-60.
12. Adir J, Narang PK, Josselson J et al. Pharmacokinetics of bretylium in renal insufficiency. N Engl J Med 1979;300:1390-1.
13. Dollery CT, Emslie-Smith D, McMichael J. Bretylium tosylate in the treatment of hypertension. Lancet 1960;1:296-9.
14. Anderson JL, Patterson E, Conlon M et al. Kinetics of antifibrillatory effects of bretylium: correlation with myocardial drug concentrations. Am J Cardiol 1980;46:583-92.
15. Kuntzman R, Tsai I, Chang R et al. Disposition of bretylium in man and rat. Clin Pharmacol Ther 1970;11:829-37.
16. Narang PK, Adir J, Josselson J et al. Pharmacokinetics of bretylium in man after intravenous administration. J Pharmacokinet Biopharm 1980;8:363-73.
17. Anderson JL, Patterson E, Wagner JG et al. Oral and intravenous bretylium disposition. Clin Pharmacol Ther 1980;28:468-78.
18. Koch-Weser J. Bretylium. N Engl J Med 1979;300:473-7.
19. Gillis RA, Clancy MM, Anderson RJ. Deleterious effects of bretylium in cats with digitalis-induced ventricular tachycardia. Circulation 1973;47:974-83.
20. Jelliffe RW, Buell J, Kalaba R et al. An improved method of digitoxin therapy. Ann Intern Med 1970;72:453-64.
21. Rasmussen K, Jervell J, Storsten L et al. Digitoxin kinetics in patients with impaired renal function. Clin Pharmacol Ther 1972;13:6-14.
22. Biller JA, Yeager AM, eds. The Harriet Lane handbook. 9th ed. Chicago: Yearbook Medical Publishers, 1981.
23. Smith TW, Haber B. Digitalis (3rd of 4 parts). N Engl J Med 1973;289:1063-72.
24. Gold H, Cattell McK, Modell W et al. Clinical studies on digitoxin with further observations on its use in the single average full dose method of digitalization. J Pharmacol Exp Ther 1944;82:187-95.
25. Perrier D, Mayersohn M, Marcus FI. Clinical pharmacokinetics of digitoxin. Clin Pharmacokinet 1977;2:292-311.
26. Bresnahan JF, Vliestra RE. Digitalis glycosides. Mayo Clin Proc 1979;54:675-84.
27. Rosen MR, Wit AL, Hoffman BF. Electrophysiology and pharmacology of cardiac arrhythmias. IV. cardiac antiarrhythmic and toxic effects of digitalis. Am Heart J 1975;89:391-9.
28. Jelliffe RW. An improved method of digoxin therapy. Ann Intern Med 1968;69:703-17.
29. Jelliffe RW, Brooker G. A nomogram for digoxin therapy. Am J Med 1974;57:63-8.
30. Steiness E, Svendsen O, Rasmussen F. Plasma digoxin after parenteral administration: local reaction after intramuscular injection. Clin Pharmacol Ther 1974;16:430-3.
31. American Hospital Formulary Service: Current drug therapy; cardiac glycosides. Am J Hosp Pharm 1978;35:1495-507.
32. Doherty JE, de Soyza N, Kane JJ et al. Clinical pharmacokinetics of digitalis glycosides. Prog Cardiovas Dis 1978;21:141-58.
33. Iisalo E. Clinical pharmacokinetics of digoxin. Clin Pharmacokinet 1977;2:1-16.
34. Sim SK. Digoxin tablets - a review of the bioavailability problems. Am J Hosp Pharm 1976;33:44-8.
35. Caldwell JH, Cline CT. Biliary excretion of digoxin in man. Clin Pharmacol Ther 1976;19:410-5.
36. Ewy GA, Marcus FI, Fillmore SJ et al. Digitalis intoxication - diagnosis, management and prevention. Cardiol Clin 1974;6:153-74.
37. Fisch C, Knoebel SB. Recognition and therapy of digitalis toxicity. Prog Cardiovasc Dis 1970;13:71-96.
38. Epstein SE, Henry WL, Clark CE et al. Asymmetric septal hypertrophy. Ann Intern Med 1974;81:650-80.
39. Deglin S, Deglin J, Chung EK. Direct current shock and digitalis therapy. Drug Intell Clin Pharm 1977;11:76-80.
40. Green LH, Smith TW. The use of digitalis in patients with pulmonary disease. Ann Intern Med 1977;87:459-65.
41. Mason DT, Awan NA. Recent advances in digitalis research. Am J Cardiol 1979;43:1056-9.
42. Maroko PR, Kjekshus JK, Sobel BE et al. Factors influencing infarct size following experimental coronary artery occlusions. Circulation 1971;43:67-82.
43. Fenster PE, Powell JR, Graves PE et al. Digitoxin-quinidine interaction: pharmacokinetic evaluation. Ann Intern Med 1980;93:698-701.
44. Hager WD, Fenster P, Mayersohn M et al. Digoxin-quinidine interaction; pharmacokinetic evaluation. N Engl J Med 1979;300:1238-41.

45. Slaughter RL, Schneider PJ, Visconti JA. Appropriateness of the use of serum digoxin and digitoxin assays. Am J Hosp Pharm 1978;35:1376-9.

46. Weintraub M. Interpretation of the serum digoxin concentration. Clin Pharmacokinet 1977;2:205-19.

47. Stone PH, Antman EM, Muller JE et al. Calcium channel blocking agents in the treatment of cardiovascular disorders. part II: hemodynamic effects and clinical application. Ann Intern Med 1980;90:886-904.

48. McAuley BJ, Schroeder JS. The use of diltiazem hydrochloride in cardiovascular disorders. Pharmacotherapy 1982;2:121-33.

49. Sasyniuk BI, Kus T. Cellular electrophysiologic changes induced by disopyramide phosphate in normal and infarcted hearts. J Int Med Res 1976;4(Suppl 1):20-5.

50. Kotter V, Linderer T, Schroder R. Effects of disopyramide on systemic and coronary hemodynamics and myocardial metabolism in patients with coronary artery disease: comparison with lidocaine. Am J Cardiol 1980;46:469-75.

51. Podrid PJ, Schoeneberger A, Lown B. Congestive heart failure caused by oral disopyramide. N Engl J Med 1980;302:614-7.

52. Yu PN. Editorial: disopyramide phosphate (Norpace): a new antiarrhythmic drug. Circulation 1979;59:236-7.

53. Niarchos AP. Disopyramide: serum level and arrhythmia conversion. Am Heart J 1976;92:57-64.

54. Heel RC, Brogden RN, Speight TM et al. Disopyramide: a review of its pharmacological properties and therapeutic use in treating cardiac arrhythmias. Drugs 1978;15:331-68.

55. Hinderling PH, Garrett ER. Pharmacokinetics of the antiarrhythmic diospyramide in healthy humans. J Pharmacokinet Biopharm 1976;4:199-230.

56. Koch-Weser J. Disopyramide. N Engl J Med 1979;300:957-62.

57. Karim A. The pharmacokinetics of norpace. Angiology 1975;26:85-98.

58. Meffin PJ, Robert EW, Winkle RA et al. Role of concentration-dependent plasma protein binding in disopyramide disposition. J Pharmacokinet Biopharm 1979;7:29-46.

59. Johnston A, Henry JA, Warrington SJ et al. Pharmacokinetics of oral disopyramide phosphate in patients with renal impairment. Br J Clin Pharmacol 1980;10:245-8.

60. Hulting J, Rosenhamer G. Anti-arrhythmic and haemodynamic effects of intravenous and oral disopyramide in patients with ventricular arrhythmia. J Int Med Res 1976;4(Suppl 1):90-5.

61. Warrington SJ, Hamer J. Some cardiovascular problems with disopyramide. Postgrad Med J 1980;56:229-33.

62. Dhurandhar RW, Nademanee K, Goldman AM. Ventricular tachycardia-flutter associated with disopyramide therapy: a report of three cases. Heart Lung 1978;7:783-7.

63. Rosen MR, Hoffman BF, Wit AL. Electrophysiology and pharmacology of cardiac arrhythmias. V. cardiac antiarrhythmic effects of lidocaine. Am Heart J 1975;89:526-36.

64. Lazzara R, Hope RR, El-Sherif N et al. Effects of lidocaine on hypoxic and ischemic cardiac cells. Am J Cardiol 1978;41:872-9.

65. Benowitz NL, Meister W. Clinical pharmacokinetics of lignocaine. Clin Pharmacokinet 1978;3:177-201.

66. Lie KI, Wellens HJ, van Capelle FJ et al. Lidocaine in the prevention of primary ventricular fibrillation. N Engl J Med 1974;291:1324-6.

67. Rowland M, Thomson PD, Guichard A et al. Disposition kinetics of lidocaine in normal subjects. Ann NY Acad Sci 1971;179:383-98.

68. Boyes RN, Scott DB, Jebson PJ et al. Pharmacokinetics of lidocaine in man. Clin Pharmacol Ther 1971;12:105-16.

69. Thomson PD, Melmon KL, Richardson JA et al. Lidocaine pharmacokinetics in advanced heart failure, liver disease, and renal failure in humans. Ann Intern Med 1973;78:499-508.

70. Blumer J, Strong JM, Atkinson AJ. The convulsant potency of lidocaine and its N-dealkylated metabolites. J Pharmacol Exp Ther 1973;186:31-6.

71. Burney RG, DiFazio CA, Peach MJ et al. Anti-arrhythmic effects of lidocaine metabolites. Am Heart J 1974;88:765-9.

72. LeLorier J, Grenon D, Latour Y et al. Pharmacokinetics of lidocaine after prolonged intravenous infusions in uncomplicated myocardial infarction. Ann Intern Med 1977;87:700-2.

73. Ribner HS, Isaacs ES, Frishman WH. Lidocaine prophylaxis against ventricular fibrillation in acute myocardial infarction. Prog Cardiovasc Dis 1979;21:287-313.

74. Gupta PK, Lichstein E, Chadda KD. Lidocaine-induced heart block in patients with bundle branch block. Am J Cardiol 1974;33:187-92.

75. Morganroth J, Pearlman AS, Dunkman WB et al. Ethmozin: a new antiarrhythmic agent developed in the USSR. Efficacy and tolerance. Am Heart J 1979;98:621-8.

76. Opie LH. Calcium antagonists. Lancet 1980;1:806-10.

77. Leonard RG, Talbert RL. Calcium-channel blocking agents. Clin Pharm 1982;1:17-33.

78. Hoffman BF, Rosen MR, Wit AL. Electrophysiology and pharmacology of cardiac arrhythmias. VII. cardiac effects of quinidine and procaine amide. B. Am Heart J 1975;90:117-7.

79. Greenspan AM, Horowitz LN, Spielman SR et al. Large dose procainamide therapy for ventricular tachyarrhythmia. Am J Cardiol 1980;46:453-62.

80. Giardina E-GV, Heissenbuttel RH, Bigger JT. Intermittent intravenous procaine amide to treat ventricular arrhythmias. Ann Intern Med 1973;78:183-93.

81. Hoffman BF, Rosen MR, Wit AL. Electrophysiology and pharmacology of cardiac arrhythmias. VII. cardiac effects of quinidine and procaine amide. Am Heart J 1975;89:804-8.

82. Drayer DE, Lowenthal DT, Woosley RL et al. Cumulation of N-acetylprocainamide, an active metabolite of procainamide, in patients with impaired renal function. Clin Pharmacol Ther 1977;22:63-9.

83. Koch-Weser J. Serum procainamide levels as the therapeutic guides. Clin Pharmacokinet 1977;2:389-402.

84. Connolly SJ, Kates RE. Clinical pharmacokinetics of N-acetylprocainamide. Clin Pharmacokinet 1982;7:206-20.

85. Koch-Weser J, Klein SW. Procainamide dosage schedules, plasma concentrations, and clinical effects. JAMA 1971;215:1454-60.

86. Karlsson E. Clinical pharmacokinetics of procainamide. Clin Pharmacokinet 1978;3:97-107.

87. Lalka D, Wyman MG, Goldreyer BN et al. Procainamide accumulation kinetics in the immediate postmyocardial infarction period. J Clin Pharmacol 1978;18:397-401.

88. Koch-Weser J. Pharmacokinetics of procainamide in man. Ann NY Acad Sci 1971;179:370-82.

89. Gibson TP, Atkinson AJ, Matusik E et al. Kinetics of procainamide and N-acetylprocainamide in renal failure. Kidney Int 1977;12:422-9.

90. Dhingra RC, Rosen KM. Procainamide and the sinus node. Chest 1979;76:620-1.

91. Lawson DH, Jick H. Adverse reactions to procainamide. Br J Clin Pharmacol 1977;4:507-11.

92. Prince RA, Brown BT, Jacknowitz AI: Agranulocytosis with procainamide therapy - report of a case. Am J Hosp Pharm 1977;34:1362-5.

93. Henningsen NC, Cederberg A, Hanson A et al. Effects of long-term treatment with procaine amide: a prospective study with special regard to ANF and SLE in fast and slow acetylators. Acta Med Scand 1975;198:475-82.

94. Wit AL, Hoffman BF, Rosen MR. Electrophysiology and pharmacology of cardiac arrhythmias. IX. cardiac electrophysiologic effects of beta adrenegic receptor stimulation and blockade. part C. Am Heart J 1975;90:795-803.

95. Kelly KL. Beta-blockers in hypertension: a review Am J Hosp Pharm 1976;33:1284-90.

96. Frishman W, Silverman R. Clinical pharmacology of the newer beta-adrenergic blocking drugs. part 2. physiologic and metabolic effects. Am Heart J 1979;97:797-807.

97. Berglund G, Andersson O, Hansson L et al. Propranolol given twice daily in hypertension. Acta Med Scand 1973;194:513-5.

98. Federman J, Vlietstra RE. Antiarrhythmic drug therapy. Mayo Clin Proc 1979;54:531-42.

99. Thadani U, Parker JO. Propranolol in the treatment of angina pectoris. comparison of duration of action in acute and sustained oral therapy. Circulation 1979;59:571-9.

100. Routledge PA, Shand DG. Clinical pharmacokinetics of propranolol. Clin Pharmacokinet 1979;4:73-90.

101. Nies AS, Shand DG. Clinical pharmacology of propranolol. Circulation 1975;52:6-15.

102. Wilkinson GR, Shand DG. A physiological approach to hepatic drug clearance. Clin Pharmacol Ther 1975;18:377-90.

103. Johnsson G, Regardh CG. Clinical pharmacokinetics of β-adrenoreceptor blocking drugs. Clin Pharmacokinet 1976;1:233-63.

104. Greenblatt DJ, Koch-Weser J. Adverse reactions to β-adrenergic receptor blocking drugs: a report from the Boston collaborative drug surveillance program. Drugs 1974;7:118-29.

105. Miller RR, Olson HG, Amsterdam EA et al. Propranolol-withdrawal rebound phenomenon. N Engl J Med 1975;293:416-8.

106. Waal-Manning HJ. Can β-blockers be used in diabetic patients? Drugs 1979;17:157-60.

107. Bauer JH, Brooks CS. The long-term effect of propranolol therapy on renal function. Am J Med 1979;66:405-10.

108. Luchi RJ, Chahine RA, Raizner AE. Coronary artery spasm. Ann Intern Med 1979;91:441-9.

109. Johnsson G. Use of β-adrenoreceptor blockers in combination with β-stimulators in patients with obstructive lung disease. Drugs 1976;11(Suppl 1):171-7.

110. Conn HL, Luchi RJ. Some cellular and metabolic considerations relating to the action of quinidine as a prototype antiarrhythmic agent. Am J Med 1964;37:685-99.

111. Covinsky JO, Russo J, Kelly KL et al. Relative bioavailability of quinidine gluconate and quinidine sulfate in healthy volunteers. J Clin Pharmacol 1979;19:261-9.

112. Ochs HR, Greenblatt DJ, Woo E. Clinical pharmacokinetics of quinidine. Clin Pharmacokinet 1980;5:150-68.

113. Greenblatt DJ, Pfeifer HJ, Ochs HR et al. Pharmacokinetics of quinidine in humans after intravenous, intramuscular and oral administration. J Pharmacol Exp Ther 1977;202:365-78.

114. Carliner NH, Fisher ML, Crouthamel WG et al. Relation of ventricular premature beat suppression to serum quinidine concentration determined by a new and specific assay. Am Heart J 1980;100:483-9.

115. Guentert TW, Holford NHG, Coates PE et al. Quinidine pharmacokinetics in man: choice of a disposition model and absolute bioavailability studies. J Pharmacokinet Biopharm 1979;7:315-30.

116. Drayer DE, Lowenthal DT, Restivo KM et al. Steady-state serum levels of quinidine and active metabolites in cardiac patients with varying degrees of renal function. Clin Pharmacol Ther 1978;24:31-9.

117. Ueda CT, Hirschfeld DS, Scheinman MM et al. Disposition kinetics of quinidine. Clin Pharmacol Ther 1976;19:30-6.

118. Ueda CT, Dzindzio BS. Quinidine kinetics in congestive heart failure. Clin Pharmacol Ther 1978;23:158-64.

119. Kessler KM, Humphries WC, Black M et al. Quinidine pharmacokinetics in patients with cirrhosis or receiving propranolol. Am Heart J 1978;96:627-35.

120. Reynolds EW, Vander Ark CR. Quinidine syncope and the delayed repolarization syndromes. Mod Concepts Cardiovasc Dis 1976;45:117-22.

121. Romankiewicz JA, Reidenberg M, Drayer D et al. The noninterference of aluminum hydroxide gel with quinidine sulfate absorption: an approach to control quinidine-induced diarrhea. Am Heart J 1978;96:518-20.

122. Gerstenblith T, Katabi G, Stein I et al. Quinidine utilization in cardiac arrhythmias: report of study involving sulfate and polygalacturonate salts. NY State J Med 1966;66:701-6.

123. Harrison DC, Winkle R, Sami M et al. Encainide: a new and potent antiarrhythmic agent. Am Heart J 1980;100:1046-54.

124. Anderson JL, Stewart JR, Perry BA et al. Oral flecainide for the treatment of ventricular arrhythmias. N Engl J Med 1981;305:473-7.

125. Zipes DP, Troup PJ. New antiarrhythmic agents. Am J Cardiol 1978;41:1005-22.

126. Rosen MR, Wit AL, Hoffman BF. Electrophysiology and pharmacology of cardiac arrhythmias. VI. cardiac effects of verapamil. Am Heart J 1975;89:665-73.

127. Stone PH, Antman EM, Muller JE et al. Calcium channel blocking agents in the treatment of cardiovascular disorders. part II: hemodynamic effects and clinical applications. Ann Intern Med 1980;93:886-904.

128. Singh BN, Roche AHG. Effects of intravenous verapamil in hemodynamics in patients with heart disease. Am Heart J 1977;94:593-9.

129. Krikler D. Verapamil in cardiology. Eur J Cardiol 1974;2:3-10.

130. Schomerus M, Spiegelhalder B, Stieren B et al. Physiological disposition of verapamil in man. Cardiovasc Res 1976;10:605-12.

131. Frishman W. Clinical pharmacology of the new beta-adrenergic blocking drugs. part 9. nadolol: a new long-acting beta-adrenoreceptor blocking drug. Am Heart J 1980;99:124-8.

132. Blanford MF. Nadolol (Corgard®-Squibb). Drug Intell Clin Pharm 1980;14:825-30.

133. Dasta JF. Metoprolol (Lopressor®-Geigy). Drug Intell Clin Pharm 1979;13:320-2.

134. Avery GS, ed. Drug treatment: principles and practice of clinical pharmacology and therapeutics. 2nd ed. New York: ADIS Press, 1980;653-4.

135. Heel RC, Brogden RN, Speight TM et al. Atenolol: a review of its pharmacological properties and therapeutic efficacy in angina pectoris and hypertension. Drugs 1979;17:425-60.

136. Kupersmith J, Antman EM, Hoffman BF. In vivo electrophysiological effects of lidocaine in canine acute myocardial infarction. Circ Res 1975;36:84-91.

137. Wit AL, Rosen MR, Hoffman BF. Electrophysiology and pharmacology cardiac arrhythmias. VIII. cardiac effects of diphenylhydantoin. B. Am Heart J 1975;90:397-404.

138. El-Sherif N, Lazzara R. Re-entrant ventricular arrhythmias in the late myocardial infarction period: mechanism of action of diphenylhydantoin. Circulation 1978;57:465-72.

139. Fisher WR, Truitt DH. The common hyperlipoproteinemias: an understanding of disease mechanisms and their control. Ann Intern Med 1976;85:497-508.

140. Martz BL. Drug management of hypercholesterolemia. Am Heart J 1979;97:389-98.

141. Cathcart-Rake WF, Dujovne CA. The treatment of hyperlipoproteinemias. Ration Drug Ther 1979;13(7):1-4.

142. Samuel P. Drug treatment of hyperlipidemia. Am Heart J 1980;100:573-7.

143. Blum CB, Havlik RJ, Morganroth J. Cholestyramine: an effective, twice-daily dosage regimen. Ann Intern Med 1976;85:287-9.

144. Kepler JA, ed. American hospital formulary service. Washington, DC: American Society of Hospital Pharmacists, 1959-82.

145. Anon. Lipid-lowering drugs. Med Lett Drugs Ther 1980;22:65-6.

146. Levy RI, Rifkind BM. Lipid lowering drugs and hyperlipidaemia. Drugs 1973;6:12-45.

147. Hofmann AF, Poley JR. Cholestyramine treatment of diarrhea associated with ileal resection. N Engl J Med 1969;281:397-402.

148. Burbige EJ, Milligan FD. Pseudomembranous colitis: association with antibiotics and therapy with cholestyramine. JAMA 1975;231:1157-8.

149. Pieroni RE, Fisher JG. Use of cholestyramine resin in digitoxin toxicity. JAMA 1981;245:1939-40.

150. West RJ, Lloyd JK, Leonard JV. Long-term follow-up of children with familial hypercholesterolaemia treated with cholestyramine. Lancet 1980;2:873-5.

151. Gugler R, Kurten JW, Jensen CJ et al. Clofibrate disposition in renal failure and acute and chronic liver disease. Eur J Clin Pharmacol 1979;15:341-7.

152. Gugler R. Clinical pharmacokinetics of hypolipidaemic drugs. Clin Pharmacokinet 1978;3:425-39.

153. Coronary Drug Project Research Group. Clofibrate and niacin in coronary heart disease. JAMA 1975;231:360-81.

154. Committee of Principal Investigators. A co-operative trial in the primary prevention of ischaemic heart disease using clofibrate. Br Heart J 1978;40:1069-118.

155. Heel RC, Brogden RN, Pakes GE et al. Colestipol: a review of its pharmacological properties and therapeutic efficacy in patients with hypercholesterolaemia. Drugs 1980;19:161-80.

156. Kane JP, Malloy MJ, Tun P et al. Normalization of low-density-lipoprotein levels in heterozygous familial hypercholesterolemia with a combined drug regimen. N Engl J Med 1981;304:251-8.

157. Illingworth DR, Rapp JH, Phillipson BE et al. Colestipol plus nicotinic acid in treatment of heterozygous familial hypercholesterolaemia. Lancet 1981;1:296-8.

158. Cathcart-Rake WF, Dujovne CA. The treatment of hyperlipoproteinemias. Ration Drug Ther 1979;13(7):1-4.

159. Samuel P. Drug treatment of hyperlipidemia. Am Heart J 1980;100:573-7.

160. Gilman AG, Goodman LS, Gilman A, eds. Goodman & Gilman's the pharmacological basis of therapeutics. 6th ed. New York: Macmillan, 1980.

161. Gugler R. Clinical pharmacokinetics of hypolipidaemic drugs. Clin Pharmacokinet 1978;3:425-39.

162. Levy RI, Rifkind BM. Lipid lowering drugs and hyperlipidaemia. Drugs 1973;6:12-45.

163. Levy RI, Morganroth J, Rifkind BM. Treatment of hyperlipidemia. N Engl J Med 1974;290:1295-301.

164. Coronary Drug Project Research Group. Clofibrate and niacin in coronary heart disease. JAMA 1975;231:360-81.

165. Heel RC, Brogden RN, Speight TM et al. Probucol: a review of its pharmacological properties and therapeutic use in patients with hypercholesterolaemia. Drugs 1978;15:409-28.

166. Levy RI, Morganroth J, Rifkind BM. Treatment of hyperlipidemia. N Engl J Med 1974;290:1295-301.

167. Swartz SL, Williams GH, Hollerberg NK et al. Endocrine profile in the long-term phase of converting-enzyme inhibition. Clin Pharmacol Ther 1980;28:499-508.

168. Koffer H, Vlasses PH, Ferguson RK et al. Captopril in diuretic-treated hypertensive patients. JAMA 1980;244:2532-5.

169. McKinstry DN, Kripalani KJ, Migdalof BH et al. The effect of repeated administration of captopril (CP) on its disposition in hypertensive patients. Clin Pharmacol Ther 1980;27:270-1.

170. McKinstry DN, Singhvi SM, Kripalani KJ et al. Disposition and cardiovascular-endocrine effects of an orally active angiotensin-converting enzyme inhibitor, SQ 14,225, in normal subjects. Clin Pharmacol Ther 1978;23:121-2.

171. Kripalani KJ, McKinstry DN, Singhvi SM et al. Disposition of captopril in normal subjects. Clin Pharmacol Ther 1980;27:636-41.

172. Wilkin JK, Hammond JJ, Kirkendall WM. The captopril-induced eruption. A possible mechanism: cutaneous kinin potentiation. Arch Dermatol 1980;116:902-5.

173. Ferguson RK, Vlasses PH, Koplin JR et al. Captopril in severe treatment-resistant hypertension. Am Heart J 1980;99:579-85.

174. McNeil JJ, Anderson A, Christophidis N et al. Taste loss associated with oral captopril treatment. Br Med J 1979;2:1555-6.

175. Matri AE, Larabi MS, Kechrid C et al. Fatal bone-marrow suppression associated with captopril. Br Med J 1981;283:277-8.

176. Baker KM, Johns DW, Ayers CR et al. Ischemic cardiovascular complications concurrent with administration of captopril. Hypertension 1980;2:73-4.

177. Warren SE, O'Connor DT. Hyperkalemia resulting from captopril administration. JAMA 1980;244:2551-2.

178. Grossman A, Eckland D, Price P et al. Captopril: reversible renal failure with severe hyperkalemia. Lancet 1980;1:712.

179. Farrow PR, Wilkinson R. Reversible renal failure during treatment with captopril. Br Med J 1979;1:1680.

180. Bennett WM, Muther RS, Parker RA et al. Drug therapy in renal failure: dosing guidelines for adults. part II. Ann Intern Med 1980;93:286-325.

181. Lilja M, Jounela AJ, Juustila H et al. Antihypertensive effects of clonidine. Clin Pharmacol Ther 1979;25:864-9.

182. Frisk-Holmberg M. The effectiveness of clonidine as an antihypertensive in a two-dose regimen. Acta Med Scand 1980;207:43-5.

183. Jain AK, Ryan JR, Vargas R et al. Efficacy and acceptability of different dosage schedules of clonidine. Clin Pharmacol Ther 1977;21:382-7.

184. Wing LMH, Reid JL, Davies DS et al. Pharmacokinetic and concentration-effect relationships of clonidine in essential hypertension. Eur J Clin Pharmacol 1977;12:463-9.

185. Davies DS, Wing LMH, Reid JL et al. Pharmacokinetics and concentration-effect relationships of intravenous and oral clonidine. Clin Pharmacol Ther 1977;21:593-601.

186. Frisk-Holmberg M, Edlund PO, Paalzow L. Pharmacokinetics of clonidine and its relation to the hypotensive effect in patients. Br J Clin Pharmacol 1978;6:227-32.

187. Dollery CT, Davies DS, Draffan GH et al. Clinical pharmacology and pharmacokinetics of clonidine. Clin Pharmacol Ther 1976;19:11-7.

188. Keranen A, Nykanen S, Taskinen J. Pharmacokinetics and side-effects of clonidine. Eur J Clin Pharmacol 1978;13:97-101.

189. Holland OB, Fairchild C, Gomez-Sanchez CE. Effect of guanabenz and hydrochlorothiazide on blood pressure and plasma renin activity. J Clin Pharmacol 1981;21:133-9.

190. Ram CVS, Kaplan NM. Individual titration of diazoxide dosage in the treatment of severe hypertension. Am J Cardiol 1979;43:627-30.

191. Hutcheon DE, Barthalmus KS. Antihypertensive action of diazoxide. Br Med J 1962;2:159-61.

192. Pearson RM, Breckenridge AM. Renal function, protein binding and pharmacological response to diazoxide. Br J Clin Pharmacol 1976;3:169-75.

193. O'Malley K, Velasco M, Pruitt A et al. Decreased plasma protein binding of diazoxide in uremia. Clin Pharmacol Ther 1975;18:53-8.

194. Koch-Weser J. Hypertensive emergencies. N Engl J Med 1977;290:211-14.

195. Sellers EM, Koch-Weser J. Influence of intravenous injection rate on protein binding and vascular activity of diazoxide. Ann NY Acad Sci 1973;226:319-32.

196. Sadee W, Segal J, Finn C. Diazoxide urine and plasma levels in humans by stable-isotope dilution-mass fragmentography. J Pharmacokinet Biopharm 1973;1:295-305.

197. Charles MA, Danforth E. Nonketoacidotic hyperglycemia and coma during intravenous diazoxide therapy in uremia. Diabetes 1971;20:501-3.

198. Pearson RM. Pharmacokinetics and response to diazoxide in renal failure. Clin Pharmacokinet 1977;2:198-204.

199. Walter IE, Khandelwal J, Falkner F et al. The relationship of plasma guanethidine levels to adrenergic blockade. Clin Pharmacol Ther 1975;18:571-80.

200. McMartin C, Simpson P. The absorption and metabolism of guanethidine in hypertensive patients requiring different doses of the drug. Clin Pharmacol Ther 1971;12:73-77.

201. Rahn KH, Goldberg LI. Comparison of antihypertensive efficacy, intestinal absorption, and excretion of guanethidine in hypertensive patients. Clin Pharmacol Ther 1969;10:858-66.

202. Hengstmann JH, Falkner FC. Disposition of guanethidine during chronic oral therapy. Eur J Clin Pharmacol 1979;15:121-25.

203. Dunn MI, Dunlap JL. Guanadrel: a new antihypertensive drug. JAMA 1981;245:1639-42.

204. O'Malley K, Segal JL, Israili ZH et al. Duration of hydralazine action in hypertension. Clin Pharmacol Ther 1975;18:581-6.

205. Koch-Weser J. Hypertensive emergencies. N Engl J Med 1977;290:211-4.

206. Zacest R, Koch-Weser J. Relation of hydralazine plasma concentration to dosage and hypotensive action. Clin Pharmacol Ther 1972;13:420-5.

207. Shepherd AMM, Ludden TM, McNay JL et al. Hydralazine kinetics after single and repeated oral doses. Clin Pharmacol Ther 1980;28:804-11.

208. Ludden TM, Shepherd AMM, McNay JL et al. Hydralazine kinetics in hypertensive patients after intravenous administration. Clin Pharmacol Ther 1980;28:736-42.

209. Shen DD, Hosler JP, Schroder RL et al. Pharmacokinetics of hydralazine and its acid-labile hydrazone metabolites in relation to acetylator phenotype. J Pharmacokinet Biopharm 1980;8:53-68.

210. Reece PA, Cozamanis I, Zacest R. Kinetics of hydralazine and its main metabolites in slow and fast acetylators. Clin Pharmacol Ther 1980;28:769-78.

211. Talseth T. Studies on hydralazine. III. bioavailability of hydralazine in man. Eur J Clin Pharmacol 1976;10:395-401.

212. Talseth T. Elimination rate and steady-state concentration in patients with impaired renal function. Eur J Clin Pharmacol 1976;10:311-7.

213. Strandberg I, Boman G et al. Acetylator phenotype in patients with hydralazine-induced lupoid syndrome. Acta Med Scand 1976;200:367-71.

214. Wright JM, McLeod PJ, McCullough W. Antihypertensive efficacy of a single bedtime dose of methyldopa. Clin Pharmacol Ther 1976;20:733-7.

215. Bennett WM, Muther RS, Parker RA et al. Drug therapy in renal failure: dosing guidelines for adults, part II. Ann Intern Med 1980;93:286-325.

216. Frolich ED. Inhibition of adrenergic function in the treatment of hypertension. Arch Intern Med 1974;133:1033-48.

217. Koch-Weser J. Hypertensive emergencies. N Engl J Med 1977;290:211-4.

218. Kwan KC, Foltz EL, Breault GO et al. Pharmacokinetics of methyldopa in man. J Pharmacol Exp Ther 1976;198:264-77.

219. Stenbaek O, Myhre E, Rugstad E et al. Pharmacokinetics of methyldopa in healthy man. Eur J Clin Pharmacol 1977;12:117-23.

220. Walson PD. Metabolic disposition and cardiovascular effects of methyldopa in unanesthetized Rhesus monkeys. J Pharmacol Exp Ther 1975;195:151-8.

221. Johnson P, Kitchin AH, Lowther CP et al. Treatment of hypertension with methyldopa. Br Med J 1966;1:133-7.

222. Lowenthal DT, Onesti G, Mutterperl R et al. Long-term clinical effects, bioavailability, and kinetics of minoxidil in relation to renal function. J Clin Pharmacol 1978;18:500-8.

223. Shen D, O'Malley K, Gibaldi M et al. Pharmacodynamics of minoxidil as a guide for individualizing dosage regimens in hypertension. Clin Pharmacol Ther 1975;17:593-8.

224. Gottlieb TB, Thomas RC, Chidsey CA. Pharmacokinetic studies of minoxidil. Clin Pharmacol Ther 1972;13:436-41.

225. Hall D, Charocopos F, Froer KL et al. ECG changes during long-term minoxidil therapy for severe hypertension. Arch Intern Med 1979;139:790-4.

226. Marquez-Julio A, Uldall PR. Pericardial effusions associated with minoxidil. Lancet 1977;2:816-7.

227. Sobota JT, Martin WB, Carlson RG et al. Minoxidil: right atrial cardiac pathology in animals and in man. Circulation 1980;62:376-87.

228. Gordillo-Paniagua G, Velasquez-Jones L, Martini R et al. Sodium nitroprusside treatment of severe arterial hypertension in children. J Pediatr 1975;87:799-802.

229. Woosley RL, Shand DG. Pharmacokinetics of antiarrhythmic drugs. Am J Cardiol 1978;41:986-95.

230. AMA Committee on Hypertension. The treatment of malignant hypertension and hypertensive emergencies. JAMA 1974;228(13):1673-9.

231. Cottrell JE, Patel K, Turndorf H et al. Intracranial pressure changes induced by sodium nitroprusside in patients with intracranial mass lesions. J Neurosurg 1978;48:329-31.

232. Creiss L, Tremblay NAG, Davies DW. The toxicity of sodium nitroprusside. Can Anaesth Soc J 1976;23:480-5.

233. Grahm RM, Pettinger WA. Prazosin. N Engl J Med 1979;300:232-6.

234. Curtis JR, Bateman FJA. Use of prazosin in management of hypertension in patients with chronic renal failure and in renal transplant recipients. Br Med J 1975;4:432-4.

235. Dynon MK, Jarrott B, Drummer O et al. Pharmacokinetics of prazosin in normotensive subjects after low oral doses. Clin Pharmacokinet 1980;5:583-90.

236. Stokes GS, Weber MA. Prazosin: preliminary report and comparative studies with other antihypertensive agents. Br Med J 1974;2:298-300.

237. Bateman DN, Hobbs DC, Twomey TM et al. Prazosin, pharmacokinetics and concentration effect. Eur J Clin Pharmacol 1979;16:177-81.

238. Chau NP, Flouvat BL, Le Roux E et al. Prazosin kinetics in essential hypertension. Clin Pharmacol Ther 1980;28:6-11.

239. Jaillon P. Clinical pharmacokinetics of prazosin. Clin Pharmacokinet 1980;5:365-76.

240. Baughman RA, Arnold S, Benet LZ et al. Altered prazosin pharmacokinetics in congestive heart failure. Eur J Clin Pharmacol 1980;17:425-8.

241. Brogden RN, Heel RC, Speight TM et al. Prazosin: a review of its pharmacological properties and therapeutic efficacy in hypertension. Drugs 1977;14:163-97.

242. Weber KT, Kinasewitz GT, West JS et al. Long-term vasodilator therapy with trimazosin in chronic cardiac failure. N Engl J Med 1980;303:242-50.

243. Ueda CT. Quinidine. In: Evans WE et al. eds. Applied pharmacokinetics. San Francisco. Applied Therapeutics. 1980:436-63.

244. Stitzel RE. The biological fate of reserpine. Pharmacol Rev 1977;28:179-205.

245. Zsoter TT, Johnson GE, DeVeber GA et al. Excretion and metabolism of reserpine in renal failure. Clin Pharmacol Ther 1973;14:325-30.

246. McMahon FG. Management of Essential Hypertension. Mount Kisco, New York: Futura Publishing Co., Inc., 1978 p 344-7.

247. Hypertension-Stroke Cooperative Study Group. Effect of antihypertensive treatment on stroke recurrence. JAMA 1974;229:409-18.

248. Glueck CJ. Colestipol and probucol. Ann Intern Med 1982;96:475-82.

249. Hall WD. Evaluating and managing hypertensive crises. Drug Ther Hosp Ed 1981;6:25-32.

250. Abrams J. Nitroglycerin and long-acting nitrates. N Engl J Med 1980;302:1234-7.

251. Abrams J. Nitrate tolerance and dependence. Am Heart J 1980;99:113-23.

252. Warren SE, Francis GS. Nitroglycerin and nitrate esters. Am J Med 1978;65:53-62.

253. Sporl-Radun S, Betzien G, Kaufmann B et al. Effects and pharmacokinetics of isosorbide dinitrate in normal man. Eur J Clin Pharmacol 1980;18:237-44.

254. Anon. Oral isosorbide dinitrate for angina. Med Lett Drugs Ther 1979;21:88.

255. Markis JE, Gorlin R, Mills RM et al. Sustained effect of orally administered isosorbide dinitrate on exercise performance of patients with angina pectoris. Am J Cardiol 1979;43:265-71;

256. Aronow WS. Clinical use of nitrates. I. nitrates as anti-anginal drugs. II. nitrates in congestive heart failure. Mod Concepts Cardiovasc Dis 1979;48:31-5, 37-42.

257. Mason DT, ed. Symposium on vasodilator and inotropic therapy of heart failure. Am J Med 1978;65:101-216.

258. Gould L, Reddy CVR, eds. Vasodilator therapy for cardiac disorders. Mount Kisco, N.Y.: Futura Publishing, 1979.

259. Abrams J. Pharmacology of nitroglycerin and long-acting nitrates and their usefulness in the treatment of chronic congestive heart failure. In: Gould L, Reddy CVR, eds. Vasodilator therapy for cardiac disorders. Mount Kisco, N.Y.: Futura Publishing, 1979;129-67.
260. Copelan HW. Burning sensation and potency of nitroglycerin sublingually. JAMA 1972;219:176-9.
261. Baaske DM, Amann AH, Wagenknecht DM et al. Nitroglycerin compatibility with intravenous fluid filters, containers, and administration sets. Am J Hosp Pharm 1980;37:201-5.
262. Amann AH, Baaske DM, Wagenknecht DM. Plastic I.V. container for nitroglycerin. Am J Hosp Pharm 1980;37:618.
263. Armstrong PW, Armstrong JA, Marks GS. Blood levels after sublingual nitroglycerin. Circulation 1979;59:585-8.
264. Chatterjee K, Parmley WW. The role of vasodilator therapy in heart failure. Prog Cardiovasc Dis 1977;19:301-25.
265. Cohn JN, Franciosa JA. Vasodilator therapy of cardiac failure. N Engl J Med 1977;297:27-31, 254-8.
266. Chatterjee K, Ports TA, Brundage BH et al. Oral hydralazine in chronic heart failure: sustained beneficial hemodynamic effects. Ann Intern Med 1980;92:600-4.
267. Franciosa JA, Cohn JN. Sustained hemodynamic effects without tolerance during long-term isosorbide dinitrate treatment of chronic left ventricular failure. Am J Cardiol 1980;45:648-54.
268. Colucci WS, Wynne J, Holman BL et al. Long-term therapy of heart failure with prazosin: a randomized double blind trial. Am J Cardiol 1980;45:337-44.
269. Orlando JR, Danahy DT, Lurie M et al. Effect of trimazosin on hemodynamics in chronic heart failure. Clin Pharmacol Ther 1978;24:531-6.
270. Ader R, Chatterjee K, Ports T et al. Immediate and sustained hemodynamic and clinical improvement in chronic heart failure by an oral angiotensin-converting enzyme inhibitor. Circulation 1980;61:931-7.
271. Hill NS, Antman EM, Green LH et al. Intravenous nitroglycerin: a review of pharmacology, indications, therapeutic effects and complications. Chest 1981;79:69-76.
272. Awan NA, Mason DT. Oral vasodilator therapy with prazosin in severe congestive heart failure. Am Heart J 1981;101:695-700.
273. Faxon DP, Halperin JL, Creager MA et al. Angiotensin inhibition in severe heart failure: acute central and limb hemodynamic effects of captopril with observations on sustained oral therapy. Am Heart J 1981;101:548-56.
274. Scriabine A, ed. Pharmacology of antihypertensive drugs. New York: Raven Press, 1980.
275. McCaughan D. The long-term effects of probucol on serum lipid levels. Arch Intern Med 1981;141:1428-32.
276. Leary WP, Asmal AC, Williams PC. Evaluation of the efficacy and safety of guanabenz versus clonidine. S Afr Med J 1979;55:83-5.
277. Anon. Gemfibrozil for hypercholesterolemia. Med Lett Drugs Ther 1982;24:59-60.

28:00 CENTRAL NERVOUS SYSTEM DRUGS

28:08 ANALGESICS AND ANTIPYRETICS

General References, Narcotic Agents: 1-4
Nonnarcotic Agents: 5,6

Acetaminophen

Various

Pharmacology. An analgesic and antipyretic similar to aspirin and other nonsteroidal anti-inflammatory agents. It has the same potency as aspirin in inhibiting brain prostaglandin synthetase, but very little activity as an inhibitor of the peripheral enzyme. This explains the very weak anti-inflammatory action of acetaminophen.[7]

Administration and Adult Dose. PO 325-650 mg q 4-6 hr, to maximum of 3.9 g/day.

Pediatric Dose. 10-15 mg/kg q 4-6 hr, to maximum of 5 doses/day; or (up to 3 months) 40 mg/dose; (4-11 months) 80 mg/dose; (12-23 months) 120 mg/dose; (2-3 yr) 160 mg/dose; (4-5 yr) 240 mg/dose; (6-8 yr) 320 mg/dose; (9-10 yr) 400 mg/dose.

Dosage Forms. **Cap** 325, 500 mg; **Drp** 80 mg/0.8 ml, 120 mg/2.5 ml; **Elxr** 120 mg/5ml; **Syrup** 120, 165 mg/5 ml; **Chew Tab** 80 mg; **Tab** 325, 500, 650 mg; **Supp** 120, 125, 325, 650 mg.

Pharmacokinetics and Biopharmaceutics. *Plasma Levels.* No good correlation has been shown between plasma concentrations and intensity of analgesic action.[7] Plasma concentrations over 200 mcg/ml at 4 hr (or 50 mcg/ml at 12 hr) following acute overdosage are associated with severe hepatic damage, whereas toxicity is unlikely if levels are under 150 mcg/ml at 4 hr (or 30–35 mcg/ml at 12 hr).[8] See Notes.

Fate. Rapidly absorbed from GI tract; less than 50% protein bound. Extensively metabolized in the liver to inactive conjugates of glucuronic and sulfuric acids (saturable), and to a hepatotoxic intermediate metabolite (first-order) by P-450 mixed-function oxidase. The intermediate is detoxified by glutathione (saturable). Only 2–3% is excreted unchanged in urine.[7,9,10]

$t_{1/2}$. 2.75–3.25 hr;[11] increased slightly in chronic hepatic disease.[12] Half-life may exceed 12 hr in acute acetaminophen poisoning.[9,13]

Adverse Reactions. In acute overdosage, potentially fatal hepatic necrosis and possible renal tubular necrosis can occur, but clinical and laboratory evidence of hepatotoxicity may be delayed for several days. (See Plasma Levels.)[8] Toxic hepatitis has also been associated with the chronic ingestion of 5–8 g/day for several weeks.[14] Occasionally erythematous or urticarial skin reactions occur; methemoglobinemia reported rarely.

Precautions. Use with caution in patients with G6PD deficiency.

Notes. Does not cause the GI erosion and bleeding associated with aspirin; has no effect on platelet function.[15] Management of acute overdosage includes emesis or gastric lavage, if no more than a few hours have elapsed since ingestion. Administration of activated charcoal is not recommended, because it may interfere with the absorption of acetylcysteine which has been used in the treatment of severe acute overdosage. Potentially dangerous acetaminophen levels (see Plasma Levels) can be managed by the administration of 140 mg/kg acetylcysteine diluted 1:3 in cola, grapefruit juice, soft drinks or plain water; follow with 70 mg/kg q 4 hr for 17 doses. If administered within 10–16 hr of ingestion, this therapy may minimize the expected hepatotoxicity.[8]

Aspirin

Various

Pharmacology. An analgesic, antipyretic and anti-inflammatory agent. Anti-inflammatory properties are related to impairment of prostaglandin biosynthesis. Unlike other nonsteroidal anti-inflammatory agents, its antiplatelet effect is irreversible (due to transacetylation of platelet cyclo-oxygenase) for the life of the platelet (8–11 days). Salicylates without acetyl groups (eg, sodium salicylate) have no useful antiplatelet effect.[16] Low doses (1–2 g/day) decrease urate excretion while high doses (> 5 g/day) induce uricosuria.[17]

Administration and Adult Dose. PO for minor pain 325–975 mg q 4 hr, to maximum of 4 g/day. PO for rheumatoid arthritis 3–6 g/day in divided doses. PO for acute rheumatic fever 5–8 g/day in 1 g divided doses.

Dosage Individualization. Uremia and/or reduced albumin levels are likely to produce higher unbound drug levels which may increase pharmacologic or toxic effects.[18]

Pediatric Dose. PO as antipyretic 65 mg/kg/day in 4–6 divided doses, to maximum of 3.6 g/day. See Precautions.

Dosage Forms. Cap 325 mg; EC Tab 325, 650 mg; SR Tab 650 mg; Tab 65, 81, 325, 487.5, 500, 650 mg; Supp 65, 130, 195, 325, 650, 1200 mg.

Patient Instructions. This drug is to be taken with food, milk or a full glass of water to minimize stomach upset; report any symptoms of GI ulceration or bleeding.

Pharmacokinetics and Biopharmaceutics. *Onset and Duration.*
PO onset of analgesia 30 min.[19]

Plasma Levels.   200–300 mcg/ml are therapeutic for rheumatic
diseases, often accompanied by mild toxic symptoms.[19] "Salicylism" is
manifested by tinnitus in the range of 200–400 mcg/ml;[20] severe or fatal toxicity may result from levels greater than 900 mcg/ml 6 hr following acute ingestion.[21]

Fate.   Rapidly absorbed from GI tract, and rapidly hydrolyzed to salicylic
acid (salicylate) which is also pharmacologically active.[19] A single
analgesic-antipyretic dose produces peak salicylate levels of 30–60 mcg/ml.
About 95% of salicylate is bound to plasma proteins in normals; 74–83%
protein bound in uremia.[18] Salicylate is metabolized primarily in the liver to
four metabolites (salicyluric acid, phenolic- and acyl- glucuronides, and gen-
tisic acid). In low doses and acidic urine, 5% free salicylate is excreted unchanged in urine, with up to 85% at high doses and alkaline urine.[19,22]

$t_{1/2}$. (Aspirin) 14–20 min;[23] (salicylate) dose-dependent: 2.4 hr with 0.25 g;
5 hr with 1 g; 6.1 hr with 1.3 g; 19 hr with 10–20 g.[24]

Adverse Reactions.   See Plasma Levels. Hearing impairment, visual
disturbances, nausea and vomiting, and mental confusion are reported. GI
upset and occult bleeding are frequent with rare acute hemorrhage from
gastric erosion. Rare hepatotoxicity occurs, particularly in children with
rheumatic fever or rheumatoid arthritis, and adults with SLE or pre-existing
liver disease;[25,26] the syndrome of asthma, angioedema and nasal polyps
may be provoked in susceptible patients. Large doses may prolong PT; a
single analgesic dose may suppress platelet aggregation leading to prolonged bleeding time.[15]

Precautions.   Use with caution in patients with gastric ulcer, bleeding
tendencies or hypoprothrombinemia, during anticoagulant therapy or with a
history of asthma. See Drug Interactions chapter. Because of the association with Reye syndrome, the use of salicylates in children with influenza or
chickenpox is not recommended.[127]

Parameters to Monitor.   Occult GI blood loss should be monitored
(periodic hematocrit, stool guaiac) in patients who ingest salicylates
regularly. Plasma salicylate level determinations are recommended in the
higher dose regimens, due to the wide variation among patients in plasma
levels produced. Utilizing tinnitus as an index of maximum salicylate
tolerance is *not* recommended in aged patients or those with pre-existing
hearing impairment.[20]

Notes.   Most buffered formulations do not produce a significant decrease
in gastric acidity.[27] Recent evidence suggests that newer enteric coatings
allow the use of EC tablets to reduce GI bleeding while maintaining reliable
absorption.[28] Those developing bronchospasm to aspirin may develop a
similar reaction to other nonsteroidal anti-inflammatory agents.[29] See Antiplatelet Drugs Comparison Chart 20:12.04.

Codeine Salts   Various

Pharmacology.   Codeine is 3-methoxy morphine and shares the general
pharmacologic properties of morphine. See Morphine.

Administration and Adult Dose.   PO, SC or IM for analgesia 15–60 mg
qid. PO or SC for antitussive action 5–15 mg q 4 hr.

Pediatric Dose.   PO or SC for analgesia 3 mg/kg/day, in 6 divided doses.
PO for antitussive action 1–1.5 mg/kg/day in divided doses.

Dosage Forms. **Tab** 15, 30, 60 mg; **Hyp Tab** 15, 30, 60 mg; **Inj** 30, 60 mg/ml. Formulated as phosphate or sulfate salt.

Patient Instructions. This drug may cause drowsiness. Until the extent of this effect is known, caution should be used when driving, operating machinery or performing other tasks requiring mental alertness. Avoid excessive concurrent use of alcohol and other drugs which cause drowsiness. Prolonged use of this drug may cause constipation.

Pharmacokinetics and Biopharmaceutics. *Onset and Duration.* PO, SC onset 15-30 min; duration 4-6 hr.[30]

   Fate. Well absorbed from GI tract and metabolized in the liver to norcodeine and morphine. A single PO 15 mg dose produces plasma levels of 26-33 ng/ml in 2 hr and 13-22 ng/ml in 5 hr.[31] 7% plasma protein bound.[26] Primarily urinary excretion of inactive forms; 3-16% excreted unchanged in urine.[32]

Adverse Reactions. Sedation, dizziness, nausea, vomiting, constipation and respiratory depression are most frequent.

Precautions. See Morphine for parenteral codeine precautions.

Notes. Low toxicity and potential for addiction.

Diflunisal

Dolobid®

Diflunisal is a difluorophenyl derivative of salicylic acid with anti-inflammatory, analgesic, antipyretic and uricosuric properties. This agent appears to be most useful in the treatment of osteoarthritis, but is also an effective analgesic for sprains and strains and minor surgery. Diflunisal seems to be better tolerated and requires less frequent dosing than aspirin. The usual dose is 1 g initially, then 500 mg bid. Available as 250, 500 mg tablets.[33]

Ibuprofen

Motrin®

Pharmacology. A nonsteroidal anti-inflammatory agent with analgesic and antipyretic properties. Effective inhibitor of cyclo-oxygenase; reversibly alters platelet function and prolongs bleeding time.

Administration and Adult Dose. **PO for rheumatoid arthritis and osteoarthritis** 300-600 mg tid or qid, to maximum of 2.4 g/day. Therapeutic response should occur within 2 weeks, at which time dose should be adjusted to lowest effective level. See Notes.

Pediatric Dose. Not recommended in children 14 yr and under.

Dosage Forms. **Tab** 300, 400, 600 mg.

Patient Instructions. This drug may be taken with a small amount of food, milk or antacid to minimize stomach upset. Report any symptoms of GI ulceration or bleeding, blurred vision or other eye symptoms, skin rash, weight gain or edema. Dizziness may occur; until the extent of this effect is known, use appropriate caution.

Pharmacokinetics and Biopharmaceutics. *Fate.* Rapidly absorbed from GI tract with peak plasma levels of 15-25 mcg/ml attained in 45-90 min following a single 200 mg dose; absorption is slowed after meals and peak plasma levels are about half those seen on an empty stomach.[34,35] 99% of drug is protein bound at plasma levels of 20 mcg/ml; metabolized to at least two inactive metabolites; 45–60% of a daily dose is excreted in the urine as metabolites and 8% as unchanged drug.[35]

   $t_{1/2}$. 1.9 hr.[36]

Adverse Reactions. Gastric distress, occult blood loss, diarrhea and vomiting, dizziness and skin rash occasionally observed; GI ulceration, fluid retention and hyperuricemia reported. Rarely, reversible decreased visual acuity and changes in color vision reported; a slight rise in the Ivy bleeding time occurs. Elevation of liver enzymes, lymphopenia, agranulocytosis and aplastic anemia have been reported rarely.[37,38]

Contraindications. Pregnancy; children 14 yr and under; syndrome of nasal polyps, angioedema and bronchospastic reactivity to aspirin or other nonsteroidal anti-inflammatory agents.

Precautions. Use with caution in patients with a history of cardiac decompensation.

Parameters to Monitor. Occult blood loss, visual disturbances and weight gain should be monitored.

Indomethacin   Indocin®

Pharmacology. See Ibuprofen.

Administration and Adult Dose. **PO for rheumatoid arthritis, rheumatoid (ankylosing) spondylitis and osteoarthritis of the hip** 25 mg bid or tid initially. Increase in 25 mg/day increments at weekly intervals until satisfactory response or total dose of 150–200 mg/day is reached. **PO for acute gouty arthritis** 50 mg tid. Reduce dosage whenever possible to attempt eventual cessation of drug. SR Cap 75 mg 1–2 times/day can be substituted for all uses except gouty arthritis, based on non-SR dose.

Pediatric Dose. Not recommended in children 14 yr and under.

Dosage Forms. **Cap** 25, 50 mg; **SR Cap** 75 mg.

Patient Instructions. This drug is to be taken with food, milk or an antacid to minimize stomach upset; report any symptoms of GI ulceration or bleeding. Dizziness or headache may occur; until the extent of these effects is known, use appropriate caution. Do not take with aspirin unless directed otherwise.

Pharmacokinetics and Biopharmaceutics. *Fate.* Rapidly and well absorbed from GI tract, with peak plasma levels reached within 2 hr.[39] 97% of drug is plasma protein bound;[40] extensive O-demethylation and N-deacylation to inactive metabolites. 21–42% excreted fecally as metabolites, with about 10–20% excreted unchanged in urine.[40]

   $t_{1/2}$. 2.6–11.2 hr.[39]

Adverse Reactions. Frontal lobe headache, drowsiness, dizziness, mental confusion and GI distress are very frequent, especially with doses greater than 100 mg/day; occasional peripheral neuropathy, occult bleeding and peptic ulcer occur. Rarely, pancreatitis, corneal opacities, hepatotoxicity, aplastic anemia, agranulocytosis, thrombocytopenia and allergic reactions are reported.[41] The syndrome of asthma, angioedema and nasal polyps may be provoked in susceptible patients. May aggravate psychiatric disorders, epilepsy or parkinsonism.

Contraindications. Pregnancy; lactation; children 14 yr and under; history of recurrent or active GI lesions; syndrome of nasal polyps, angioedema and bronchospastic reactivity to aspirin or other nonsteroidal anti-inflammatory agents.

Precautions. Careful instructions to, and observations of, the patient are essential. Use with great care in the elderly. May mask the signs and symptoms of infection. Blurred vision warrants a thorough ophthalmologic examination. Headache, which persists despite dosage reduction, and corneal deposits and retinal disturbances (including those of the macula) necessitate cessation of drug use. See Drug Interactions chapter.

Parameters to Monitor. Periodic ophthalmologic examination and CBCs during prolonged therapy.

Notes. The clinical efficacy of indomethacin in the treatment of rheumatoid arthritis has not been impressive in controlled trials and should not generally be used as an alternative to aspirin.[41] Other nonsteroidal anti-inflammatory agents (eg, naproxen, ibuprofen) are preferable due to their proven efficacy and lower toxicity.

Meperidine Hydrochloride   Demerol®, Various

Pharmacology. See Morphine.

Administration and Adult Dose. PO, SC or IM for analgesia 50–150 mg (or **very slow IV** 50–100 mg, preferably diluted) q 3–4 hr prn. Oral doses are about half as effective as a parenteral dose.[42] Reduce dosage when given concomitantly with phenothiazines and other drugs that potentiate the depressant effects of meperidine. See Notes.

Pediatric Dose. PO, SC or IM for analgesia 6 mg/kg/day in 6 divided doses, to maximum of 100 mg/dose. See Notes.

Dosage Forms. Syrup 10 mg/ml; Tab 50, 100 mg; Inj 25, 50, 75, 100 mg/ml.

Pharmacokinetics and Biopharmaceutics. *Onset and Duration.* PO onset about 20 min, duration 3 hr;[42] SC or IM onset about 10 min, duration 2–4 hr.[43]

Fate. Good absorption by parenteral route; hydrolyzed and also metabolized in the liver to normeperidine (an active metabolite), which is also hydrolyzed. About 50% of an oral dose undergoes first-pass metabolism.[42] After a single IM 100 mg dose, mean plasma levels of 670 ng/ml and 650 ng/ml are attained in 1 and 2 hr respectively.[44,45] An average of 2% unchanged drug and 6% (range 1–21%) normeperidine is excreted in urine.[45]

$t_{1/2}$. α phase 12 min, β phase 3.2 hr, increasing to 7 hr in patients with cirrhosis or acute liver disease.[45,46] Normeperidine has a half-life of 14–21 hr in normals, increasing to 35 hr in renal failure.[47]

Adverse Reactions. See Morphine. The metabolite normeperidine has excitant effects which may precipitate tremors, myoclonus or seizures. Factors which predispose to seizures include doses greater than 100 mg q 2 hr for greater than 24 hr, renal failure and history of seizures.[47] Local irritation and induration occur with repeated SC injection.

Contraindications. Patients who have received MAO inhibitors within 14 days.

Precautions. See Morphine and Drug Interactions chapter.

Parameters to Monitor. Signs of respiratory depression.

Notes. 80–100 mg of meperidine by the parenteral route is approximately equivalent to 10 mg of morphine.[43] IM is preferred route.

Methadone   Dolophine®, Various

Pharmacology. A synthetic narcotic analgesic qualitatively similar to morphine. Analgesic activity of *l*-methadone is 8–50 times that of the *d* isomer. *d*-Methadone lacks addiction liability, but possesses antitussive activity. Because methadone is a long-acting narcotic agent, it can be substituted for short-acting narcotic agents for maintenance and detoxification. Methadone abstinence syndrome is similar to morphine; however, onset is slower and course more prolonged.

Administration and Adult Dose. **IM or SC for pain** 2.5–10 mg q 3–4 hr. **PO for pain** 5–15 mg q 4–6 hr. **PO for maintenance and detoxification treatment** 5–20 mg initially, followed by supplementary doses of 5–10 mg if withdrawal is not suppressed or signs reappear. After stabilization, 10–40 mg/day in single (for maintenance) or divided (for detoxification) doses is adequate for most patients. Detoxification by dosage reduction of 20% per day is usually well tolerated in hospitalized patients.[48]

Pediatric Dose. **PO or SC for pain** 0.7 mg/kg/24 hr or 20 mg/M^2/24 hr, in 4–6 divided doses.

Dosage Forms. **Tab** 5, 10 mg; **Dispersible Tab** 40 mg; **Soln** 1 mg/ml; **Inj** 10 mg/ml.

Pharmacokinetics and Biopharmaceutics. *Onset and Duration.* (Analgesia) onset SC or IM 10–20 min, PO 30–60 min; duration PO, SC or IM 4–5 hr after a single dose, may be longer with multiple doses.[48,49]
      Plasma Levels. Best rehabilitation in methadone maintenance patients has been associated with plasma levels above 211 ng/ml.[50] There is no good correlation between plasma levels and analgesia.[51]
      Fate. About 50% absorbed orally;[43,51] 71–87% plasma protein bound.[51] Following a single dose, 30% is metabolized to form pyrrolidines and pyrroline which are excreted in urine and bile; 21% is excreted unchanged in the urine.[43,51] Extent of metabolism appears to increase with chronic therapy, resulting in a 15–25% decline in plasma levels after 8–10 days of therapy.[50,51] Urinary methadone excretion is increased by urine acidification.[51]
      $t_{1/2}$. α phase 14.3 hr; β phase 54.8 hr, 22.2 hr with chronic administration.[52]

Adverse Reactions. See Morphine. Methadone administered frequently and for prolonged periods may have cumulative effects on respiration.[53]

Precautions. See Morphine and Drug Interactions chapter.

Parameters to Monitor. See Morphine Adverse Reactions. During methadone maintenance, monitor for signs of withdrawal which include lacrimation, rhinorrhea, diaphoresis, yawning, restlessness, insomnia, dilated pupils and piloerection.[48]

Notes. For treatment of narcotic addiction in detoxification or maintenance programs, methadone may be dispensed only by approved pharmacies. Maintenance therapy (treatment for longer than 3 weeks) may be undertaken only by approved methadone programs; this does not apply to addicts hospitalized for other medical conditions.

Morphine Sulfate

Various

Pharmacology. Narcotic agents interact with stereospecific opiate receptors in the CNS and other tissues. Analgesia is produced primarily through an alteration in emotional response to pain. The relief of pain is fairly specific; other sensory modalities are essentially unaffected and mental processes are not impaired (unlike anesthetics), except when given in large doses or to unusually susceptible individuals. They also possess antitussive effects, usually at doses less than those required for analgesia.

Administration and Adult Dose. **PO for analgesia** 8–20 mg q 4 hr; **SC or IM for analgesia** 5–15 mg q 4 hr (10 mg/70 kg is optimal initial dose); **IV for analgesia** 4–10 mg, dilute and inject slowly over 4–5 min period. **IV infusion** 40–95 mg/hr.[54]

Pediatric Dose. SC or IM 0.1–0.2 mg/kg/dose, to maximum of 15 mg; may repeat q 4 hr. IV use one-half the IM dose.

Dosage Forms. **Soln** 10, 20 mg/5 ml; **Tab** 10, 15, 30 mg; **Inj** 8, 10, 15 mg/ml.

Pharmacokinetics and Biopharmaceutics. *Onset and Duration.* Following single SC 10 mg dose, onset 15–30 min, duration 4–5 hr.[43]
Plasma Levels. It is speculated that moderate analgesia requires plasma levels of at least 50 ng/ml.[55]
Fate. Rapid absorption parenterally with rapid disappearance from plasma, especially after IV administration; inactivated in the liver, primarily by conjugation with glucuronic acid. After an IM dose of 10 mg, peak levels of about 56 ng/ml are reached within 20 min. Well absorbed from GI tract, but first-pass conjugation is so rapid that significant levels of free morphine are not found in either plasma or urine. Mostly excreted in urine with 3.4% (oral) and about 9% (parenteral) of dose excreted unchanged.[56,57]
$t_{1/2}$. 2.1–2.9 hr.[56,57]

Adverse Reactions. Respiratory and circulatory depression are major adverse effects, the former occurring with therapeutic doses. Dose-related signs of intoxication include miosis, drowsiness, decreased rate and depth of respiration, bradycardia and hypotension. Sedation, dizziness, nausea, vomiting, sweating and constipation occur frequently. Euphoria, dysphoria, dry mouth, biliary tract spasm, postural hypotension, syncope, tachy- and bradycardia, urinary retention and possible allergic-type reactions are reported occasionally. The majority of allergic-type reactions consist of skin rash, and wheal and flare over vein which may occur with IV injection; these are due to direct stimulation of histamine release, are not truly allergic and are not a sign of more serious reactions. True allergy is very rare.

Contraindications. Contraindications are relative rather than absolute, such that Precautions should be closely observed.

Precautions. Use with caution and in reduced dosage when giving concurrently with other CNS depressant drugs. Use with caution in pregnancy; the presence of head injury, other intracranial lesions or pre-existing increase in intracranial pressure; patients having an acute asthmatic attack; the presence of chronic obstructive pulmonary disease, cor pulmonale; decreased respiratory reserve; pre-existing respiratory depression, hypoxia or hypercapnia; patients whose ability to maintain blood pressure is already compromised; patients with atrial flutter or other supraventricular tachycardias; patients with prostatic hypertrophy or urethral stricture; elderly or debilitated patients; and in patients with acute abdominal pain, when administration of drug might obscure the diagnosis or clinical course. Do not administer IV unless a narcotic antagonist and facilities for assisted or controlled respiration are immediately available. See Drug Interactions chapter.

Parameters to Monitor. Signs of respiratory or cardiovascular depression should be monitored.

Notes. Brompton's mixture, which is usually prepared as a combination of morphine and cocaine in an alcohol and syrup base, has been used for many years in the management of chronic pain. Evidence for the superiority of Brompton's or other mixtures over plain morphine solution is questionable.[58,59]

Naproxen   Naprosyn®
Naproxen Sodium   Anaprox®

Pharmacology. A propionic acid derivative similar to ibuprofen and fenoprofen.

Administration and Adult Dose. PO for rheumatoid arthritis and osteoarthritis (base) 250-375 mg bid initially; (sodium) 275 mg bid or 275 mg q AM and 550 mg q evening initially. If no improvement has occurred after 4 weeks of therapy, other drug therapy should be considered. **PO for mild to moderate pain and dysmenorrhea** (sodium) 550 mg, followed by 275 mg q 6-8 hr. Daily doses greater than 1 g (base) or 1.375 g (sodium) are not recommended.

Pediatric Dose. Safety and efficacy not established. For children under 50 kg, doses of 5 mg/kg/day have been given investigationally.[60]

Dosage Forms. Tab 250, 375, 500 mg (base); 275, 500 mg (sodium salt).

Patient Instructions. This drug may be taken with food, milk or an antacid to minimize stomach upset; report any symptoms of GI ulceration or bleeding. It may cause drowsiness. Until the extent of this effect is known, caution should be used when driving, operating machinery or performing other tasks requiring mental alertness. Avoid excessive concurrent use of alcohol and other drugs which cause drowsiness.

Pharmacokinetics and Biopharmaceutics. *Plasma Levels.* Trough concentrations above 50 mcg/ml are associated with response in rheumatoid arthritis.[203]
    Fate. Readily and completely absorbed orally; more rapid with the sodium salt. 99.6% bound to plasma proteins at concentrations of 23-49 mcg/ml. About 95% of the drug is excreted in the urine, 10% as unchanged drug and the rest as inactive metabolites. Some enterohepatic recirculation may take place.[62-64] Plasma levels vary considerably between different individuals receiving similar doses. Plasma levels tend to plateau at and above a dose of 250 mg bid. As dosage is increased, binding sites become saturated and more drug is available for renal clearance.[61]
    $t_{1/2}$. 12-15 hr.[61]

Adverse Reactions. GI side effects include indigestion, abdominal discomfort, nausea, vomiting and heartburn; these have been generally less frequent than with aspirin and indomethacin. Episodes of GI bleeding have been reported and are at times severe and occasionally fatal. CNS side effects occur occasionally, and include headache, drowsiness, vertigo and tinnitus. Rarely, visual disturbances, thrombocytopenia, agranulocytosis and jaundice are observed.[65] Interstitial nephritis and nephrotic syndrome have been reported.[66,67]

Contraindications.   Patients exhibiting the syndrome of nasal polyps, angioedema and bronchospasm induced by aspirin or other nonsteroidal anti-inflammatory agents.

Precautions.   Pregnancy. Pre-existing ulcer disease or history of GI bleeding. Because of the high protein binding of naproxen, potential exists for displacement of other highly protein bound drugs such as warfarin, aspirin, sulfonylureas and hydantoins; however, clinically significant interactions have not been reported. GI effects and inhibition of platelet aggregation may be important in predisposing patients receiving anticoagulants to bleeding episodes.

Notes.   Aspirin remains the standard therapy for the treatment of rheumatoid arthritis. Naproxen appears to compare favorably with aspirin in efficacy.[65] Naproxen offers an alternative to the more toxic anti-inflammatory agents such as indomethacin and phenylbutazone in patients intolerant to aspirin. Naproxen 750 mg/day has shown greater subjective antirheumatic activity than fenoprofen 2.4 g/day and ibuprofen 2.4 g/day.[65] Naproxen and/or its metabolites may cause a false elevation in the assay for urinary 17-ketogenic steroids. Measurements of 17-hydroxycorticosteroids are apparently unaltered.

Oxaprozin (Investigational - Wyeth)

Oxaprozin is an alkanoic acid nonsteroidal anti-inflammatory agent with analgesic and antipyretic properties. It is effective in the treatment of rheumatoid arthritis and other inflammatory conditions. A unique property of this drug is its long half-life (40 hr) allowing single daily dosage. Adverse effects appear to be similar to other available nonsteroidal anti-inflammatory agents and generally less frequent than with aspirin. Dosage is usually 1.2 g in a single daily dose.[68,69]

Pentazocine Salts   Talwin®, Talwin® Nx

Pharmacology.   A narcotic analgesic with weak opioid antagonist activity. Unlike pure narcotic agonists (and nalbuphine), pentazocine (and butorphanol) increases cardiac workload, making it unacceptable in patients with myocardial infarction.[3] Naloxone is added to tablets to eliminate IV abuse potential.

Administration and Adult Dose.   PO 50–100 mg q 3–4 hr, to maximum of 600 mg/day; **SC or IM** (excluding patients in labor) 30–60 mg, or **IV** 30 mg q 3–4 hr, to maximum of 360 mg/day. Based on duration of analgesic effect, dosing q 2.5 hr has been recommended.[70]

Pediatric Dose.   Not recommended in children under 12 yr.

Dosage Forms.   **Tab** (hydrochloride) 50 mg with naloxone 0.5 mg (Talwin® Nx); **Inj** (lactate) 30 mg/ml (Talwin®).

Patient Instructions.   This drug may cause dizziness; until the extent of this effect is known, use appropriate caution; report any mental changes.

Pharmacokinetics and Biopharmaceutics.   *Onset and Duration.* PO onset 15–30 min, duration 3 hr; SC or IM onset 15–20 min, duration 2–3 hr; IV onset 2–3 min, duration 1 hr.[71]
    Fate.   Well absorbed after parenteral administration; 11–32% of an oral dose is bioavailable, dependent almost entirely on first-pass metabolism.[72]

Peak plasma levels are attained in about 2.5 hr (oral), about 45 min (IM) and about 30 min (IV).[73] Extensively metabolized in the liver, but rate of metabolism is highly variable. Data suggest that urban living and/or smoking habits may increase the rate of metabolism.[74] 60-70% of dose is recovered in urine, of which 3-24% (higher amount in acidic urine and/or after IV use) is unchanged drug.[71,75]

$t_{1/2}$. 2.1 hr (IM).[71]

Adverse Reactions. Sedation, sweating, dizziness, nausea, euphoria and hallucinations are most frequent. Occasionally, insomnia, anxiety, constipation, dry mouth, syncope, visual blurring, flushing, decreased blood pressure and tachycardia are reported. Also, after oral use, rare GI distress, anorexia and vomiting are reported. After parenteral use, diaphoresis, sting on injection, respiratory depression, transient apnea in newborn from use in mother during labor, shock, urinary retention and alterations in uterine contractions during labor occur rarely. Other rarely reported effects include muscle tremor and toxic epidermal necrolysis. Local skin reactions, and ulceration and fibrous myopathy at the injection site have been reported with long-term parenteral use.[70,75]

Contraindications. Children under 12 yr.

Precautions. See Morphine. Also, use cautiously in patients with myocardial infarction because pentazocine increases cardiac workload. There are reports of dependence and withdrawal symptoms following extended use.[76]

Notes. Oral use is about one-third as potent as IM pentazocine use[77] and to achieve comparable plasma levels, 75 mg orally is approximately equivalent to 40 mg IM.[71] 30-60 mg parenteral pentazocine is approximately equivalent to 10 mg of morphine and 75-100 mg of meperidine.[76] Effects of pentazocine are antagonized by naloxone only (ie, not by nalorphine or levallorphan).

Phenylbutazone   Azolid®, Butazolidin®, Various

Pharmacology. See Ibuprofen. In doses of 600 mg/day, it also has mild uricosuric activity; low doses decrease urate excretion.

Administration and Adult Dose. **PO for rheumatoid arthritis, ankylosing spondylitis, acute osteoarthritis or painful shoulder** 300-600 mg/day in 3-4 divided doses initially, then maintain at the minimum effective dose to a maximum of 400 mg/day; discontinue drug after a week in the absence of a favorable response. **PO for gouty arthritis** 400 mg initially, then 100 mg q 4-6 hr for no longer than one week. **PO for acute superficial thrombophlebitis** 600 mg/day in divided doses for 2-3 days, then 300 mg/day for no longer than a total of 7-10 days.

Pediatric Dose. Not recommended in children 14 yr and under.

Dosage Forms. Cap 100 mg; Tab 100 mg.

Patient Instructions. This drug is to be taken with food, milk or an antacid to minimize stomach upset. Dizziness may occur; until the extent of this effect is known, use appropriate caution. Report fever, sore throat, oral lesions, salivary gland enlargement, skin rash, itching, weight gain, fluid accumulation, black tarry stools or blood in the stool.

Pharmacokinetics and Biopharmaceutics. *Fate.* Generally well absorbed from GI tract, although bioavailability problems among brands have been reported.[78] Azolid®, Butazolidin®, and generic products from Chelsa and Cord appear to be bioequivalent. Slow but extensive hepatic metabolism to oxyphenbutazone (having anti-inflammatory and sodium-retaining activity) and γ-hydroxyphenylbutazone (having uricosuric, but no anti-inflammatory or sodium-retaining activity). 99% of phenylbutazone, 95% of oxyphenbutazone and a great amount of γ-hydroxyphenylbutazone are protein bound.[79] Following 3–4 days of an 800 mg/day oral dose, highly variable steady-state phenylbutazone levels (reflecting highly individual variations in metabolic rate) of 60–150 mcg/ml are attained. Increased dosage does not produce significant increases in the plasma level.[80] After an oral dose, urinary excretion of unchanged phenylbutazone is negligible, oxyphenbutazone is about 3% and γ-hydroxyphenylbutazone is about 4%.[81]

Adverse Reactions.   Frequent effects include nausea, vomiting and GI distress. Sodium and water retention, edema, dizziness and exacerbation of peptic ulcer occur occasionally. Rarely, agranulocytosis, aplastic anemia, thrombocytopenia, hepatotoxicity, nephritis, exfoliative dermatitis, Stevens-Johnson syndrome and erythema multiforme are observed.

Contraindications.   Children 14 yr and under; senile patients; history or symptoms of dyspepsia, GI inflammation or ulceration; blood dyscrasias, renal, hepatic or cardiac dysfunction; hypertension; thyroid disease; systemic edema; polymyalgia rheumatica and temporal arteritis; concomitant use with long-term anticoagulant therapy.

Precautions.   Careful instructions to, and observations of, the patient (especially the elderly) are essential to prevent serious, life-threatening adverse reactions. In elderly patients, restrict treatment to one week and discontinue drug if clinical edema appears; in patients under 60 yr, clinical edema unresponsive to dosage reduction is an indication to discontinue the drug. Serious and even fatal blood dyscrasias may occur suddenly or after many days or weeks following withdrawal of drug. Any significant change in total white cell count, decrease in granulocytes, appearance of immature forms or fall in hematocrit requires immediate cessation of drug and complete hematologic investigation. Use with caution in pregnancy and lactation, and in patients receiving antidiabetic and sulfonamide agents. See Drug Interactions chapter.

Parameters to Monitor.   The following should be accomplished at regular intervals: a detailed history of the disease and adverse reactions; a complete physical examination including a check of the patient's weight; and a weekly (especially in the elderly) or q 2 week CBC. Blurred vision may warrant a complete ophthalmologic examination.

Piroxicam   Feldene®

Piroxicam is an oxicam enolic acid nonsteroidal anti-inflammatory agent chemically and pharmacokinetically distinct from earlier compounds. Recent studies show piroxicam to be effective in patients with rheumatoid arthritis, osteoarthritis and ankylosing spondylitis. Some reports suggest superiority of piroxicam over other available nonsteroidal anti-inflammatory agents for these conditions. The half-life of the drug is about 41 hours which allows a single daily dosage regimen. Piroxicam is 98% protein bound and largely metabolized with only 10% excreted unchanged in the urine. Adverse effects appear to be similar to other available nonsteroidal anti-inflammatory agents, although some studies suggest that GI complaints and bleeding may be more frequent. Dosage is usually 20 mg in a single daily dose. Available as 10 and 20 mg capsules.[201,202]

Propoxyphene Hydrochloride
Darvon®, Various

Propoxyphene Napsylate
Darvon-N®

Pharmacology. Structurally similar to methadone. Pharmacologic actions similar to narcotic analgesics; however, analgesic effects may be inferior. Possesses little antitussive activity.

Administration and Adult Dose. PO (hydrochloride) 65 mg q 4 hr prn; PO (napsylate) 100 mg q 4 hr prn.

Pediatric Dose. Not recommended.

Dosage Forms. Cap 32, 65 mg (hydrochloride); **Tab** 100 mg (napsylate); **Susp** 10 mg/ml (napsylate).

Patient Instructions. This drug may cause drowsiness and/or dizziness; until the extent of this effect is known, caution should be used when driving, operating machinery or performing other tasks requiring mental alertness. Avoid excessive use of alcohol while taking this drug.

Pharmacokinetics and Biopharmaceutics. *Onset and Duration.*
PO onset about 1 hr.[82]
   Plasma Levels. Plasma concentrations over 2 mcg/ml, or over 1 mcg/ml when combined with other depressants, can cause death.[83]
   Fate. Rapid absorption of the hydrochloride from the GI tract and extensive first-pass hepatic metabolism to norpropoxyphene (activity unknown). Following a single 130 mg dose, peak propoxyphene plasma levels are reached in 2 hr and peak norpropoxyphene levels in 4 hr; propoxyphene and norpropoxyphene account for 20–25% of urinary excretion, of which 1–5% is unchanged drug.[84] The napsylate is relatively water insoluble and more slowly absorbed than the hydrochloride; however, it has been shown that the two salts exhibit similar plasma concentration-time curves and similar systemic availabilities when compared on an equimolar basis.[85]
   $t_{1/2}$. (Propoxyphene) 11.8 hr; (norpropoxyphene) 36.6 hr.[86]

Adverse Reactions. Dizziness, sedation, nausea and vomiting are most frequent. Occasionally constipation, euphoria, dysphoria, minor visual disturbances and skin rashes are observed. Chronic ingestion of doses exceeding 800 mg/day has caused toxic psychosis and convulsions.

Precautions. Pregnancy. Depressant effects may be additive with other CNS depressants; chronic administration can produce primarily psychic, but with high doses, also physical drug dependence.[87]

Notes. Clinical effectiveness is no greater than aspirin or codeine and may be inferior to these analgesics. A 32 mg dose of the hydrochloride lacks substantial evidence of efficacy beyond a placebo effect; higher doses of propoxyphene probably yield more analgesia.[82] Propoxyphene napsylate has been used successfully as an alternative to methadone for maintenance and detoxification of narcotic dependence. Usual starting doses are 800–1,200 mg/day in 2–4 divided doses.[88]

Narcotic Analgesics Comparison Chart[a]

DRUG	DOSAGE FORMS	EQUIVALENT IM DOSE[b] (MG)	ORAL/PARENTERAL EFFICACY RATIO	DURATION OF ANALGESIA (HOURS)	CARDIAC WORKLOAD	PARTIAL ANTAGONIST ACTIVITY
Alphaprodine Nisentil®	Inj 40, 60 mg/ml	45	—	1–2	↓	no
Butorphanol Stadol®	Inj 1, 2 mg/ml	2	1/16	3–4	↑	yes
Codeine Various	Inj 30, 60 mg/ml Hyp Tab 15, 30, 60 mg Tab 15, 30, 60 mg	120 [30]	1/2–2/3	3–6	↓	no
Hydromorphone Dilaudid® Various	Inj 1, 2, 3, 4, 10 mg/ml Tab 1, 2, 3, 4 mg Supp 3 mg	1.5 [1]	1/5	4–5	↓	no
Meperidine Demerol® Various	Inj 25, 50, 75, 100 mg/ml Tab 50, 100 mg Syrup 10 mg/ml	100 [50]	1/3–1/2	2–4	↓	no
Methadone Dolophine® Various	Inj 10 mg/ml Tab 5, 10 mg Dispersible Tab 40 mg Soln 1 mg/ml	10 [3]	1/2	3–5	↓	no
Morphine Various	Inj 8, 10, 15 mg Tab 10, 15, 30 mg Soln 10, 20 mg/5 ml	10 [9]	1/6	4–5	↓	no

Continued

Narcotic Analgesics Comparison Chart[a]

DRUG	DOSAGE FORMS	EQUIVALENT IM DOSE[b] (MG)	ORAL/PARENTERAL EFFICACY RATIO	DURATION OF ANALGESIA (HOURS)	CARDIAC WORKLOAD	PARTIAL ANTAGONIST ACTIVITY
Nalbuphine Nubain®	Inj 10 mg/ml	10	1/6	3–6	↓	yes
Oxycodone	Tab 5 mg with acetaminophen 325 mg (Percocet-5®, Various); 5 mg with aspirin 325 mg (Percodan®); 2.5 mg with aspirin 325 mg (Percodan-Demi®)	15 [5]	1/2	3–4	↓	no
Pentazocine Talwin® Talwin® Nx	Inj 30 mg/ml Tab 50 mg with naloxone 0.5 mg	50 [25]	1/3	2–3	↑	yes

a. From references 1-4, 43, 49, 204.
b. Doses in brackets are oral/ doses equivalent to about 30 mg of oral codeine; due to individual variability in absorption, equivalent doses may differ between patients.

Nonsteroidal Anti-Inflammatory Agents Comparison Chart[a]

DRUG	DAILY DOSAGE RANGE FOR RHEUMATOID ARTHRITIS	HALF-LIFE (HOURS)	PERCENT PROTEIN BOUND	INTERACTION WITH ORAL ANTICOAGULANTS[b]
Aspirin Various	3.6–6 g divided q 4 hr	2–25 (dose-dependent)	95 (salicylate)	Likely
Diflunisal Dolobid®	500 mg bid for mild-moderate pain	10	99	Possible
Fenoprofen Nalfon®	2.4–3.2 g in 4 divided doses	2.5	99	Possible
Ibuprofen Motrin®	1.6–2.4 g in 3–4 divided doses	1.9	99	Unlikely
Indomethacin Indocin®	75–150 mg in 3 divided doses	7	97	Possible
Meclofenamate Meclomen®	200–400 mg in 3–4 divided doses	3	?	Likely
Naproxen Anaprox® Naprosyn®	500–750 mg in 2 divided doses	13	99	Unlikely
Oxaprozin (Investigational-Wyeth)	1.2 g once daily	40	99	Unlikely

Continued

Nonsteroidal Anti-Inflammatory Agents Comparison Chart[a]

DRUG	DAILY DOSAGE RANGE FOR RHEUMATOID ARTHRITIS	HALF-LIFE (HOURS)	PERCENT PROTEIN BOUND	INTERACTION WITH ORAL ANTICOAGULANTS[b]
Phenylbutazone Azolid® Butazolidin® Various	300–400 mg in 3–4 divided doses	72	99	Very Likely
Piroxicam Feldene®	20 mg once daily	41	98	Unknown
Sulindac Clinoril®	300–400 mg in 2 divided doses	18 (active sulfide metabolite)	93 (sulindac) 98 (sulfide)	Likely
Tolmetin Tolectin®	1.2–2 g in 3–4 divided doses	1	99	Unlikely
Zomepirac Zomax®	200–400 mg divided q 4–6 hr for mild-moderate pain	4	98	Possible

a. Adapted from references 5, 6, 89, 90, 201, 202.
b. Refers to alteration in prothrombin time only; all of these agents cause gastritis and interfere with platelet function.

28:10 NARCOTIC ANTAGONISTS

Naloxone Hydrochloride   Narcan®

Pharmacology. An allyl derivative of hydromorphone which is a competitive narcotic antagonist. It is essentially free of narcotic agonist properties and is used in the reversal of overdoses with narcotic drugs.

Administration and Adult Dose. **IV (preferred), IM or SC for known or suspected narcotic overdose** 0.4 mg initially, may repeat q 2-3 min for 2-3 doses. Dosing may be repeated prn, with the frequency of repeat doses based on clinical evaluation of the patient; repeat doses up to 0.1 mg/kg have been recommended if there is no response to the first dose;[91] a trial of at least 3 doses should precede the determination that no narcotic is present. The duration of therapy is dependent on the narcotic that has been taken.[92]

Pediatric Dose. **IV, IM or SC for known or suspected narcotic overdose** 0.01 mg/kg initially, may be repeated like the adult dose. This dose has been given IM or into the umbilical vein to reverse neonatal respiratory depression resulting from narcotic use during labor.[93,94]

Dosage Forms. Inj 0.02, 0.4 mg/ml.

Pharmacokinetics and Biopharmaceutics. *Onset and Duration.* Onset IV within 2 min, slightly longer when given IM or SC; duration reported up to several hr, but practical duration probably 1 hr or less.[95,96]

  Fate. 59-67% metabolized by hepatic conjugation and renal elimination of the conjugated compound.[97]

  $t_{1/2}$. 60-90 min in adults;[98,99] about 3 hr in neonates.[99]

Precautions. Administration to narcotic-dependent persons (including neonates of dependent mothers) may precipitate acute withdrawal symptoms.

Parameters to Monitor. Respiratory rate, pupil size (may not be useful in mixed drug overdoses), heart rate, blood pressure, symptoms of acute narcotic withdrawal syndrome.

Notes. Effective in reversing agonist-antagonist narcotics (eg, butorphanol, nalbuphine, pentazocine) as well as diphenoxylate and propoxyphene-induced respiratory depression. Naloxone can be routinely given to patients with coma of unknown etiology.

28:12 ANTICONVULSANTS

General References: 100-103

Class Instructions. It is important to take this drug as directed. Discontinuing this medication could result in increased seizure activity. This drug may cause drowsiness; until the extent of this effect is known, caution should be used when driving, operating machinery or performing other tasks requiring mental alertness. Avoid excessive concurrent use of alcohol and other drugs which cause drowsiness. Report any difficulty in walking, slurring of speech or abnormal sleepiness. Report to your physician if you should become pregnant.

Carbamazepine

Tegretol®

Pharmacology. An anticonvulsant whose effects resemble those of phenytoin. Chemically related to the tricyclic antidepressants; electrophysiological effects responsible for anticonvulsant activity are unknown.

Administration and Adult Dose. PO for epilepsy 200 mg bid initially. Increase gradually in 200 mg/day increments to optimum effect, to maximum of 1.2 g/day. For doses of 800 mg/day or greater, tid or qid dosing is recommended. The average patient requires 450–700 mg/M^2/day. **PO for trigeminal neuralgia** 100 mg bid initially. Increase by up to 200 mg/day in increments of 100 mg q 12 hr, to maximum of 1.2 g/day. Adjust to minimum effective maintenance dose, usually 400–800 mg/day.

Pediatric Dose. PO 225 mg/M^2/day in 2 divided doses initially; 450–700 mg/M^2/day in 2–4 divided doses for maintenance to maximum of 1 g/day. See also Phenobarbital Notes.

Dosage Forms. Tab 200 mg.

Patient Instructions. Sore throat, fever or oral lesions may be an early sign of a severe, but rare blood disorder and should be reported immediately. See also Class Instructions.

Pharmacokinetics and Biopharmaceutics. *Onset and Duration.* Steady-state plasma levels may be reached in 2–4 days.[100]

    Plasma Levels. 4–12 mcg/ml; level-related side effects include vertigo, dizziness, drowsiness, ataxia and diplopia (rare below 6 mcg/ml, frequent above 8.5 mcg/ml).[100-102]

    Fate. About 70% of an oral dose is absorbed slowly, with peak plasma concentrations reached in 6–18 hr. V_d is 0.79–1.8 L/kg; Cl is 0.025–0.096 L/hr/kg. 60–73% bound to plasma proteins; slightly lower in patients with hepatic disease. After multiple doses, about 15% is converted to a possibly active metabolite, carbamazepine-10, 11-epoxide (see Notes). About 2% of drug is excreted unchanged in the urine. Combined treatment with other anticonvulsants (eg, phenytoin, phenobarbital) may decrease plasma half-life necessitating more frequent dosing.[100,103]

    $t_{1/2}$. 30–60 hr after a single dose. 5–20 hr after multiple dosing, suggesting self-induction of metabolism.[100,104]

Adverse Reactions. When dosage is increased by small increments over 7–10 days, side effects are minimized. See Plasma Levels. Water intoxication has occasionally been reported and may be related to elevated levels.[102] Occasionally headache, nausea, stomatitis and rashes occur; rare aplastic anemia, renal damage and lenticular opacities are reported (the onset of aplastic anemia is reported to occur from 3 weeks to 2 yr after therapy is begun).

Contraindications. History of previous bone marrow depression.

Precautions. Pregnancy. Because of structural relationship to tricyclic antidepressants, MAO inhibitors should be discontinued a minimum of 14 days before carbamazepine therapy is begun — see also Drug Interactions chapter. Abrupt withdrawal of the drug in patients with epilepsy may precipitate status epilepticus.

Parameters to Monitor. Plasma levels should be monitored at least twice during the first month of therapy because of the possibility of self-induction of metabolism;[103] then, any time toxicity or lack of efficacy is suspected.[101] Baseline CBC and renal function tests should be performed.

Notes. It has been suggested that the carbamazepine-10, 11-epoxide metabolite may contribute to the clinical effect as well as to side effects.[100]

Clonazepam   Clonopin®

Pharmacology. As with other benzodiazepines, appears to enhance the effectiveness of the inhibitory neurotransmitter γ-aminobutyric acid. Suppresses the spread of seizure activity produced by epileptogenic foci, but does not abolish abnormal discharge.

Administration and Adult Dose. PO initial dose should not exceed 1.5 mg/day in 3 divided doses. Then, adjust in 0.5–1 mg/day increments q 3 days to optimum effect, to maximum of 20 mg/day.

Pediatric Dose. PO (up to 10 yr or 30 kg) initial dose is 10–30 mcg/kg/day in 2–3 divided doses. Then, adjust in 0.25–0.5 mg/day increments q 3 days until a maintenance dose of 100–200 mcg/kg/day is reached, or optimum effect is attained. See also Phenobarbital Notes.

Dosage Forms. Tab 0.5, 1, 2 mg.

Patient Instructions. See Class Instructions.

Pharmacokinetics and Biopharmaceutics. *Onset and Duration.* With daily oral doses, steady-state plasma levels are reached in 4–12 days.[100]
   Plasma Levels. 20–70 ng/ml. Very few controlled trials have been performed to evaluate the relationship between plasma levels and therapeutic effect.[104,105] Level-related side effects include drowsiness, ataxia, dizziness and dysphoria (greater than 60 ng/ml); and increased frequency of seizures (greater than 100 ng/ml).[100,103]
   Fate. 47–85% bound to plasma proteins.[103,105] V_d is 2–6 L/kg; Cl is about 0.05 L/hr/kg.[100,103] Steady-state plasma levels may be reduced when other anticonvulsants (eg, phenytoin, phenobarbital) are added to the regimen.[100,105] 98% is converted to two inactive metabolites and 2% is excreted unchanged in the urine.[100]
   $t_{1/2}$. 19–60 hr (average 36).[103]

Adverse Reactions. See Plasma Levels. Frequent drowsiness and ataxia occur, which may diminish with time; behavioral and psychiatric problems occur occasionally. Rarely, transient changes in liver function tests, anemia, thrombocytopenia, leukopenia and respiratory depression are observed.

Contraindications. Significant liver disease; acute narrow angle glaucoma.

Precautions. Pregnancy. May increase the frequency of generalized seizures in patients with mixed seizure disorders. Abrupt withdrawal of the drug in patients with epilepsy may precipitate status epilepticus.

Parameters to Monitor. Plasma level monitoring is controversial because of limited information relating therapeutic effects and adverse reactions to plasma levels.[100]

Notes. Although a parenteral preparation is not yet available in the US, evidence suggests that clonazepam may be more effective than diazepam in status epilepticus; single IV doses of 1–4 mg are usually sufficient, although some patients may require multiple injections.[105]

Ethosuximide   Zarontin®

Pharmacology. A succinimide anticonvulsant that is very selective in suppressing the spike-and-wave EEG pattern of absence seizures.

Administration and Adult Dose. **PO** initial dose is 500 mg/day, then adjust q 4–7 days in 250 mg/day increments to optimum effect, to maximum of 1.5 g/day.

Pediatric Dose. **PO** (under 6 yr) 250 mg/day initially, then adjust q 4–7 days by 250 mg/day to optimum effect, to maximum of 1.5 g/day; (over 6 yr) same as adult dose, given in 2 divided doses. The optimal daily dose for most children is 20–40 mg/kg/day. See also Phenobarbital Notes.

Dosage Forms. **Cap** 250 mg; **Syrup** 50 mg/ml.

Patient Instructions. This drug may be taken with food, milk or an antacid to minimize stomach upset. See also Class Instructions.

Pharmacokinetics and Biopharmaceutics. *Onset and Duration.* Steady-state plasma concentrations are reached in 8–10 days.[106]
  Plasma Levels. (Therapeutic) 40–100 mcg/ml.[103]
  Fate. Well absorbed orally; not significantly protein bound. V_d is 0.6–0.7 L/kg; Cl is 0.012–0.016 L/hr/kg.[103] About 80% is converted to three inactive metabolites. 20% is excreted unchanged in the urine at steady-state.[100,106]
  $t_{1/2}$. (Adults) 56 hr; (children) 24 hr.[106]

Adverse Reactions. Frequent dose-related side effects are GI upset, drowsiness and dizziness; these may diminish with time. Occasionally, parkinson-like symptoms, photophobia and agitation are seen; rarely, Stevens-Johnson syndrome, SLE, leukopenia, thrombocytopenia and aplastic anemia are reported.

Precautions. Pregnancy. May increase the frequency of generalized seizures in patients with mixed seizure disorders. Abrupt withdrawal of the drug may precipitate petit mal status.

Parameters to Monitor. Plasma levels are suggested, although therapeutic range is based on only a few controlled studies.[100] Periodic CBC should be performed.

Phenobarbital   Various

Pharmacology. A barbiturate anticonvulsant that limits the spread of seizure activity and increases the threshold for electrical stimulation of the motor cortex. Anticonvulsant activity is unrelated to sedation. See also Phenobarbital 28:24.

Administration and Adult Dose. **PO for epilepsy** 1–5 mg/kg/day initially, then slowly adjust to optimum effect; usual dose is 100–200 mg/day. Because of a long half-life, the drug can be taken once daily, usually at bedtime. Some investigators have suggested using double the initial maintenance dose for the first 4 days in order to reach steady-state plasma levels more quickly (about 3–4 days).[107] **IM for status epilepticus** 4–6 mg/kg (200–600 mg). See Phenobarbital 28:24 for sedative dosage. **SC not recommended.**

Dosage Individualization. Dosage reduction may be necessary in severe chronic liver disease or in renal impairment.[100,108]

Pediatric Dose. **PO for epilepsy** 3–6 mg/kg/day, adjust to individual requirements. **IM** 3.5 mg/kg/dose. See Notes.

Patient Instructions. See Class Instructions.

Dosage Forms. **Drops** 16 mg/ml; **Elxr** 4 mg/ml; **Tab** 8, 16, 32, 65, 100 mg; **Inj** 30, 65, 130, 163 mg/ml; **Pwdr for Inj** 65, 120, 130, 325 mg.

Pharmacokinetics and Biopharmaceutics. *Onset and Duration.*

Steady-state plasma concentrations are achieved in 1.5–4 weeks.[107] IM 20–60 min required for peak effect.[109]

Plasma Levels. (Anticonvulsant) 15–45 mcg/ml.[112]

Fate. About 80% oral absorption, although variable, with 20–45% bound to plasma proteins. V_d is 0.6–1.01 L/kg; Cl is 0.003–0.013 L/hr/kg.[103] Peak plasma levels after oral dosage occur in 8–18 hr.[110,111] There is much individual variation in metabolism and elimination; about 65% is converted to the inactive metabolite para-hydroxyphenobarbital. 35% is excreted unchanged in the urine; acidic urine may increase, and alkaline urine decrease half-life.[100,106]

$t_{1/2}$. (Adults) 2–5 days; (children) 1.6–2.9 days.[100] In one study, half-life increased to 5.4 days in chronic liver disease, while remaining unchanged in acute liver disease.[108]

Adverse Reactions. Most frequent dose-related side effect is sedation, to which tolerance usually develops. Children and the elderly may become paradoxically excited and hyperactive. Occasionally, skin rashes, disturbances in motor function and megaloblastic anemia may occur. Rarely, Stevens-Johnson syndrome, exfoliative dermatitis, photosensitivity, hepatitis and jaundice have been reported. SC administration may result in necrosis or sloughing; IV administration may cause injury to adjacent nerves and extravasation can produce tissue necrosis.[112]

Contraindications. Respiratory disease where dyspnea or obstruction is present; marked renal impairment.

Precautions. Pregnancy. Use with caution in presence of porphyria or severe cardiac disease and in patients with pulmonary or cardiovascular disease. Severe liver disease might be expected to decrease metabolism to the drug's inactive metabolite, although information is limited. In patients with renal disease increased toxicity has been observed.[100] See Drug Interactions chapter. Abrupt withdrawal of the drug in patients with epilepsy may precipitate status epilepticus.

Parameters to Monitor. Plasma levels should be obtained at the onset of therapy to see if they are adequate. This is unnecessary if a clear therapeutic effect is indicated by cessation of epilepsy. Plasma levels should then be obtained during therapy after steady-state is achieved and any time toxicity or lack of efficacy is suspected.[101]

Notes. Febrile seizures in infants may be controlled by phenobarbital, but not with phenytoin.[107] Do not mix with other injectables. In overdosage, excretion may be enhanced by alkalinizing the urine. Children with epilepsy who have had no seizures for 4 years while taking anticonvulsants have about a 70% chance of remaining free of seizures after drugs are withdrawn. Recurrence rate is lowest in children who have had few seizures and those with a normal or mildly abnormal electroencephalogram at the time of drug discontinuation.[113]

Phenytoin   Dilantin®, Various

Pharmacology. A hydantoin anticonvulsant which exerts its effects without general CNS depression by limiting maximal seizure activity. It also reduces the spread of focal seizure activity through promotion of neuronal sodium outflow.

Administration and Adult Dose. PO 4–6 mg/kg/day. Usual initial dose is PO 100 mg tid, then adjust in increments of 50–100 mg/day q 2 weeks. Due to dose-related kinetics, small increases in dose may produce greater than proportional increases in plasma levels. Using plasma levels as a guide, many patients can be dosed once or twice daily to increase compliance.[100] Of the currently marketed phenytoin products, only Dilantin Kapseals® are classified as "extended" and approved for once-a-day use. **PO loading dose** 1 g in divided doses (400 mg, 300 mg, 300 mg) over a 4 hr period, followed in about 24 hr by a daily dose of 300–400 mg can be used to achieve therapeutic plasma levels in 8–24 hr.[114] **IV loading dose** 1 g (or calculated dose based on V_d) can be given at a rate no greater than 50 mg/min to achieve a rapid onset. When direct IV administration is impractical, the loading dose can be added to a volume control set and diluted with 0.45% or 0.9% sodium chloride solution to a concentration of 20–30 mg/ml.[115] Phenytoin is also stable in lactated Ringer's injection over a concentration range of 0.4–4.55 mg/ml.[116] **IM administration not recommended** because of slow, erratic absorption and painful local reactions. If no other route is available, some investigators suggest a 50% increase in IM dosage with respect to the PO dose, to prevent a fall in plasma concentration; follow by a PO dose 50% less than original PO dose for the same period of time the patient received the IM dose.[100] However, firm recommendations are lacking with regard to proper IM dosage.[117]

Dosage Individualization. In chronic uremia, phenytoin is displaced from plasma proteins, thus decreasing total plasma concentration and increasing the free fraction of drug.[101,118,119] Dosage modification is unnecessary because the concentration of unbound drug remains unchanged. Therefore, lower plasma concentrations are required to maintain therapeutic effects similar to those of nonuremics. The effect is more dramatic in uremics with reduced albumin concentrations. Dosage increase may be necessary in pregnancy because of enhanced clearance.[120]

Pediatric Dose. PO 5–7 mg/kg/day in 1–2 doses, adjust to individual requirements. **PO loading dose** 500–600 mg, followed in about 24 hr by a daily dose of 200 mg has been used.[114] See also Phenobarbital Notes.

Dosage Forms. (Phenytoin) **Chew Tab** 50 mg; **Susp** 30, 125 mg/5 ml. (Phenytoin sodium) **Cap** 30, 100 mg; **Inj** 50 mg/ml.

Patient Instructions. This drug may be taken with food or milk to minimize stomach upset. Shake oral suspension prior to each dose. See also Class Instructions.

Pharmacokinetics and Biopharmaceutics. *Onset and Duration.* Without a loading dose, steady-state plasma levels are not achieved for 5–15 days.[106]
    Plasma Levels. 10–20 mcg/ml;[100,101] level-related side effects include nystagmus (greater than 20 mcg/ml),[106] ataxia (greater than 30 mcg/ml), and somnolence (greater than 40 mcg/ml).[103]
    Fate. Absorption rate is slow and variable; usually 90% is absorbed from properly designed dosage forms.[106] Differences in bioavailability be-

tween pharmaceutical preparations may occur; brand or batch changes may cause alterations in plasma levels.[121] Evidence suggests that chewable tablets and capsules are bio-equivalent.[105] Continuous NG feedings may interfere with PO absorption.[205] IM absorption is slow and erratic.[117] V_d is 0.5-0.8 L/kg;[103] 87-93% (average 90) is bound to plasma proteins;[100,106] free fraction is 10% in normals, 20% in uremics with normal serum albumin and 20-35% in uremics with reduced albumin concentrations.[119] The major inactive metabolite of phenytoin is 5-(p-hydroxyphenyl)-5-phenylhydantoin (HPPH). 60-75% of the daily dose is excreted in urine as HPPH, and 1-5% of the drug is excreted in urine unchanged.[100]

$t_{1/2}$. Highly variable, due to dose-related saturation kinetics. Half-life increases as plasma levels increase and ranges from 8-60 hr (average 22);[100,103] half-life is decreased in uremia; about 8 hr with serum creatinine greater than 5 mg/dl;[118,122] and unchanged in acute liver disease in one study.[123]

Adverse Reactions. See Plasma Levels. Frequently nausea and vomiting are seen with high oral doses. Gum hyperplasia occurs frequently.[124] Occasional megaloblastic anemia due to folate deficiency occurs (see Notes) and chronic therapy may result in metabolic bone disease (osteomalacia). Rarely, pseudolymphoma and SLE are reported.[124] When given IV at a rate exceeding 50 mg/min, hypotension, cardiovascular collapse and CNS depression may occur. This is partially due to the propylene glycol solvent.[125]

Precautions. Pregnancy. Do not administer IV at a rate exceeding 50 mg/min. Patients with liver disease have highly variable plasma clearance rates for phenytoin.[100] Abrupt drug withdrawal in patients with epilepsy may precipitate status epilepticus. See Drug Interactions chapter.

Parameters to Monitor. Obtain levels at the onset of therapy to see if they are adequate. This is unnecessary if a clear therapeutic effect is indicated by cessation of epilepsy. Plasma levels should then be taken during therapy after steady-state is achieved and any time toxicity or lack of efficacy is suspected.[101] Frequently observe for nystagmus and ataxia.

Notes. Parenteral phenytoin forms a precipitate and/or microcrystals in dextrose-containing solutions; microcrystals are slowly formed in saline solutions.[126] Prolonged phenytoin therapy may result in folic acid deficiency; whether such patients should be treated with folic acid is controversial; lowering of plasma phenytoin concentrations has been reported when patients were given folic acid.[124,206] Failure to agitate the oral suspension prior to each dose may produce initial under-dosing, followed progressively by overdosing as the liquid is used. Phenytoin has antiarrhythmic properties and appears to be particularly useful in digitalis glycoside-induced arrhythmias.[43] Phenytoin is not useful in infantile febrile seizures.[107]

Primidone   Mysoline®

Pharmacology. See Phenobarbital.

Administration and Adult Dose. PO 250 mg/day initially, then adjust weekly in increments of 250 mg/day, in divided doses, to optimum effect; maintenance dose is 10-25 mg/kg/day, to maximum of 2 g/day.[128]

Pediatric Dose. PO (under 8 yr) 125 mg/day initially, then adjust weekly in increments of 125 mg/day to optimum effect; maintenance dose is 5-20 mg/kg/day;[128] (over 8 yr) same as adult dose. See also Phenobarbital Notes.

Dosage Forms. **Susp** 50 mg/ml; **Tab** 50, 250 mg.

Patient Instructions. See Class Instructions.

Pharmacokinetics and Biopharmaceutics. *Plasma Levels.* For primidone 5-10 mcg/ml.[129] The therapeutic significance of the plasma levels of primidone in relation to its two active metabolites is not well understood.[100,101] See also Phenobarbital.

Fate. 60-80% of an oral dose is absorbed. Primidone is converted in the liver to two active metabolites, phenylethylmalonamide (PEMA) and phenobarbital. Formation of PEMA is rapid; phenobarbital may not be detected in the plasma until 3-4 days after therapy is initiated. Almost no primidone is excreted unchanged in the urine.[100,107]

$t_{1/2}$. (Primidone) 5-10 hr; (PEMA) 24-48 hr.[129] See also Phenobarbital.

Adverse Reactions. Sedation and ataxia are frequent, but tend to diminish with continued therapy. Occasionally nausea, vomiting, folic acid deficiency and megaloblastic anemia are seen. Rarely, leukopenia, thrombocytopenia, SLE and lymphadenopathy occur.[107]

Precautions. Pregnancy. Use with caution in porphyria. Abrupt withdrawal of the drug in patients with epilepsy may precipitate status epilepticus.

Parameters to Monitor. Firm recommendations concerning plasma monitoring are lacking; however, determination of both primidone and phenobarbital levels are suggested.[100,129]

Valproic Acid   Depakene®
Divalproex   Depakote®

Pharmacology. A carboxylic acid whose mechanism of action may be related to increased brain levels of the inhibitory neurotransmitter γ-aminobutyric acid (GABA). There is evidence that this increase results from competitive inhibition of enzymes which catabolize GABA.

Administration and Adult Dose. PO 15 mg/kg/day initially in 3-4 divided doses; however, some authors recommend 7-10 mg/kg/day initially to minimize GI and sedative side effects.[130] Increase dose by 5-10 mg/kg/day at weekly intervals to optimum effect, to maximum of 60 mg/kg/day.

Pediatric Dose. PO same as adult dose. Average daily doses used in one trial were (under 3 yr) 54 mg/kg; (4-7 yr) 43 mg/kg; (8-11 yr) 33 mg/kg; (over 12 yr) 23 mg/kg.[131] See also Phenobarbital Notes.

Dosage Forms. **Cap** 250 mg; **Syrup** 250 mg/5 ml (as sodium) (Depakene®). **EC Tab** 250, 500 mg (Depakote®).

Patient Instructions. This drug may be taken with food or milk to minimize stomach upset. See also Class Instructions.

Pharmacokinetics and Biopharmaceutics. *Onset and Duration.* Steady-state plasma levels are achieved in 3-4 days.[103]

Plasma Levels. Therapeutic levels appear to range from 50-100 mcg/ml; levels greater than 100-150 mcg/ml may be associated with a higher prevalence of altered behavior, confusion and reduced seizure control.[103,130,132]

Fate. Rapidly and completely absorbed; absorption may be delayed if taken with a meal.[133] 80-95% (average 90) bound to plasma proteins. When plasma levels exceed 100 mcg/ml, the free drug fraction increases as binding sites become saturated.[103,130,133] At very high plasma concentrations, the unbound fraction may be greater than 50%.[133] Decreased protein binding has been demonstrated in patients with cirrhosis from acute viral hepatitis.[133] Four major metabolic pathways have been identified; the 3-oxo-valproic acid metabolite appears to have activity equal to valproic acid.[133] 2–7% of valproic acid is excreted unchanged in the urine.[130,133]

$t_{1/2}$. (Adults and children over 3 yr) 8–20 hr (ave 12); (children under 3 yr) 10–67 hr (longest in children under 2 months). In patients with acute viral hepatitis half-life was prolonged to 25.1 hr from an average of 14.9 hr.[133]

Adverse Reactions. See Plasma Levels. Anorexia, nausea and vomiting, and sedation are frequent. Hepatotoxicity occurs occasionally and is usually transient and asymptomatic;[130] some patients develop toxic hepatitis, and fatalities resulting from hepatic failure have been reported. In some patients who develop isolated increases in hepatic enzymes (SGOT, SGPT), reversion to normal may occur with a dosage reduction of *at least* 10 mg/kg/day.[207] The drug should be discontinued in all patients who develop changes in albumin, prothrombin time or alkaline phosphatase. Rarely tremor, ataxia, diplopia, asterixis, alopecia and curly hair, as well as thrombocytopenia and altered platelet function have been reported.

Precautions. Pregnancy. Use with caution in patients with pre-existing hepatic disease. Absence status has occurred in patients also receiving clonazepam. See Drug Interactions chapter.

Parameters to Monitor. Plasma level monitoring may be useful in reducing toxicity.[103] Liver function tests, platelet counts and bleeding time should be performed before initiating therapy and at frequent intervals thereafter.

Notes. Eliminated partly as ketone bodies which may cause a false-positive test for ketones in the urine. Altered thyroid function tests of unknown significance are reported.

Anticonvulsants Comparison Chart[a]

DRUG	SEIZURE TYPE AND DRUGS OF CHOICE				DOSAGE AND PLASMA LEVELS		THERAPEUTIC PLASMA LEVELS (MCG/ML)
	GRAND MAL & FOCAL MOTOR	PSYCHOMOTOR	PETIT MAL	MYOCLONIC	AVERAGE DAILY DOSE (MG/KG) ADULT	CHILD	
Phenytoin	A,E	A,E	—	—	4–6	5–7	10–20
Phenobarbital	A,E	C,E	D,E	—	1–5	3–6	15–45
Primidone	C,E	B,E	—	C	10–25	5–20	5–10
Carbamazepine	C,E	A,E	—	—	17–25	450–700 mg/M²/day	4–12
Clonazepam	—	—	B,E	A[b]	0.1–0.2	0.1–0.2	0.02–0.07
Ethosuximide	—	—	A,E	—	20–30	20–60	40–100
Valproic Acid	C,E	—	B,E	B,E	15–30	15–30	50–100

a. This table is a guide to the selection of the most appropriate anticonvulsant for the seizure type listed, but is not an all-inclusive guide to therapy. Consult references 100, 101, 103, 107, 128, 130 for further information.

b. Other benzodiazepines may be drugs of first and second choice.

Key:
A Drug of choice.
B Drug of second choice, if patient unable to tolerate or unresponsive to first choice.
C Drug of third choice, if patient unable to tolerate or unresponsive to second choice.
D Drug of little value and in some cases may make seizure type worse.
E Drug useful in combination with one or more other anticonvulsants.

28:16 PSYCHOTHERAPEUTIC AGENTS

General References: 154-156

Class Instructions. This drug may cause drowsiness. Until the extent of this effect is known, caution should be used when driving, operating machinery or performing other tasks requiring mental alertness. Avoid excessive concurrent use of alcohol and other drugs which cause drowsiness. This drug may also cause dry mouth, blurring of vision or constipation.

28:16.04 ANTIDEPRESSANTS

Monoamine Oxidase Inhibitors

Pharmacology. The antidepressant action of monoamine oxidase inhibitors (MAOIs) is presumably due to increased concentrations of catecholamines and indolamines, resulting from decreased metabolism by MAO in the CNS.

Administration and Adult Dose. See MAOIs Comparison Chart for oral dosage range. Phenelzine dose is 1 mg/kg/day.[134] Doses should be initiated at the lower limit and titrated upward depending on tolerance to side effects. Dosage schedule should remain divided, usually bid or tid.

Dosage Individualization. Initial dosage and rate of upward dosage titration should be reduced if the patient has taken a tricyclic antidepressant within 7-10 days.

Pediatric Dose. Not recommended in children under 16 yr.

Dosage Forms. See MAOIs Comparison Chart.[134,136]

Patient Instructions. This drug usually takes 2 weeks for significant response and up to 4 weeks for full therapeutic benefit to occur. Nausea and vomiting, sweating, severe occipital headache and stiff neck may be a sign of a serious adverse effect and should be reported immediately. Avoid concurrent use of diet pills, cough and cold remedies and restrict consumption of aged foods high in tyramine (see Tyramine in Food and Beverages in the Dietary Considerations chapter). See also Class Instructions.

Pharmacokinetics and Biopharmaceutics. *Onset and Duration.* Onset 2 weeks, while maximum improvement occurs after 4 weeks.[134,135] Central MAO inhibition reaches its peak within 2-4 weeks.
   Fate. Termination of drug action is dependent upon MAO regeneration, because the drugs or their active metabolites chemically combine with MAO.

Adverse Reactions. Autonomic effects are frequent and are not necessarily dose-dependent; these include postural hypotension, dry mouth and constipation. Drowsiness is more frequent with phenelzine, while overstimulation and agitation is more likely with tranylcypromine. Occasionally delayed ejaculation, edema, skin rash, urinary retention and blurred vision occur.[134,135] Of special concern is hypertensive crisis resulting from concurrent use of sympathomimetic amines or ingestion of high tyramine-content food and drinks.[136]

Contraindications. Patients over 60 yr; patients with confirmed or suspected cerebrovascular defect; cardiovascular disease; hypertension;

pheochromocytoma; history of liver disease or abnormal liver function tests.

Precautions. Combinations with sympathomimetic drugs, tricyclic antidepressants and other MAOIs should be avoided; postural hypotension may be increased when phenothiazine, tricyclic antidepressant or antihypertensive drugs are co-administered—see Drug Interactions chapter. Avoid diets high in tyramine content—see Tyramine in Food and Beverages in the Dietary Considerations chapter. Like other antidepressant drugs, MAOIs may switch bipolar patients to a hypomanic or manic state. The possibility of suicide should always be considered in depressed patients and adequate precautions taken.

Parameters to Monitor. Inhibition of platelet MAO (a minimum of 60–80% inhibition) correlates with clinical response.[136,137]

Notes. MAOIs are second-line drugs to tricyclic antidepressants for major depressive disorders and drugs of choice for atypical depressions and some phobic disorders.[134,136,138] Phenelzine is the preferred MAOI, because it has been more recently and thoroughly studied in terms of indications, efficacy, dosage and safety.[134]

Monoamine Oxidase Inhibitors Comparison Chart

DRUG	USUAL EFFECTIVE DAILY DOSAGE RANGE (MG)	DOSAGE FORMS	COMMENTS
Phenelzine Nardil®	60–90	Tab 15 mg	Most sedating MAOI; hydrazine
Tranylcypromine Parnate®	20–40	Tab 10 mg	Most stimulating MAOI; nonhydrazine
Isocarboxazid Marplan®	20–40	Tab 10 mg	Mild stimulating effect; hydrazine

Tricyclic Antidepressants (TCAs)

Pharmacology. TCAs are not general CNS stimulants, but rather have a very specific effect on neurotransmitters. Blockade of norepinephrine and serotonin reuptake at presynaptic terminals is the likely mechanism of antidepressant activity. TCAs differ greatly in their effect on neurotransmitters—see Tricyclics and Related Antidepressants Comparison Chart.

Administration and Adult Dose. See Tricyclics and Related Antidepressants Comparison Chart for **PO** dosage ranges. Initiate dosing at lower limit of range. Use divided dosing schedule to assess tolerance to side effects, then once daily dosing at bedtime can be used. "Long-acting" forms (eg, imipramine pamoate) offer no advantages.[139] **IM** rarely used (eg, surgical patient NPO for 1–2 days).

Dosage Individualization. Initial dose and rate of titration should be reduced in patients with cardiovascular or hepatic disease and in adolescent or geriatric patients.

Pediatric Dose. Not recommended in children under 12 yr. Imipramine, however, is indicated for childhood enuresis. **PO for enuresis** (under 12 yr) 25–50 mg/day; (over 12 yr) up to 75 mg/day.

CLINICAL DRUG DATA

Dosage Forms. See Tricyclics and Related Antidepressants Comparison Chart.

Patient Instructions. See Class Instructions. These drugs usually take 2 weeks for significant response and up to 4 weeks for full therapeutic benefit.

Pharmacokinetics and Biopharmaceutics. *Onset and Duration.* Peak plasma levels do not correlate with onset of therapeutic effect. Physiologic symptoms of depression (eg, insomnia, anorexia, decreased energy) should show some response after 1 week, while mood (eg, pessimism, hopelessness, anhedonia) often requires 2–4 weeks for response.

Plasma Levels. Nortriptyline has a well established therapeutic range and shows a curvilinear relationship of plasma levels and response ("therapeutic window").[140] Other tricyclic antidepressants show a linear relationship, but their therapeutic ranges are not well-established. See Tricyclics and Related Antidepressants Comparison Chart.

Fate. Oral absorption is variable due to first-pass metabolism (protriptyline 15%, imipramine 53% and doxepin 73%).[141,142] Major metabolites are desmethyl (for tertiary amines) and hydroxy compounds; rate may be genetically determined.[143]

$t_{1/2}$. See Tricyclics and Related Antidepressants Comparison Chart.

Adverse Reactions. Sedation is frequent; anticholinergic effects (dry mouth, blurred vision, constipation, urinary retention, aggravation of narrow angle glaucoma and prostatic hypertrophy) and postural hypotension may occur. See Tricyclics and Related Antidepressants Comparison Chart for relative differences in frequency of common adverse reactions. Occasionally fine hand tremor, hypomanic or manic episodes in bipolar patients and cardiac effects (ECG changes, first degree heart block, arrhythmias) occur. Cholestatic jaundice and blood dyscrasias are rare.

Contraindications. Pregnancy; congestive heart failure; angina pectoris; cardiovascular disease; cardiac arrhythmias.

Precautions. Use with caution in the elderly, or in patients with epilepsy, glaucoma, prostatic hypertrophy, renal or liver disease. Many drug interactions—see Drug Interactions chapter. 10–25% of manic-depressive patients may be "switched" into a manic or hypomanic state by antidepressants; concurrent lithium therapy may prevent this switch.[144]

Notes. Ingestion of 1–2 g of a tricyclic antidepressant constitutes a life-threatening medical emergency.[145] Quantities dispensed to depressed patients with suicidal ideation should be limited.

Amoxapine   Asendin®

Amoxapine is a dibenzoxazepine compound with antidepressant activity comparable to the tricyclic antidepressants. A majority of controlled studies show amoxapine to have a more rapid onset of effect than TCAs. Sedative and anticholinergic effects are much less than with TCAs. Usual dosage for an acute depressive episode is 300–400 mg/day to a maximum of 600 mg/day. Usual daily maintenance dosage is 150–300 mg/day. Amoxapine can be dosed once daily. Available in 25, 50, 100 and 150 mg tablets.[146]

Maprotiline
Ludiomil®

Pharmacology. Tetracyclic compound representing a new chemical class of drugs with antidepressant activity. Maprotiline selectively inhibits the re-uptake of norepinephrine with no effect on serotonin.

Administration and Adult Dose. See Tricyclics and Related Antidepressants Comparison Chart for **PO** dosage range. Initiate dosing at lower limit of range in divided schedule, then titrate upward to 3 mg/kg/day.[147] Once daily dosing at bedtime can be used to take advantage of its sedative effect, with no change in efficacy or steady-state plasma levels.[148]

Dosage Individualization. Initial dose and rate of titration should be reduced in patients with cardiovascular or hepatic disease and in geriatric patients.

Pediatric Dose. Safety and efficacy in children under 18 yr not established.

Dosage Forms. See Tricyclics and Related Antidepressants Comparison Chart.

Patient Instructions. See Class Instructions.

Pharmacokinetics and Biopharmaceutics. *Onset and Duration.* Delayed onset similar to tricyclics, although some, but not all, studies suggest it may have a more rapid onset.[149]
   Plasma Levels. Although therapeutic and toxic levels are not established, 200–300 ng/ml often correlates with clinical response.[150]
   Fate. Peak plasma levels occur 9–16 hr after a single oral dose. V_d is 22.6 L/kg; 88% protein-bound. Principal metabolite is desmethylmaprotiline, with minor metabolites from hydroxylation and oxidation. Desmethylmaprotiline and maprotiline-N-oxide are active.[150]
   $t_{1/2}$. See Tricyclics and Related Antidepressants Comparison Chart.

Adverse Reactions. Side effects are similar in nature and frequency to TCAs; however, the severity of these effects and number of study drop-outs due to these effects tend to be less with maprotiline.[150] See Tricyclic Antidepressants Adverse Reactions and the Tricyclics and Related Antidepressants Comparison Chart.

Contraindications. Pregnancy; congestive heart failure; angina pectoris; cardiovascular disease; cardiac arrhythmias.

Precautions. Use with caution in the elderly, patients with hepatic or renal disease, glaucoma or prostatic hypertrophy and patients with seizure disorders. Drug interactions are probably similar to those of the TCAs; maprotiline neither inhibits nor induces microsomal enzymes.[148]

Notes. As the first tetracyclic antidepressant compound, maprotiline is of significant interest, but no striking advantages are yet apparent compared to TCAs. In overdosage, delirium and seizures are more frequent with maprotiline, but cardiac arrhythmias are less severe compared to tricyclic antidepressants.[150]

Mianserin (Investigational - Organon)
Tolvon®

Mianserin is a tetracyclic compound with antidepressant activity comparable to amitriptyline and imipramine. Unlike all currently available antidepressants, it has virtually no anticholinergic activity and does not produce postural hypotension or adverse ECG effects. Mianserin does possess sedative activity. Usual initial adult dose is 30 mg/day adjusted to clinical response. 40–80 mg/day is adequate for most depressive disorders and a maximum of 120 mg/day has been used. Once daily dosing at bedtime may be used.[151]

Nomifensine   Merital®

Nomifensine is a tetrahydroisoquinoline compound with antidepressant activity similar to TCAs. Its biochemical effects are unique in that it is a potent dopamine agonist, weakly blocks norepinephrine reuptake and has minimal effect on serotonin. Of most importance is that nomifensine virtually lacks anticholinergic and cardiotoxic effects and has little sedative effect. Precise dosing ranges have not been established, but early studies show a range of 50–200 mg/day.[152]

Trazodone   Desyrel®

Trazodone is a triazolopyridine compound with antidepressant activity similar to tricyclic antidepressants. Trazodone inhibits reuptake of serotonin centrally. Compared to tricyclic antidepressants, trazodone has much lower anticholinergic activity, is less cardiotoxic and has a moderate sedative effect. Usual dosage is 200–400 mg/day to a maximum of 600 mg/day. Trials using trazodone as an antianxiety drug employ doses of 50–200 mg/day.[153] Available as 50 and 100 mg tablets.

Tricyclics and Related Antidepressants Comparison Chart[d]

DRUG CLASS DRUG	USUAL DAILY ADULT DOSAGE RANGE (MG) (A) ACUTE (M) MAINTENANCE	DOSAGE FORMS	HALF-LIFE (HOURS)	THERAPEUTIC PLASMA LEVELS (NG/ML)	BIOCHEMICAL EFFECTS[a] (N) NOREPINEPHRINE (S) SEROTONIN	RELATIVE FREQUENCY OF SIDE EFFECTS SEDATION	ANTI-CHOLINERGIC
TRICYCLICS **Amitriptyline** Elavil® Endep® Amitril® Various	(A) 150–300 (M) 75–150	Tab 10, 25, 50, 75, 100, 150 mg Inj 10 mg/ml	15–19	125–250[b]	(N) 0 (S) +	High	High
Nortriptyline Pamelor® Aventyl®	(A) 100–200 (M) 75–150	Cap 10, 25, 75 mg Soln 10 mg/5 ml Tab 10, 25 mg	18–28	50–150	(N) + (S) +	Moderate	Moderate
Protriptyline Vivactil®	(A) 30–60 (M) 20–40	Tab 5, 10 mg	74	>70	(N) c (S) c	Very Low	Low
Imipramine Tofranil® Presamine® Antipress® Imavate® Janimine® Various	(A) 150–300 (M) 75–150	Cap 75, 100, 125, 150 mg Tab 10, 25, 50 mg Inj 12.5 mg/ml	15–19	180–250[b]	(N) + (S) +	Moderate	Moderate

Continued

Tricyclics and Related Antidepressants Comparison Chart[d]

DRUG CLASS DRUG	USUAL DAILY ADULT DOSAGE RANGE (MG) (A) ACUTE (M) MAINTENANCE	DOSAGE FORMS	HALF-LIFE (HOURS)	THERAPEUTIC PLASMA LEVELS (NG/ML)	BIOCHEMICAL EFFECTS[a] (N) NOREPINEPHRINE (S) SEROTONIN	RELATIVE FREQUENCY OF SIDE EFFECTS SEDATION	RELATIVE FREQUENCY OF SIDE EFFECTS ANTI-CHOLINERGIC
Desipramine Norpramin® Pertofrane®	(A) 150–300 (M) 75–150	Cap 25, 50 mg Tab 25, 50, 75, 100, 150 mg	18–28	c	(N) + (S) 0	Low	Low
Trimipramine Surmontil®	(A) 150–300 (M) 75–150	Cap 25, 50 mg	c	c	(N) + (S) 0	Moderate	Moderate
Dothiepin (Investig- ational- Marion)	(A) 150–300 (M) 75–150	—	16–20	c	(N) c (S) c	Moderate	Low
Doxepin Sinequan® Adapin®	(A) 150–300 (M) 75–150	Cap 10, 25, 50, 75, 100, 150 mg Soln 50 mg/5 ml	15–19	>110[b]	(N) c (S) c	High	Moderate
TETRACYCLICS **Maprotiline** Ludiomil®	(A) 150–300 (M) 75–150	Tab 25, 50 mg	29–31	200–300	(N) + (S) 0	Moderate	Moderate
DIBENZOXAZEPINES **Amoxapine** Asendin®	(A) 300–600 (M) 150–300	Tab 50, 100, 150 mg	c	c	(N) + (S) +	Low	Very Low

a. Blocks reuptake of (N) Norepinephrine, (S) Serotonin.
b. Includes active metabolites.
c. Not well established.
d. From references 136, 146, 150, 154.

28:16.08 TRANQUILIZERS

Neuroleptic Drugs

Pharmacology. The antipsychotic efficacy is most likely related to blockade of postsynaptic dopaminergic receptors in the mesolimbic area of the brain, although other neurotransmitter systems may also be involved.

Administration and Adult Dose. See Neuroleptic Drugs Comparison Chart for oral dosage ranges. Initiate therapy with divided doses until therapeutic dosage found, then, for most patients, once daily dosing at bedtime is preferred. For maintenance therapy, decrease acute dosage by 25% q 1-3 months, with a target maintenance dose being 20-30% of the acute treatment dose.[157] **Rapid IM** neuroleptization is indicated for rapid control of aggressive, combative, psychotic patients; one to four IM injections of 2.5-10 mg of haloperidol, fluphenazine or thiothixene is usually sufficient.[158] **IM depot** fluphenazine decanoate is indicated only for drug-responsive patients with an established history of noncompliance.

Dosage Individualization. Doses in the lower range are sufficient for most elderly patients and the rate of dosage titration should be slower.[157]

Pediatric Dose. As with adults, dosage is primarily determined by titration and adjustment to the individual. No precise dosage ranges exist, but in general, initial dosage is lower and should be increased more gradually in children.

Dosage Forms. See Neuroleptic Drugs Comparison Chart.

Patient Instructions. See Class Instructions. These drugs usually take several weeks for significant clinical response and up to 6 weeks for full therapeutic response.

Pharmacokinetics and Biopharmaceutics. *Onset and Duration.* Onset of antipsychotic activity is variable, with significant response requiring days to weeks.[157]

    Plasma Levels. Not used clinically.[159]

    Fate. During chronic PO chlorpromazine therapy, peak plasma levels occur within 3 hr. Oral SR products have poor bioavailability. Peak plasma levels can be delayed up to 6 hr after IM administration. IM injection of chlorpromazine gives plasma levels several times higher than an equivalent PO dose, while haloperidol can be used in a PO:IM ratio of 1-1.5:1.[160,161] Prior to extensive hepatic metabolism, a significant portion of chlorpromazine is metabolized crossing the intestinal wall to the portal circulation. Phenothiazines have many active metabolites, while haloperidol has inactive metabolites.[162] Chlorpromazine is 95-98% protein bound.[160]

    $t_{1/2}$. Plasma half-lives have no clinical correlation to biologic half-lives for neuroleptic drugs. Chlorpromazine plasma half-life has been reported as 2-31 hr, thioridazine 4-10 hr, thiothixene 34 hr and haloperidol 13-35 hr. Of more clinical importance than half-life is the attainment of steady-state CNS levels and tissue saturation which allows once daily dosing.

Adverse Reactions. See Neuroleptic Drugs Comparison Chart for relative frequency of the common adverse reactions. Frequently sedation, extrapyramidal effects (eg, parkinsonism, dystonic reactions, akathisia), anticholinergic effects (eg, dry mouth, blurred vision, constipation, urinary retention) and postural hypotension occur. Occasionally weight gain, amenorrhea, galactorrhea, ejaculatory disturbance, photosensitivity and skin rash. Rarely cholestatic jaundice, seizures, thermoregulatory impairment, agranulocytosis, quinidine-like effect and skin or eye pigmentation occur. Tardive dyskinesia is a long-term adverse effect, sometimes irreversible and untreatable.[163]

Contraindications.   Coma; circulatory collapse or severe hypotension; bone marrow depression; history of blood dyscrasias.

Precautions.   Use cautiously in patients with myasthenia gravis, Parkinson's disease, seizure disorders or hepatic disease. See Drug Interactions chapter.

Notes.   No neuroleptic drug has been shown to possess greater safety or efficacy for any subgroup of schizophrenic patients or any target symptom.[157] See also Prochlorperazine (56:20) for anti-emetic uses.

Neuroleptic Drugs Comparison Chart[a]

DRUG CLASS DRUG	ORAL DOSAGE RANGE (MG/DAY)	ORAL EQUIVALENT ANTI-PSYCHOTIC DOSE	DOSAGE FORMS	RELATIVE FREQUENCY OF SIDE EFFECTS			
				SEDATION	ANTI-CHOLINERGIC	EXTRA-PYRAMIDAL	POSTURAL HYPOTENSION
PHENOTHIAZINES							
Chlorpromazine Thorazine® Various	50–1200	100	Soln 30, 100 mg/ml Syrup 10 mg/5 ml Tab 10, 25, 50, 100, 200 mg Inj 25 mg/ml Supp 25, 100 mg SR cap not recommended	High	Moderate	Moderate	High
Thioridazine Mellaril®	50–800	100	Soln 30, 100 mg/ml Susp 25, 100 mg/5 ml Tab 10, 15, 25, 50, 100, 150, 200 mg	High	High	Low	High
Trifluoperazine Stelazine®	5–40⁺	5	Soln 10 mg/ml Tab 1, 2, 5, 10 mg Inj 2 mg/ml	Low	Low	High	Low

Continued

Neuroleptic Drugs Comparison Chart[a]

DRUG CLASS DRUG	ORAL DOSAGE RANGE (MG/DAY)	ORAL EQUIVALENT ANTI-PSYCHOTIC DOSE	DOSAGE FORMS	SEDATION	ANTI-CHOLINERGIC	EXTRA-PYRAMIDAL	POSTURAL HYPOTENSION
				RELATIVE FREQUENCY OF SIDE EFFECTS			
Perphenazine Trilafon®	12–64	8	Soln 16 mg/5 ml Tab 2, 4, 8, 16 mg Inj 5 mg/ml	Low	Low	High	Low
Fluphenazine Prolixin® Permitil®	2–20	2	Elxr 0.5 mg/ml Soln 5 mg/ml Tab 0.25, 1, 2.5, 5, 10 mg Inj 2.5 mg/ml	Low	Low	Very High	Low
Fluphenazine Decanoate Fluphenazine Enanthate Prolixin®	12.5–100 (IM)	0.67 (IM)	Inj 25 mg/ml	Low	Low	Very High	Low
THIOXANTHENES **Thiothixene** Navane®	5–60	4	Cap 1, 2, 5, 10, 20 mg Soln 5 mg/ml Inj 2 mg/ml	Low	Low	High	Low

Continued

Neuroleptic Drugs Comparison Chart[a]

DRUG CLASS DRUG	ORAL DOSAGE RANGE (MG/DAY)	ORAL EQUIVALENT ANTI-PSYCHOTIC DOSE	DOSAGE FORMS	RELATIVE FREQUENCY OF SIDE EFFECTS			
				SEDATION	ANTI-CHOLINERGIC	EXTRA-PYRAMIDAL	POSTURAL HYPOTENSION
BUTYROPHENONES **Haloperidol** Haldol®	2–100	2	Soln 2 mg/ml Tab 0.5, 1, 2, 5, 10, 20 mg Inj 5 mg/ml	Low	Very Low	Very High	Low
DIBENZOXAZEPINES **Loxapine** Loxitane® Daxolin®	20–250	15	Cap 5, 10, 25, 50 mg Soln 25 mg/ml Inj 50 mg/ml	Low	Low	High	Low
DIHYDROINDOLONES **Molindone** Moban® Lidone®	50–400	10	Cap 5, 10, 25 mg Soln 20 mg/ml Tab 5, 10, 25, 50, 100 mg	Low	Low	High	Low

a. From references 154, 157.

28:16.12 OTHER PSYCHOTHERAPEUTIC AGENTS

Lithium Carbonate

Eskalith®, Lithane®,
Lithobid®, Lithonate®,
Lithotabs®, Various

Lithium Citrate

Lithonate-S®

Pharmacology. The mechanism of antimanic effect is unknown; lithium may substitute for Na^+, K^+, Mg^{++} and Ca^{++} at various cellular sites and alter the synthesis and function of various neurotransmitters.

Administration and Adult Dose. Individualize dosing according to plasma levels and clinical response. Acute manic episodes typically require 1.2-2.4 g/day, while maintenance therapy requires 900 mg-1.5 g/day.[164]

Dosage Individualization. Dosage must be more carefully adjusted in patients with decreased renal function (eg, renal disease and the elderly) and in patients receiving thiazide diuretics.

Pediatric Dose. Not recommended in children under 12 yr.

Dosage Forms. **Cap** 300 mg (8 mEq); **Tab** 300 mg; **SR Tab** 300, 450 mg; **Syrup** 8 mEq/5 ml (as citrate).

Patient Instructions. This drug may be taken with food, milk or antacid to minimize stomach upset. Report immediately if signs of toxicity occur, such as persistent diarrhea, vomiting, hand tremor, drowsiness or slurred speech, or prior to beginning any diet. In hot weather, ensure adequate water and salt intake.

Pharmacokinetics and Biopharmaceutics. *Onset and Duration.* Onset 7-10 days.[165]
   Plasma Levels. For acute mania or hypomania 0.8-1.5 mEq/L. For prophylaxis 0.6-1.2 mEq/L.[164,166] Levels above 1.5 mEq/L are regularly associated with some signs of toxicity and levels above 2.0 result in serious toxicity. See Adverse Reactions.
   Fate. Virtually total absorption within 8 hr after oral administration, with peak levels occurring in 2-4 hr. Distribution is throughout total body water, but tissue uptake is not uniform. Not protein bound or metabolized, but freely filtered through the glomerulus with about 80% being reabsorbed.[167]
   $t_{1/2}$. 18-20 hr; up to 36 hr in the elderly.[168]

Adverse Reactions. **Dose-related:** (therapeutic plasma levels) nausea, vomiting, diarrhea, polyuria, polydipsia, fine hand tremor, muscle weakness; (1.5-2.0 mEq/L) coarse hand tremor, persistent GI effects, muscle hyperirritability, slurred speech, confusion; (over 2.0 mEq/L) stupor, seizures, increased deep tendon reflexes, irregular pulse, hypotension, coma.
   Non-dose-related: Nontoxic goiter, nephrogenic diabetes insipidus-like syndrome, folliculitis, acneiform eruptions, cogwheel rigidity, leukocytosis. Possible long-term adverse effect is histochemical evidence of renal damage.[164,169]

Contraindications. Fluctuating renal function; significant renal impairment.

Precautions. Use with caution in patients with significant cardiac disease, organic brain disease or the elderly. See Drug Interactions chapter.

Parameters to Monitor. Pre-lithium workup should include thyroid function tests, serum creatinine and BUN, CBC (for baseline white count), urinalysis (for base-line specific gravity), electrolytes and ECG (if over 40 yr).[164] During therapy, obtain plasma levels (drawn 8–12 hr after last dose) q 2 weeks during initiation and monthly during maintenance.

28:24 SEDATIVES AND HYPNOTICS

General References: 170-172

Class Instructions. This drug causes drowsiness and may produce sleep. Do not exceed prescribed dosage and use caution when driving, operating machinery or performing other tasks requiring mental alertness. Avoid concurrent use of alcohol and other drugs which cause drowsiness or sleep.

Benzodiazepines

Pharmacology. Benzodiazepines have a more specific anxiolytic effect than other sedatives such as barbiturates. Benzodiazepines facilitate gamma aminobutyric acid (GABA)-mediated transmission and mimic the actions of glycine at its receptor sites. Barbiturates share the GABA effect, but have negligible effects on the glycine receptor.[173] Benzodiazepines are the preferred agents in alcohol withdrawal—see Notes.

Administration and Adult Dose. See Benzodiazepines Comparison Chart. Optimal oral dosing requires individual titration to clinical response. The long-acting drugs can be dosed once daily at bedtime, while the short-acting drugs require multiple daily dosing—see Benzodiazepines Comparison Chart. Dosing schedule should be determined by the individual patient's degree of dysfunction from daytime anxiety versus insomnia. **PO for alcohol withdrawal** chlordiazepoxide 25–100 mg or diazepam 5–20 mg q 6 hr (not prn) for agitation, tremor and anxiety. Many patients need PO chlordiazepoxide 100–200 mg the first day; occasionally 300 mg or more is necessary; unusual cases may require up to 1600 mg the first day. **IV for extreme agitation of withdrawal** chlordiazepoxide 12.5 mg/min or diazepam 2.5 mg/min slow push until patient is calm. After the first day, dose can be decreased by 25% daily and discontinued on the 5th day. Published withdrawal protocols are only guidelines; dosage may need to be adjusted upward for withdrawal breakthrough or decreased for toxicity. Higher doses may be necessary in heavy smokers; lower doses may be needed in patients with severe liver disease and decreased serum albumin; **IM not recommended** because of slow, erratic absorption, pain and muscle damage.[174] See Fate and Notes.

Dosage Individualization. Patients with liver disease or elderly patients may have reduced clearance and/or enhanced CNS sensitivity which requires dosage reduction. Alcoholic patients with reduced serum proteins may require a lower dosage due to decreased protein binding.

Pediatric Dose. PO (diazepam) 1–2.5 mg tid-qid. Most benzodiazepines are not recommended in children due to insufficient clinical experience.

Dosage Forms. See Benzodiazepines Comparison Chart.

Patient Instructions. See Class Instructions.

Pharmacokinetics and Biopharmaceutics. *Fate.* Oral diazepam and chlordiazepoxide administration gives faster and more complete drug absorption than IM injection.[175] Lorazepam is the first benzodiazepine with rapid and reliable IM absorption.[176] Midazolam and flunitrazepam may also offer good IM absorption.[177] See also Benzodiazepines Comparison Chart.

Adverse Reactions. Frequent effects include drowsiness, dizziness, ataxia and disorientation; these effects rarely require drug discontinuation and are easily managed by dosage reduction. Occasionally, agitation and excitement may occur; this "paradoxical rage reaction" is usually attributed to the long-acting drugs and a short-acting drug is preferred for patients with a history of aggressive, hostile behavior.[178] Hypotension and respiratory depression are occasionally observed with parenteral therapy. Rarely, hepatic disease and blood dyscrasias occur.[179]

Contraindications. Acute narrow angle glaucoma.

Precautions. Pregnancy; impaired hepatic function. Abrupt drug withdrawal may result in rebound insomnia, an abstinence syndrome similar to barbiturate withdrawal, seizures or, rarely, psychosis.[180] See Drug Interactions chapter.

Notes. Benzodiazepines are preferred over barbiturates, phenothiazines or paraldehyde for alcohol withdrawal because they are equally efficacious, provide superior anticonvulsant activity and are less toxic. No evidence suggests superiority of any benzodiazepine over others in withdrawal efficacy, although chlordiazepoxide has been most well studied and is most often used. Pharmacokinetic differences may be important in some patients (eg, oxazepam may be preferred in severe liver disease).[174]

Alprazolam   Xanax®

Alprazolam is a triazolobenzodiazepine used as an anxiolytic and antidepressant. Compared to diazepam, it has as quick an onset of effect, an earlier peak plasma level and a much shorter duration of action. Studies in mixed anxious-depressed outpatients have shown alprazolam to be more effective than diazepam. An antidepressant action separate from anxiolytic activity cannot be established at this time, because alprazolam has not been evaluated in major depressive disorders. Adverse effects are similar to other benzodiazepines, but may be less severe (eg, sedation and ataxia, which are dose-related). Alprazolam is 3–5 times more potent than diazepam; initial oral dose is 0.25–0.5 mg tid, which can be increased up to 4 mg/day. The lower dosage range is recommended for anxiety, while the higher doses are recommended for neurotic depression and mild anxious depression.[181] It is available in tablets of 0.25, 0.5 and 1 mg.

Flurazepam   Dalmane®

Pharmacology. The hypnotic effect is probably related to its facilitation of gamma aminobutyric acid-mediated neurotransmission, but the exact mechanism is unknown.

Administration and Adult Dose. See Benzodiazepines Comparison Chart. A PO 30 mg initial dose is preferred for young healthy patients, because 15 mg may be less effective.[182] Elderly patients, particularly over 70 yr, should be given an initial dose of 15 mg PO at bedtime.[183,184]

Pediatric Dose. Not recommended in children under 15 yr.

Dosage Forms. See Benzodiazepines Comparison Chart.

Patient Instructions. See Class Instructions, 28:24. Patients should be advised that the full benefit of hypnotic effect may not be seen until after several nights' use.

Pharmacokinetics and Biopharmaceutics. *Onset and Duration.* Clinical effect increases on the second and third night of continuous use and persists for several nights after drug discontinuation.

Fate. Rapidly absorbed after oral administration and rapidly metabolized to N_1-hydroxyethyl flurazepam and N-desalkylflurazepam. Flurazepam levels are too low to detect within a few hours after ingestion.[182] The hydroxyethyl metabolite is measurable only in the early hours after ingestion; the major active metabolite is N-desalkylflurazepam.[185]

$t_{1/2}$. (N-desalkylflurazepam) 47–100 hr, reaching steady-state in 7–10 days.[185]

Adverse Reactions. Unwanted morning drowsiness or hangover are frequent; prevalence of hangover is about 5% with the 30 mg dose in young patients, rising to 39% with the 30 mg dose in patients over 70 yr.[183,184] Occasional effects include impairment of motor function and intellectual performance, dry mouth, nightmares, delirium and confusion.[182]

Precautions. Pregnancy; impaired hepatic function. See Drug Interactions chapter.

Notes. Flurazepam is preferred to nonbenzodiazepine hypnotics, because it is much safer in overdose, interferes less with sleep physiology and remains effective beyond one week of continuous use.[182,186] There are no differences which indicate flurazepam over other benzodiazepines for insomnia, but others have not been as well studied for this indication.

Triazolam   Halcion®

Triazolam is a triazolobenzodiazepine compound with hypnotic efficacy equal to flurazepam. It differs from flurazepam, because it has a rapid onset of effect and very short half-life. Its short-term efficacy is established, but efficacy beyond 2–4 weeks has not been established. Of some concern are reports of rebound insomnia when triazolam is discontinued after only several days' use. Common adverse effects include drowsiness, dry mouth and ataxia which are dose-related; less common is anterograde amnesia. Triazolam is 30–60 times more potent than flurazepam; initial oral hypnotic dose is 0.25–0.5 mg; in geriatric or debilitated patients the dosage range is 0.125–0.25 mg.[186] Available as 0.25 and 0.5 mg tablets.

Benzodiazepines and Related Drugs Comparison Chart[a]

DRUG	ORAL DOSAGE RANGE	DOSAGE FORMS	PEAK ORAL PLASMA LEVELS (HOURS)	HALF-LIFE (HOURS)	MAJOR ACTIVE METABOLITES (HALF-LIFE IN HOURS)
ANXIOLYTICS					
LONG-ACTING					
Diazepam Valium®	6–40 mg/day	Tab 2, 5, 10 mg Inj 5 mg/ml SR Cap 15 mg	1–2	20–50	Desmethyldiazepam (30–60)
Chlordiazepoxide Librium® Libritabs® Various	15–100 mg/day	Cap 5, 10, 25 mg Inj 100 mg Tab 5, 10, 25 mg	2–4	5–30	Desmethylchlordiazepoxide; demoxepam; desmethyl-diazepam
Clorazepate Tranxene®	15–60 mg/day	Cap 3.75, 7.5, 15 mg Tab 11.25, 22.5 mg	b	30–60[a]	Desmethyldiazepam
Prazepam Centrax®	20–60 mg/day	Cap 5, 10 mg Tab 10 mg	6	78	3-Hydroxyprazepam; desmethyldiazepam
SHORT-ACTING					
Halazepam Paxipam®	60–160 mg/day	Tab 20, 40 mg	1–3	7	n-3-Hydroxyhalazepam; desmethyldiazepam
Oxazepam Serax®	30–120 mg/day	Cap 10, 15, 30 mg Tab 15 mg	1–2	5–10	None

Continued

Benzodiazepines and Related Drugs Comparison Chart[a]

DRUG	ORAL DOSAGE RANGE	DOSAGE FORMS	PEAK ORAL PLASMA LEVELS (HOURS)	HALF-LIFE (HOURS)	MAJOR ACTIVE METABOLITES (HALF-LIFE IN HOURS)
Lorazepam[c] Ativan®	2–6 mg/day	Tab 0.5, 1, 2 mg	2	10–20	None
Alprazolam[f] Xanax®	0.75–4 mg/day	Tab 0.25, 0.5, 1 mg	0.7–1.6	12–19	α-Hydroxyalprazolam
HYPNOTICS					
LONG-ACTING					
Flurazepam Dalmane®	15–60 mg	Cap 15, 30 mg	d	d	Desalkylflurazepam (50–100)
Flunitrazepam[c] Rohypnol® (Investigational-Roche)	1–2 mg	e	<1	—	7-Aminoflunitrazepam (23) N-desmethylflunitrazepam (31)
SHORT-ACTING					
Temazepam Restoril®	15–30 mg	Cap 15, 30 mg	2–3	9–12	None
Triazolam[f] Halcion®	0.125–0.5 mg	Tab 0.25, 0.5 mg	0.5–1.5	2.3	α-Hydroxytriazolam

Continued

Benzodiazepines and Related Drugs Comparison Chart[a]

DRUG	ORAL DOSAGE RANGE	DOSAGE FORMS	PEAK ORAL PLASMA LEVELS (HOURS)	HALF-LIFE (HOURS)	MAJOR ACTIVE METABOLITES (HALF-LIFE IN HOURS)
Midazolam[c] (Investigational-Roche)	5–10 mg	e	0.4–0.7	1.8	None

a. From references 177, 181, 187-191.
b. Hydrolyzed to desmethyldiazepam before absorption.
c. Also used as an IV anesthetic; well absorbed IM.
d. Rapidly and completely metabolized to desalkylflurazepam.
e. Not commercially available in US.
f. Not a true benzodiazepine, but a closely related triazolobenzodiazepine.

Chloral Hydrate
Noctec®, Somnos®, Various

Pharmacology. A halogenated aliphatic alcohol, rapidly reduced to trichloroethanol which is responsible for CNS depression.

Administration and Adult Dose. **PO or PR for sleep** 500 mg–1 g hs, to maximum of 2 g. **PO or PR for sedation** 250 mg tid after meals, to maximum of 2 g/day. **PO for alcohol withdrawal** 500 mg–1 g q 6 hr (often given with paraldehyde).

Pediatric Dose. **PO or PR for sleep** 50 mg/kg to maximum of 1 g/dose. Sedative dose is one-half the hypnotic dose, given in divided doses.

Dosage Forms. See Sedatives and Hypnotics Comparison Chart.

Patient Instructions. Capsules should be taken with a full glass of liquid; syrup should be mixed in a half glass of water, juice or ginger ale. See also Class Instructions.

Pharmacokinetics and Biopharmaceutics. *Onset and Duration.* Onset 30–60 min.
   Fate. Rapidly and well absorbed from GI tract; rapidly reduced to active metabolite trichloroethanol, with a smaller fraction oxidized to the inactive trichloroacetic acid. Metabolites and their glucuronides excreted in urine.[192]
   $t_{1/2}$. (Trichloroethanol) 8 hr.[193]

Adverse Reactions. Occasionally, gastric irritation and nausea occur; rarely, excitement, delirium, disorientation, erythematous and urticarial allergic reactions are reported.

Contraindications. Marked hepatic and renal impairment.

Precautions. Pregnancy; gastritis; severe cardiac disease. See Drug Interactions chapter.

Notes. Chloral hydrate is a useful agent for prn use, but loses its hypnotic efficacy by the second week of use.[194] Unlike barbiturates, chloral hydrate causes no significant enzyme induction and there is no significant effect on REM sleep or difficulty with REM rebound for most patients.[195]

Phenobarbital
Various

Pharmacology. A "long-acting" barbiturate which depresses a wide range of cellular functions in many organ systems, although its central depressant action is desired for sedative-hypnotic effect. See also Phenobarbital, 28:12.

Administration and Adult Dose. See Sedatives and Hypnotics Comparison Chart. **PO hypnotic dose,** although rarely indicated, is 100–200 mg. See Phenobarbital, 28:12 for anticonvulsant dosage.

Dosage Individualization. Dosage reduction may be necessary in severe chronic liver disease or in renal impairment.[100,108]

Pediatric Dose. **PO for sedation** 2 mg/kg/day in 4 divided doses.

Dosage Forms. See Sedatives and Hypnotics Comparison Chart.

Patient Instructions. See Class Instructions.

Pharmacokinetics and Biopharmaceutics. *Onset and Duration.*
PO onset of sedation 20–60 min; duration 6–8 hr.[196]
   Plasma Levels. (Anticonvulsant) 15–45 mcg/ml.[196]
   Fate. About 80% oral absorption, although variable, with 20–45% bound to plasma proteins. V_d is 0.6–1.01 L/kg; Cl is 0.003–0.013 L/hr/kg.[192] Peak plasma levels after oral dosage occur in 8–18 hr.[110,111] There is much individual variation in metabolism and elimination; about 65% is converted to the inactive metabolite para-hydroxyphenobarbital. 35% is excreted unchanged in the urine; acidic urine may increase, and alkaline urine decrease half-life.[108,193]
   $t_{1/2}$. (Adults) 2–5 days; (children) 1.6–2.9 days.[193] In one study, half-life increased to 5.4 days in chronic liver disease, while remaining unchanged in acute liver disease.[197]

Adverse Reactions. Most frequent dose-related side effect is sedation, to which tolerance usually develops. Children and the elderly may become paradoxically excited and hyperactive. Occasionally skin rashes, disturbances in motor function and megaloblastic anemia may occur. Rarely, Stevens-Johnson syndrome, exfoliative dermatitis, photosensitivity, hepatitis and jaundice have been reported. SC administration may result in necrosis or sloughing; IV administration may cause injury to adjacent nerves and extravasation can produce tissue necrosis.[196]

Contraindications. Respiratory disease where dyspnea or obstruction is present; marked renal impairment.

Precautions. Pregnancy. Use with caution in presence of porphyria or severe cardiac disease and IV in patients with pulmonary or cardiovascular disease. Severe liver disease might be expected to decrease metabolism to the drug's inactive metabolite, although information is limited. In patients with renal disease, increased toxicity has been observed.[193] See Drug Interactions chapter.

Parameters to Monitor. Plasma levels should be obtained at the onset of therapy to see if they are adequate. This is unnecessary if a clear therapeutic effect is indicated by cessation of epilepsy. Plasma levels should then be obtained during therapy after steady-state is achieved and any time toxicity or lack of efficacy is suspected.[101]

Notes. Febrile seizures in infants may be controlled by phenobarbital, but not with phenytoin.[107] Do not mix with other injectables. In overdosage, excretion may be enhanced by alkalinizing the urine.

Secobarbital   Seconal®, Various

Pharmacology. A "short-acting" barbiturate, capable of producing all levels of CNS depression.

Administration and Adult Dose. **PO for sleep** 100 mg; **PO for preoperative sedation** 200–300 mg 1–2 hr before surgery. **IM for sedation** 1–2 mg/kg. **IV for preanesthesia basal sleep** up to 250 mg, at a rate not to exceed 50 mg/15 sec.

Pediatric Dose. **PO for sedation** 2 mg/kg/day in 4 divided doses; **PO for preoperative sedation** 50–100 mg.

Dosage Forms. See Sedatives and Hypnotics Comparison Chart.

Patient Instructions. See Class Instructions.

Pharmacokinetics and Biopharmaceutics. *Onset and Duration.*
Oral or rectal onset 10–30 min; duration 6–8 hr.[196]
   Fate. Well absorbed following oral, rectal or parenteral administration; 52–57% plasma protein bound.[198] Metabolized to active and inactive compounds; less than 0.1% excreted in urine unchanged.[111]
   $t_{1/2}$. See Sedatives and Hypnotics Comparison Chart.

Adverse Reactions. CNS depression, sedation and morning hangover are dose-related. Rarely, hypersensitivity reactions (eg, skin rashes, Stevens-Johnson syndrome, photosensitivity, blood dyscrasias) occur.

Contraindications. See Phenobarbital. Also, parenteral secobarbital is contraindicated in obstetric deliveries.

Precautions. See Phenobarbital. Although secobarbital is not harmful in renal disease, the parenteral polyethylene glycol vehicle may irritate the kidneys.

Notes. Refrigerate injection; do not mix with other injectables. Hypnotic efficacy is significantly reduced after 1–2 weeks of continuous use.[194,199]

Sedatives and Hypnotics Comparison Chart

DRUG CLASS DRUG	ORAL DOSE	DOSAGE FORMS	HALF-LIFE (HOURS)[a]
SEDATIVES			
BARBITURATES			
Phenobarbital Various	15–30 mg bid-qid	Drops 16 mg/ml Elxr 4 mg/ml Tab 8, 16, 32, 65, 100 mg Inj 30, 65, 130, 163 mg/ml Pwdr for Inj 65, 120, 130, 325 mg	48–120
Amobarbital Amytal® Various	30–50 mg bid-tid	Cap 65, 200 mg Elxr 44 mg/5 ml Tab 15, 30, 50, 100 mg Pwdr for Inj 250, 500 mg	14–42
PROPANEDIOLS			
Meprobamate Equanil® Miltown®	400 mg tid-qid	Cap 400 mg Tab 200, 400, 600 mg SR Cap 200, 400 mg	6–16
HYPNOTICS			
BARBITURATES			
Pentobarbital Nembutal® Various	100–200 mg	Cap 30, 50, 100 mg Elxr 20 mg/5 ml Supp 30, 60, 120, 200 mg Inj 50 mg/ml	21–42

Continued

Sedatives and Hypnotics Comparison Chart

DRUG CLASS DRUG	ORAL DOSE	DOSAGE FORMS	HALF-LIFE (HOURS)[a]
Secobarbital Seconal® Various	100–200 mg	Cap 50, 100 mg Elxr 22 mg/5 ml Supp 30, 60, 120, 200 mg Inj 50 mg/ml	19–34
CHLORAL DERIVATIVES **Chloral Hydrate** Noctec® Various	500 mg–1.5 g	Cap 250, 500 mg Supp 325, 500, 650 mg Syrup 250, 500 mg/5 ml	8 (Trichloroethanol)
Triclofos Triclos®	1.5 g	Soln 100 mg/ml Tab 750 mg	8 (Trichloroethanol)
PIPERIDINEDIONES **Glutethimide** Doriden®	500 mg–1 g	Cap 500 mg Tab 250, 500 mg	5–22
Methyprylon Noludar®	200–400 mg	Cap 300 mg Tab 50, 200 mg	4
ACETYLINIC ALCOHOLS **Ethchlorvynol** Placidyl®	500 mg–1 g	Cap 100, 200, 500, 750 mg	6

Continued

Sedatives and Hypnotics Comparison Chart

DRUG CLASS DRUG	ORAL DOSE	DOSAGE FORMS	HALF-LIFE (HOURS)[a]
QUINAZOLINE			
Methaqualone[b]	150–300 mg (tablets)	Tab 150, 300 mg	18–42
Quaalude®	200–400 mg (capsules)	Cap (hydrochloride)	
Parest®		200, 400 mg	
Mequin®			
OTHER			
L-Tryptophan	7.5–15 g	Tab 125, 200, 250, 500, 667 mg	—
Trofan®			
Tryptacin®			
Various			

a. From references 193, 200.
b. In the U.S., withdrawn by the manufacturer.

References, 28:00 Central Nervous System Drugs

1. Miller RR. Dosage and choice of parenteral strong analgesics. Am J Hosp Pharm 1974;31:780-2.

2. Beaver WT. The pharmacologic basis for the choice of an analgesic. I. potent analgesics. Pharmacol for Physicians 1970;4(10):1-7.

3. Miller RR. Evaluation of nalbuphine hydrochloride. Am J Hosp Pharm 1980;37:942-9.

4. Ameer B, Salter FJ. Drug therapy reviews: evaluation of butorphanol tartrate. Am J Hosp Pharm 1979;36:1683-91.

5. Hovander G. Recently approved alternatives to aspirin. Drug Intell Clin Pharm 1979;13:673-9.

6. Evens RP. Drug therapy reviews: antirheumatic agents. Am J Hosp Pharm 1979;36:622-33.

7. Koch-Weser J. Acetaminophen. N Engl J Med 1976;295:1297-1300.

8. Cote J, Moriarty RW, Rumack BH. Facing toxic overdose of acetaminophen. Patient Care 1979;13:16-33.

9. Slattery JT, Levy G. Acetaminophen kinetics in acutely poisoned patients. Clin Pharmacol Ther 1979;25:184-94.

10. Mitchell JR, Thorgeirsson SS, Potter WZ et al. Acetaminophen-induced hepatic injury: protective role of glutathione in man and rationale for therapy. Clin Pharmacol Ther 1974;16:676-84.

11. Albert KS. Pharmacokinetics of orally administered acetaminophen in man. J Pharmacokinet Biopharm 1974;2:381-93.

12. Finlayson NDC, Prescott LF, Adjepon-Yamoah KK et al. Antipyrine, lidocaine, and paracetamol metabolism in chronic liver disease (abstract). Gastroenterology 1974;67:790.

13. Prescott LF, Roscoe P, Wright N et al. Plasma-paracetamol half-life and hepatic necrosis in patients with paracetamol overdosage. Lancet 1971;1:519-22.

14. Barker JD, de Carle DJ, Anuras S. Chronic excessive acetaminophen use and liver damage. Ann Intern Med 1977;87:299-301.

15. Mielke CH, Heiden D, Britten AF et al. Hemostasis, antipyretics, and mild analgesics: acetaminophen vs aspirin. JAMA 1976;235:613-6.

16. Fuster V, Chesebro JH. Antithrombotic therapy: role of platelet-inhibitor drugs (3 parts) Mayo Clin Proc 1981;56:102-12;185-95;265-73.

17. Yu TF, Gutman AB. Study of the paradoxical effects of salicylate in low, intermediate and high dosage on the renal mechanisms for excretion of urate in man. J Clin Invest 1959;38:1298-1315.

18. Borga O, Odar-Cederlof I, Ringberger V-A et al. Protein binding of salicylate in uremic and normal plasma. Clin Pharmacol Ther 1976;20:464-75.

19. Davison C. Salicylate metabolism in man. Ann NY Acad Sci 1971;179:249-68.

20. Mongan E, Kelly P, Nies K et al. Tinnitus as an indication of therapeutic serum salicylate levels. JAMA 1973;226:142-5.

21. Done AK. Aspirin-overdosage: incidence, diagnosis, and management. Pediatrics 1978;62(suppl):890-7.

22. Levy G, Tsuchiya T, Amsel LP. Limited capacity for salicyl phenolic glucuronide formation and its effect on the kinetics of salicylate elimination in man. Clin Pharmacol Ther 1972;13:258-68.

23. Rowland M, Riegelman S, Harris PA et al. Absorption kinetics of aspirin in man following oral administration of an aqueous solution. J Pharm Sci 1972;61:379-85.

24. Levy G. Pharmacokinetics of salicylate elimination in man. J Pharm Sci 1965;54:959-67.

25. Levy G, Yaffe SJ. Clinical implications of salicylate-induced liver damage. Am J Dis Child 1975;129:1385-6.

26. Jusko WJ, Gretch M. Plasma and tissue protein binding of drugs in pharmacokinetics. Drug Metab Rev 1976;5:43-140.

27. Anon. Is all aspirin alike? Med Lett Drugs Ther 1974;16:57-9.

28. Lanza FL, Royer GL, Nelson RS. Endoscopic evaluation of the effects of aspirin, buffered aspirin, and enteric-coated aspirin on gastric and duodenal mucosa. N Engl J Med 1980;303:136-8.

29. Szczeklik A, Gryglewski RJ, Czerniawska-Mysik G et al. Aspirin-induced asthma. J Allergy Clin Immunol ·1976;58:10-8.

30. Kepler JA, ed. American Hospital Formulary Service. Washington, DC: American Society of Hospital Pharmacists, 1959-82.

31. Schmerzler E, Yu W, Hewitt MI et al. Gas chromatographic determination of codeine in serum and urine. J Pharm Sci 1966;55:155-7.

32. Way EL, Adler TK. The pharmacologic implications of the fate of morphine and its surrogates. Pharmacol Rev 1968;12:383-446.

33. Brogden RN et al. Diflunisal: a review of its pharmacological properties and therapeutic use in pain and musculoskeletal strains and sprains and pain in osteoarthritis. Drugs 1980;19:84-106.

34. Adams SS, Cliffe EE, Lessel B et al. Some biological properties of 2-(4-isobutylphenyl)-propionic acid. J Pharm Sci 1967;56:1686.

35. Mills RFN, Adams SS, Cliffe EE et al. The metabolism of ibuprofen. Xenobiotica 1973;3:589-98.

36. Kaiser DG, Vangiessen GJ, GLC determination of ibuprofen in plasma. J Pharm Sci 1974;63:219-21.

37. Gryfe CI, Rubenzahl S. Agranulocytosis and aplastic anemia possibly due to ibuprofen. Can Med Assoc J 1976;114:877.

38. Stempel DA, Miller JJ. Lymphopenia and hepatotoxicity with ibuprofen. J Pediatr 1977;90:657-8.

39. Alvan G, Orme M,¡Bertilsson L et al. Pharmacokinetics of indomethacin. Clin Pharmacol Ther 1975;18:364-73.

40. Duggan DE, Hogans AF, Kwan KC. The metabolism of indomethacin in man. J Pharmacol Exp Ther 1972;181:563-75.

41. O'Brien WM. Indomethacin: a survey of clinical trials. Clin Pharmacol Ther 1968;9:94-107.

42. Mather LE, Tucker GT. Systemic availability of orally administered meperidine. Clin Pharmacol Ther 1976;20:535-40.

43. Gilman AG, Goodman LS, Gilman A, eds. Goodman and Gilman's the pharmacological basis of therapeutics. 6th ed. New York: Macmillan, 1980.

44. Fochtman FW, Winek CL. Therapeutic serum concentrations of meperidine (Demerol®). J Forensic Sci 1969;14:213-8.

45. Klotz U, McHorse TS Wilkinson GR et al. The effect of cirrhosis on the disposition and elimination of meperidine in man. Clin Pharmacol Ther 1974;16:667-75.

46. McHorse TS, Wilkinson GR, Johnson RF et al. Effect of acute viral hepatitis in man on the disposition and elimination of meperidine. Gastroenterology 1975;68:775-80.

47. Tang R, Shimomura SK, Rotblatt M. Meperidine-induced seizures in sickle cell patients. Hosp Formul 1980;15:764-72.

48. Fultz JM, Senay EC. Guidelines for the management of hospitalized narcotic addicts. Ann Intern Med 1975;82:815-8.

49. DiBlasi M, Washburn CJ. Using analgesics effectively. Am J Nurs 1979;79:74-8.

50. Holmstrand J, Anggard E, Gunne L-M. Methadone maintenance: plasma levels and therapeutic outcome. Clin Pharmacol Ther 1978;23:175-80.

51. Berkowitz BA. The relationship of pharmacokinetics to pharmacological activity: morphine, methadone and naloxone. Clin Pharmacokinet 1976;1:219-30.

52. Verebely K, Volavka J, Mule S et al. Methadone in man: pharmacokinetic and excretion studies in acute and chronic treatment. Clin Pharmacol Ther 1976;18:180-90.

53. Olsen GD, Wendel JA, Livermore JD et al. Clinical effects and pharmacokinetics of racemic methadone and its optical isomers. Clin Pharmacol Ther 1977;21:147-57.

54. Holmes AH. Morphine IV infusion for chronic pain. Drug Intell Clin Pharm 1978;12:556-7.

55. Berkowitz BA, Ngai SH, Yang JC et al. The disposition of morphine in surgical patients. Clin Pharmacol Ther 1975;17:629-35.

56. Stanski DR, Greenblatt DJ, Lowenstein E. Kinetics of intravenous and intramuscular morphine. Clin Pharmacol Ther 1978;24:52-9.

57. Brunk SF, Delle M. Morphine metabolism in man. Clin Pharmacol Ther 1974;16:51-7.

58. Melzack R, Mount BM, Gordon JM. The Brompton mixture versus morphine solution given orally: effects on pain. Can Med Assoc J 1979;120:435-8.

59. Twycross RG. Value of cocaine in opiate-containing elixirs. Br Med J 1977;4:1348.

60. Ansell BM, Hanna DB, Stoppard M. Naproxen absorption in children. Curr Med Res Opin 1975;3:46-50.

61. Runkel R, Forchielli E, Sevelius H et al. Nonlinear plasma level response to high doses of naproxen. Clin Pharmacol Ther 1974;15:261-6.

62. Runkel R, Chaplin M, Boost G et al. Absorption, distribution, metabolism, and excretion of naproxen in various laboratory animals and human subjects. J Pharm Sci 1972;61:703-8.

63. Segre EJ. Naproxen metabolism in man. J Clin Pharmacol 1975;15:316-23.

64. Runkel R, Forchielli E, Boost G et al. Naproxen-metabolism, excretion and comparative pharmacokinetics. Scand J Rheumatology (Suppl)1973;2:29-36.

65. Brogden RN, Pinder RM, Sawyer PR et al. Naproxen: a review of its pharmacological properties and therapeutic efficacy and use. Drugs 1975;9:326-63.

66. Brezin JH, Katz SM, Schwartz AB et al. Reversible renal failure and nephrotic syndrome associated with nonsteroidal anti-inflammatory drugs. N Engl J Med 1979;301:1271-3.

67. Cartwright KC, Trotter TL, Cohen ML. Naproxen nephrotoxicity. Ariz Med 1979;36:124-6.

68. Janssen FW et al. Metabolism and kinetics of oxaprozin in normal subjects. Clin Pharmacol Ther 1980;27:352-62.

69. Reynolds WJ et al. Oxaprozin: a once-daily treatment regimen in rheumatoid arthritis. J Rheumatol 1979;6:345-50.

70. Anon. Reevaluation of parenteral pentazocine. Med Lett Drugs Ther 1976;18:46-7.

71. Berkowitz B. Influence of plasma levels and metabolism on pharmacological activity: pentazocine. Ann NY Acad Sci 1971;179:269-81.

72. Ehrnebo M, Boreus LO, Lonroth U. Bioavailability and first-pass metabolism of oral pentazocine in man. Clin Pharmacol Ther 1977;22:888-92.

73. Burt RAP, Beckett AH. The absorption and excretion of pentazocine after administration by different routes. Br J Anesth 1971;43:427-35.

74. Keeri-Szanto M, Pomeroy JR. Atmospheric pollution and pentazocine metabolism. Lancet 1971;1:947-9.

75. Oh SJ, Rollins JL, Lewis I. Pentazocine-induced fibrous myopathy. JAMA 1975;231:271-3.

76. Brogden RN, Speight TM, Avery GS. Pentazocine: a review of its pharmacologic properties, therapeutics, efficacy and dependence liability. Drugs 1973;5:6-91.

77. Beaver WT. A Clinical comparison of the effects of oral and intramuscular administration of analgesics: Pentazocine and phenazocine. Clin Pharmacol Ther 1968;9:582-97.

78. DiSanto AR. Phenylbutazone. J Am Pharm Assoc 1976;NS16:365-7.

79. Koch-Weser J, Sellers EM. Binding of drugs to serum albumin (2 parts). N Engl J Med 1976;294:311-6; 526-31.

80. Burns JJ, Rose RK, Chenkin T et al. The physiological disposition of phenylbutazone (Butazolidin) in man and a method for its estimation in biological material. J Pharmacol Exp Ther 1953;109:346-57.

81. Burns JJ, Rose RK, Goodwin S et al. The metabolic fate of phenylbutazone (Butazolidin) in man. J Pharmacol Exp Ther 1955;113:481-9.

82. Miller RR, Feingold A, Paxinos J. Propoxyphene hydrochloride: a critical review. JAMA 1970;213:996-1006.

83. McBay AJ, Hudson P. Propoxyphene overdose deaths. JAMA 1975;233:1257.

84. Verebely K, Inturrisi CE. Disposition of propoxyphene and norpropoxyphene in man after a single oral dose. Clin Pharmacol Ther 1974;15:302-9.

85. Poust RI, Jaffe JM. Propoxyphene. J Am Pharm Assoc 1976;NS16:97-100.

86. Wolen RL, Ziege EA, Gruber CM. Determination of propoxyphene and norpropoxyphene by chemical ionization mass fragmentography. Clin Pharmacol Ther 1975;17:15-20.

87. Anon. Darvon and Darvon-N. Med Lett Drugs Ther 1972;14:37-8.

88. Tennant FS, Russell BA, Casas SK et al. Heroin detoxification: a comparison of propoxyphene and methadone. JAMA 1975;232:1019-22.

89. Baragar FD, Smith TC. Drug interaction studies with sodium meclofenamate (Meclomen®). Curr Ther Res (Suppl)1978;23:S51-9.

90. Muschek LD, Grindel JM. Review of the pharmacokinetics and metabolism of zomepirac in man and animals. J Clin Pharmacol 1980;20:223-9.

91. Moore RA, Rumack BH, Conner CS et al. Naloxone: underdosage after narcotic poisoning. Am J Dis Child 1980;134:156-8.

92. Anon. Diagnosis and management of reactions to drug abuse. Med Lett Drugs Ther 1980;22:73-6.

93. Gerhardt T, Bancalari E, Cohen H et al. Use of naloxone to reverse narcotic respiratory depression in the newborn infant. J Pediatr 1977;90:1009-12.

94. Fischer CG, Cook DR. Respiratory and narcotic antagonistic effects of naloxone in infants. Anesth Analg 1974;53:849-52.

95. Longnecker DE, Grazis PA, Eggers GWN. Naloxone for antagonism of morphine-induced respiratory depression. Anesth Analg 1973;52:447-52.

96. Evans JM, Hogg MIJ, Lunn JN et al. Degree and duration of reversal by naloxone of effects of morphine in conscious subjects. Br Med J 1974;2:589-91.

97. Fishman J, Roffwarg H, Hellman L. Disposition of naloxone-7, 8-^{3}H in normal and narcotic-dependent men. J Pharmacol Exp Ther 1973;187:575-80.

98. Ngai SH, Berkowitz BA, Yang JC et al. Pharmacokinetics of naloxone in rats and in man: basis for its potency and short duration of action. Anesthesiology 1976;44:398-401.

99. Moreland TA, Brice JEH, Walker CHM et al. Naloxone pharmacokinetics in the newborn. Br J Clin Pharmacol 1980;9:609-12.

100. Hvidberg EF, Dam M. Clinical pharmacokinetics of anticonvulsants. Clin Pharmacokinet 1976;1:161-88.

101. Eadie MJ. Plasma level monitoring of anticonvulsants. Clin Pharmacokinet 1976;1:52-66.

102. Penry JK, Newmark ME. The use of antiepileptic drugs. Ann Intern Med 1979;90:207-18.

103. Morselli PL, Franco-Morselli R. Clinical pharmacokinetics of antiepileptic drugs in adults. Pharmacol Ther 1980;10:65-101.

104. Diehl LW, Muller-Oerlinghausen B, Riedel E. The importance of individual pharmacokinetic data for treatment of epilepsy with carbamazepine. Int J Clin Pharmacol Biopharm 1976;14:144-8.

105. Pinder RM, Brogden RN. Speight TM et al. Clonazepam: a review of its pharmacological properties and therapeutic efficacy in epilepsy. Drugs 1976;12:321-61.

106. Anderson RJ, Gambertoglio JG, Schrier RA. Clinical Use of Drugs in Renal Failure. Springfield: Charles C Thomas, 1976.

107. Woodbury DM, Penry JK, Buchanan RA et al. Antiepileptic drugs. New York: Raven Press, 1972.

108. Alvin J, McHorse T, Hoyumpa A et al. The effect of liver disease in man on the disposition of phenobarbital. J Pharmacol Exp Ther 1975;192:224-35.

109. Lombroso CT. The treatment of status epilepticus. Pediatrics 1974;53:536-40.

110. Lous P. Plasma levels and urinary excretion of three barbituric acids after oral administration to man. Acta Pharmacol Toxicol 1954;10:147-65.

111. Parker KD, Elliott HW, Wright JA et al. Blood and urine concentrations of subjects receiving barbiturates, meprobamate, glutethimide, or diphenylhydantoin. Clin Toxicol 1970;3:131-45.

112. Gugler R, Azarnoff DL. The clinical use of plasma drug concentrations. Ration Drug Ther 1976;10(11):1-7.

113. Emerson R, D'Souza BJ, Vining EP et al. Stopping medication in children with epilepsy. N Engl J Med 1981;304:1125-9.

114. Wilder BJ, Serrano EE, Ramsay RE. Plasma diphenylhydantoin levels after loading and maintenance doses. Clin Pharmacol Ther 1973;14:797-801.

115. Cloyd JC, Gumnit RJ, McLain LW. Status epilepticus: the role of intravenous phenytoin. JAMA 1980;244:1479-81.

116. Pfeifle CE, Adler DS, Gannaway WL. Phenytoin sodium solubility in three intravenous solutions. Am J Hosp Pharm 1981;38:358-62.

117. Perrier D, Rapp R, Young B et al. Maintenance of therapeutic phenytoin plasma levels via intramuscular administration. Ann Intern Med 1976;85:318-21.

118. Odar-Cederlof I, Borga O. Kinetics of diphenylhydantoin in uraemic patients: consequences of decreased plasma protein binding. Eur J Clin Pharmacol 1974;7:31-7.

119. Winter ME, Katcher BS, Koda-Kimble MA, eds. Basic clinical pharmacokinetics. San Francisco: Applied Therapeutics, 1980.

120. Hooper WD, Bochner F, Eadie MJ et al. Plasma protein binding of diphenylhydantoin: effects of sex hormones, renal and hepatic disease. Clin Pharmacol Ther 1974;15:276-82.

121. Feldman S, Phenytoin. J Am Pharm Assoc 1975; NS15:647-50.

122. Letteri JM, Melik H, Louis S et al. Diphenylhydantoin metabolism in uremia. N Engl J Med 1971;285:648-52.

123. Blaschke TF, Meffin PJ, Melmon KL et al. Influence of acute viral hepatitis on phenytoin kinetics and protein binding. Clin Pharmacol Ther 1975;17:685-91.

124. Reynolds EH. Chronic antiepileptic toxicity: a review. Epilepsia 1975;16:319-52.

125. Louis S, Kutt H, McDowell F. The cardiocirculatory changes caused by Dilantin and its solvent. Am Heart J 1967;74:523-29.

126. Cloyd JC, Bosch DE, Sawchuk RJ. Concentration-time profile of phenytoin after admixture with small volumes of intravenous fluids. Am J Hosp Pharm 1978;35:45-8.

127. Anon. Surgeon general's advisory on the use of salicylates and Reye syndrome. Morbid Mortal Wkly Rep 1982;31:289-90.

128. Millichap JG. Drug treatment of convulsive disorders. N Engl J Med 1972;286:464-9.

129. Kutt H. Pharmacodynamic and pharmacokinetic measurements of antiepileptic drugs. Clin Pharmacol Ther 1974;16:243-50.

130. Browne TR. Drug therapy: valproic acid. N Engl J Med 1980;302:661-66.

131. Jeavons PM, Clark JE, Maheshwari MC. Treatment of generalized epilepsies of childhood and adolescence with sodium valproate. Devel Med Child Neurol 1977;19:9-25.

132. Coulter DL, Wu H, Allen RJ. Valproic acid therapy in childhood epilepsy. JAMA 1980;244:785-8.

133. Gugler R, von Unruh GE. Clinical pharmacokinetics of valproic acid. Clin Pharmacokinet 1980;5:67-83.

134. Robinson DS, Nies A, Ravaris L et al. Clinical pharmacology of phenelzine. Arch Gen Psychiatry 1978;35:629-35.

135. Tyrer P, Gardner M, Lambourn J et al. Clinical and pharmacokinetic factors affecting response to phenelzine. Br J Psychiatry 1980;136:359-65.

136. Gelenberg AJ. Prescribing antidepressants. Drug Ther 1979;9:95-112.

137. Stern SL, Rush AJ, Mendels J. Toward a rational pharmacotherapy of depression. Am J Psychiatry 1980;137:545-52.

138. Paykel ES, Parker RR, Penrose RJJ et al. Depressive classification and prediction of response to phenelzine. Br J Psychiatry 1979;134:572-81.

139. Anon. Antidepressant Drugs, The Medical Letter reference handbook. New Rochelle, New York: The Medical Letter, 1975:54-6.

140. Risch SC, Huey LY, Janowsky DS. Plasma levels of tricyclic antidepressants and clinical efficiency: review of the literature, parts I and II. J Clin Psychiatry 1979;40:4-16, 58-69.

141. Ziegler VE, Biggs JT, Wylie LT et al. Protriptyline kinetics. Clin Pharmacol Ther 1978;23:580-4.

142. Gram LF, Christiansen J. First-pass metabolism of imipramine in man. Clin Pharmacol Ther 1975;17:555-63.

143. Taska RJ. Clinical laboratory aids in the treatment of depression. Curr Concepts Psychiatry 1977;3:12-20.

144. Bunney WE. Psychopharmacology of the switch process in affective illness. In: DiMascio A, Kollam KF, eds. Psychopharmacology: a generation of progress. New York: Raven Press, 1978;1249-59.

145. Bailey DN, Dyke C van, Langou RA et al. Tricyclic antidepressants: plasma levels and clinical findings in overdose. Am J Psychiatry 1978;135:1325-8.

146. Rickels K, Case G, Werblowsky J et al. Amoxapine and imipramine in the treatment of depressed outpatients: a controlled study. Am J Psychiatry 1981;138:20-4.

147. Coopen A, Montgomery SA, Gupta RK et al. A double-blind comparison of lithium carbonate and maprotiline in the prophylaxis of the affective disorders. Br J Psychiatry 1976;128:479-85.

148. Pinder RM, Brogden RN, Speight TM et al. Maprotiline: a review of its pharmacological properties and therapeutic efficacy in mental depressive states. Drugs 1977;13:321-52.

149. Trick KLK. Double-blind comparison of maprotiline with amitriptyline in the treatment of depressive illness. Int Pharmacopsychiatry 1975;10:193-8.

150. Stimmel GL. Maprotiline (Ludiomil®). Drug Intell Clin Pharm 1980;14:585-90.

151. Brogden RN, Heel RC, Speight TM et al. Mianserin: a review of its pharmacological properties and therapeutic efficacy in depressive illness. Drugs 1978;16:273-301.

152. Fields ED. Nomifensine maleate. Drug Intell Clin Pharm 1982;16:547-52.

153. Rawls WN. Trazodone. Drug Intell Clin Pharm 1982;16:7-13.

154. Klein DF, Gittleman R, Quitkin F et al, eds. Diagnosis and drug treatment of psychiatric disorders: adults and children. 2nd ed. Baltimore: Williams and Wilkins, 1980.

155. Jarvick ME. Psychopharmacology in the practice of medicine. New York: Appleton-Century-Crofts, 1977.

156. Eisdorfer C, Fann WE. Psychopharmacology of aging. New York: Spectrum Publications, 1980.

157. Kessler KA, Waletzky JP. Clinical use of the antipsychotics. Am J Psychiatry 1981;138:202-9.

158. Donlon PT, Hopkins J, Tupin JP. Overvic\. efficacy and safety of the rapid neuroleptization method with injectable haloperidol. Am J Psychiatry 1979;136:273-8.

159. May PRA, Van Putten T. Plasma levels of chlorpromazine in schizophrenia: a critical review of the literature. Arch Gen Psychiatry 1978;35:1081-7.

160. Curry SH, Davis JM, Janowski DS, et al. Factors affecting chlorpromazine plasma levels in psychiatric patients. Arch Gen Psychiatry 1970;22:209-16.

161. Mason AS, Granacher RP. Basic principles of rapid neuroleptization. Dis Nerv Syst 1976;37:547-51.

162. DiMascio A, Shader RI. Butyrophenones in Psychiatry. New York: Raven Press, 1972;11-23.

163. Anon. Tardive dyskinesia: summary of a Task Force Report of the American Psychiatric Association. Am J Psychiatry 1980;137:1163-72.

164. Stimmel GL. Affective disorders. J Contin Educ Hosp Clin Pharm 1979;1:27-39.

165. Goodwin FK, Zis AP. Lithium in the treatment of mania. Arch Gen Psychiatry 1979;36:840-4.

166. Grof P. Some practical aspects of lithium treatment. Arch Gen Psychiatry 1979;36:891-3.

167. Schou M. Biology and pharmacology of the lithium ion. Pharmacol Rev 1957;9:17-58.

168. Amidsen A. Serum level monitoring and clinical pharmacokinetics of lithium. Clin Pharmacokinet 1977;2:73-92.

169. Ramsey TA, Cox M. Lithium and the kidney: a review. Am J Psychiatr 1982;139:443-9.

170. Greenblatt DJ, Miller RR. Rational use of psychotropic drugs. I. Hypnotics. Am J Hosp Pharm 1974; 31:990-5.

171. Kales A, Kales JD. Sleep disorders: recent findings in the diagnosis and treatment of disturbed sleep. N Engl J Med 1974;290:487-99.

172. National Academy of Sciences Institute of Medicine. Sleeping pills, insomnia, and medical practice. Washington, DC: National Academy of Sciences, 1979. (Publication No. IOM-79-04).

173. Snyder SH, Enna SJ, Young AB. Brain mechanisms associated with therapeutic actions of benzodiazepines: focus on neurotransmitters. Am J Psychiatry 1977;134:662-5.

174. Sellers EM, Kalant H. Alcohol intoxication and withdrawal. N Engl J Med 1976;294:757-62.

175. Hillestad L, Hansen T, Melsom H, et al. Diazepam metabolism in normal man: I. Serum concentrations and clinical effects after IV, IM, and oral administration. Clin Pharmacol Ther 1974;16:479-84.

176. Greenblatt DJ, Joyce TH, Comer WH, et al. Clinical Pharmacokinetics of lorazepam. II. Intramuscular injection. Clin Pharmacol Ther 1977;21:222-30.

177. Dundee JW. New IV anaesthetics. Br J Anaesth 1979;5:641-8.

178. Brown CR. The use of benzodiazepines in prison populations. J Clin Psychiatry 1978;39:219-22.

179. Greenblatt DJ, Shader RI. Benzodiazepines (2 parts). N Engl J Med 1974;291:1011-15 and 1239-43.

180. Covi L, Lipman R, Pattison JH, et al. Length of treatment with anxiolytic sedatives and response to their sudden withdrawal. Acta Psychiatrica Scand 1973;49:51-64.

181. Evans RL. Alprazolam. Drug Intell Clin Pharm 1981;15:633-8.

182. Greenblatt DJ, Shader RI, Koch-Weser J. Flurazepam hydrochloride, a benzodiazepine hypnotic. Ann Intern Med 1975;83:237-41.

183. Marttila JK, Hammel RJ, Alexander B, et al. Potential untoward effects of longterm use of flurazepam in geriatric patients. J Amer Pharm Assoc 1977;NS17:692-5.

184. Greenblatt DJ, Allen MD, Shader RI. Toxicity of high-dose flurazepam in the elderly. Clin Pharmacol Ther 1977;21:355-61.

185. Kaplan SA, deSilva JAF, Jack ML, et al. Blood level profile in man following chronic oral administration of flurazepam hydrochloride. J Pharm Sci 1973;62:1932-5.

186. Kales A, Bixler EO, Kales JD, et al. Comparative effectiveness of nine hypnotic drugs: sleep laboratory studies. J Clin Pharmacol 1977;17:207-13.

187. Mattila MAK, Larni HM. Flunitrazepam: a review of its pharmacological properties and therapeutic use. Drugs 1980;20:353-74.

188. Eberts FS, Philopoulos Y, Reineke LM et al. Triazolam disposition. Clin Pharmacol Ther 1981;29:81-93.

189. Smith MT et al. Eur J Clin Pharmacol 1981;19:271.

190. Greenblatt DJ, Shader RI. Pharmacokinetic understanding of antianxiety drug therapy. South Med J 1978;71 (Suppl 2):2-9.

191. Greenblatt DJ, Shader RI, Koch-Weser J. Pharmacokinetics in clinical medicine: oxazepam versus other benzodiazepines. Dis Nerv Syst 1975;36(Sect 2):6-13.

192. Marshall EK Jr, Owens AH Jr. Absorption, excretion, and metabolic fate of chloral hydrate and trichloroethanol. Bull Johns Hopkins Hosp 1954;95:1-18.

193. Breimer DD. Clinical pharmacokinetics of hypnotics. Clin Pharmacokinet 1977;2:93-109.

194. Kales A, Bixler EO, Kales JD et al. Comparative effectiveness of nine hypnotic drugs: sleep laboratory studies. J Clin Pharmacol 1977;17:207-13.

195. Greenblatt DJ, Miller RR. Rational use of psychotropic drugs. I. Hypnotics. Am J Hosp Pharm 1974;31:990-5.

196. Anon. Current drug therapy-barbiturates. Am J Hosp Pharm 1976;33:333-9.

197. Hvidberg EF, Dam M. Clinical pharmacokinetics of anticonvulsants. Clin Pharmacokinet 1976;1:161-88.

198. Jusko WJ, Gretch M. Plasma and tissue protein binding of drugs in pharmacokinetics. Drug Metab Rev 1976;5:43-140.

199. Kales A, Hauri P, Bixler EO et al. Effectiveness of intermediate - term use of secobarbital. Clin Pharmacol Ther 1976;20:541-5.

200. Kadak D, Inaba T, Endrenyi L et al. Comparative drug elimination capacity in man-glutethimide, amobarbital, antipyrine, and sulfinpyrazone. Clin Pharmacol Ther 1973;14:552-60.

201. Special Symposium on Piroxicam. Eur J Rheumatol Inflammation 1981;4:275-377.

202. Ishizaki T et al. Pharmacokinetics of piroxicam, a new nonsteroidal anti-inflammatory agent, under fasting and postprandial states in man. J Pharmacokinet Biopharm 1979;7:369-81.

203. Day RO et al. Relationship of serum naproxen concentration to efficacy in rheumatoid arthritis. Clin Pharmacol Ther 1982;31:733-40.

204. Rubin TN, Tomosada WP. The pain cocktail as an adjunctive agent in the treatment of spine pain patients. Drug Intell Clin Pharm 1981;15:958-63.

205. Bauer LA. Interference of oral phenytoin absorption by continuous nasogastric feedings. Neurology 1982;32:570-72.

206. Gibberd FB, Nicholls A, Wright MG. The influence of folic acid on the frequency of epileptic attacks. Eur J Clin Pharmacol 1981;19:57-60.

207. Willmore LJ, Wilder BJ, Bruni J et al. Effect of valproic acid on hepatic function. Neurology 1978;28:961-4.

40:00 ELECTROLYTIC, CALORIC AND WATER BALANCE

40:12 REPLACEMENT SOLUTIONS

General References: 1-3

Class Instructions. Oral products should be taken with (tablets) or diluted in (liquids and powders) 3/4 to 1 glass of water or juice to avoid GI injury or laxative effect; may be taken with food or after meals if upset stomach occurs.

Phosphate Salts   Various

Pharmacology. Structural element of bones and involved in carbohydrate metabolism, energy transfer, muscle contraction and as a buffer in the renal excretion of hydrogen ion.

Administration and Adult Dose. **PO** 250–500 mg (8–16 mmol) of phosphorus qid initially, adjusted according to serum phosphate and calcium. **IV replacement** (recent and uncomplicated hypophosphatemia) 0.08 mmol/kg, to maximum of 0.2 mmol/kg; (prolonged and multiple causes) 0.16 mmol/kg, to maximum of 0.24 mmol/kg. No single dose should exceed 0.24 mmol/kg.[1] Doses should be infused over 6 hr and additional doses guided by serum levels. When serum level reaches 2 mg/dl, change to oral dosing. **IV in TPN** 5–15 mmol/L.

Dosage Individualization. Renal impairment decreases requirements. The salt form should be carefully chosen based on patient's sodium and potassium requirements. Needs are increased during alcohol withdrawal, diabetic ketoacidosis, respiratory alkalosis, aluminum antacid therapy, burns and anabolism.[1,4]

Pediatric Dose. **PO** (under 4 yr) 250 mg (8 mmol) of phosphorus qid initially; (over 4 yr) same as adult dose. **IV** same as adult dose. **IV in TPN** (infants) 1.5–2 mmol/kg/day.

Dosage Forms. See Phosphate Replacement Products Comparison Chart.

Patient Instructions. Do not take capsules whole, but dissolve contents in 3/4 glass of water before taking. Powder must be dissolved in one gallon of water before using. Chilling solution may improve palatability. See Class Instructions.

Pharmacokinetics and Biopharmaceutics. *Plasma Levels.* (As phosphorus) adults 3.0–4.5 mg/dl (0.1–0.15 mmol/dl); children 4.0–7.0 mg/dl (0.13–0.23 mmol/dl). Levels below 1 mg/dl are dangerous and require replacement.[1]

Fate. About 67% is absorbed from the GI tract.[4] Normal daily adult intake is 800–1000 mg phosphorus with about 90% excreted in urine and 10% in feces.[1]

Adverse Reactions. Occasionally diarrhea and stomach upset occur with oral dosage forms.[4] Dose-related hyperphosphatemia, metastatic calcium deposition, dehydration and hyperkalemia or hypernatremia (depending on salt used) can occur.[1]

Contraindications. Hyperphosphatemia; hypocalcemia; hyperkalemia (potassium salt); hypernatremia (sodium salt).

Precautions. Use cautiously in patients with renal impairment and in those with hypercalcemia. Dilute IV forms before use and administer slowly.

Parameters to Monitor. Serum phosphorus regularly, frequency determined by condition of patient; BUN and/or Cr_s and serum calcium periodically. Monitor serum sodium and/or potassium periodically, depending on salt form used.

Notes. Phosphate salts may precipitate in the presence of calcium salts in IV solutions; add no more than 40 mmol phosphate and 5 mEq calcium per liter.

Phosphate Replacement Products Comparison Chart[a]

PRODUCT	PHOSPHORUS MG	PHOSPHORUS MMOL	SODIUM MG	SODIUM MEQ	POTASSIUM MEQ
ORAL					
Fleet's Phospho-Soda® (per ml)	128	4.1	111	4.8	0
Neutra-Phos® Plain (per cap or 75 ml)	250	8.1	164	7.1	7.1
Neutra-Phos® K (per cap or 75 ml)	250	8.1	0	0	14.3
K-Phos® Modified Formula (per tablet)	125	4	67	2.9	1.4
K-Phos® Neutral (per tablet)	250	8.1	301	13.1	1.4
Skim Milk (per quart)	1000	32	552	24	40
INTRAVENOUS					
Potassium Phosphate Abbott (per ml)	94	3	0	0	4.4
Sodium Phosphate Abbott (per ml)	94	3	0.2	4	0

a. From reference 1 and product information.

Potassium Salts   Various

Pharmacology. The major intracellular cation; involved in electrical activity and glucose utilization.

Administration and Adult Dose. Variable, must be adjusted to needs of patient. PO 40–60 mEq/day prevents hypokalemia in most patients on long-term diuretic therapy; however, ambulatory patients with uncomplicated hypertension and most edematous patients need no supplementation.[3,5,6] IV up to 10 mEq/hr; concentration should not exceed 30 mEq/L if serum potassium exceeds 2.5 mEq/L. If serum potassium is less than 2.0 mEq/L, up to 40 mEq/hr may be given; a maximum concentration of 80 mEq/L and a maximum of 400 mEq/day should not be exceeded. Infusion into a central vein requires use of a volume control device — potassium concentration should not exceed 40 mEq/L unless the infusion site is via a large vein distal to the heart (eg, femoral vein).

Dosage Individualization. Maintenance doses should be based on serum potassium; renal impairment decreases requirements.

Pediatric Dose. PO 1–2 mEq/kg/day during diuretic therapy.

Dosage Forms. PO—see Oral Potassium Products Comparison Chart; **Inj** (potassium chloride) 2 mEq/ml; (potassium acetate) 2, 2.5 mEq/ml; (potassium phosphate)—see Phosphate Replacement Products Comparison Chart.

Patient Instructions. See Class Instructions.

Pharmacokinetics and Biopharmaceutics. *Plasma Levels.* 3.5–5 mEq/L (may vary depending on laboratory); signs of hypokalemia appear below 2.5 mEq/L; levels above 7 mEq/L are dangerous. Clinical signs of hyperkalemia (eg, hyporeflexia) are not reliable indicators of serum levels. Levels do not correlate well with total body stores; alkalosis decreases levels and acidosis increases levels.[3,5,6]

Fate. Well absorbed orally. Normal daily intake is about 100 mEq, with 85–90% excreted in urine and 10–15 mEq excreted in feces. Losses are increased in vomiting, diarrhea, aldosteronism and therapy with potassium wasting drugs. Urinary losses are decreased in renal impairment and with low sodium diets.[3]

Adverse Reactions. Bad taste, nausea, vomiting, diarrhea and abdominal discomfort may occur frequently with oral liquids. Small bowel and occasional gastric ulceration may occur with enteric-coated tablets and they should not be used.[7] Hyperkalemia may occur. Local tissue necrosis may occur if IV solution extravasates.

Contraindications. Severe renal impairment with oliguria or azotemia; untreated Addison's disease; adynamia episodica hereditaria, acute dehydration; heat cramps; hyperkalemia. Additionally, all solid dosage forms (including timed release products) are contraindicated in patients in whom delay or arrest of the tablet through the GI tract may occur.

Precautions. Use with caution (if at all) in patients receiving potassium-sparing diuretics, in patients with digitalis-induced atrioventricular conduction disturbances and in early chronic renal failure secondary to diabetes mellitus.

Parameters to Monitor. Serum potassium regularly, frequency determined by condition of patient; BUN and/or serum creatinine periodically.

Notes. Chloride salt is preferred for most uses, such as during diuretic therapy; non-chloride salt is preferred in acidosis, such as with amphotericin B, carbonic anhydrase inhibitors or mafenide. A potassium-sparing diuretic may be preferable to potassium supplementation when large supplements are needed, when aldosterone levels are elevated or when enhanced therapeutic response is desired.[3,7] See also Potassium Content of Selected Foods and Salt Substitutes in the Dietary Considerations chapter.

Oral Potassium Products Comparison Chart

PRODUCT	BRAND NAMES	POTASSIUM CONTENT
Potassium Chloride Liquid 5%	Various	5 ml = 3.3 mEq 15 ml = 10 mEq
Potassium Chloride Liquid 10%	Kaochlor® Kay Ciel® K-Lor® Klorvess® Various	5 ml = 6.7 mEq 15 ml = 20 mEq
Potassium Chloride Liquid 15%	Rum-K®	5 ml = 10 mEq 15 ml = 30 mEq
Potassium Chloride Liquid 20%	Kaon-Cl® 20% Klor-Con® Various	5 ml = 13.3 mEq 15 ml = 40 mEq
Potassium Chloride Powder	K-Lyte/Cl®	1 packet = 25 mEq
	K-Lor® Kay Ciel® Kato® Klor-Con® Various	1 packet = 20 mEq
	K-Lor®	1 packet = 15 mEq
Potassium Chloride Tablets, Effervescent	K-Lyte/Cl® 50	1 tab = 50 mEq
	K-Lyte/Cl®	1 tab = 25 mEq
	Kaochlor-Eff® Klorvess®	1 tab = 20 mEq
Potassium Chloride Capsules, Tablets, Timed Release	Kaon-Cl® 10 K-Tab® Klotrix®	1 tab = 10 mEq
	Micro-K® Slow-K®	1 cap = 8 mEq 1 tab = 8 mEq
	Kaon-Cl®	1 tab = 6.7 mEq
Potassium Acetate/ Bicarbonate/Citrate	Potassium Triplates® Tri-K®	5 ml = 15 mEq 15 ml = 45 mEq

Continued

Oral Potassium Products Comparison Chart

PRODUCT	BRAND NAMES	POTASSIUM CONTENT
Potassium Bicarbonate/	K-Lyte DS®	1 packet = 50 mEq
Citrate	K-Lyte®	1 packet = 25 mEq
Potassium Gluconate	Kaon®	5 ml = 6.7 mEq
	Various	15 ml = 20 mEq

40:18 POTASSIUM-REMOVING RESINS

General References: 3

Sodium Polystyrene Sulfonate

Kayexalate®

Pharmacology. Cation exchange resin that exchanges potassium for sodium with about 33% exchange efficiency. 15 g resin (4 *level* teaspoonfuls) binds about 20 mEq of potassium and liberates an equal amount of sodium.

Administration and Adult Dose. PO 15 g daily to qid,[4] although doses of up to 40 g qid have been recommended.[3] The total dose and duration of therapy depends on patient response. Powder should be given with, or suspended in, a sorbitol solution to prevent constipation (eg, 15 ml of 70% sorbitol).[3] **PR as enema** 30 g once or twice a day as an emulsion in 150–200 ml sorbitol solution retained for 4–10 hr if possible; alternatively, enema may be retained for 30–45 min and repeated at 1–2 hr intervals until serum potassium is in a safe range.[4]

Dosage Forms. Pwdr 454 g.

Pharmacokinetics and Biopharmaceutics. *Onset and Duration.* Onset hours to days.

Fate. Not absorbed from GI tract; takes up potassium and liberates sodium as it passes through intestine.[4]

Adverse Reactions. Anorexia, nausea and vomiting occur frequently with large doses; gastric irritation and fecal impaction (especially in the elderly) occur occasionally. These effects may be avoided by using the enema. See Drug Interactions chapter.

Precautions. Use with caution in patients who cannot tolerate any additional sodium load. If rapid potassium lowering is required, other measures should be employed.

Parameters to Monitor. Serum potassium at least daily and more frequently if indicated; electrocardiogram and patient signs may be useful in evaluating status.

Notes. Heating may alter the exchange properties of the resin. Rectal administration is less effective than oral use.

40:28 DIURETICS

General References: 8-11

Class Instructions. If divided doses are taken, the last dose should usually be taken in the afternoon or early evening to avoid having to void urine during the night. If no potassium supplement or no potassium-sparing diuretic has been prescribed, some foods high in potassium should be taken each day (see Potassium Content of Selected Foods in the Dietary Considerations chapter). Highly salted foods should be avoided, but rigid salt restriction need not be followed. Excessive water intake should be avoided. Dizziness or lightheadedness (especially upon arising from sitting or lying), muscle cramps, weakness, lethargy, dry mouth, thirst or low urine output should be reported.

Amiloride Hydrochloride   Midamor®

Amiloride is a potassium-sparing diuretic with a mechanism and site of action resembling triamterene. It has antihypertensive activity equivalent to the thiazides and a longer duration of action than triamterene. Adverse reactions are generally similar to triamterene. Dosage is 10 mg/day in 1 or 2 doses, to a maximum of 20 mg daily. It is available as 5 mg tablets and also in Moduretic® which contains hydrochlorothiazide 50 mg and amiloride 5 mg.[12]

Bumetanide   Bumex®

Bumetanide is a potent sulfonamide loop diuretic with a mechanism and site of action very similar to furosemide. Adverse reactions are similar to furosemide, except bumetanide has caused a sometimes severe myalgia with high doses in patients with renal failure. Dosage is 0.5-2 mg/day PO, IM, or IV. Doses up to 40 mg have been used in renal failure.[13,14] Available as 0.5 and 1 mg tablets and inj 0.25 mg/ml.

Ethacrynic Acid   Edecrin®

Pharmacology. Potent nonsulfonamide diuretic with a mechanism and site of action, potency and electrolyte excretion pattern similar to furosemide. Furosemide is preferable, because it is less toxic and has a broader dose-response curve.[15]

Administration and Adult Dose. PO for edema 50-100 mg/day initially, then adjust dose in 25-50 mg/day increments, according to patient requirements and response. Maintenance dosage range is 50-200 mg/day, although some patients may require up to 200 mg bid. **IV** (slowly over several minutes) 0.5-1 mg/kg (50 mg for average patient), to maximum of 100 mg in one dose. If second dose is required, change injection site. **Do not give IM or SC.**

Pediatric Dose. Contraindicated in infants. PO 25 mg in one dose; increase by 25 mg increments to desired effect and maintain on alternate day dosage or by alternating therapy with rest periods. **IV (slowly over several minutes)** 0.5-1 mg/kg in a single dose. **Do not give IM or SC.**

Dosage Forms. Tab 25, 50 mg; Inj 50 mg.

Patient Instructions. See Class Instructions. Also, take with food or milk to avoid stomach upset.

Pharmacokinetics and Biopharmaceutics. *Onset and Duration.*
PO onset 30 min; peak 2 hr; duration 6–8 hr. IV onset 5 min; peak 15–30 min; duration 2 hr.[10]

Adverse Reactions. Similar to furosemide; however, hearing loss is more frequent, more often permanent and has occurred after oral use in oliguric patients.[15,16] Nausea, abdominal pain and diarrhea are common; occasionally GI bleeding may occur.[16] Pain and thrombophlebitis may occur after IV administration.

Contraindications. Anuria (except for single dose in acute anuria); hypotension; dehydration with low serum sodium; metabolic alkalosis with hypokalemia; nursing mothers. Should be discontinued if increasing electrolyte imbalance, azotemia, and/or oliguria occurs during its use in severe renal disease, or if severe watery diarrhea occurs during its use in any patient.

Parameters to Monitor. See Furosemide.

Precautions. See Furosemide and Drug Interactions chapter.

Notes. IV injection should be used within 24 hr after reconstitution and should not be mixed or infused with whole blood or its derivatives. Drug is not a sulfonamide derivative, and therefore may be useful in patients allergic to sulfonamides.

Furosemide   Lasix®, Various

Pharmacology. Inhibits active chloride transport in the ascending limb of the loop of Henle, causing markedly enhanced excretion of chloride and its attendant sodium and water. Medullary hypertonicity is decreased, thus interfering with the countercurrent multiplier system and resulting in large volumes of dilute urine. Potassium, magnesium, calcium and phosphate excretion are also increased. IV doses increase venous capacitance independent of diuretic effect, producing rapid improvement in pulmonary edema.[17]

Administration and Adult Dose. PO for edema 20–80 mg as a single morning dose initially, increasing successive doses by 20–40 mg in 6–8 hr until response is obtained or to maximum of 600 mg/day (although doses this large probably indicate need for sodium restriction and/or addition of other diuretics to regimen). After response, effective dosage is given in 1–2 doses daily; usual maintenance dose is 40–120 mg/day. **PO for chronic renal failure** 240 mg bid, increasing to maximum of 500 mg bid.[8] **PO for hypertension** 40 mg bid. **IV** should be used only when oral administration is not feasible. Doses can be given over 1–2 min, except rate should not exceed 4 mg/min when large doses are given to patients in renal failure. **IM or IV for edema** 20–40 mg as a single dose; additional doses of 20 mg greater than previous dose may be given q 2 hr until desired response is obtained. This dose is then given in 1–2 doses daily for maintenance; change to PO as soon as feasible. **IV for acute pulmonary edema** 40 mg initially, may repeat in 1 hr with 80 mg if necessary.

Pediatric Dose. PO for edema 2 mg/kg in 1 dose initially, increasing by 1–2 mg/kg in 6–8 hr if necessary, to maximum of 6 mg/kg/day. **IM or IV** 1 mg/kg in 1 dose initially, increasing by 1 mg/kg q 2 or more hr until desired response is obtained or to maximum of 6 mg/kg/day. See Notes.

Dosage Individualization. See Hydrochlorothiazide.

Dosage Forms. **Soln** 10 mg/ml; **Tab** 20, 40, 80 mg; **Inj** 10 mg/ml.

Patient Instructions. See Class Instructions.

Pharmacokinetics and Biopharmaceutics. *Onset and Duration.*

(Venous capacitance) IV onset 5 min, duration > 1 hr. (Diuresis) PO onset 30–60 min, peak 1–2 hr, duration 6 hr; IV onset 15 min, peak 30–60 min, duration 1–2 hr; duration may be prolonged in severe renal impairment. (Hypertension) maximum effect may not occur for several days.[17,18]

Plasma Levels. No relationship between plasma levels and therapeutic effect.[19]

Fate. Much discrepancy among studies because of the lack of reliable assay techniques; 60–69% bioavailable in normals with much variability; 43–46% in uremia; absorption may be markedly impaired in patients with edematous bowel caused by CHF or nephrotic syndrome. 91–98% bound to plasma proteins; reduced in hypoalbuminemia and azotemia. Furosemide appears to be conjugated with glucuronic acid and excreted primarily in the urine by filtration and secretion as unchanged drug and glucuronide. Some studies indicate an increase in hepatic clearance in renal impairment, while others show a decrease.[20-22]

$t_{1/2}$. About 50 min in normals, increasing to about 120 min in CHF and up to several hr in renal impairment.[20]

Adverse Reactions. Dehydration, hypotension, hypochloremic alkalosis and hypokalemia are frequent, although hyperkalemia may occur when potassium supplements or potassium-sparing diuretics are also given. Hyperglycemia, glucose intolerance and hyperuricemia occur as with thiazides—see Hydrochlorothiazide.[15,16,23] Hearing loss, occasionally permanent, has been reported, usually associated with too rapid IV injection of large doses in patients with renal impairment. Rarely thrombocytopenia, neutropenia, jaundice, pancreatitis and a variety of skin reactions have been reported.

Contraindications. Anuria (except for single dose in acute anuria); pregnancy.

Precautions. Furosemide is extremely potent and profound dose-related diuresis and fluid and electrolyte disturbances can occur if the drug is used indiscriminantly. Use caution in patients with severe or progressive renal disease; discontinue if renal function worsens. Use with caution in liver disease, cirrhosis and ascites (may precipitate hepatic encephalopathy),[24] or history of diabetes or gout. Dosage of potent hypotensive agents may have to be reduced if furosemide is added to regimen. Caution should be used in patients allergic to other sulfonamides. See Drug Interactions chapter.

Parameters to Monitor. Monitor serum potassium closely, other electrolytes periodically and serum glucose, uric acid, BUN and creatinine occasionally. Observe for clinical signs of fluid or electrolyte disturbance—see Hydrochlorothiazide.

Notes. Total body potassium is not depleted during long-term use in essential hypertension with or without renal disease; potassium supplementation is not needed unless other factors warrant it.[5,16] Slightly less effective antihypertensive agent than the thiazides.[25] Furosemide has been used IV in hypercalcemia[26] and IV and PO in the treatment of SIADH;[27,28] these techniques require careful monitoring and replacement of fluid and electrolytes—consult literature for details. Furosemide is light-sensitive; oral solution must be refrigerated and protected from light; discard an open bottle after 60 days. Do not use injection if solution is yellow; slight discoloration of tablets does not affect potency.

Hydrochlorothiazide

Esidrix®, Hydrodiuril®, Oretic®, Various

Pharmacology. Thiazides increase sodium and chloride excretion by interfering with their reabsorption in the cortical diluting segment of the nephron; a mild diuresis of slightly concentrated urine results. Potassium, bicarbonate, magnesium, phosphate and iodide excretion is also increased, while calcium is decreased. Antihypertensive efficacy is primarily due to a decrease in extracellular fluid volume, although direct vasodilation may also occur. Urine output is decreased in diabetes insipidus.[4,29,30]

Administration and Adult Dose. PO for edema 25-200 mg/day in 1-3 doses initially; 25-100 mg/day or intermittently for maintenance, to a maximum of 200 mg/day. **PO for hypertension** 25-50 mg bid initially; 25-100 mg/day in one dose for maintenance, to a maximum of 200 mg/day. Use the minimum dose required for effectiveness; larger doses increase side effects with little additional benefit.

Dosage Individualization. Thiazides and related diuretics (except metolazone) are not effective as diuretics with a Cl_{cr} less than 20-30 ml/min.[4,5,29]

Pediatric Dose. PO (under 6 months) may require up to 3.3 mg/kg/day in 2 doses; (over 6 months) 2.2 mg/kg/day in 2 doses.

Dosage Forms. Tab 25, 50, 100 mg.

Patient Instructions. See Class Instructions. Also, if stomach upset occurs, take drug with meals. If persistent anorexia, nausea or vomiting occurs, consult the physician or pharmacist.

Pharmacokinetics and Biopharmaceutics. *Onset and Duration.* Onset of diuresis within 2 hr; peak in 3-6 hr; duration 6-12 hr. Onset of hypotensive effect in 3-4 days; duration one week or less after discontinuing therapy.[29]

   Plasma Levels. No relationship between levels and therapeutic effect.[19]

   Fate. 71 ± 15% oral absorption in normals;[31] increased slightly when given with food and considerably when given with an anticholinergic; decreased by one-half after intestinal shunt surgery.[32] No differences in absorption among formulations. 40-64% plasma protein bound.[19,31] More than 95% excreted unchanged by filtration and secretion.[19]

   $t_{1/2}$. α phase 5.2 hr, β phase 5.6-14.8 hr; prolonged in uncompensated CHF or renal impairment.[19,31]

Adverse Reactions. Volume depletion, hypotension and weakness may occur with high doses and salt restriction. Dilutional hyponatremia may occur in patients with excessive fluid intake; hypochloremic alkalosis may occur.[16] Hypokalemia is frequent; however, its treatment in otherwise healthy hypertensive patients is usually unnecessary.[6,16] Potassium chloride supplementation or potassium-sparing diuretic therapy is needed in older patients, those with cirrhosis, those on digitalis glycosides, those taking other potassium-wasting drugs or if serum potassium falls below 3.0 mEq/L.[2,16,29] Hyperuricemia frequently occurs, but is reversible and treatment is unnecessary unless prior personal or family history of gout exists.[16] Hyperglycemia and alterations in glucose tolerance (usually reversible), loss of diabetic control and precipitation of diabetes occur occasionally.[16] Decreased glucose tolerance may increase in prevalence after several years of therapy.[16,33] Thrombocytopenia and pancreatitis occur rarely. Elevation of serum cholesterol and triglycerides occurs, but significance is unknown.[34]

Contraindications. Anuria; pregnancy, unless accompanied by severe edema; allergy to sulfonamide derivatives.

Precautions. Use with caution in patients with renal function impairment, liver disease (may precipitate hepatic encephalopathy),[24] history of diabetes or gout. Dosage of potent hypotensive agents may have to be reduced if a thiazide is added to the regimen. See Drug Interactions chapter.

Parameters to Monitor. Serum potassium weekly to monthly initially; every 3-6 months when stable.[6,35] Other serum electrolytes periodically. Monitor all electrolytes more closely when other losses occur (eg, vomiting, diarrhea). Clinical signs of fluid or electrolyte depletion such as dry mouth, thirst, weakness, lethargy, muscle pains or cramps, hypotension, oliguria, tachycardia and GI upset.

Thiazide and Related Diuretics Comparison Chart[a]

DRUG	DAILY DOSAGE RANGE FOR EDEMA	DAILY DOSAGE RANGE FOR HYPERTENSION	MAXIMUM DAILY DOSAGE	DOSAGE FORMS	DURATION OF DIURESIS (HOURS)
Bendroflumethiazide Naturetin®	2.5–5 mg	2.5–15 mg	20 mg	Tab 2.5, 5, 10 mg	18–24
Benzthiazide Various	50–150 mg	50–100 mg	200 mg	Tab 25, 50 mg	12–18
Chlorothiazide Diuril®	1–2 g	1–2 g	2 g	Susp 50 mg/ml Tab 250, 500 mg Inj 500 mg[b]	6–12 (PO) 2 (IV)
Chlorthalidone[c] Hygroton® Various	50–200 mg daily or on alternate days	25–100 mg	200 mg	Tab 25, 50, 100 mg	48–72
Cyclothiazide Anhydron®	1–2 mg on alternate days	2 mg	6 mg	Tab 2 mg	24–36
Hydrochlorothiazide Various	25–100 mg	25–100 mg	200 mg	Tab 25, 50, 100 mg	6–12
Hydroflumethiazide Diucardin® Saluron®	25–100 mg	50–100 mg	200 mg	Tab 50 mg	10–12
Indapamide[c] Lozol®	2.5–5 mg	2.5–5 mg	5 mg	Tab 2.5 mg	up to 38

Continued

Thiazide and Related Diuretics Comparison Chart[a]

DRUG	DAILY DOSAGE RANGE FOR EDEMA	DAILY DOSAGE RANGE FOR HYPERTENSION	MAXIMUM DAILY DOSAGE	DOSAGE FORMS	DURATION OF DIURESIS (HOURS)
Methyclothiazide Aquatensen® Enduron®	2.5–5 mg	2.5–5 mg	10 mg	Tab 2.5, 5 mg	24
Metolazone[c] Diulo® Zaroxolyn®	5–10 mg[d]	2.5–5 mg	20 mg	Tab 2.5, 5, 10 mg	12–24
Polythiazide Renese®	1–4 mg	2–4 mg	4 mg	Tab 1, 2, 4 mg	24–36
Quinethazone[c] Hydromox®	50–100 mg	50–100 mg	200 mg	Tab 50 mg	18–24
Trichlormethiazide Various	1–4 mg	2–4 mg	4 mg	Tab 2, 4 mg	24

a. From references 8, 10, 29; patients unresponsive to maximal dose of one agent are unlikely to respond to another agent,[29] except as in d. below.
b. There is no therapeutic advantage in giving the drug parenterally.
c. Not a thiazide, but similar in structure and mechanism of action.
d. In high doses (up to 20 mg/day), metolazone is more effective than other thiazide-like diuretics in patients with chronic renal failure and creatinine clearances less than 20 ml/minute.[29,36]

Mannitol

Osmitrol®, Various

Pharmacology. Osmotic diuretic that inhibits sodium and chloride reabsorption in the proximal tubule and ascending loop of Henle. Sodium, potassium, calcium and phosphate excretion are increased and GFR decreases slightly. Mannitol increases serum osmolality, expanding intravascular volume and decreasing intra-ocular and intracranial pressures. It also appears to disrupt the blood-brain barrier, enhancing penetration of other drugs into the CNS.[37]

Administration and Adult Dose. Never administer IM or SC, or add to whole blood for transfusion. IV as diagnostic evaluation of acute oliguria (*after* blood pressure and CVP are normal and cardiac output is maximized) give test dose of 12.5–25 g of 20–25% solution over 3–5 min (often along with furosemide 80–120 mg IV), repeat in 1 hr if urine output is less than 50 ml/hr. If no response after 2 doses, give no more mannitol and treat for acute tubular necrosis. If response occurs, look for underlying cause of oliguria (eg, hypovolemia). **IV for prevention of acute renal failure** give test dose as above to a total dose of 50 g or more in 1 hr as a loading dose, then maintain urine output at 50 ml/hr with continuous infusion of 5% solution, 20 mEq/L sodium chloride and 1 g/L calcium gluconate. **IV for promotion of excretion of toxins** give test dose and loading doses as above, then maintain urine output at 150–500 ml/hr with continuous infusion of 5% solution, 45 mEq/L sodium chloride, 24 mEq/L sodium acetate, 1 g/L calcium gluconate, 1 g/L magnesium sulfate and 20 mEq/L potassium acetate. To alkalinize urine to enhance excretion of acidic toxins (eg, phenobarbital, myoglobin), use less chloride and more acetate as sodium salt or use sodium bicarbonate.[38] **IV for reduction of intracranial or intraocular pressure** 1.5–2 g/kg over 30–60 min as a 15–25% solution. **IV to decrease nephrotoxicity of cisplatin** 12.5 g push just prior to cisplatin, then 10 g/hr for 6 hr with 20% solution. Replace fluids with 0.45% sodium chloride with 20–30 mEq/L potassium chloride at 250 ml/hr for 6 hr. Maintain urine output greater than 100 ml/hr with mannitol infusion.[39] See Notes.

Pediatric Dose. IV for oliguria or anuria give test dose of 200 mg/kg as above; therapeutic dose 2 g/kg over 2–6 hr as a 15–20% solution. **IV for reduction of intracranial or intraocular pressure** 2 g/kg over 30–60 min as a 15–25% solution. **IV for intoxications** 2 g/kg as 5–10% solution as needed to maintain a high urinary output. See Notes.

Dosage Forms. Inj 5, 10, 15, 20, 25%; Inj as 5, 10, 15% solution with 0.45% NaCl; Inj as 5, 15% solution with 5% dextrose and 0.12% or 0.45% NaCl.

Pharmacokinetics and Biopharmaceutics. *Onset and Duration.* (Diuresis) onset 1–3 hr. (Decrease in intraocular pressure) onset in 30–60 min; duration 4–6 hr. (Decrease in intracranial pressure) onset within 15 min; peak 60–90 min; duration 3–8 hr after stopping infusion.[18,38]

   Fate. 17% absorbed orally.[18] A 200 g/70 kg IV dose increases serum osmolality to 380 mOsm/kg, expands extracellular volume by 2+ liters and decreases serum sodium to 115 mEq/L.[40] Given IV, drug is distributed in extracellular space primarily, but it can slowly penetrate intracellularly. Excreted unchanged in urine, primarily by filtration; 7–10% metabolized by liver.[38]

   $t_{1/2}$. 15 min.[38]

Adverse Reactions. Most serious are fluid and electrolyte imbalance, particularly symptoms of fluid overload such as pulmonary edema, hypertension, water intoxication and congestive heart failure. Necrosis of skin can occur if solution extravasates.

Contraindications. Patients with well established anuria due to severe renal disease or impaired renal function who do not respond to test dose; severe pulmonary congestion, frank pulmonary edema or severe congestive heart failure; severe dehydration; edema not due to renal, cardiac or hepatic disease which is associated with abnormal capillary fragility or membrane permeability; active intracranial bleeding, except during craniotomy.

Precautions. Pregnancy. Observe solution for crystals before administering (see Notes). Water intoxication may occur if fluid input exceeds urine output; masking of inadequate hydration or hypovolemia may occur by drug-induced sustaining of diuresis.

Parameters to Monitor. Monitor urine output closely and discontinue drug if it is low. Monitor serum electrolytes closely, taking care not to misinterpret low serum sodium as a sign of hypotonicity (see Fate); if serum sodium is low, measure serum osmolality.[40]

Notes. Mannitol may crystallize out of solution at concentrations above 15%—crystals may be redissolved by warming in hot water and shaking or by autoclaving; cool to body temperature before administration. Solutions of 20% or greater should be administered through an inline filter. Addition of electrolytes to solutions of 20% or greater may cause precipitation. Mannitol is also used as a urologic irrigant following transurethral prostatic resection and has been used as an osmotic cathartic prior to barium enema.[41]

Spironolactone   Aldactone®, Various

Pharmacology. A competitive aldosterone antagonist that blocks sodium-potassium exchange at the distal tubule, producing a very mild diuresis. Diuretic effect is maximal in states of hyperaldosteronism. Sodium, chloride and calcium excretion are increased, while potassium and magnesium are decreased. Antihypertensive activity is equal to thiazides and it also has a direct positive inotropic action on the heart.[4,16,42]

Administration and Adult Dose. PO for edema 25-200 mg/day (usually 100 mg) initially, adjusting dose after 5 days. If response is inadequate, a thiazide, furosemide, or ethacrynic acid should be added to the regimen. PO for essential hypertension 50-100 mg/day initially, adjusting dose after 2 weeks; up to 100 mg/day combined with a thiazide.[43] Dose of 100 mg bid has been used in low renin hypertension[44] and doses up to 400 mg/day have been used in primary aldosteronism.[45] PO for ascites 100 mg/day initially, increasing to 200-400 mg/day. Restrict sodium to 2 g/day or less and, if necessary, fluid to 1 L/day. Doses of up to 1 g/day have been used, but such high doses are expensive and are an indication for adding a thiazide or loop diuretic.[46] See Parameters to Monitor. Daily or bid dosing is as effective as multiple doses.[42,45,47] To eliminate delay in onset, a loading dose of 2 to 3 times the daily dose may be given on the first day of therapy.[42]

Pediatric Dose. PO 3.3 mg/kg/day, readjust dose after 5 days; dose may be increased up to triple this value. Restrict duration of therapy to 1 month.

Dosage Forms. Tab 25, 50, 100 mg; **Tab** 25 mg with hydrochlorothiazide 25 mg (Aldactazide®). **Tab** 50 mg with hydrochlorothiazide 50 mg (Aldactazide® 50/50).

Patient Instructions. Avoid excessive amounts of high potassium foods or salt substitutes. See also Class Instructions.

Pharmacokinetics and Biopharmaceutics. *Onset and Duration.* Onset gradual, peak 2-3 days with continued dosing;[35] onset can be hastened by giving loading dose;[42] duration 2-3 days after cessation of therapy.[35]

Fate.   Low bioavailability of unchanged drug due to extensive first-pass metabolism to active metabolite, canrenone, which accounts for 30-70% of antimineralocorticoid activity of spironolactone.[19,42,48-51] Canrenone levels are greater when spironolactone is taken with food, possibly indicating increased bioavailability.[19] Canrenone is 98% bound to plasma proteins and is in equilibrium with canrenoate; a total of less than 10% of these metabolites are excreted unchanged in urine.[42,48] Sulfur-containing metabolites probably contribute to activity.[49]

$t_{1/2}$.   (Canrenone) 13-26 hr (average 19) when given in 1 or 2 doses daily; 9-16 hr (average 12.5) when given in 4 divided doses daily.[42,47]

Adverse Reactions.   Hyperkalemia may occur, most frequently in patients with renal function impairment and those receiving potassium supplements.[52,53] Dehydration and hyponatremia occur occasionally, especially when drug is combined with other diuretics. Hyperchloremic acidosis has been reported in cirrhosis.[54] Occasionally, estrogen-like side effects occur including gynecomastia (dose and duration related and usually reversible), decreased libido and relative impotence in males; menstrual irregularities and breast tenderness in females.[52,55]

Contraindications.   Anuria; acute renal insufficiency; rapidly deteriorating renal function; serum creatinine greater than 2.5 mg/dl; serum potassium greater than 5.5 mEq/L.

Precautions.   Pregnancy. Caution in patients with renal function impairment (serum creatinine greater than 1.5 mg/dl) or hepatic disease.[16,52] Dosage of potent hypotensives may have to be decreased if spironolactone is added to the regimen. Potassium supplements should be given only to those with demonstrated hypokalemia who are taking a proximally acting diuretic and a corticosteroid concurrently with spironolactone or only for very short periods in treating cirrhosis and ascites. The drug should not be given with triamterene or amiloride. Spironolactone is tumorigenic in animals and its use should be restricted to patients in whom other therapy is inadequate or inappropriate. See Drug Interactions chapter.

Parameters to Monitor.   Serum electrolytes, particularly potassium, should be measured periodically, especially early in the course of therapy.[35] BUN and/or serum creatinine should be measured periodically. In ascites, obtain daily weight and urinary electrolytes in addition to above, maintaining weight loss at no greater than 0.5-1 kg/day and urinary Na$^+$/K$^+$ ratio at greater than 1.[46]

Notes.   Useful in patients with diabetes or gout because it causes no impairment of glucose tolerance and minimal hyperuricemia. Used in the diagnosis of primary aldosteronism and may be used in the management of the condition in patients unable to undergo surgery.[45] More expensive, yet more effective than potassium supplements.[43] Suspension of drug in cherry syrup is stable for 1 month if refrigerated.

Triamterene   Dyrenium®

Pharmacology.   Acts directly on distal tubular transport of sodium exchange for potassium and hydrogen, producing a mild diuresis that is independent of aldosterone levels. Sodium, chloride, calcium and possibly bicarbonate excretion are increased, while potassium and possibly magnesium are decreased. Antihypertensive activity is inconsistent and less pronounced than with thiazides or spironolactone.[4,16]

Administration and Adult Dose. PO initially 100 mg bid after meals if used alone; lower dose if used with another diuretic. Maintenance dosage should be adjusted to needs of the patient and may range from 100 mg/day to 100 mg every other day; maximum dosage is 300 mg/day.

Pediatric Dose. PO 4 mg/kg/day initially, may increase to 6 mg/kg/day in 1 or 2 doses after meals; maximum dose is 300 mg daily. Decrease dose if used with another diuretic.

Dosage Forms. **Cap** 50, 100 mg; **Cap** 50 mg with hydrochlorothiazide 25 mg (Dyazide®).

Patient Instructions. This drug may be taken with food or milk to minimize stomach upset. Report persistent loss of appetite, nausea or vomiting. Avoid eating excessive amounts of high potassium foods or salt substitutes. See also Class Instructions.

Pharmacokinetics and Biopharmaceutics. *Onset and Duration.* Onset 2–4 hr; full therapeutic effect may not occur for several days; duration 7–9 hr.

Fate. 30–70% absorbed orally.[56] Metabolized to para-hydroxy metabolite, which is partly further metabolized to sulfate conjugate; these two compounds, triamterene glucuronide and a small amount of free triamterene are excreted in the urine and bile.[56-58] 43–53% protein bound; V_d is 2.5 L/kg.[19]

$t_{1/2}$. 1.9–3.7 hr (average 2.8); increased in uremia.[19]

Adverse Reactions. Nausea, vomiting, diarrhea and dizziness occur frequently. Dehydration and hyponatremia with an increase in BUN occur occasionally, especially when drug is combined with other diuretics. Hyperkalemia occurs occasionally, especially in diabetics and in patients with renal function impairment; metabolic acidosis has been reported. Megaloblastic anemia can occur in alcoholic cirrhosis. Triamterene renal stones reported rarely.[8,16,53]

Contraindications. Severe or progressive renal disease or dysfunction (except possibly nephrosis); serum creatinine greater than 2.5 mg/dl; severe hepatic disease; patients with serum potassium greater than 5.5 mEq/L or developing hyperkalemia while taking the drug; concomitant potassium supplementation.

Precautions. Pregnancy. May cause elevation in serum uric acid in patients predisposed to gout. Should not be used with spironolactone or amiloride. Use with extreme caution with serum creatinine greater than 1.5 mg/dl.

Parameters to Monitor. Serum electrolytes, particularly potassium, should be measured periodically, especially early in the course of therapy;[35] BUN and/or serum creatinine should be measured periodically.

Notes. Appears to be less effective than spironolactone in sparing potassium,[53] but is less expensive.

Diuretics of Choice Comparison Chart[a]

CONDITION	ETHACRY-NIC ACID	FURO-SEMIDE	OSMOTIC	SPIRONO-LACTONE	THIAZIDES	TRIAM-TERENE/AMILORIDE	COMMENTS AND OTHER TREATMENTS	REFERENCES
Hypertension	C	B	—	D,E	A	E	Loop diuretic may be added to thiazide for a few days to overcome refractoriness	8–10
Right Heart Failure	B	B	—	E	A	E	Treat underlying pathology; digitalis	8,10
Left Heart Failure	B	B	—	—	A	—	Digitalis	8
Pulmonary Edema	A(IV)	A(IV)	—	—	—	—	Digitalis, O_2, aminophylline, morphine; consult literature	8,10
Cirrhotic Edema and Ascites	C	C	—	A,E	B	C,E	Na^+ and H_2O restriction; albumin, mannitol if severe; slow diuresis preferable	8,10,24
Acute Renal Failure	C	C	C	—	—	—	Hydration, dialysis	8,10,35
Chronic Renal Failure	C	A	—	—	—	—	Diet, dialysis	8,10,16
Nephrotic Syndrome	A	A	—	—	D	—	Corticosteroids, increase protein intake, plasma expanders, mannitol	8
Diabetes Insipidus	—	—	—	E	A	E	Thiazides most useful in nephrogenic form; long-acting agent preferred	30

Continued

Diuretics of Choice Comparison Chart[a]

CONDITION	ETHACRY-NIC ACID	FURO-SEMIDE	OSMOTIC	SPIRONO-LACTONE	THIAZIDES	TRIAM-TERENE/ AMILORIDE	COMMENTS AND OTHER TREATMENTS	REFERENCES
Drug Poisoning	C	C	C	—	—	—	Fluids; urinary acidification or alkalinization; dialysis	8,30
Hypercalcemia	—	A	—	—	—	—	Replace fluid loss; many other drugs useful	26,30
Hypercalciuria	—	—	—	—	A	—		8,30
Relative Maximal Potency[F]	>15%	>15%	10-15%	<5%	5-10%	<5%	Total diuresis is also determined by the duration of action and fluid and electrolyte balance of patient[8,16,35]	10,40

a. This table is a guide to the selection of the most appropriate diuretic for the condition listed, but is not an all-inclusive guide to therapy. Consult references 8-10, 35 for further information.

Key to Table:
A Diuretic of choice.
B Diuretic of second choice if patient unresponsive to first choice.
C Useful in some circumstances.
D May be useful alone, but low potency limits usefulness.
E Useful as an adjunct to a more potent diuretic to reduce potassium loss and possibly enhance therapeutic effect.
F Numbers refer to maximum fraction of filtered sodium that is excreted following maximally effective dose of drug.
G Mercurial diuretics and carbonic anhydrase inhibitors are essentially obsolete as diuretics.

40:40 URICOSURIC AGENTS

(SEE ALSO ANTI-GOUT AGENTS 92:00)

General References: 59-63

Probenecid   Benemid®, Various

Pharmacology. An organic acid that inhibits renal tubular reabsorption of urate, thereby increasing the urinary excretion of uric acid and lowering serum urate. Probenecid also interferes with renal tubular secretion of penicillins and cephalosporins causing an increase or prolongation in antibiotic plasma levels.

Administration and Adult Dose. PO for chronic gout 250 mg bid for 1 week, then 500 mg bid. Prophylactic colchicine, in doses of 0.5-1.5 mg/day for the first 6-12 months after initiation of treatment effectively diminishes the exacerbation of uricosuric-induced gouty attacks in patients with chronic tophaceous gout.[61,62] A liberal fluid intake and alkalinization of the urine (to prevent hematuria, renal colic, costovertebral pain and urate stone formation) is recommended, at least until serum uric acid levels normalize and tophaceous deposits disappear. If an acute gouty attack is precipitated during therapy, add colchicine to control the attack. **PO to prolong penicillin action** 2 g/day in 4 divided doses.

Dosage Individualization.   For chronic gout in renal impairment (although probably ineffective when Cl_{cr} is 30 ml/min or less), increase initial dose of 500 mg bid in 500 mg/day increments monthly to the dosage that maintains normal serum uric acid levels, to maximum of 2 g/day in divided doses.

Pediatric Dose. Contraindicated in children under 2 yr. **PO to prolong penicillin action** (under 50 kg) 25 mg/kg initially, then maintain at 40 mg/kg/day in 4 divided doses; (over 50 kg) same as adult dose.

Dosage Forms. Tab 500 mg.

Patient Instructions. This drug may be taken with food, milk or an antacid to minimize stomach upset. Drink a large amount (10-12 full glasses) of fluids each day and avoid the use of aspirin-containing products unless directed otherwise.

Pharmacokinetics and Biopharmaceutics. *Fate.* Rapidly and well-absorbed from GI tract; 93-99% protein bound, mostly to albumin.[64,65] Extensively metabolized or conjugated, such that about 40% is excreted in the urine as monoacyl glucuronide, less than 5% as unchanged drug and the remainder as hydroxylated metabolites which may have uricosuric activity.[66,67]

$t_{1/2}$. Dose-dependent (increases with increasing dose), with a range of 4-17 hr (usually 6-12 hr).[68]

Adverse Reactions. Headache, GI upset and skin rash occasionally. Exacerbation of gout and uric acid stones have been reported.[62] Nephrotic syndrome, hepatic necrosis, aplastic anemia, and hemolytic anemia (possibly related to G6PD deficiency) occur rarely.

Contraindications. Children under 2 yr; known blood dyscrasias or uric acid kidney stones; salicylates; initiation of therapy during an acute gouty attack.

Precautions. Hypersensitivity reactions require drug discontinuation. Use with caution in patients with a history of peptic ulcer; not recommended in conjunction with a penicillin in the presence of renal impairment.[63] Probenecid increases the plasma concentrations of indomethacin and conjugated sulfa drugs; salicylates antagonize the uricosuric action of probenecid. See Drug Interactions chapter.

Parameters to Monitor. Serum uric acid; pretreatment 24-hour urinary uric acid excretion.[60] When alkali is administered, periodically determine acid-base balance.[60] Occasionally determine plasma levels of sulfa drugs when co-administered with probenecid for prolonged periods.

Notes. Probenecid and other uricosuric drugs are not effective in patients with renal failure.[63] May cause a false-positive Benedict's test.

Sulfinpyrazone   Anturane®

Sulfinpyrazone, an analog of phenylbutazone, is a uricosuric agent with a mechanism and site of action resembling probenecid.[61-63] It is also an effective antiplatelet agent and may prevent some episodes of sudden death in survivors of myocardial infarction. Adverse effects are similar to probenecid with the addition of rarely reported blood dyscrasias. Dosage is 200–400 mg/day in 2 divided doses to a maximum of 800 mg/day as a uricosuric agent and 200 mg qid for prevention of sudden death, post-myocardial infarction. See also Antiplatelet Drugs Comparison Chart (20:12.04).[69,70] Available as 100 mg tablets and 200 mg capsules.

References, 40:00 Electrolytic, Caloric and Water Balance

1. Benderev K. Hypophosphatemia and phosphorus supplementation. Hosp Pharm 1980;15:611-13.
2. Beeley L. When do patients on diuretics need potassium replacement? Adverse Drug Reac Bull 1980;Number 84:304-7.
3. Rovner DR. Use of pharmacologic agents in the treatment of hypokalemia and hyperkalemia. Ration Drug Ther 1972;6(2):1-6.
4. Gilman AG, Goodman LS, Gilman A, eds. Goodman and Gilman's the pharmacological basis of therapeutics. 6th ed. New York: Macmillan, 1980.
5. Anderson RJ, Gambertoglio JG, Schrier RW, eds. Clinical use of drugs in renal failure. Springfield, IL: Charles C Thomas, 1976.
6. Wilkinson PR, Hesp R, Issler H et al. Total body and serum potassium during prolonged thiazide therapy for essential hypertension. Lancet 1975;1:759-62.
7. Kosman ME. Management of potassium problems during long-term diuretic therapy. JAMA 1974;230:743-8.
8. Anderton JL, Kincaid-Smith P. Diuretics II. clinical considerations. Drugs 1971;1:141-65.
9. Dustan HR, Tarazi RC, Bravo EL. Diuretic and diet treatment of hypertension. Arch Intern Med 1974;133:1007-13.
10. Davies DL, Wilson GM. Diuretics: mechanism of action and clinical application. Drugs 1975;9:178-226.
11. Loggie JMH, Kleinman LI, Van Maanen EF. Renal function and diuretic therapy in infants and children (3 parts). J Pediatr 1975;86:485-96,657-69,825-32.
12. Macfie HL, Colvin CL, Anderson PO. Amiloride. Drug Intell Clin Pharm 1981;15:94-8.
13. Brogden RN, Speight TM, Avery GS. Bumetanide: a preliminary report of its pharmacological properties and therapeutic efficacy in oedema. Drugs 1975;9:4-18.
14. Tuzel IH, ed. Perspectives on bumetanide. J Clin Pharmacol 1981;21:529-712.
15. Cooperman LB, Rubin IL. Toxicity of ethacrynic acid and furosemide. Am Heart J 1973;85:831-4.
16. Tweeddale MG. Diuretic drugs. In Dukes MNG, ed. Meyler's side effects of drugs. 9th ed. Amsterdam: Excerpta Medica, 1980;337-67.
17. Dikshit K, Vyden JK, Forrester JS et al. Renal and extrarenal hemodynamic effects of furosemide in congestive heart failure after acute myocardial infarction. N Engl J Med 1973;288:1087-90.
18. Kepler JA, ed. American hospital formulary service. Washington, DC: American Society of Hospital Pharmacists, 1959-82.
19. Beerman B, Groschinsky-Grind M. Clinical pharmacokinetics of diuretics. Clin Pharmacokinet 1980;5:221-45.
20. Benet LZ. Pharmacokinetics/pharmacodynamics of furosemide in man: a review. J Pharmacokinet Biopharm 1979;7:1-27.
21. Cutler RE, Blair AD. Clinical pharmacokinetics of furosemide. Clin Pharmacokinet 1979;4:279-96.

22. Odlind BG, Beermann B. Diuretic resistance: reduced bioavailability and effect of oral furosemide. Br Med J 1980;2:1577.

23. Spino M, Sellers EM, Kaplan HL et al. Adverse biochemical and clinical consequences of furosemide administration. Can Med Assoc J 1978;118:1513-8.

24. Sherlock S, Senewiratne B, Scott A et al. Complications of diuretic therapy in hepatic cirrhosis. Lancet 1966;1:7446-53.

25. Anderson J, Godfrey BE, Hill DM et al. A comparison of the effects of hydrochlorothiazide and of furosemide in the treatment of hypertensive patients. Q J Med 1971;NS40:541-60.

26. Suki WN, Yium JJ, Von Minden M et al. Acute treatment of hypercalcemia with furosemide. N Engl J Med 1970;283:836-40.

27. Hantman D, Rossier B, Zohlman R et al. Rapid correction of hyponatremia in the syndrome of inappropriate secretion of antidiuretic hormone. Ann Intern Med 1973;78:870-5.

28. Decaux G, Waterlot Y, Genette F et al. Treatment of the syndrome of inappropriate secretion of antidiuretic hormone with furosemide. N Engl J Med 1981;304:329-30.

29. Anderson PO et al. Current drug therapy—thiazide diuretics. Am J Hosp Pharm 1975;32:473-80.

30. Martinez-Maldonado M, Eknoyan G, Suki WN. Diuretics in nonedematous states — physiological basis for the clinical use. Arch Intern Med 1973;131:797-808.

31. Benet LZ, Sheiner LB. Design and optimization of dosage regimens; pharmacokinetic data. In Gilman AG, Goodman LS, Gilman A, eds. Goodman and Gilman's the pharmacological basis of therapeutics. 6th ed. New York: Macmillan, 1980;1675-737.

32. Backman L, Beerman B, Groschinsky-Grind M et al. Malabsorption of hydrochlorothiazide following intestinal shunt surgery. Clin Pharmacokinet 1979;4:63-8.

33. Amery A, Bulpitt C, de Schaepdryver A et al. Glucose intolerance during diuretic therapy. Lancet 1978;1:681-3.

34. Grimm RH, Leon AS, Hunninghake DB et al. Effects of thiazide diuretics on plasma lipids and lipoproteins in mildly hypertensive patients. Ann Intern Med 1981;94:7-11.

35. Frazier HS, Yager H. The clinical use of diuretics (2 parts) N Engl J Med 1973;288:246-9,455-9.

36. Stern A. Metolazone, a diuretic agent. Am Heart J 1976;91:262-3.

37. Gunby P. Mannitol opens pathway for brain tumor chemotherapy. JAMA 1981;245:1802. News.

38. Nissenson AR, Weston RE, Kleeman CR. Mannitol. West J Med 1979;131:277-84.

39. Hoffman DM, Grossano D. Use of mannitol diuresis to reduce cis-platinum nephrotoxicity. Drug Intell Clin Pharm 1978;12:489-90.

40. Gennari FJ, Kassirer JP. Osmotic diuresis. N Engl J Med 1974;291:714-20.

41. Palmer KR, Khan AN. Oral mannitol: a simple and effective bowel preparation for barium enema. Br Med J 1979;4:1038.

42. Sadee W, Schroder R, Leitner E et al. Multiple dose kinetics of spironolactone and canrenoate-potassium in cardiac and hepatic failure. Eur J Clin Pharmacol 1974;7:195-200.

43. Ramsay LE, Hettiarachchi J, Fraser R et al. Amiloride, spironolactone, and potassium chloride in thiazide-treated hypertensive patients. Clin Pharmacol Ther 1980;27:533-43.

44. Karlberg BE, Kagedal B, Tegler L et al. Controlled treatment of primary hypertension with propranolol and spironolactone. Am J Cardiol 1976;37:642-9.

45. Brown JJ, Davies DL, Ferriss JB et al. Comparison of surgery and prolonged spironolactone therapy in patients with hypertension, aldosterone excess, and low plasma renin. Br Med J 1972;2:729-34.

46. Eggert RC. Spironolactone diuresis in patients with cirrhosis and ascites. Br Med J 1970;4:401-3.

47. Karim A, Zagarella J, Hutsell TC et al. Spironolactone. III. Canrenone—maximum and minimum steady-state plasma levels. Clin Pharmacol Ther 1976;19:177-82.

48. Karim A, Zagarella J, Hribar J et al. Spironolactone. I. Disposition and metabolism. Clin Pharmacol Ther 1976;19:158-69.

49. Ramsay L, Shelton J, Harrison I et al. Spironolactone and potassium canrenoate in normal man. Clin Pharmacol Ther 1976;20:167-77.

50. Huston GJ, Turner P. Antagonism of fludrocortisone by spironolactone and canrenone. Br J Clin Pharmacol 1976;3:201-4.

51. Ramsay L, Asbury M, Shelton J et al. Spironolactone and canrenoate-K: relative potency at steady state. Clin Pharmacol Ther 1977;21:602-9.

52. Greenblatt DJ, Koch-Weser J. Adverse reactions to spironolactone: a report from the Boston Collaborative Drug Surveillance Program. JAMA 1973;225:40-3.

53. Anon. Potassium-sparing diuretics: spironolactone v. triamterene and amiloride. Drug Ther Bull 1972;10:30-2.

54. Gabow PA, Moore S, Schrier RW. Spironolactone-induced hyperchloremic acidosis in cirrhosis. Ann Intern Med 1979;90:338-40.

55. Loriaux DL, Menard R, Taylor A et al. Spironolactone and endocrine dysfunction. Ann Intern Med 1976;85:630-6.

56. Pruitt AW, Winkel JS, Dayton PG. Variations in the fate of triamterene. Clin Pharmacol Ther 1977;21:610-9.

57. Pruitt AW, Dayton PG, Steinhorst J. Fate of triamterene in man. Clin Res 1974;22:77a.

58. Lehmann K. Separation, isolation and identification of metabolic products of triamterene. Arzneim Forsch 1965;15:812-6.

59. Rodnan GP, Robin JA, Tolchin SF et al. Allopurinol and gouty hyperuricemia: efficacy of a single daily dose. JAMA 1975;231:1143-7.

60. Boss GR, Seegmiller JE. Hyperuricemia and gout: classification, complications and management. N Engl J Med 1979;300:1459-68.

61. Simkin PA. Management of gout. Ann Intern Med 1979;90:812-6.

62. Mangini RJ. Drug therapy reviews: pathogenesis and clinical management of hyperuricemia and gout. Am J Hosp Pharm 1979;36:497-504.

63. Yu TF. Milestones in the treatment of gout. Am J Med 1974;56:676-85.

64. Jusko WJ, Gretch M. Plasma and tissue protein binding of Drugs in pharmacokinetics. Drug Metab Rev 1976;5:43-140.

65. Koch-Weser J, Sellers EM. Binding of drugs to serum albumin (2 parts). N Engl J Med 1976;294:311-6,526-31.

66. Israili ZH, Perel JM, Cunningham RF et al. Metabolites of probenecid. Chemical, physical, and pharmacological studies. J Med Chem 1972;15:709-13.

67. Perel JM, Cunningham RF, Fales HM et al. Identification and renal excretion of probenecid metabolites in man. Life Sci 1970;9:1337-43.

68. Dayton PG, Yu TF, Chen W et al. The physiological disposition of probenecid, including renal clearance, in man, studied by an improved method for its estimation in biological material. J Pharmacol Exp Ther 1963;140:278-86.

69. Margulies EH, White AM, Sherry S. Sulfinpyrazone: a review of its pharmacological properties and therapeutic use. Drugs 1980;20:179-97.

70. Hood WB. More on sulfinpyrazone after myocardial infarction. N Engl J Med 1982;306:988-9.

48:00 EXPECTORANTS AND COUGH PREPARATIONS

General References: 1-3

Class Instructions. Antitussives. This drug should not be used to suppress productive cough; see your physician or pharmacist if cough persists. **Expectorants.** This drug should be taken with a large quantity of fluid to ensure proper drug action; see your physician or pharmacist if cough persists.

Codeine Salts   Various

See Section 28:08

Dextromethorphan Hydrobromide   Various

Pharmacology. The nonanalgesic, nonaddictive d-isomer of the codeine analog of levorphanol. With usual antitussive doses, the cough threshold is elevated centrally without noted effect on the respiratory, cardiovascular or GI systems.

Administration and Adult Dose. PO as cough suppressant 10–30 mg tid-qid, to maximum of 120 mg/day.

Pediatric Dose. PO as cough suppressant 1 mg/kg/day in 3-4 divided doses.

Dosage Forms. Elxr 1.5, 2, 3 mg/ml; **Lozenges** 5, 7.5, 10 mg; **Syrup** 0.5, 1, 1.5, 2, 3 mg/ml; available in many combination products in variable concentrations.

Patient Instructions. See Class Instructions for antitussive use.

Pharmacokinetics and Biopharmaceutics. *Onset and Duration.* Duration about 4 hr.

Adverse Reactions. Mild and infrequent drowsiness and GI upset.[3] Intoxication, bizarre behavior, CNS depression and respiratory depression can occur with extremely high doses. Naloxone may be effective in reversing these effects.[4,5]

Notes. Approximately equipotent with codeine in antitussive effectiveness.[1]

Guaifenesin

2/G®, Robitussin®,
Various

Pharmacology.   The proposed expectorant action of guaifenesin is through an increased output of respiratory tract fluid, enhancing the flow of less viscid secretions, promoting ciliary action and facilitating the removal of inspissated mucus. Evidence of the effectiveness of guaifenesin is largely subjective and not established clinically.[6-8]

Administration and Adult Dose.   PO as expectorant 200–400 mg q 4 hr, to a maximum of 2.4 g/day has been proposed.[1]

Pediatric Dose.   PO as expectorant 12 mg/kg/day in 6 divided doses.

Dosage Forms.   **Cap** 200 mg; **Syrup** 20 mg/ml; **Tab** 100, 200 mg.

Patient Instructions.   See Class Instructions for expectorant use.

Adverse Reactions.   Occasional drowsiness, nausea and possibly vomiting.

Notes.   May produce a color interference with certain laboratory determinations of 5-hydroxyindoleacetic acid (5-HIAA) and vanilmandelic acid (VMA).[9] May lower serum uric acid;[10] may have a mild, transitory antiplatelet action (without affecting bleeding time) which is of little clinical importance.[11]

References, 48:00 Expectorants and Cough Preparations

1. Anon. Establishment of a monograph for OTC cold, cough, allergy, bronchodilator and antiasthmatic products. Fed Regist 1976;41:38312-424.
2. Anon. Over-the-counter cough remedies. Med Lett Drugs Ther 1979;21:103-4.
3. Cormier JF, Bryant BG. Cold and allergy products. In: Penna RP, ed. Handbook of nonprescription drugs. 6th ed. American Pharmaceutical Association. Washington, DC, 1979:73-114.
4. Committee on Drugs. Use of codeine- and dextromethorphan-containing cough syrups in pediatrics. Pediatrics 1978;62:118-22.
5. Shaul WL, Wandell M, Robertson WO. Dextromethorphan toxicity: reversal by naloxone. Pediatrics 1977;59:117-9.
6. Boyd EM, Sheppard EP, Boyd CE. The pharmacological basis of the expectorant action of glyceryl guaiacolate. Appl Ther 1967;9:55-9.
7. Hirsch SR, Viernes PF, Kory RC. The expectorant effect of glyceryl guaiacolate in patients with chronic bronchitis. Chest 1973;63:9-14.
8. Heilborn H, Pegelow K-O, Odeblad E. Effect of bromhexine and guaiphenesine on clinical state, ventilatory capacity and sputum viscosity in chronic asthma. Scand J Resp Dis 1976;57:88-96.
9. Hansten PD. Drug interactions. 4th ed. Philadelphia: Lea & Febiger, 1979.
10. Ramsdell CM, Kelley WN. The clinical significance of hypouricemia. Ann Intern Med 1973;78:239-42.
11. Buchanan GR, Martin V, Levine PH et al. The effects of "anti-platelet" drugs on bleeding time and platelet aggregation in normal human subjects. Am J Clin Pathol 1977;68:355-9.

56:00 GASTROINTESTINAL DRUGS

General References: 1,2

56:04 ANTACIDS AND ADSORBENTS

General References: 1,3,4

Activated Charcoal   Various

Pharmacology. A nonspecific GI adsorbent used in the management of acute poisonings.

Administration and Adult Dose. **PO or via lavage tube** dispersed in liquid, 30–120 g, as soon as possible after ingestion of poison.[5] If syrup of ipecac-induced emesis is contemplated, delay administration of activated charcoal until after emesis; repeat administration of activated charcoal after gastric lavage.

Pediatric Dose. Same as adult dose.

Dosage Forms. Pwdr.

Patient Instructions. This material will cause the stools to turn black.

Pharmacokinetics and Biopharmaceutics. *Onset and Duration.* Onset immediate; duration continual while it remains in the GI tract.
   Fate. Eliminated unchanged in the feces.

Adverse Reactions. Stools will turn black; gritty consistency may cause emesis in some patients.

Parameters to Monitor. Passage of activated charcoal in the stools.

Notes. A suspension of activated charcoal in 70% sorbitol[6] may increase patient acceptance of the drug. Substances *not* readily adsorbed by activated charcoal include mineral acids, alkalis, boric acid, DDT, ferrous sulfate, malathion and many water insoluble compounds.[7]

Antacids   Various

Pharmacology. Antacids are weakly basic inorganic compounds whose primary action is to buffer stomach acid. Buffering action partially inactivates pepsin and increases lower esophageal sphincter pressure. Gastric juice and acid secretion may be increased by gastrin release due to the elevated pH. All antacids increase urine pH by 1–2 units. Aluminum salts bind phosphate in the GI tract, decreasing serum phosphate levels. Magnesium antacids generally induce diarrhea, while aluminum antacids can produce constipation.

Administration and Adult Dose. **PO for peptic ulcer disease** 100–160 mEq buffering capacity per dose, given 1 and 3 hr after meals and at bedtime for 4–6 weeks until healing is complete. Additional prn doses may be taken if pain persists.[4,5] **PO, NG for prophylaxis of stress ulceration** titrate hourly to ensure gastric pH of 3.5 or greater at the end of each hour; doses of up to 120 ml q 1 hr have been used.[3] **PO for phosphate binding in renal failure** (aluminum hydroxide or carbonate) titrate dose based on serum phosphate. See Antacid Products Comparison Chart.

Pediatric Dose. **PO for peptic ulcer disease** (up to 12 yr) maximum dose of 5–15 ml as often as q 1 hr.

Dosage Forms. See Antacid Products Comparison Chart.

Patient Instructions. Ulcer pain may not be relieved initially; however, it is necessary to take this medication for a full 4–8 weeks to ensure ulcer healing. Diarrhea may occur with magnesium-containing antacids; this may be minimized by alternating doses with aluminum antacids. Antacids may interfere with other medications; take any other medications 1–2 hours before or after antacids unless otherwise directed. If tablets are used, chew thoroughly before swallowing.

Pharmacokinetics and Biopharmaceutics. *Onset and Duration.* Onset of buffering is immediate; duration is 20–40 min taken on an empty stomach and 2–3 hr if ingested after meals.[1]
   Fate. Antacids are absorbed to varying degrees. Calcium carbonate is significantly absorbed and can result in hypercalcemia and/or systemic alkalosis; magnesium is 15–30% absorbed; aluminum hydroxide is slightly absorbed. Calcium, magnesium and aluminum are excreted renally with normal renal function.[9-11] The unabsorbed portion is excreted in the feces.

Adverse Reactions. Calcium carbonate can cause rebound acid secretion, metabolic alkalosis and hypercalcemia ("milk-alkalai syndrome") which can lead to nephrolithiasis. Magnesium-containing antacids frequently cause diarrhea; hypermagnesemia can occur in patients with renal impairment. Aluminum hydroxide and carbonate antacids occasionally cause constipation and can result in hypophosphatemia; encephalopathy has been reported in dialysis patients receiving aluminum antacids.[10,12]

Precautions. Use with caution in patients with renal impairment, edema, hypertension or CHF. See Drug Interactions chapter.

Parameters to Monitor. Observe for diarrhea and relief of epigastric pain. Obtain periodic serum magnesium in patients with renal impairment and serum phosphate during chronic use.

Notes. Tablet formulations are generally not as effective as liquids; however, thoroughly chewed magnesium-containing antacid tablets might be effective.[13]

Antacid Products Comparison Chart[a]

ANTACID	ACID NEUTRALIZING CAPACITY[b]		SODIUM CONTENT[b]	
	MEQ/TABLET	MEQ/5 ML	MG/TABLET	MG/5 ML	MEQ/5 ML

ANTACID	MEQ/TABLET	MEQ/5 ML	MG/TABLET	MG/5 ML	MEQ/5 ML
Aluminum Carbonate Gel, Basic					
Basaljel®	14.0	14.0	2.1	2.4	0.1
Aluminum Hydroxide Gel					
AlternaGel®	—	12.0	—	1.95	0.08
Amphojel®	9.0 (300 mg tablet)	6.5	1.4 (300 mg tablet)	6.9	0.3
Aluminum Hydroxide with Magnesium Hydroxide					
Aludrox®	11.5	14.0	1.6	1.15	0.05
Creamalin®	—	—	41.0	—	—
Maalox®	8.5 (#1 tablet)	13.5	0.84 (#1 tablet)	1.35	0.06
Maalox® Therapeutic Concentrate	—	28.3	—	1.25	0.05
WinGel®	—	—	2.5	2.5	0.11
Aluminum Hydroxide with Magnesium Hydroxide and Calcium Carbonate					
Camalox®	18.0	18.0	1.5	2.5	0.11
Aluminum Hydroxide with Magnesium Hydroxide and Simethicone					
Di-Gel®	—	12.3	10.6	8.5	0.37
Gelusil®	11.0	12.0	0.8	0.7	0.03
Gelusil II®	21.0	24.0	2.1	1.3	0.06
Maalox Plus®	8.5	13.5	1.0	1.35	0.06
Mylanta®	11.5	12.7	0.77	0.68	0.03
Mylanta II®	23.0	25.4	1.3	1.14	0.05

Continued

Antacid Products Comparison Chart[a]

ANTACID	ACID NEUTRALIZING CAPACITY[b]		SODIUM CONTENT[b]		
	MEQ/TABLET	MEQ/5 ML	MG/TABLET	MG/5 ML	MEQ/5 ML
Calcium Carbonate with Glycine					
Titralac®	7.5	19.0	0.3	11.0	0.48
Magaldrate					
Riopan® and Riopan Plus® (with Simethicone)	13.5	13.5	0.3	0.3	0.01

a. From reference 1 and product literature.
b. Product formulations, and hence neutralizing capacity and sodium content, are subject to change by manufacturer.

56:08 ANTI-DIARRHEA AGENTS

General References: 14, 15

Diphenoxylate Hydrochloride with Atropine Sulfate

Lomotil®, Various

Pharmacology. Diphenoxylate is a narcotic-like agent that slows GI motility; atropine is added in subtherapeutic amounts to decrease abuse potential.

Administration and Adult Dose. PO 1–2 tablets or 5–10 ml 3–6 times daily for 24–48 hr initially to control diarrhea, then 1 tablet or 5 ml bid-tid prn.

Pediatric Dose. Use liquid only. PO (2–5 yr) 4 ml tid; (5–8 yr) 4 ml qid; (8–12 yr) 4 ml 5 times daily. Not recommended under 2 yr.

Dosage Forms. Syrup 2.5 mg diphenoxylate and 25 mcg atropine/5 ml; Tab 2.5 mg diphenoxylate and 25 mcg atropine.

Patient Instructions. This drug may cause blurred vision, drowsiness or dizziness. Until the severity of these reactions is known, caution should be used when performing tasks that require mental alertness.

Pharmacokinetics and Biopharmaceutics. *Onset and Duration.* Onset 45–60 min; duration 3–4 hr.
  Fate. Diphenoxylate is well absorbed from the GI tract and metabolized to an active metabolite, diphenoxylic acid. Both drug and metabolite attain peak plasma levels in 2 hr; their conjugates are excreted primarily in the urine.[16]
  $t_{1/2}$. (Diphenoxylate) 2.5 hr; (diphenoxylic acid) 12–24 hr.[16]

Adverse Reactions. Drowsiness, dizziness and headache occur occasionally. Anticholinergic symptoms such as dry mouth, blurred vision, fever or tachycardia may occur with high doses (over 12–15 tablets) in adults, or occasionally with usual doses in children.

Contraindications. Children under 2 yr; advanced liver disease.

Precautions. Use with caution in children due to variable response and potential for toxicity, and in patients with acute ulcerative colitis or cirrhosis.

Parameters to Monitor. Frequency and volume of bowel movements; observe for signs of atropine toxicity.[14]

Notes. Diphenoxylate 2.5 mg has equivalent efficacy to 5 ml of paregoric. Taste of syrup may be unpleasant.

Loperamide

Imodium®

Pharmacology. A synthetic antidiarrheal, structurally similar to haloperidol that causes a dose-related inhibition of colonic motility without significant opiate activity.

Administration and Adult Dose. PO 4 mg initially, then 2 mg prn, to maximum of 16 mg/day.[15]

Pediatric Dose. Not recommended.

Dosage Forms. Cap 2 mg.

Pharmacokinetics and Biopharmaceutics. *Onset and Duration.*
Onset 45–60 min; duration 4–6 hr.
   Fate. Absorption from GI tract is insignificant; less than 2% of a dose is recovered in the urine.[18]
   $t_{1/2}$. 7–15 hr (average 11).[15]

Adverse Reactions. Abdominal cramping occurs occasionally; nausea, dizziness and dry mouth are rare.

Precautions. Use with caution in patients with ulcerative colitis.

Parameters to Monitor. Frequency and volume of bowel movements.

Notes. Adverse reactions may be less frequent than with diphenoxylate with atropine.

56:12 CATHARTICS AND LAXATIVES

General References: 17,19,20

Bisacodyl
Dulcolax®, Various

Pharmacology. A cathartic structurally similar to phenolphthalein that produces its effect by direct contact with colonic mucosa. Net water and electrolyte absorption may also be inhibited.

Administration and Adult Dose. PO 5–20 mg; PR 10–20 mg. Dosage is variable, and should be adjusted based on response.

Pediatric Dose. PO (over 6 yr) 5 mg; PR (under 2 yr) 5 mg; (over 2 yr) 10 mg.

Dosage Forms. EC Tab 5 mg; Supp 10 mg.

Patient Instructions. Tablets should be swallowed whole (not chewed or crushed) and should not be taken within 1 hour of antacids or dairy products.

Pharmacokinetics and Biopharmaceutics. *Onset and Duration.*
Onset PO 4–8 hr; PR 15 min–1 hr.[17]
   Fate. Absorption is less than 5% by oral or rectal route. Rapidly converted by intestinal and bacterial enzymes to its active desacetyl metabolite.[21]

Adverse Reactions. Abdominal cramps occur occasionally; excessive use of suppositories can cause rectal irritation.

Contraindications. Acute surgical abdomen; fecal impaction; intestinal obstruction; abdominal pain of unknown origin; intestinal perforation.[17]

Notes. Useful for preoperative or radiographic bowel preparation. Cathartic effect can be overcome by the application of a local anesthetic.[17]

Docusate Sodium
Docusate Calcium

Colace®, Doxinate®, Various
Surfak®

Pharmacology. An anionic surfactant that lowers the surface tension of the oil-water interface of the stool, allowing fecal material to be penetrated by water and fat, thereby softening the stool. The emulsifying action also enhances the absorption of many fat-soluble drugs.[17,22]

Administration and Adult Dose. PO (sodium or calcium salt) 50–500 mg/day in single or divided doses.[17]

Pediatric Dose. PO (sodium salt) 5 mg/kg/day in 3–4 divided doses.

Dosage Forms. (Sodium salt) **Cap** 50, 60, 100, 240, 250, 300 mg; **Soln** 10, 50 mg/ml; **Syrup** 4 mg/ml; **Tab** 50, 100, 250 mg. (Calcium salt) **Cap** 50, 240 mg.

Patient Instructions. This drug should be taken with a full glass of fluid; liquid or solution should be taken in milk, fruit juice or infant formula to mask bitter taste.

Pharmacokinetics and Biopharmaceutics. *Onset and Duration.* Onset of effect on stools 1–3 days after first dose with continuous use.
   Fate. May be partially absorbed in the duodenum and jejunum and secreted in the bile.[17,19]

Adverse Reactions. Occasional abdominal cramps.

Contraindications. Undiagnosed abdominal pain; intestinal obstruction. Theoretically, absorption of mineral oil is enhanced by these drugs and therefore long-term concurrent use with mineral oil should be avoided.[17]

Precautions. Concurrent use with oxyphenisatin (removed from US market) or danthron may cause chronic active hepatitis by enhancing their absorption.[23-25] Concurrent use with aspirin results in greater mucosal damage than when either agent is given separately.[17]

Parameters to Monitor. Frequency and consistency of stools; ease of defecation.

Notes. Surfactant cathartic useful for hard dry stools and in lessening the strain of defecation. Use of 200 mg or less daily in the hospital setting may be ineffective in altering the prevalence of constipation.[17,22,25] These agents may change intestinal morphology, cellular function and cause fluid and electrolyte accumulation in the colon.[17,22]

Hydrocolloid Mucilloid

Metamucil®,
Effersyllium®,
Various

Pharmacology. Bulk forming cathartic which absorbs water and provides an emollient mass.

Administration and Adult Dose. PO for constipation 4–12 g (1 level teaspoonful to 1 level tablespoonful) or 1–2 packets bid-qid, stirred in a full glass of water, followed by an additional glass of liquid. PO for diarrhea—see Notes.

Pediatric Dose. PO (over 6 yr) 1.25–5 g daily-tid with fluid as above.

Dosage Forms. Pwdr 210, 420 g; **Pwdr** (effervescent) 6.4, 7 g packets.

Patient Instructions. Mix with a full glass of water before taking and follow with another glass of liquid.

Pharmacokinetics and Biopharmaceutics. *Onset and Duration.* Onset 12–24 hr, but 2–3 days may be required for full effect.[27,28]

Adverse Reactions. Flatulence and defecation of soft bulky stools occurs frequently. Serious side effects are rare, but intestinal obstruction has been reported.[17]

Contraindications. Acute surgical abdomen; fecal impaction; intestinal obstruction; abdominal pain of unknown origin; intestinal perforation.[17]

Precautions. Use with caution in patients who require fluid restriction, because constipation may occur unless fluid intake is adequate. Use effervescent Metamucil® formulation (packet) with caution in patients who require sodium restriction. The noneffervescent formulation of Metamucil® should be used cautiously in diabetics because it contains 50% dextrose (14 kcal/7 g).

Notes. Useful in lessening the strain of defecation and for inpatients who are on low residue diets and/or constipating medications. May relieve symptoms in patients with diverticular disease.[2] Large doses may be used to "firm up" effluent from an ileostomy or ascending colostomy or diarrhea caused by tube feedings.

Lactulose   Cephulac®, Chronulac®

Pharmacology. A synthetic derivative of lactose which is metabolized by colonic bacteria to lactic and small amounts of acetic and formic acids, resulting in acidification of colonic contents and decreased ammonia absorption.[20]

Administration and Adult Dose. PO as a cathartic 15–30 ml (10–20 g), to maximum of 60 ml; **PO for hepatic encephalopathy** 15–60 ml (10–40 g) 3–6 times daily, titrated to produce about 3+ stools per day with a pH < 5.5.[21]

Dosage Individualization. Elderly patients may require reduced doses.[19]

Pediatric Dose. PO as a cathartic (infants) 2.5–10 ml/day in divided doses; (older children) 5–30 ml/day in single or divided doses.

Dosage Forms. Syrup 10 g/15 ml.

Patient Instructions. In the treatment of hepatic encephalopathy, 3–4 loose stools per day are common, but a worsening of diarrhea should be reported.

Pharmacokinetics and Biopharmaceutics. *Onset and Duration.* (Catharsis) onset 12–24 hr; duration 24–36 hr. (Hepatic encephalopathy) onset and duration variable.[21]
   Fate. After oral administration, 3% is absorbed and most reaches the colon unabsorbed and unchanged. The small amount absorbed is excreted in the urine unchanged.[19]

Adverse Reactions. Flatulence, belching and abdominal discomfort are frequent initially. Hypokalemia and metabolic acidosis may result from diarrhea.

Contraindications. Patients requiring a low galactose diet.

Precautions. Concurrent use with neomycin may be less effective than use alone in hepatic encephalopathy. Use with caution in diabetics due to small amounts of free lactose and galactose in the drug.

Parameters to Monitor. Observe for changes in hepatic encephalopathy, number of stools per day and stool pH (maintain at about pH 5).[20] Periodically obtain serum potassium and bicarbonate levels during prolonged use.

Magnesium Salts   Various

Pharmacology. A saline cathartic that inhibits fluid and electrolyte absorption by increasing osmotic forces in the gut lumen; it has also been suggested that part of its action may be due to cholecystokinin release which stimulates small bowel motility and inhibits fluid and electrolyte absorption from the jejunum and ileum.[17]

Administration and Adult Dose. PO (citrate) 200–300 ml; (sulfate) 20–30 ml of 50% solution (10–15 g) in a full glass of water; (milk of magnesia) 15–30 ml.

Pediatric Dose. PO (citrate) 4 ml/kg/dose; (sulfate) 250 mg/kg/dose in a one-half glass or more of water; (milk of magnesia) 0.5 ml/kg/dose.

Dosage Forms. **Soln** (citrate) 77 mEq magnesium/dl; (sulfate) 50%; **Susp** (milk of magnesia) 15, 30, 180, 320, 640 ml (also available as a concentrate with 10 ml = 30 ml of susp); **Pwdr** (citrate and sulfate) 454 g.

Patient Instructions. Milk of magnesia and magnesium sulfate should be taken with at least one full glass of liquid; magnesium sulfate may be taken with fruit juice to partially mask its bitter taste.

Pharmacokinetics and Biopharmaceutics. *Onset and Duration.* Onset 2–8 hr.[27]
   Fate. Slow absorption of 15–30% of a dose from the GI tract. Absorbed magnesium is rapidly excreted in the urine in normal renal function.[17]

Adverse Reactions. Chronic use in patients with renal impairment may lead to hypermagnesemia, CNS depression and hypotension. Excessive use can lead to electrolyte abnormalities; dehydration may occur if taken with insufficient fluids.[17]

Contraindications. Acute surgical abdomen, fecal impaction, intestinal obstruction; abdominal pain of unknown origin; intestinal perforation; nausea; vomiting.[17]

Precautions. Use with caution in patients with impaired renal function.

Parameters to Monitor. Periodic serum magnesium levels in patients with impaired renal function.

Notes. Magnesium salts are useful for preparing the bowel for radiologic examination and surgical procedures. The following amounts of various magnesium salts are approximately equivalent to 80 mEq of magnesium: 100 ml citrate; 2.4 g (30 ml) milk of magnesia; and 10 g sulfate. The sulfate salt is the most potent cathartic, but is the least palatable; its use is mainly limited to the treatment of poisonings.[17]

56:20 EMETICS AND ANTIEMETICS

Apomorphine Hydrochloride   Various

Pharmacology.   A morphine derivative which induces vomiting by stimulation of the chemoreceptor trigger zone (CTZ) in the CNS.

Administration and Adult Dose. **SC for emesis** 0.1 mg/kg to maximum of 10 mg. Repeat dosing is *not* recommended. Precede use with 240 ml water PO. Hypodermic tablet requires dissolution in sterile water immediately prior to use. Reconstituted solution is unstable and should not be used if a green or brown color or a precipitate develops.

Pediatric Dose.   **SC for emesis** 0.1 mg/kg or 3 mg/M^2.

Dosage Forms.   Hyp Tab 6 mg.

Pharmacokinetics and Biopharmaceutics. *Onset and Duration.* Onset 2–15 min; duration up to 40 min.[29,30]

Adverse Reactions.   Prolonged or violent emesis; CNS depression and respiratory depression possibly requiring reversal with naloxone may occur. Excessive doses may cause cardiac depression and death.

Contraindications.   Overdose with alcohol, sedative-hypnotics and other drugs with CNS depression as a major symptom; impending shock or unconsciousness; convulsions or impending convulsions; ingestion of corrosive or caustic substances. Use in petroleum distillate ingestion is controversial.

Precautions.   Use cautiously in children, debilitated persons, patients with cardiac disease or persons predisposed to nausea and vomiting.

Parameters to Monitor.   Onset and frequency of emesis; signs of CNS or respiratory depression; presence of poison in the vomitus.

Notes.   Apomorphine depressant and emetic effects may be terminated by the narcotic antagonist naloxone which should be immediately available whenever apomorphine is used; patients who fail to vomit with apomorphine should be considered for gastric lavage. Apomorphine is difficult to prepare, potentially more toxic, and only marginally more rapid in onset than syrup of ipecac; therefore, it is not the emetic of choice in most patients. It has the advantage of being useful in uncooperative patients and not being inhibited by co-administration of activated charcoal. An experimental stable solution of apomorphine has been described.[31]

Benzquinamide Hydrochloride   Emete-Con®

Pharmacology.   A nonphenothiazine antiemetic whose exact mechanism of action is unknown (probably supression of the chemoreceptor trigger zone).

Administration and Adult Dose.   **IM as an antiemetic** 50 mg (0.5–1 mg/kg); may repeat in 1 hr then q 3–4 hr as needed; inject deep into a large muscle. **IV as an antiemetic** 25 mg (0.2–0.4 mg/kg) given slowly (1 ml/min) with subsequent doses given IM.

Pediatric Dose.   Not recommended.

Dosage Forms. Inj 50 mg.

Pharmacokinetics and Biopharmaceutics. *Onset and Duration.*
Onset usually within 15 min; duration variable, but probably less than 6 hr.[32]
   Fate. Primarily inactivated by hepatic metabolism with only 5–10%
eliminated unchanged in the urine.[33]
   $t_{1/2}$. 40–60 min.[33]

Adverse Reactions. Drowsiness is the most frequent reaction. Also
reported are extrapyramidal reactions and delirium.[34,35] IM administration
is preferred because of sudden increases in blood pressure and cardiac arrhythmias associated with IV use.

Precautions. May mask signs of drug overdose or organic causes of
nausea and vomiting.

Parameters to Monitor. Frequency of vomiting, signs of CNS depression.

Notes. Reconstituted solution is stable for 14 days at room temperature.
Ineffective when administered orally for cancer chemotherapy-related
nausea and vomiting.[36]

Delta-9-Tetrahydrocannabinol (Investigational - NCI)

Delta-9-tetrahydrocannabinol (THC) is the most active antinauseant component of cannabis products. Its mechanism is unknown, but it is at least as
effective as the phenothiazines in cancer chemotherapy-induced nausea
and vomiting. Response is accompanied by a "high" which some patients,
especially the elderly, may find unpleasant; sedation is also frequent. Optimum dosage has not been defined, probably partly because of the poor
bioavailability of presently available oral dosage forms. The National
Cancer Institute (NCI) has recommended a starting dose of 5 mg/M^2 of body
surface area q 4 hr, starting 6–8 hr before chemotherapy and continuing for
12 hr after it is discontinued; dosage can be increased to 7.5 mg/M^2 if
necessary. The drug is available in 2.5 and 5 mg capsules from NCI to approved investigators and pharmacies only.[37]

Ipecac Syrup   Various

Pharmacology. A mixture of plant alkaloids, including emetine and
cephaeline, which induces emesis through stimulation of the stomach and
the chemoreceptor trigger zone in the CNS.

Administration and Adult Dose. PO for emesis 30 ml, followed by 240
ml or more of water; may repeat once in 20–30 min if no effect.

Pediatric Dose. PO for emesis (6 mo–1 yr) 10 ml; (1–5 yr) 15 ml given as
above; (over 5 yr) same as adult dose. Give with at least 120 ml of water.

Dosage Forms. Syrup 70 mg/ml (should not be confused with fluidextract
of ipecac which is 14 times more potent).

Patient Instructions. This drug should be taken with at least one or more
glasses of water. Save vomitus in a bowl for later inspection. Do not take
without first consulting poison information center or physician.

Pharmacokinetics and Biopharmaceutics. *Onset and Duration.* Onset about 15–20 min; duration usually about 25 min, but may last several hr.[29,38]

Adverse Reactions. Mild drowsiness and diarrhea may occur after emesis.[29] Protracted vomiting with GI damage and cardiotoxicity, manifested by tachycardia and ECG abnormalities has occurred after toxic doses of fluidextract.[39] Acute toxicity is unlikely with normal doses of the syrup.

Contraindications. Present or anticipated CNS depression; convulsions or anticipated convulsions; ingestion of corrosives or caustics. Use in petroleum distillate ingestion is controversial.

Precautions. Do not administer activated charcoal until emesis has occurred; do not administer milk unless water is unavailable as milk may delay the onset of emesis.[40] If emesis does not occur, gastric lavage should be considered as an alternative.

Parameters to Monitor. Onset and frequency of emesis; presence of poison in the vomitus.

Notes. Syrup of ipecac is the emetic of choice in most toxic ingestions and is useful for inducing emesis at home. Appears effective in anti-emetic drug ingestions,[38,41] although the prescribing information for some phenothiazine drugs specifically recommends against its use in phenothiazine poisoning.

Prochlorperazine Salts   Compazine®

Pharmacology. A phenothiazine tranquilizer which is used mainly for its antiemetic properties (several other phenothiazines are also used as antiemetics—see Antiemetic Agents Comparison Chart). It suppresses the chemoreceptor trigger zone in the CNS; not effective for the treatment of motion sickness or vertigo.

Administration and Adult Dose. PO as an antiemetic 5–10 mg tid-qid; PR as an antiemetic 25 mg bid; IM as an antiemetic (deep in upper outer quadrant of buttock) 5–10 mg q 4–6 hr, to maximum of 40 mg/day. IM presurgically (given as above) 5–10 mg 1–2 hr before induction, may repeat once before or after surgery; IV presurgically 5–10 mg 15–30 min before induction or as infusion (20 mg/L) started 15–30 min before induction. SC not recommended.

Dosage Individualization. Use the lower end of the recommended dosage range in elderly patients.

Pediatric Dose. Not to be used in surgery or in patients under 9 kg or 2 yr. PO or PR as an antiemetic 0.4 mg/kg/day in 3–4 divided doses; IM as an antiemetic (deep in upper outer quadrant of buttock) 0.13 mg/kg. SC not recommended.

Dosage Forms. Inj 5 mg/ml; Supp 2.5, 5, 25 mg; Syrup 1 mg/ml; Tab 5, 10 mg. Larger dose tablets are available for psychiatric use.

Patient Instructions. This drug may cause drowsiness. Until the extent of this effect is known, caution should be used when driving, operating machinery or performing other tasks requiring mental alertness. Avoid excessive concurrent use of alcohol or other drugs which cause drowsiness.

Pharmacokinetics and Biopharmaceutics. *Onset and Duration.*
PO onset 30–40 min; PR onset 60 min; IM onset 10–20 min. Duration for all
routes 3–4 hr.[19]
   Fate. Primarily eliminated by liver metabolism.[42]

Adverse Reactions. Extrapyramidal reactions, especially dystonias and
dyskinesias occur occasionally (other extrapyramidal reactions are less
likely because of the short duration of therapy when used as an antiemetic).
Anticholinergic effects such as dry mouth, mydriasis, cycloplegia, urinary
retention, decreased GI motility and tachycardia have been reported.[43,44]
SC use can cause local reactions at injection site.

Contraindications. Pediatric surgery; children under 9 kg or 2 yr; comatose or greatly depressed states due to CNS depressants; bone marrow
depression.

Precautions. Antiemetic action may mask signs and symptoms of overdose with other drugs and may mask the diagnosis and treatment of other
conditions such as intestinal obstruction, brain tumor or Reye syndrome.
Use with caution in conditions in which the drug's anticholinergic effects
might be detrimental, in children with acute illnesses or dehydration or in
patients with a history of allergy to phenothiazine derivatives (eg, blood
dyscrasias, jaundice). Avoid getting the concentrate or injection solutions
on hands or clothing, due to possibility of contact dermatitis.

Notes. The injectable form should not be mixed with other agents in the
same syringe; the solution should be protected from light; slight yellowish
discoloration will not alter potency, but markedly discolored solution
should be discarded. Protect suppositories from heat.

Antiemetic Agents Comparison Chart[a]

DRUG	INITIAL DOSE[b] ADULT	INITIAL DOSE[b] PEDIATRIC	INDICATIONS NAUSEA AND VOMITING	INDICATIONS MOTION SICKNESS	INDICATIONS VERTIGO
PHENOTHIAZINES					
Chlorpromazine Thorazine® Various	PO 10–25 mg; IM 25 mg; PR 100 mg	(>6 mo) PO, IM 0.55 mg/kg; PR 1.1 mg/kg	X		
Perphenazine Trilafon®	PO 2–4 mg; IM 5 mg	—	X		
Prochlorperazine Compazine® Various	PO, IM 5–10 mg; PR 25 mg	(>9 kg or 2 yr) PO, PR 0.4 mg/kg; IM 0.13 mg/kg	X		
Promethazine Phenergan® Various	PO, PR 25 mg; IM 12.5–25 mg	PO, PR, IM 0.25–0.5 mg/kg	X	X	
Thiethylperazine Torecan®	PO, IM 10 mg	—	X		
Triflupromazine Vesprin®	PO 20–30 mg; IM 5–15 mg; IV 1–3 mg	(>2½ yr) PO, IM 0.07 mg/kg	X		
ANTIHISTAMINES					
Buclizine Bucladin®	PO 50 mg	—	X	X	

Continued

Antiemetic Agents Comparison Chart[a]

| DRUG | INITIAL DOSE[b] | | INDICATIONS | | |
	ADULT	PEDIATRIC	NAUSEA AND VOMITING	MOTION SICKNESS	VERTIGO
Cyclizine Marezine®	PO, IM 50 mg	(6–10 yr) PO 25 mg	X	X	
Dimenhydrinate Dramamine® Various	PO, IM, IV 50 mg; PR 100 mg	(8–12 yr) PO 25–50 mg; IM 1.2 mg/kg	X	X	X
Diphenhydramine Benadryl® Various	PO 50 mg; IM, IV 10–50 mg	(>9 kg) PO 12.5–25 mg; IM, IV 1.25 mg/kg	c	X	c
Meclizine Antivert® Bonine® Various	PO 25–50 mg	—	X	X	
MISCELLANEOUS **Benzquinamide** Emete-Con®	IM 50 mg; IV 25 mg	—	X		
Diphenidol Vontrol®	PO 25 mg; IM 20–40 mg; IV 20 mg	(>6 mo or 12 kg) PO 0.9 mg/kg; IM 0.4 mg/kg	X		X

Continued

Antiemetic Agents Comparison Chart[a]

| | INITIAL DOSE[b] | | INDICATIONS | | |
DRUG	ADULT	PEDIATRIC	NAUSEA AND VOMITING	MOTION SICKNESS	VERTIGO
Droperidol Inapsine®	IM 5 mg IV 0.5 mg	—	c		
Haloperidol Haldol®	PO, IM 1–2 mg	—	c		
Metoclopramide Reglan®	PO, IM 5–20 mg IV 1–2 mg/kg	—	X		
Scopolamine Transderm-Scōp® Various	PO 0.6–1.2 mg; SR Patch 1.5 mg[d]	—		X	
Trimetho-benzamide Tigan® Various	PO 250 mg; PR 200 mg; IM 200 mg	PO 5 mg/kg; PR 4 mg/kg	X		

a. From references 45–52.
b. Initial dose only, check prescribing information for subsequent dosing.
c. Not an FDA approved use, but appears effective.
d. Provides continuous drug release for 3 days; a total of 0.5 mg is released.

56:40 MISCELLANEOUS GASTROINTESTINAL DRUGS

Carbenoxolone Sodium (Investigational-Merrell Dow)

Biogastrone®, Duogastrone®

Carbenoxolone is a semisynthetic derivative of glycyrrhizic acid which is derived from licorice. Its precise mechanism of action is unknown, but it appears to increase the rate of healing of gastric ulcers; its efficacy in duodenal ulcers is questionable. Severe side effects can occur, related to the drug's mineralocorticoid activity: rapid weight gain due to sodium and water retention, congestive heart failure and hypertension may occur; hypokalemia, while less frequent, may be severe. The side effects can be treated with thiazide diuretics or amiloride, but spironolactone may inhibit the ulcer healing activity of carbenoxolone and thiazides can increase potassium loss. The usual dose is 100 mg tid for one week, then 50 mg tid until ulcer healing is complete, but no longer than 12 weeks. It is available in 50 mg tablets and 50 mg delayed-release capsules abroad.[53,54]

Chenodiol

Chenix®

Chenodiol is a bile acid used to dissolve gallstones. Its efficacy is somewhat limited with a 41% partial and 13% complete dissolution of gallstones with a dose of 750 mg/day for 2 years. A high recurrence rate has been noted and neither the need for surgery nor biliary symptoms are decreased during therapy. The drug appears to be more effective in patients who are below their ideal body weight, who have small stones or a serum cholesterol $\geq$ 227 mg/dl and in women. Highly radiopaque (high calcium) stones are resistant to therapy and nonvisualization of the gallbladder with cholecystography is associated with a poor success rate. Mild diarrhea occurs frequently and low density lipoproteins are increased about 10% over baseline during therapy. Increases in hepatic enzymes (SGOT and SGPT) occur occasionally, usually during the first three months of therapy. These elevations are usually mild and transient and are reversible on discontinuation of the drug. The usual dose is 750 mg/day, although a dose of 12–15 mg/kg/day may be optimal. The severity of diarrhea is minimized if the dose is gradually increased to this level over a period of weeks.[76-78]

Cimetidine

Tagamet®

Pharmacology.   Histamine H_2-receptor antagonist that reduces acid secretion by parietal cells in the stomach.

Administration and Adult Dose.   PO, IM or slow IV infusion for acute duodenal ulcer, active benign gastric ulcer or hypersecretory conditions 300 mg qid, to maximum of 2.4 g/day. Treatment of duodenal ulcer should continue for 4-6 weeks. Higher doses may be necessary in severe hypersecretory states such as Zollinger-Ellison syndrome. PO for prophylaxis of recurrent duodenal ulcer 300 or 400 mg hs.

Dosage Individualization.   In renal failure with Cr_s > 3.5 mg/dl, reduce dose to 300 mg q 12 hr; an extra dose should be given after hemodialysis,[55,56] but not peritoneal dialysis.[57] Greater dosage reductions are necessary in severe hepatic disease.[58]

Pediatric Dose. PO, IM or slow IV infusion (newborn) 10-20 mg/kg/day in divided doses;[59] (older children) 20-40 mg/kg/day in 4 divided doses.

Dosage Forms. Tab 200, 300 mg; Syrup 300 mg/5 ml; Inj 150 mg/ml.

Patient Instructions. Take prescribed dose for full length of treatment, even if epigastric pain goes away.

Pharmacokinetics and Biopharmaceutics. *Onset and Duration.* Onset 0.5-1 hr; duration 4-6 hr.[55]

Plasma Levels. 0.5-1 mcg/ml to inhibit 50% and 3.9 mcg/ml to inhibit 90% pentagastrin stimulated acid secretion.[60] 1.25 mcg/ml associated with mental changes in critically ill patients, but troughs as low as 0.25-0.5 mcg/ml may affect mental status in hepatic impairment.[58,61]

Fate. 70-80% absorbed orally; peak levels of 1-5 mcg/ml after 300 mg oral dose.[61] V_d is 0.4-0.6 L/kg; CNS penetration is enhanced in liver disease.[58,61] About 77% excreted unchanged in the urine.[58]

$t_{1/2}$. 2 hr;[55,58] 2.9 hr in liver disease;[58] 4-5 hr in renal failure;[56-58] 6.7 hr in renal and liver disease.[58]

Adverse Reactions. Rashes occasionally reported; severe bradycardia has been reported.[62] Mental status changes such as hallucinations, confusion, delirium and encephalopathy have been reported, primarily with IV use in the elderly, renal or hepatic impaired patients. Leukopenia, thrombocytopenia, gynecomastia and oligospermia reported rarely.[58,62] Serum creatinine and liver enzymes may rise during treatment, although renal and hepatic function are usually unaffected.

Precautions. Pregnancy; clinical experience is limited in children. Microsomal metabolism of many drugs may be inhibited—see Drug Interactions chapter.

Parameters to Monitor. Improvement in ulcer symptomatology, although this probably does not correlate with endoscopic evidence of healing;[63] CBC, serum creatinine and liver enzymes periodically.[62]

Notes. Cimetidine is no more effective, and is probably less effective, than antacids in prophylaxis or treatment of acute GI bleeding in critically ill patients;[64] effectiveness in chronic gastric ulceration is disputed.[55] Use as a supplement to oral enzymes in patients with cystic fibrosis and pancreatic exocrine insufficiency may improve digestion.[65] False-positive Hemoccult® results may occur in gastric aspirates after oral tablet use.

Metoclopramide

Reglan®

Pharmacology. Increases motility of the GI tract, probably by sensitizing gut muscle to the action of acetylcholine. It also has dopamine blocking activity and increases prolactin secretion.[66]

Administration and Adult Dose. PO for GI hypomotility 10 mg qid, 30 min before meals and hs for 2-8 weeks. IV to aid radiologic examination or facilitate small bowel intubation 10 mg over 1-2 min. IV for prophylaxis of vomiting due to cisplatin chemotherapy 2 mg/kg 30 min before cisplatin and q 2 hr for 2 doses, then q 3 hr for 3 doses. If emesis is suppressed after initial 2 doses, reduction of subsequent doses to 1 mg/kg may be tried. Doses should be diluted in 50 ml of fluid and infused over at least 15 minutes.[67] See Notes.

Dosage Individualization. A preliminary report indicates that the dose should be decreased by 60% in severe renal impairment.[68]

Pediatric Dose. IV to aid **radiologic examination** (under 6 yr) 0.1 mg/kg; (6–14 yr) 2.5–5 mg.

Dosage Forms. Tab 10 mg; Inj 5 mg/ml.

Patient Instructions. This drug may cause drowsiness or fatigue. Until the extent of this effect is known, use caution in driving or operating machinery.

Pharmacokinetics and Biopharmaceutics. *Onset and Duration.* Onset PO 10–30 min, IV 1–3 min; duration 3 hr.[69] Peak GI effects occur about 2 hr after oral administration, but may be delayed with delayed gastric emptying.
   Fate. Bioavailability is 58–73% after oral administration due to a first-pass effect. After 10 mg in oral solution, peak levels of 40 ng/ml are attained in 2 hr in normals; absorption may be delayed in patients with delayed gastric emptying. V_d is about 2–3 L/kg. The drug is metabolized to various conjugates and 16–21% is excreted unchanged in the urine after IV administration.[69-71]
   $t_{1/2}$. α phase 4 min; β phase about 4.8 hr.[70] In severe renal impairment, half-life increases to 14 hr.[68]

Adverse Reactions. Drowsiness, lassitude and fatigue occur frequently. Dizziness and weakness occur occasionally; extrapyramidal side effects such as opisthotonos, clonic convulsions and oculogyric crisis occur less frequently, but may be striking in children.[72] Potentiation of extrapyramidal side effects may occur with phenothiazines or butyrophenones. Diarrhea occurs frequently with large IV doses.

Contraindications. Concurrent use of MAO inhibitors, tricyclic antidepressants or sympathomimetics.

Precautions. Pregnancy.

Notes. Metoclopramide is stable in D5W, D5NS, Ringer's and Lactated Ringer's solutions for 48 hr at room temperature; unless it is to be used immediately, dilutions should be protected from light. High-dose metoclopramide is more effective than phenothiazines in cisplatin-induced nausea and vomiting. It has also been used orally in gastroesophageal reflux.

Ranitidine   Zantac®

Ranitidine is a histamine H_2-receptor antagonist pharmacologically and therapeutically similar to cimetidine. Ranitidine does not appear to inhibit hepatic microsomal enzymes or to have antiandrogenic effects. It does cross the blood-brain barrier, but mental confusion has not been reported. Its half-life is 2.3–3 hr and it has been successfully used in twice daily dosing regimens. Dosage in duodenal ulcer is 150 mg bid.[73] It is also indicated in pathological hypersecretory states. Available as 150 mg tablets.

Sucralfate   Carafate®

Sucralfate is the aluminum salt of a sulfated disaccharide which is not absorbed from the GI tract. It forms a barrier on ulcers, protecting them against gastric acid, pepsin and bile. It also directly inhibits the action of pepsin and bile. Sucralfate appears to be most effective in duodenal ulcers and to be about as effective as cimetidine in duodenal and gastric ulcers. Side effects are very uncommon, with constipation reported occasionally and GI distress rarely. The drug may interfere with tetracycline absorption because of its aluminum content. Antacids may be taken, but not within one-half hour of a dose. The adult dose is 1 g qid on an empty stomach 1 hour before meals and at bedtime for 4–8 weeks. It is available in 1 g tablets.[74,75,79]

References, 56:00 Gastrointestinal Drugs

1. Penna RP, ed. Handbook of nonprescription drugs. 6th ed. Washington, DC: American Pharmaceutical Association, 1979.

2. Spiro HM. Clinical gastroenterology. 2nd ed. New York: Macmillan, 1977.

3. Hastings PR, Skillman JJ, Bushnell LS et al. Antacid titration in the prevention of acute gastrointestinal bleeding. N Engl J Med 1978;298:1041-5.

4. Peterson WL, Sturdevant RAL, Frankl HD et al. Healing of duodenal ulcer with an antacid regimen. N Engl J Med 1977;297:341-5.

5. Greensher J, Mofenson HC, Picchioni AL et al. Activated charcoal update. JACEP 1979;8:261-3.

6. Mayersohn M, Perrier D, Picchioni AL. Evaluation of a charcoal-sorbitol mixture as an antidote for oral aspirin overdose. Clin Toxicol 1977;11:515-33.

7. Hayden JW, Comstock EG. Use of activated charcoal in acute poisoning. Clin Toxicol 1975;8:515-33.

8. Morrissey JF, Barreras RF. Antacid therapy. N Engl J Med 1974;290:550-4.

9. Levy G, Lampman T, Kamath BL. Decreased serum salicylate concentrations in children with rheumatic fever treated with antacid. N Engl J Med 1975;293:323-5.

10. Kachny WD, Hegg AP, Alfrey AL. Gastrointestinal absorption of aluminum from aluminum containing antacids. N Engl J Med 1977;296:1389-90.

11. Ivanovich P, Fellow H, Rich C. The absorption of calcium carbonate. Ann Intern Med 1967;66:917-23.

12. Alfrey AC, Le Gendre GR, Kaehny WD. The dialysis encephalopathy syndrome. N Engl J Med 1976;294:184-8.

13. Svensson CK, Wiser TH. Lack of efficacy of antacid tablets—fact or fiction? Drug Intell Clin Pharm 1981;15:120-1.

14. Barowsky H. Schwartz SA. Method for evaluating diphenoxylate hydrochloride. JAMA 1962;180:1058-61.

15. Heel RC, Brogden RN, Speight TM et al. Loperamide: a review of its pharmacological properties and therapeutic efficacy in diarrhea. Drugs 1978;15:33-52.

16. Karin A, Raney RE, Evensen KL. Pharmacokinetics and metabolism of diphenoxylate in man. Clin Pharmacol Ther 1972;13:407-19.

17. Pietrusko RG. Use and abuse of laxatives. Am J Hosp Pharm 1977;34:291-300.

18. Heykants J, Michiels M, Knaeps A et al. Loperamide (R 18553), a novel type of antidiarrheal agent. part 5: the pharmacokinetics of loperamide in rats and man. Arzneim Forsch 1974;24:1649-53.

19. Kepler JA, ed. American hospital formulary service. Washington, DC: American Society of Hospital Pharmacists, 1959-82.

20. Conn HO, Lieberthal MM, eds. The hepatic coma syndromes and lactulose. Baltimore: Williams and Wilkins, 1979.

21. Gilman AG, Goodman LS, Gilman A, eds. Goodman and Gilman's the pharmacological basis of therapeutics. 6th ed. New York: Macmillan, 1980.

22. Anon. Safety of stool softeners. Med Lett Drugs Ther 1977;19:45-6.

23. Godfrey H. Dangers of dioctyl sodium sulfosuccinate in mixtures. JAMA 1971;215:643.

24. Goldstein GB, Lam KC, Mistilis SP. Drug-induced active chronic hepatitis. Am J Dig Dis 1973;18:177-84.

25. Tolman KG, Hammar S, Sannella JJ. Possible hepatotoxicity of Doxidan®. Ann Intern Med 1976;84:290-2.

26. Goodman J, Pang J, Bessman AN. Dioctyl sodium sulfosuccinate—an ineffective prophylactic laxative. J Chron Dis 1976;29:59-63.

27. Anon. USP Dispensing Information. Rockville, MD: United States Pharmacopeal Convention, 1981.

28. Anon. Laxatives and dietary fiber. Med Lett Drugs Ther 1973;15:98-100.

29. MacLean WC. A comparison of ipecac syrup and apomorphine in the immediate treatment of ingestion of poisons. J Pediatr 1973;82:121-4.

30. Corby DG, Decker WJ, Moran MJ et al. Clinical comparison of pharmacologic emetics in children. Pediatrics 1968;42:361-4.

31. deCastro FJ, Jaeger RW, Peters A et al. Apomorphine: clinical trial of stable solution. Clin Toxicol 1978;12:65-8.

32. Klein RL, Graves CL, Kim YI et al. Inhibition of apomorphine-induced vomiting by benzquinamide. Clin Pharmacol Ther 1970;11:530-7.

33. Hobbs DC, Connolly AG. Pharmacokinetics of benzquinamide in man. J Pharmacokinet Biopharm 1978;6:477-85.

34. Grove WR, Bender JF, Fortner CL et al. A benzquinamide-induced extrapyramidal reaction. Drug Intell Clin Pharm 1976;10:638-9.

35. Chapin JW, Wingard DW. Physostigmine reversal of benzquinamide-induced delirium. Anesthesiology 1977;46:364-5.

36. Moertel CG, Schutt AJ, Hahn RG et al. Oral benzquinamide in the treatment of nausea and vomiting. Clin Pharmacol Ther 1975;18:554-7.

37. Anderson PO, McGuire GG. Delta-9-tetrahydrocannabinol as an antiemetic. Am J Hosp Pharm 1981;38:639-46.

38. Manoguerra AS, Krenzelok EP. Rapid emesis from high-dose ipecac syrup in adults and children intoxicated with antiemetics or other drugs. Am J Hosp Pharm 1978;35:1360-2.

39. Miser JS, Robertson WO. Ipecac poisoning. West J Med 1978;128:440-3.

40. Varipapa RJ, Oderda GM. Effect of milk on ipecac-induced emesis. N Engl J Med 1977;296:112-3.

41. Thoman ME, Verhulst HL. Ipecac syrup in antiemetic ingestion. JAMA 1966;196:433-4.

42. Anderson RJ, Gambertoglio JG, Schrier RW. Clinical use of drugs in renal failure. Springfield: Charles C Thomas, 1976:197.

43. Drugs for psychiatric disorders. Med Lett Drugs Ther 1980;22:77-84.

44. Side effects of antipsychotic drugs and their treatment. In: Klein DF, Gittelman R, Quitkin F et al. Diagnosis and drug treatment of psychiatric disorders. 2nd ed. Baltimore: Williams and Wilkins, 1980:172-214.

45. Shirkey HC, ed. Pediatric therapy. 6th ed. St. Louis: CV Mosby, 1980.

46. Frytak S, Moertel CG. Management of nausea and vomiting in the cancer patient. JAMA 1981;245:393-6.

47. Mellencamp E, Wang RIH. The patient with nausea II. Motion sickness. Drug Ther 1977;7(May):49-54.

48. Mellencamp E, Wang RIH. The patient with nausea III. Cancer, pregnancy or surgery. Drug Ther 1977; 7(June):102-12.

49. Schwinghammer T. Antiemetics: choosing from the alternatives. Hosp Formul 1980;15:38-51.

50. Barton MD, Libonati M, Cohen PJ. The use of haloperidol for treatment of postoperative nausea and vomiting—a double-blind placebo-controlled trial. Anesthesiology 1975;42:508-12.

51. Loeser EA, Bennett G, Stanley TH et al. Comparison of droperidol, haloperidol and prochlorperazine as postoperative anti-emetics. Can Anaesth Soc J 1979;26:125-7.

52. Diamond MJ, Keeri-Szanto M. Reduction of post-operative vomiting by preoperative administration of oral metoclopramide. Can Anaesth Soc J 1980;27:36-9.

53. Pinder RM, Brogden RN, Sawyer PR et al. Carbenoxolone: a review of its pharmacological properties and therapeutic efficacy in peptic ulcer disease. Drugs 1976;11:245-307.

54. Anon. Carbenoxolone sodium for gastric ulcer. Med Lett Drugs Ther 1975;17:67-8.

55. Burland WL, Simkins MA, eds. Cimetidine: the proceedings of the second international symposium on H_2 receptor antagonists. Amsterdam: Oxford/Excerpta Medica, 1977.

56. Ma KW, Brown DC, Masler DS et al. Effects of renal failure on blood levels of cimetidine. Gastroenterology 1978;74:473-477(part 2).

57. Vaziri ND, Ness RL, Barton CH. Peritoneal dialysis clearance of cimetidine. Am J Gastroenterol 1979;71:572-6.

58. Schentag JJ, Cerra FB, Calleri GM et al. Age, disease and cimetidine disposition in healthy subjects and chronically ill patients. Clin Pharmacol Ther 1981;29:737-43.

59. Chhattriwalla Y, Colon AR, Scanlon JW. The use of cimetidine in the newborn. Pediatrics 1980;65:301-2.

60. Gugler R, Fuchs G, Dieckmann M et al. Cimetidine plasma concentration-response relationships. Clin Pharmacol Ther 1981;29:744-8.

61. Kimelblatt BJ, Cerra FB, Calleri G et al. Dose and serum concentration relationships in cimetidine-associated mental confusion. Gastroenterology 1980;78:791-5.

62. Sawyer D, Conner CS, Scalley R. Cimetidine: adverse reactions and acute toxicity. Am J Hosp Pharm 1981;38:188-97.

63. Collen MJ, Hanan MR, Maher JA et al. Cimetidine vs placebo in duodenal ulcer therapy. Dig Dis Sci 1980;25:744-9.

64. Bivins BA, Rogers EL, Rapp RP et al. Clinical failures with cimetidine. Surgery 1981;88:417-24.

65. Hubbard VS, Dunn GD, Lester LA. Effectiveness of cimetidine as an adjunct to supplemental pancreatic enzymes in patients with cystic fibrosis. Am J Clin Nutr 1980;33:2281-6.

66. Schulze-Delrieu K. Metoclopramide. Gastroenterology 1979;77:768-79.

67. Gralla RJ, Itri LM, Pisko SE et al. Antiemetic efficacy of high-dose metoclopramide: randomized trials with placebo and prochlorperazine in patients with chemotherapy-induced nausea and vomiting. N Engl J Med 1981;305:905-9.

68. Bateman DN, Gokal R. Metoclopramide in renal failure. Lancet 1980;1:982.

69. Bateman DN, Kahn C, Mashiter K et al. Pharmacokinetic and concentration-effect studies with intravenous metoclopramide. Br J Clin Pharmacol 1978;6:401-7.

70. Graffner C, Lagerstrom P-O, Lundborg P et al. Pharmacokinetics of metoclopramide intravenously and orally determined by liquid chromatography. Br J Clin Pharmacol 1979;8:469-74.

71. Teng L, Bruce RB, Dunning LK. Metoclopramide metabolism and determination by high-pressure liquid chromatography. J Pharm Sci 1977;66:1615-8.

72. Pinder PM, Brogden RN, Sawyer PR et al. Metoclopramide: a review of its pharmacological properties and clinical use. Drugs 1976;12:81-131.

73. Fourth European Congress of Gastrointestinal Endoscopy. Proceedings of the first International Symposium on Ranitidine. Scand J Gastroenterol 1981;16(suppl 69):1-131.

74. McGraw BF, Caldwell EG. Sucralfate. Drug Intell Clin Pharm 1981;15:578-80.

75. Marks IN. Current therapy in peptic ulcer. Drugs 1980;20:283-99.

76. Schoenfield LJ, Lachin JM et al. Chenodiol (chenodeoxycholic acid) for dissolution of gallstones: the national cooperative gallstone study. Ann Intern Med 1981;95:257-82.

77. Ruppin DC, Dowling RH. Is recurrence inevitable after gallstone dissolution by bile acid therapy? Lancet 1982;1:181-5.

78. Hoffmann AF. Gallstone-dissolving drugs. Drug Ther (hosp) 1982;April:87-103.

79. Garnett WR. Sucralfate—alternative therapy for peptic-ulcer disease. Clin Pharm 1982;1:307-14.

68:00 HORMONES AND SYNTHETIC SUBSTITUTES

68:04 ADRENALS

General References: 1-3

Class Instructions. These drugs may be taken with food, milk or antacid to minimize stomach upset. Single daily doses or alternate-day doses should be taken in the morning prior to 9 AM. Multiple doses should be taken at evenly spaced intervals during the day. Report unusual weight gain, lower extremity swelling, muscle weakness, face swelling, menstrual irregularities, prolonged sore throat, fever, cold, infection or serious injury. Patients on chronic steroid therapy should carry appropriate identification. Do not discontinue this medication without medical approval; tell any new physician that you are taking a corticosteroid.

Beclomethasone Dipropionate Beconase®, Beclovent®, Vancenase®, Vanceril®

Pharmacology. Potent glucocorticoid—see Prednisone.

Administration and Adult Dose. **Inhal for asthma** 336–504 mcg (8–12 inhalations) divided into 2–3 doses, to maximum of 840 mcg/day (20 inhalations). In severe cases, start with 504–672 mcg/day (12–16 inhalations); after patient is symptom-free for 30 days and pulmonary function tests normalized, decrease daily dose by 84 mcg (2 inhalations) at weekly intervals until minimum dose necessary to control patient has been defined. **Intranasal for nasal congestion** not responsive to maximally tolerated doses of antihistamine-decongestant combination 42 mcg/nostril bid-qid (168–336 mcg/day total dose) for several days, then decrease dose (if symptoms do not recur) to minimum amount necessary to control stuffiness.[4-7]

Pediatric Dose. Same as adult dose; safety and efficacy of nasal inhalation in children not established.

Dosage Forms. **Inhal** (Beclovent®, Vanceril®) 42 mcg/inhalation (200 doses/inhaler); **Nasal Inhal** (Beconase®, Vancenase®) 42 mcg/inhalation (200 doses/inhaler).

Patient Instructions. To use oral inhaler, add 6-inch paper extension tube to inhaler mouthpiece. Tilt head up, place mouthpiece with extension into mouth and while breathing normally actuate inhaler; inhale and hold breath for 5 seconds. Medication is for preventive therapy only and should not be used to treat an acute asthmatic attack; use at regularly scheduled intervals as prescribed. Allow at least 10 seconds between inhalations. Patients concurrently using inhaled sympathomimetics should use the bronchodilator several minutes before the beclomethasone aerosol to prevent bronchospasm induced by beclomethasone and to enhance penetration of the steroid into the bronchial tree. Rinse mouth with water or mouthwash after each use to reduce *Candida* growth. Report hoarseness or sore throat. If long-term systemic corticosteroid therapy has been recently discontinued (within several months), report immediately if trauma, surgery or infections occur. See also Class Instructions.

Pharmacokinetics and Biopharmaceutics. *Onset and Duration.* Clinical effect usually evident in several days to 2 weeks.

Fate. About 90% of an inhaled dose is absorbed from GI tract, because most of inhaled drug is swallowed.[8] Rapid absorption from respiratory and GI tissues. Plasma levels are very low with usual doses and their significance is not known. Drug and free and conjugated metabolites appear in feces. Less than 10% of drug and metabolites are excreted in urine.

Adverse Reactions. Deaths due to adrenal insufficiency during and after transfer from systemic corticosteroids to aerosol may occur. After oral use, localized growth of *Candida* in the mouth occurs frequently, but clinically apparent infections are less common. Hoarseness and dry mouth occur occasionally; minimal suppression of pituitary-adrenal function from aerosol use at usual doses occurs to about the same degree as alternate-day prednisone.[9] After intranasal use, irritation and burning of the nasal mucosa and sneezing occur occasionally; intranasal and pharyngeal *Candida* infections, nasal ulceration and epistaxis occur rarely.[4]

Contraindications. Status asthmaticus or other acute episodes of asthma in which intensive measures are required; beclomethasone-exacerbated symptoms.

Precautions. During stress or severe asthmatic attacks, patients withdrawn from systemic corticosteroids should resume them (in large doses) immediately and contact their physician.

Parameters to Monitor. For treatment of asthma, frequency of asthmatic symptoms during day; nocturnal use of prn sympathomimetic inhaler. For nasal congestion, relief of symptoms.

Notes. Oral inhalation is indicated only for patients (including those already receiving oral corticosteroids) who require chronic treatment with corticosteroids in conjunction with other asthmatic therapy. Patients needing chronic steroids should be continued on therapeutic doses of theophylline.[10] The nasal inhalation provides effective, prompt relief of nasal congestion when maximally tolerated doses of oral sympathomimetics are inadequate.

Dexamethasone

Decadron®, Hexadrol®, Various

Dexamethasone is a potent, long-acting glucocorticoid lacking sodium-retaining activity with low to moderate doses—see Oral Corticosteroids Comparison Chart. Dexamethasone is used in several special situations such as cerebral edema, septic shock and in the "dexamethasone suppression test" to screen for Cushing's disease and depression. Clear evidence of efficacy in improving the outcome of septic shock is lacking; however, some clinicians believe that corticosteroids may be effective if given in the early stages of bacteremic septic shock. The dose in cerebral edema is 10 mg IV (as sodium phosphate) initially, followed by 4 mg IM or IV q 6 hr; after 2–4 days of therapy, dosage may be tapered over 5–7 days. In septic shock, doses of 6 mg/kg IV, repeated q 4–6 hr for no longer than 48 hr; however, repeating doses more than 1–2 times is seldom justified. It should be noted that Decadron® injection contains 8 mg/ml of creatinine which can complicate the evaluation of creatinine clearance; Hexadrol® injection and some generic products contain no creatinine. The dexamethasone suppression test is performed by administering 1 mg orally at 11 PM and measuring serum cortisol at 8 AM and 4 PM the next day. A cortisol concentration of greater than 5 mcg/dl in either sample is abnormal. Dexamethasone is available in tablets of 0.25, 0.5, 0.75, 1.5 and 4 mg; an elixir of 0.1 mg/ml; and as an injection containing 4, 10 or 24 mg/ml.[11-13]

Flunisolide   Nasalide®

Flunisolide is a potent corticosteroid that is available as a 0.025% solution for nasal inhalation. It is indicated for symptomatic relief of seasonal or perennial rhinitis when effectiveness or tolerance of conventional treatment is unsatisfactory. Efficacy of flunisolide is equivalent to beclomethasone nasal inhalation in perennial and seasonal rhinitis and superior to cromolyn sodium in seasonal rhinitis; it may be less effective in patients with nonallergic rhinitis than in those with a demonstrable allergic component. Irritation and stinging of the nasal mucosa occurs occasionally; intranasal and pharyngeal *Candida* colonization, nasal ulceration, sneezing and epistaxis occur rarely. The usual dose is 2 sprays (50 mcg) in each nostril bid, increasing to tid if needed, to a maximum of 8 sprays/nostril/day. The usual children's dose is 1 spray/nostril tid to 2 sprays/nostril bid, to a maximum of 4 sprays/nostril/day; not recommended in children under 6 years. It is available in a 25 ml pump spray bottle containing 6.25 mg of drug.[14]

Methylprednisolone Sodium Succinate   Solu-Medrol®, Various

Methylprednisolone sodium succinate is an injectable glucocorticoid that is about 1.25 times as potent as prednisone and prednisolone—see Oral Corticosteroids Comparison Chart. It is commonly used when oral therapy is not possible and in situations in which large parenteral doses are necessary. Side effects are similar to prednisone in equivalent doses. Clear evidence of efficacy in improving the outcome of septic shock is lacking; however, some clinicians believe that corticosteroids may be effective if given in the early stages of bacteremic septic shock. The dose in septic shock and other serious conditions is 30 mg/kg IV over 10–20 min, repeated q 4–6 hr for no longer than 48 hr; however, repeating doses more than 1–2 times is seldom justified in septic shock. The drug is available in 40, 125, 500 and 1000 mg vials.[11,12]

Prednisone   Deltasone®, Orasone®, Various

Pharmacology.   A synthetic glucocorticoid with minimal sodium-retaining activity. At the cellular level, glucocorticoids appear to act by controlling the rate of protein synthesis. Clinically, these drugs are used primarily for their anti-inflammatory and immunosuppressant effects.

Administration and Adult Dose.   Total daily dose is variable, depending on the clinical disorder and patient response.[1,15] Daily divided high-dose therapy for initial control of more severe disease states may be necessary until satisfactory control is obtained, usually 4–10 days for many allergic and collagen diseases. Administration of short-acting preparation given as a single dose in the morning (eg, 6–8 AM) is likely to produce fewer side effects and less pituitary-adrenal suppression than either a divided daily dose regimen with the same agent or an equivalent dose of a long-acting agent.[2,16] Alternate-day therapy (ie, total 48-hr dose administered every other morning) further reduces the prevalence and degree of steroid side effects. However, it may not be uniformly effective in treating all disease states[2,16,17,137] unless large doses are used (eg, 40–60 mg every other day for adults requiring chronic steroid therapy for asthma). Adrenal suppression may not occur with single daily doses given either in the morning or evening if the dose is not more than 15 mg of prednisone,[18] but Cushing's syndrome may still occur.[3] Protocols for withdrawal from glucocorticoid therapy have been published.[1,19]

Common initial doses are: PO for arthritis 10 mg/day; **PO for collagen diseases** 1 mg/kg/day; **PO for rheumatic carditis** 40 mg/day; **PO for nephrotic syndrome** 60 mg/day; **PO for skin disorders** 40 mg/day, up to 120 mg/day in pemphigus; **PO for ulcerative colitis** 60–120 mg/day; **PO for thrombocytopenia** 0.5 mg/kg/day; **PO for organ transplantation** 50–100 mg/day;[15] **PO for acute asthma exacerbations** in adults and adolescents 40 mg 2–6 times/day for 3–5 days,[20] hospitalized patients may need a parenteral preparation q 4 hr. In all cases, reduce dose to minimal effective maintenance dose as soon as possible.

Pediatric Dose. Dose depends on disease state and patient response. **Common initial doses are: PO** 2 mg/kg/day; **PO for nephrosis** (1.5–4 yr) 30–40 mg/day; (4–10 yr) 60 mg/day; (over 10 yr) 80 mg/day. **PO for asthma exacerbations** (infants) 10 mg 2–6 times/day depending on severity (status asthmaticus, q 4 hr); (2–5 yr) 20 mg 2–6 times/day for 3–5 days; (6–10 yr) 30 mg 2–6 times/day for 3–5 days; (over 10 yr) 40 mg 2–6 times/day for 3–5 days.[20]

Dosage Forms. **Tab** 1, 2.5, 5, 10, 20, 50 mg.

Patient Instructions. See Class Instructions. If a dose is missed and the proper schedule is *every other day*, take it as soon as possible and resume the schedule unless it is past noon. In that case, wait until the next morning and resume every other day dosing. If the proper schedule is *once a day*, take the dose as soon as possible. If not remembered until the next day do not double that day's dose; skip the missed dose. If the proper schedule is *several times a day*, take the dose as soon as possible and resume the normal schedule. If not remembered until the next dose is due, then take that regular dose and skip the missed dose; resume the normal dosing schedule.[21]

Pharmacokinetics and Biopharmaceutics. *Onset and Duration.* See Oral Corticosteroids Comparison Chart.

Plasma Levels. Therapeutic effects are not directly correlated with plasma concentration; however, the half-life of the effect on serum corticosterone is 1.5–2 times the plasma half-life.[22,23]

Fate. Bioavailability differences between products have been reported;[24] 70–95% protein bound depending on plasma concentration;[15] V_d of prednisolone is 1 L/kg. Prednisone and cortisone must be metabolized in the liver to their active forms, prednisolone and hydrocortisone, respectively;[26] liver disease does not impair conversion to active metabolites. In fact, patients with liver disease and hypoalbuminemia are more likely to suffer major side effects of prednisone as a result of decreased protein binding and delayed clearance of prednisolone.[27-29] Prednisolone is eliminated primarily by hepatic metabolism, with greater than 90% of metabolites found in the urine. About 7–15% of a dose of prednisone or prednisolone is excreted as unchanged prednisolone in urine.

$t_{1/2}$. (Prednisone) 3.3–3.8 hr;[27] (prednisolone) 2.1–4 hr; may exhibit dose-dependent kinetics—with increasing doses, values of V_d, plasma clearance and $t_{1/2}$ may increase.[15]

Adverse Reactions. Prolonged therapy may lead to suppression of pituitary-adrenal function. Too rapid a withdrawal of long-term therapy can cause acute adrenal insufficiency (eg, fever, myalgia, arthralgia and malaise); suppressed patients are unable to respond to stress. Therapy with prednisone (other adrenocorticoids vary in propensity for certain adverse effects), depending on dose and duration, can result in fluid and electrolyte disturbances (with possible edema and hypertension), hyperglycemia and glycosuria, spread of herpes conjunctivitis, activation of tuberculosis, peptic ulcers (although one review found no association between steroid therapy alone and peptic ulcer),[30] osteoporosis, myopathy, behavioral disturbances,[31] poor wound healing, ocular cataracts, arrest of growth, pseudotumor cerebri (primarily in children)[1] and Cushing's syndrome (moon face, buffalo hump, central obesity, easy bruising, acne, hirsutism and striae).[15] Acute onset reactions in one study occurred in 11.4% of patients and included psychiatric reactions, GI reactions, hyperglycemia, infections and leukocytosis.[31]

Contraindications. Systemic fungal infections (except as maintenance therapy in adrenal insufficiency).

Precautions. Pregnancy; breast feeding; diabetes mellitus; osteoporosis; peptic ulcer; esophagitis; tuberculosis and other acute and chronic bacterial, viral and fungal infections; hypertension or other cardiovascular diseases; immunizations; hypoalbuminemia; psychosis; suppression of TB skin test reactions. See Drug Interactions chapter.

Parameters to Monitor. Observe for psychotic personality changes and signs or symptoms of Cushing's syndrome. With short-term, high-dose therapy, frequently monitor serum potassium and glucose, blood pressure and stool guaiac. With long-term therapy, monitor these parameters occasionally and perform periodic eye examinations. The 24-hr urinary free cortisol is the most sensitive measurement of HPA axis suppression.

Notes. Other more expensive glucocorticoids offer minimal advantages over prednisone in most clinical situations.[16,32] Patients who have received daily steroid therapy for asthma for less than 3 weeks *do not* require dose tapering.

Oral Corticosteroids Comparison Chart[a]

DURATION AND DRUG	EQUIVALENT ANTI-INFLAMMATORY DOSE (MG)	RELATIVE ANTI-INFLAMMATORY POTENCY	RELATIVE MINERALO-CORTICOID ACTIVITY	DOSAGE FORMS	PLASMA HALF-LIFE (HOURS)	COMMENTS
SHORT-ACTING (biologic activity less than 12 hr)						
Cortisone Various	25	0.8	0.8	Tab 5, 10, 25 mg	0.5	Must be hydroxylated to active species (hydrocortisone)
Hydrocortisone Various	20	1	1	Tab 5, 10, 20 mg Susp 2 mg/ml	1.5	Daily secretion in man = 20 mg
INTERMEDIATE-ACTING (biologic activity 12–36 hr)						
Prednisone Various	5	4	0.8	Tab 1, 2.5, 5, 10, 20, 50 mg	3.6	Must be hydroxylated to active species (prednisolone)
Prednisolone Various	5	4	0.8	Tab 1, 2.5, 5 mg	3	Minimal sodium-retaining activity
Methylpred-nisolone Medrol® Various	4	5	0.5	Tab 2, 4, 8, 16, 24, 32 mg	3.3	Minimal sodium-retaining activity

Continued

Oral Corticosteroids Comparison Chart[a]

DURATION AND DRUG	EQUIVALENT ANTI-INFLAMMATORY DOSE (MG)	RELATIVE ANTI-INFLAMMATORY POTENCY	RELATIVE MINERALO-CORTICOID ACTIVITY	DOSAGE FORMS	PLASMA HALF-LIFE (HOURS)	COMMENTS
Triamcinolone Aristocort® Kenacort® Various	4	5	0	Tab 1, 2, 4, 8, 16 mg Syrup 400, 800 mcg/ml	3.3+	May cause a higher frequency of muscle wasting
LONG-ACTING (biologic activity 36–54 hr)						
Betamethasone Celestone®	0.6	25	0	Tab 600 mcg Syrup 120 mcg/ml	—	Minimal sodium retaining activity, but with high doses retention may occur
Dexamethasone Decadron® Hexadrol® Various	0.75	30	0	Tab 250, 500, 750 mcg, 1.5, 4 mg Elxr 100 mcg/ml	Males 3.4 Females 2.4	
MINERALOCORTICOID (biologic activity 12–24 hr)						
Fludrocortisone Florinef®	—	10	125	Tab 100 mcg	—	Mineralocorticoid useful in Addison's disease

a. From references 1, 3, 25, 33–35.

68:12 CONTRACEPTIVES

(SEE ALSO ESTROGENS 68:16 AND PROGESTOGENS 68:32)

General References: 36-41

Class Instructions. Estrogens, Progestogens and Combinations. Report immediately if any of the following occur: new severe or persistent headache; blurred vision; calf, chest or abdominal pain; or any abnormal vaginal bleeding. This (oral) drug may be taken with food, milk or an antacid to minimize stomach upset.

Oral Contraceptives
(Estrogen-Progestogen Combinations)

Pharmacology. These drugs cause inhibition of ovulation, endometrial changes which are hostile to egg implantation and cervical mucus changes which are hostile to sperm migration.

Administration and Adult Dose. PO for contraception 1 tablet daily beginning on the fifth day after onset of menses and continued for 20–21 days, depending on the product; stop for 7 days and restart the next cycle of 20–21 tablets. Combination 28-day products (7 inert tablets) are taken 1 tablet daily continuously. **PO for contraception postpartum** start 2–4 weeks postpartum; lactation may increase period of infertility. **PO for contraception postabortion** start immediately if gestation is terminated at 12 weeks or less; start in 1 week if gestation terminated at 13–28 weeks.[39] **PO for dysfunctional uterine bleeding (anovulatory cycles)** (any combination agent) 1 tablet qid for 5–7 days for acute bleeding, then 1 tablet daily cyclically as for contraception for 3 months to prevent further bleeding.[36] **PO for dysmenorrhea or endometriosis** 1 tablet cyclically as for contraception for 3–9 months to induce a pseudopregnant state—use minimal estrogen, maximal progestin combination (eg, Ovral®, Demulen®, Norlestrin® 2.5 mg).[36] **PO for emergency postcoital contraception** 2 tablets of Ovral® taken as soon as possible after coitus, and 2 more tablets taken 12 hr later, but within 72 hr after coitus.[58] See Notes.

Dosage Forms. See Oral Contraceptive Agents Comparison Chart.

Patient Instructions. See Class Instructions. **Contraception.** If one dose is missed, take it as soon as it is remembered or take 2 tablets the next day; if 2 doses are missed, take 2 tablets daily for the next 2 days. If more than 2 doses are missed and bleeding occurs, consider as a normal period and restart cycle; also use an alternative form of contraception for the remainder of the cycle. Report if no menses occur for 2 months. **Acute anovulatory bleeding.** Expect heavy and severely cramping flow 2–4 days after stopping pills with normal periods thereafter.

Pharmacokinetics and Biopharmaceutics. *Onset and Duration.* Onset of contraception after one week of regimen. Dysfunctional uterine bleeding should decrease within 12–24 hr of starting regimen.

Fate. Well absorbed and widely distributed. Mestranol is converted to ethinyl estradiol in vivo.[112] Ethinyl estradiol and progestogens are slowly inactivated by liver and undergo enterohepatic circulation. Conjugated to glucuronides and sulfates which are excreted in the urine and feces.[112]

$t_{1/2}$. (Mestranol) 40–60 hr;[113] (ethinyl estradiol) 27–52 hr;[112] (norgestrel) 27–55 hr;[42] (norethindrone) 70 hr.[113]

Adverse Reactions.   See Hormone Excess and Deficiency Symptomatology and Adverse Reactions of Oral Contraceptives Comparison Charts.

Contraindications.   Presence or history of thrombophlebitis or thromboembolic disorders; known or suspected pregnancy; presence or history of carcinoma of breast, genitals or other estrogen-dependent tumors; cerebral vascular or coronary artery disease; markedly impaired liver function; undiagnosed abnormal genital bleeding; heavy smoking (over 15 cigarettes/day) in women 35 yr or older.[37,38,40,41]

Precautions.   Use with caution in patients with hyperlipidemia, diabetes, conditions which may be aggravated by fluid retention (eg, hypertension, convulsions, migraine and cardiac or renal dysfunction), severe varicosities, in adolescents in whom regular menses are not established and during lactation. Oral contraceptives may be less effective, resulting in increased breakthrough bleeding and/or pregnancy, when given with rifampin, phenobarbital, ampicillin, penicillin V, phenytoin, chloramphenicol, tetracycline, primidone, nitrofurantoin or neomycin.[43,44] Caffeine elimination may be impaired by oral contraceptives.[45] Antipyrine clearance (dependent on cytochrome P-450) is impaired by oral contraceptives.[46] See Drug Interactions chapter.

Parameters to Monitor.   Complete pretreatment physical examination with special reference to blood pressure, breast, abdomen, pelvis and Pap smear. Repeat examination every year.

Notes.   Initial selection of an oral contraceptive should approximate as closely as possible the patient's natural hormone balance.[47] Ortho-Novum® 1/50, Norinyl® 1 + 50 and Lo-Ovral® are balanced agents that are often selected as the initial contraceptive. Certain combination contraceptives (ie, Ovral®) are effective as postcoital contraceptives. Compared to estrogens, Ovral® is cheaper, causes less nausea and vomiting, and takes 12 hours rather than 5 days for a course of therapy.[58]

Ortho-Novum® 10/11 is a new "biphasic" birth control pill in which the daily hormone dose changes with the cycle to mimic the normal hormonal pattern of the menstrual cycle. Lower daily doses are given early in the cycle, while slightly higher doses later in the cycle decrease spotting and breakthrough bleeding. This preparation reduces the total dose per cycle to less than most conventional oral contraceptives. Tablets given on days 1–10 contain 0.5 mg norethindrone and 35 mcg ethinyl estradiol; days 11–21 contain 1 mg norethindrone and 35 mcg ethinyl estradiol.[52]

Oral Contraceptive Agents Comparison Chart[a]

PRODUCT	DOSAGE[b] CYCLE	ESTROGEN[c]	PROGESTOGEN[d]	POTENCY[e] ESTROGENIC[h]	PROGESTATIONAL[f]	ANDROGENIC	BREAKTHROUGH BLEEDING[g] AND SPOTTING(%)
COMBINATION AGENTS CONTAINING LESS THAN 50 MCG OF ESTROGEN							
Loestrin®1/20	21,28	Ethinyl Estradiol 20 mcg	Norethindrone Acetate 1 mg	+	+ +	+ +	25.2
Loestrin® 1.5/30	21,28	Ethinyl Estradiol 30 mcg	Norethindrone Acetate 1.5 mg	+	+ + +	+ + +	30.9
Brevicon® ModiCon®	21,28	Ethinyl Estradiol 35 mcg	Norethindrone 0.5 mg	+ +	+	+	14.6
Lo-Oval®	21,28	Ethinyl Estradiol 30 mcg	Norgestrel 0.3 mg	+	+	+ +	9.8
Ovcon®35	21,28	Ethinyl Estradiol 35 mcg	Norethindrone 0.4 mg	+ +	+	+	19
COMBINATION AGENTS CONTAINING 50 MCG OF ESTROGEN							
Norinyl® 1 + 50 Ortho-Novum® 1/50	21,28	Mestranol 50 mcg	Norethindrone 1 mg	+ +	+ +	+	10.6
Demulen®	21,28	Ethinyl Estradiol 50 mcg	Ethynodiol Diacetate 1 mg	+	+ +	+	13.4
Norlestrin ®1/50	21,28	Ethinyl Estradiol 50 mcg	Norethindrone Acetate 1 mg	+ +	+ +	+ +	13.6

Continued

Oral Contraceptive Agents Comparison Chart[a]

PRODUCT	DOSAGE[b] CYCLE	ESTROGEN[c]	PROGESTOGEN[d]	POTENCY[e] ESTROGENIC[h]	PROGESTATIONAL[f]	ANDROGENIC	BREAKTHROUGH BLEEDING[g] AND SPOTTING(%)
Norlestrin® 2.5/50	21,28	Ethinyl Estradiol 50 mcg	Norethindrone Acetate 2.5 mg	+	+++	++++	5.1
Oral®	21	Ethinyl Estradiol 50 mcg	Norgestrel 0.5 mg	++	+++	+++	4.5
Ovcon®-50	21,28	Ethinyl Estradiol 50 mcg	Norethindrone 1 mg	++	++	++	11.9
COMBINATION AGENTS CONTAINING GREATER THAN 50 MCG ESTROGEN							
Ortho-Novum® 1/80 Norinyl® 1 + 80	21,28	Mestranol 80 mcg	Norethindrone 1 mg	++	+	++	7.2
Ovulen®	20,21,28	Mestranol 100 mcg	Ethynodiol Diacetate 1 mg	+++	++	+	6.1
Ortho-Novum® 2 mg Norinyl® 2 mg	20	Mestranol 100 mcg	Norethindrone 2 mg	++	++	+++	28.8
Ortho-Novum® 10	21	Mestranol 60 mcg	Norethindrone 10 mg	N/A	++++	++++	3.8
Enovid-E®	20,21	Mestranol 100 mcg	Norethynodrel 2.5 mg	+++	+	0	10.9

Continued

Oral Contraceptive Agents Comparison Chart[a]

PRODUCT	DOSAGE[b] CYCLE	ESTROGEN[c]	PROGESTOGEN[d]	POTENCY[e] ESTROGENIC[h]	POTENCY[e] PROGESTATIONAL[f]	POTENCY[e] ANDROGENIC	BREAKTHROUGH BLEEDING[g] AND SPOTTING (%)
Enovid® 5 mg	20	Mestranol 75 mcg	Norethynodrel 5 mg	+ + + +	+ +	0	7.4
PROGESTOGEN ONLY							
Micronor® Nor-Q.D.®	Con- tinuous	None	Norethindrone 0.35 mg	+	+ + +	+	42.3
Ovrette®	Con- tinuous	None	Norgestrel 0.075 mg	0	+	+	34.9

a. Adapted from reference 47.
b. 28-day cycles contain 7 placebo tablets to complete the 28-day cycle.
c. Estrogen equivalent potency: ethinyl estradiol is 1.5–1.75 times as potent as mestranol, because mestranol must be demethylated to its active form, ethinyl estradiol. Inhibition of ovulation requires 50 mcg of ethinyl estradiol versus 80 mcg mestranol.
d. Norethynodrel has estrogenic properties; norgestrel has estrogen antagonist properties; norethindrone, norethindrone acetate and ethynodiol diacetate have weak estrogenic properties, but also have estrogen antagonist properties. Relative progestogenic potency: norgestrel > ethynodiol diacetate > norethindrone acetate > norethindrone > norethynodrel.
e. Potency designations are based on laboratory tests of individual components. Applicability of these methods for combination products used clinically has been questioned.
f. Progestational potency as measured by delay of menses test.
g. Prevalence of bleeding decreases from the first cycle to third cycle by 50–66% per cycle; these figures represent data submitted to FDA on prevalence of bleeding on third cycle of use.
h. Overall estrogenic effect as modified by anti-estrogenic/estrogenic effect of progestational component.

Adverse Reactions of Oral Contraceptives Comparison Chart[a]

REACTION	CLINICAL INFORMATION	CAUSAL FACTORS
Myocardial Infarction	Increased risk 2.8 x that of nonuser; risk is concentrated in females over 35 yr, smokers and presence of other predisposing factors (eg, ↑ lipids, ↑ BP); risk may persist after discontinuation in long-term users [48]	May be related to progestin/estrogen ratio: progestogens decrease HDL, estrogens increase HDL
Thromboembolism and Thrombophlebitis	Increased risk 4–11 x that of nonuser; risk concentrated in smokers, older females and duration of use > 5 yr. Risk decreased with estrogen < 50 mcg	Related to estrogen dose (estrogens decrease antithrombin III and increase coagulation factors and platelet aggregation)
Hepatic Tumors	Both benign and malignant tumors reported. Risk greater with duration of use > 5 yr. Shock can result from rupture of mass. Surgical intervention may be needed, because not always reversible with discontinuation of pill	Unknown, although mestranol and higher hormone formulations implicated
Breast Disease	No increase in breast cancer shown; improvement in fibrocystic disease and fibroadenoma with > 2 yr use	Protection secondary to progestin component. Does not prevent breast cancer
Endometrial Cancer; Cervical Cancer	Sequentials implicated in endometrial cancer; no increased prevalence with combinations, but increased cervical erosions and eversions; no increased cervical cancer risk	Progestin component protective against adenomatous hyperplasia (which may be precursor to adeno cancer)
Congenital Abnormalities	Increased risk of heart and limb defects in offspring following use early in pregnancy. Risk < 1/1000	Both estrogen and progestin are teratogenic

Adverse Reactions of Oral Contraceptives Comparison Chart[a]

REACTION	CLINICAL INFORMATION	CAUSAL FACTORS
Postpill Amenorrhea	Prevalence 0.2–2.6% after pill use; check for pituitary tumor if presence of galactorrhea	Presence of irregular menses prior to starting pill; unrelated to duration or dose
Metabolic	Abnormal glucose tolerance found in predisposed individuals (eg, sub-clinical or gestational diabetes), rare cases of diabetic ketoacidosis	Hyperinsulinemia with relative insulin resistance caused by progestogens with synergistic effect of estrogen
	Elevated triglycerides; may precipitate pancreatitis in patients with underlying hyperlipidemia	
Gallbladder Disease	Twofold increase in gallstones in users compared to nonusers	Estrogens increase cholesterol saturation
Infertility	Little risk of permanent sterility. Conception rate after discontinuation may temporarily lag behind that of nonusers for a few months	Risk concentrated in older women with long history of contraceptive use

a. From references 37, 38, 40, 41, 48.

Hormone Excess and Deficiency Symptomatology Comparison Chart[a]

CONDITION	SYMPTOMATOLOGY
Estrogen Excess	Estrogen excess may also be a result of progestogen deficiency. Symptoms include nausea, vomiting, vertigo, leukorrhea, increase in leiomyoma size, uterine cramps, breast tenderness with fluid retention, cystic breast changes, cholasma, edema and fluid retention resulting in abdominal or leg pain with cyclic weight gain, headaches on pill days, ill-fitting contact lenses and hypertension
Estrogen Deficiency	Estrogen deficiency may also be a result of progestogen excess. Symptoms include irritability, nervousness, decreased libido, hot flashes, early and midcycle breakthrough bleeding and spotting (days 1–7), atrophic vaginitis, dyspareunia, no withdrawal bleeding with continued contraceptive use, decreased amount of withdrawal bleeding
Progestogen Excess	Progestogen excess may also be a result of estrogen deficiency. Symptoms include increased appetite and weight gain on non-pill days, tiredness, fatigue, weakness, depression, decreased libido, decreased length of menstrual flow, *Candida* vaginitis, headaches on non-pill days, breast tenderness on non-pill days
Progestogen Deficiency	Progestogen deficiency may also be a result of estrogen excess. Symptoms include late breakthrough bleeding (days 8–21), heavy menstrual flow and clots, dysmenorrhea, delayed onset of menses following last pill
Androgen Excess	Symptoms include increased appetite and weight gain, oily scalp, acne, hirsutism

a. Adapted from reference 47.

68:16 ESTROGENS

General References: 49-51

Diethylstilbestrol   Various
Diethylstilbestrol Diphosphate   Stilphostrol®

Pharmacology. Diethylstilbestrol (DES) is a nonsteroidal stilbene derivative with estrogenic activity and shares actions and uses of other estrogens. See Conjugated Estrogens.

Administration and Adult Dose. PO for postmenopausal symptoms and prevention of osteoporosis use smallest effective dose in the range

0.25–1 mg/day, in cycles of 21–25 days/month;[49,50,65] administer as with conjugated estrogens. **PO for dysfunctional uterine bleeding** 2 mg q 2 hr until bleeding stops. **PO for suppression of postpartum lactation** most effective when given before lactation begins: 5 mg/day for 5 days. **PO for prostatic cancer** 1–3 mg/day.[53] **PO for breast cancer** 10–20 mg/day.[54] **PO for emergency postcoital contraception** within 72 hr of unprotected intercourse 25 mg bid for 5 days.[55] **Vag Supp for atrophic vaginitis** 0.1–1 mg/day. **IV for prostatic cancer** (DES phosphate) 250–500 mg 1–2 times/week.

Dosage Forms. Tab 0.1, 0.25, 0.5, 1, 5, 50 mg; Inj 50 mg/ml; Vag Supp 0.1, 0.5 mg.

Patient Instructions. See Class Instructions, 68:12.

Adverse Reactions. See Conjugated Estrogens.

Contraindications. See Conjugated Estrogens.

Precautions. See Conjugated Estrogens.

Parameters to Monitor. See Conjugated Estrogens.

Notes. High-dose postcoital DES is associated with a high frequency of nausea and vomiting, so pretreatment with an antiemetic is desirable. DES phosphate 1.6 mg contains 1 mg DES.

Estradiol and its Esters

Estinyl®, Estrace®,
Various

Pharmacology. Estradiol is the most potent of the naturally occurring estrogens and is the major estrogen secreted during the reproductive years. Estradiol and its derivatives share the actions of other estrogens. See Conjugated Estrogens.

Administration and Adult Dose. **PO for postmenopausal symptoms and prevention of osteoporosis** use smallest effective dose in the range of (ethinyl estradiol) 0.02–0.05 mg/day or (micronized estradiol) 1–2 mg/day in cycles of 21–25 days/month; administer as with conjugated estrogens.[49,50,65] **PO for dysfunctional uterine bleeding** 0.05–0.1 mg/day for 3 weeks with addition of progestogen the third week. **PO for suppression of postpartum lactation** most effective when given before lactation begins (ethinyl estradiol) 0.1–0.15 mg/day for 5–7 days. **PO for palliation of prostatic cancer** (ethinyl estradiol) 0.05–2 mg/day. **PO for palliation of breast cancer** (ethinyl estradiol) 1 mg tid. **PO for emergency postcoital contraception** within 72 hr of unprotected intercourse (ethinyl estradiol) 2.5 mg bid for 5 days.[56] **IM for postmenopausal symptoms and prevention of osteoporosis** when oral or vaginal therapy does not provide expected response, is poorly tolerated or when noncompliance occurs (estradiol benzoate) 0.5–1.5 mg 2–3 times/week; (estradiol cypionate) 1–5 mg q 2–4 weeks; (estradiol valerate) 5–10 mg q 2–4 weeks.[50] **IM for dysfunctional uterine bleeding** (estradiol valerate) 20 mg initially, then 5 mg q 2 weeks with addition of progestogen. **IM for suppression of postpartum lactation** (estradiol valerate) 10–30 mg immediately after delivery. **IM for palliation of prostatic cancer** (polyestradiol phosphate) 40 mg q 2–3 weeks.

Dosage Forms. Tab (ethinyl estradiol) 0.02, 0.05, 0.5 mg; (micronized estradiol) 1, 2 mg; Inj (estradiol cypionate in oil) 1, 5 mg/ml; (estradiol valerate in oil) 10, 20, 40 mg/ml; (polyestradiol phosphate) 20 mg/ml.

Pharmacokinetics and Biopharmaceutics. *Onset and Duration.*
Onset of depot products variable following IM injection. Duration (cypionate) 14–28 days; (valerate) 14–21 days; (polyestradiol phosphate) 14–28 days.[57]

Fate. Estradiol is not orally active because of extensive and rapid first-pass metabolism with the exception of the micronized product in which decreased particle size augments absorption. Addition of ethinyl radical results in an orally active compound that is 15–20 times more active than estradiol.

$t_{1/2}$. (Ethinyl estradiol) 27–52 hr.[112]

Adverse Reactions. Pain at injection site occurs frequently. See Conjugated Estrogens.

Contraindications. See Conjugated Estrogens.

Precautions. See Conjugated Estrogens.

Parameters to Monitor. See Conjugated Estrogens.

Notes. Estradiol has been advocated as the estrogen replacement of choice because it is the principal estrogen of the reproductive years; however, advantages over other estrogens for this use have not been established. See Conjugated Estrogens.

Estrogens, Conjugated
Estrogens, Esterified

Premarin®, Various
Evex®, Menest®, Various

Pharmacology. Hormones capable of producing characteristic effects on specific tissues (such as breast) and causing proliferation of vaginal and uterine mucosa. Estrogens increase calcium deposition in bone and accelerate epiphyseal closing following initial growth stimulation.

Administration and Adult Dose. PO for postmenopausal symptoms and prevention of osteoporosis use smallest effective dose in the range 0.3–1.25 mg/day, in cycles of 21–25 days/month; for patients with intact uterus, monthly administration of progestogen is recommended to induce endometrial sloughing and possibly decrease the risk of endometrial cancer. For women experiencing migraine or other symptoms during the withdrawal period, a 5 day/week regimen or a shorter withdrawal period may be employed. PO for dysfunctional uterine bleeding 2.5–5 mg/day for 7–10 days, then decrease to 1.25 mg/day for 2 weeks with addition of progestogen the third week. PO to decrease progression of postmenopausal osteoporosis 1.25 mg/day cyclically.[49,60] PO to prevent postpartum lactation (most effective given immediately postpartum before lactation begins) 3.75 mg q 4 hr for 5 doses or 1.25 mg q 4 hr for 5 days. PO for palliation of prostatic cancer 1.25–2.5 mg tid.[57] PO for palliation of breast cancer (patients should be at least 5 yr postmenopause) 10 mg tid. PO for emergency postcoital contraception (within 72 hr of unprotected intercourse) 10 mg tid for 5 days.[56] Vaginally for postmenopausal symptoms and/or atrophic vaginitis 1.25–2.5 mg/day.[49,50] IV for rapid cessation of dysfunctional uterine bleeding 25 mg of conjugated estrogen q 6–12 hr until bleeding stops.[59]

Dosage Forms. Tab 0.3, 0.625, 1.25, 2.5 mg; Inj 25 mg; Vag Crm 0.625 mg/g.

Patient Instructions. See Class Instructions, 68:12.

Pharmacokinetics and Biopharmaceutics. *Fate.* GI absorption of oral estrogens is complete, with wide distribution and concentration in fat. Inactivation of estrogens occurs mainly in the liver with degradation to less active estrogenic products such as estrone. Metabolites are conjugated with sulfate and glucuronic acid and excreted in urine.[112] Vaginal creams are readily absorbed and produce plasma levels of estradiol and estrone approaching those attained after oral ingestion (mostly in the form of estrone).[81]

Adverse Reactions. Nausea, vomiting, breast tenderness and spotting occur frequently—see Hormone Excess and Deficiency Symptomatology Comparison Chart. Increased risk of endometrial cancer with longer duration of use (over 3 yr), with higher doses and with unopposed estrogen stimulation.[62] Small increase in breast cancer risk with over 15 yr of usage.[63] Increased risk of myocardial infarction in men taking greater than 3 mg/day of DES. Hypercalcemia occurs occasionally in patients with breast cancer. Thromboembolism, thrombophlebitis, diabetes, hypertension and gall bladder disease may occur—see Adverse Reactions of Oral Contraceptives Comparison Chart.

Contraindications. Pregnancy; history or presence of estrogen-dependent breast and uterine cancer (except in appropriate patients treated for metastatic disease); undiagnosed abnormal genital bleeding; history or presence of thromboembolism or severe thrombophlebitis; active or severe chronic liver disease.

Precautions. Use with caution in patients with disease states which may be exacerbated by increased fluid retention (eg, asthma, epilepsy, migraine and cardiac or renal dysfunction); in women with strong family history of breast cancer or presence of fibrocystic disease, fibroadenoma or abnormal mammogram; in women with fibromyomata, diabetes, hyperlipidemia, severe liver disease or history of jaundice during pregnancy; and in young patients in whom bone growth is not complete. Estrogen can increase thyroid binding globulin and cause false elevations in T_4 and false depression of resin T_3 uptake, while the thyroid index and the patient remain normal; see Drug Interactions chapter.

Parameters to Monitor. Signs and symptoms of side effects, especially abnormal bleeding. Pretreatment physical examination with reference to blood pressure, breasts, pelvic and Pap smear. Baseline laboratory should include glucose, triglycerides and cholesterol, liver function tests and calcium. Repeat examination every year.

Notes. Conjugated estrogens contain a mixture of 50-65% sodium estrone sulfate and 20-35% sodium equilin sulfate obtained from the urine of pregnant mares. Esterified estrogens are a combination of 75-85% sodium estrone sulfate and 6.5-15% sodium equilin sulfate. Postmenopausal women most likely to develop osteoporosis are whites, while blacks seem to be spared.[60] Estrogens may be efficacious in prevention of fractures resulting from osteoporosis.[60,64,65]

Estrone and its Esters   Ogen®, Theelin®

Pharmacology. Estrone is the major estrogen produced in the postmenopausal period. It is one-half as potent as estradiol and shares the actions of other estrogens. See Conjugated Estrogens.

Administration and Adult Dose. PO for postmenopausal symptoms and prevention of osteoporosis use smallest effective dose in the range of (piperazine estrone sulfate) 0.625-2.5 mg/day in cycles of 21-25 days/month; administer as with conjugated estrogens.[49,50,65] **PO for suppression of postpartum lactation** most effective when given before lactation begins (piperazine estrone sulfate) 4.5 mg q 4 hr for 4 doses. **PO for palliation of prostatic cancer** (piperazine estrone sulfate) 3-6 mg tid. **PO for emergency postcoital contraception** within 72 hr of unprotected intercourse (piperazine estrone sulfate) 5 mg tid for 5 days.[56] **Vaginally for postmenopausal symptoms and/or atrophic vaginitis** (piperazine estrone sulfate) 3-8 mg/day. **IM for postmenopausal symptoms and prevention of osteoporosis** when oral or vaginal therapy does not provide expected response, is poorly tolerated or when noncompliance occurs (estrone) 0.1-2 mg weekly.

Dosage Forms. **Tab** (piperazine estrone sulfate) 0.625, 1.25, 2.5, 5 mg. **Inj** (estrone) 2, 5 mg/ml. **Vag Crm** (estropipate) 1.5 mg/g.

Patient Instructions. See Class Instructions, 68:12.

Pharmacokinetics and Biopharmaceutics. *Fate.* Estrone is not orally active due to enzymatic degradation in the gut and liver. Addition of piperazine moiety increases oral efficacy and stability. Estrone is hydroxylated to α-hydroxyestrone, estriol and 2-hydroxyestrone.[112]

Adverse Reactions. See Conjugated Estrogens.

Contraindications. See Conjugated Estrogens.

Precautions. See Conjugated Estrogens.

Parameters to Monitor. See Conjugated Estrogens.

Notes. See Conjugated Estrogens. Estropipate is the new U.S. Adopted Name for piperazine estrone sulfate.

Estrogens Comparison Chart[a]

DRUG	EQUIPOTENT PHYSIOLOGIC DOSE[b]	DOSAGE FORMS	COMMENTS
STEROIDAL AGENTS			
Conjugated Estrogens Premarin® Various	0.625 mg	Tab 0.3, 0.625, 1.25, 2.5 mg Vag Crm 0.625 mg/g Inj 25 mg	Expensive; nausea is rare; contains mainly estrone
Esterified Estrogens Evex® Menest® Various		Tab 0.3, 0.625, 1.25, 2.5 mg	
Ethinyl Estradiol Estinyl®	0.02 mg	Tab 0.02, 0.05, 0.5 mg	Moderate cost; some nausea with oral; pain at site of injection; variable onset with duration of 14-28 days with depot injections; estradiol is the major estrogen secreted during the reproductive years
Estradiol, Micronized Estrace®	1 mg	Tab 1, 2 mg	
Estradiol Cypionate Depo-Estradiol®		Inj 1, 5 mg/ml in oil	
Estradiol Valerate Delestrogen®		Inj 10, 20, 40 mg/ml in oil	
Polyestradiol Phosphate Estradurin®		Inj 20 mg/ml	

Continued

Estrogens Comparison Chart[a]

DRUG	EQUIPOTENT PHYSIOLOGIC DOSE[b]	DOSAGE FORMS	COMMENTS
Estrone Theelin® Various		Inj 2, 5 mg/ml Vag Crm 0.2 mg/3.5 g	No advantage over conjugated/esterified; except tasteless and no urine odor; estrone is the major estrogen of the postmenopausal years
Estropipate Ogen® Various	1.25 mg	Tab 0.625, 1.25, 2.5, 5 mg Vag Crm 1.5 mg/g	
NONSTEROIDAL AGENTS			
Chlorotrianisene Tace®	12	Cap 12, 25, 72 mg	Expensive; weak estrogenic activity, metabolized by liver to a more active compound. Long duration of action because of storage in adipose tissue. Infrequently used because of long duration of activity.
Diethylstilbestrol Various	0.25 mg	Tab 0.1, 0.25, 0.5, 1, 5 mg Vag Supp 0.1, 0.5 mg	Inexpensive; frequent nausea, drug of choice for prostatic cancer, postcoital contraception, and breast cancer; may be less desirable for estrogen replacement because of its relationship to carcinogenicity
Diethylstilbestrol Diphosphate Stilphostrol®		Tab 50 mg Inj 50 mg/ml	
Dienestrol Various		Vag Crm 0.01% Vag Supp 0.7 mg	

a. Potency of estrogens: estradiol > estrone > estriol.
b. See monographs or product information for exact dosing regimens for various uses.

68:20 INSULINS AND ANTIDIABETIC AGENTS

General References: 66,67

Glyburide

Diabeta®,
Micronase®

Glyburide is a "second-generation" sulfonylurea with a mechanism of action similar to the older sulfonylureas; in addition, it probably produces a release of an insulinotropic hormone from the gut which stimulates pancreatic beta cells. Second-generation agents have a greater milligram potency than earlier agents, but their maximal effect is essentially the same. The frequency of side effects in general is lower with the newer agents. Most notably absent are the flushing reaction with alcohol, hyponatremia, and a lack of drug-drug interactions with phenylbutazone, salicylates and warfarin. Because of their potency, it is important that these agents be taken with meals and avoided in elderly or debilitated patients. Other "second-generation" agents include glipizide, gliclazide, glisoxepide, glibornuride, gliquidone and the nonsulfonylureas, glymidine and glycodiazine. Glyburide is relatively short-acting with low doses, but intermediate acting at higher doses. It is primarily metabolized to inactive metabolites, but a clinically insignificant amount of a compound with 1/6th the potency of the parent drug is also formed. Essentially no drug is excreted unchanged in the urine, and dosage modification is unnecessary in renal impairment. For the purpose of conversion among sulfonylureas, equivalent doses are approximately as follows: tolbutamide 500 mg, chlorpropamide 125 mg, glyburide 5 mg and glipizide 5 mg. The usual dose of glyburide is 2.5–20 mg/day, to a maximum of 30 mg/day. It is available as a 5 mg tablet.[66,75-78]

Sulfonylurea Agents

Pharmacology. These agents acutely enhance insulin secretion from the pancreatic beta cells and potentiate insulin action on several extrahepatic tissues. Chronically, sulfonylureas increase peripheral utilization of glucose, suppress hepatic gluconeogenesis and possibly increase the sensitivity and/or number of peripheral insulin receptors. In addition, acetohexamide has significant uricosuric activity.[66,68]

Administration and Adult Dose. See Sulfonylurea Agents Comparison Chart.

Dosage Individualization. Dosing alterations of all sulfonylureas may be necessary in patients with severe hepatic dysfunction. With renal disease, especially in geriatric patients, there is an increased duration of action with chlorpropamide and acetohexamide.

Dosage Forms. See Sulfonylurea Agents Comparison Chart.

Patient Instructions. Approved diets should be consistent on a day-to-day basis. Medication should be taken the same time each morning. Factors which might alter blood glucose levels (eg, infection, fasting states) as well as any side effects should be reported.

Pharmacokinetics and Biopharmaceutics. See Sulfonylurea Agents Comparison Chart.
   Plasma Levels. Vary due to rates and completeness of absorption, differing rates of metabolism, renal clearance and degree of protein binding.[66]

$t_{1/2}$. See Sulfonylurea Agents Comparison Chart—acetohexamide and chlorpropamide half-lives may be prolonged in patients with renal failure.[66,69,70]

Adverse Reactions. Anorexia, nausea, vomiting, diarrhea, allergic skin reactions and hypoglycemic reactions (especially with chlorpropamide) occur occasionally. Hematologic disorders, mild disulfiram-like reaction to alcohol, hypothyroidism (with long-term use), hyponatremia (most common with chlorpropamide; may occur with tolbutamide), hepatic damage, cholestatic jaundice and bone marrow suppression occur rarely.

Contraindications. Pregnancy; insulinopenic diabetes; juvenile, unstable or brittle diabetes; diabetes complicated by acidosis, ketosis, diabetic coma, major surgery, severe infection or severe trauma.

Precautions. Although controversial, the data of University Group Diabetes Program (UGDP) suggests that obese patients with mild adult-onset diabetes who are not insulin-dependent are more likely to die from cardiovascular complications when taking fixed doses of tolbutamide than if they relied on diet alone or on insulin.[71] Criticism of the UGDP study has been made.[72] Displacement from protein occurs with high-dose salicylates, phenylbutazone, sulfonamides, MAO inhibitors, phenytoin and bishydroxycoumarin. Drugs which impair glucose tolerance include oral contraceptives, corticosteroids, thiazides, furosemide, thyroid hormones (large doses) and niacin.[72] Acute ingestion of alcohol produces hypoglycemia, but chronically, it increases metabolism of sulfonylureas.[66] See also Drug Interactions chapter.

Parameters to Monitor. Clinical symptoms of hyperglycemia (mainly polyphagia, polyuria, polydipsia, numbing and/or tingling of feet) and/or hypoglycemia (hunger, nervousness, warmth, sweating, palpitations, headaches, confusion, drowsiness, anxiety, blurred vision and/or paresthesias of lips). Urine glucose should be measured frequently as a routine; blood glucose should be measured frequently initially; methods are available for home glucose monitoring—see Glucose Testing Systems Comparison Chart. Long-term diabetic control may best be monitored using hemoglobin A_{1c}.[73,74]

Sulfonylurea Agents Comparison Chart[a]

DRUG	DOSAGE FORMS	DAILY DOSAGE[b]	FATE	HALF-LIFE (HOURS)	DURATION (HOURS)
Acetohexamide Dymelor®	Tab 250, 500 mg	250 mg–1.5 g in 2 doses	60% converted to active metabolites; excreted by kidney	Parent 1.6 Metabolite 5.3	8–12+
Chlorpropamide Diabinese®	Tab 100, 250 mg	100–500 mg in 1 dose	Metabolized, as well as 20% excreted unchanged	25–42 (average 33; urine pH dependent)	24–72
Glipizide Glibenese®	Tab 5 mg	2.5–25 mg in 1–2 doses	Converted to inactive metabolites	3.3	6–12
Glyburide Diabeta® Micronase®	Tab 2.5, 5, 7.5 mg	2.5–20 mg in 1–2 doses	Converted mostly to inactive metabolites	10	10–15
Tolazamide Tolinase®	Tab 100, 250 mg	100 mg–1 g in 1–2 doses	Slow absorption and onset; metabolized to partially active metabolites	7	10–15
Tolbutamide Orinase®	Tab 500 mg	500 mg–2 g in 2–3 doses	Converted to inactive metabolites	5.6	6–12

a. From references 66-68, 70, 76, 78-81.
b. Except for chlorpropamide, divided doses should be used when higher doses are required; highest dose listed represents the maximum recommended daily dosage.

Glucose Testing Systems Comparison Chart[a]

PRODUCT AND MANUFACTURER	EQUIPMENT	PROCEDURE[b]	RANGE	INTERFERING SUBSTANCES	COMMENTS
BLOOD[c]					
Glucose Oxidase					
Chemstrip® bG	Color chart or Accu-Check® bG reflectometer.	Apply 1 large drop of blood to strip; wait 60 s; wipe off blood with cotton swab	20–800 mg/dl	Not known	Good accuracy when used by patients; strips may be saved and read up to 2 weeks later with little loss of accuracy
Dextrostix®	Dextrometer® reflectometer	Apply 1 large drop of blood to strip; wait 60 s; wash off blood with water; read in 1–2 s	0–250 mg/dl visually; 0–399 mg/dl with Dextrometer®	Not known	Visual accuracy inadequate; should be used with a reflectometer
StatTek®	StatTek® reflectometer	Same as Chemstrip® bG	50–350 mg/dl with meter; 350–800 mg/dl visually	Not known	Accuracy comparable to Dextrometer® method

Continued

Glucose Testing Systems Comparison Chart[a]

PRODUCT AND MANUFACTURER	EQUIPMENT	PROCEDURE[b]	RANGE	INTERFERING SUBSTANCES	COMMENTS
Visidex®	Color charts (green = 20–180 mg/dl; orange = 200–800 mg/dl)	Same as Dextrostix®; if glucose > 180 mg/dl on green chart, wait 30 s longer and read orange chart	20–800 mg/dl	Not known	Screening method of choice; may give false low readings over 1.5 g/dl
URINE **Glucose Oxidase** Diastix® Mega-Diastix® (for the visually impaired)	Color chart	Dip in urine or pass through urine stream; read in 30 s	0–2 g/dl	False negative: ascorbic acid (over 75 mg/dl); ketones (over 40 mg/dl)	Semiquantitative; not suitable for adjustment of insulin dosage or sliding scale regimens; useful in diet or oral hypoglycemic controlled diabetics
Tes-Tape®	Color chart	Dip in urine; read in 60 s; if over 0.5 g/dl, wait another 60 s, then read	0–2 g/dl	False negative: ascorbic acid, levodopa, methyldopa, salicylates	

Continued

Glucose Testing Systems Comparison Chart[a]

PRODUCT AND MANUFACTURER	EQUIPMENT	PROCEDURE[b]	RANGE	INTERFERING SUBSTANCES	COMMENTS
Copper Reduction (Benedict's)					
Clinitest®	Dropper, test tube, color chart	Add 5 drops of urine to 10 drops water; add Clinitest® tablet; wait until 15 s after reaction stops; shake gently; then read	0–2 g/dl	False positive: ascorbic acid, cephalosporins, chloral hydrate, isoniazid, levodopa, methyldopa, nalidixic acid, PAS, penicillin in huge doses, probenecid, salicylates, other sugars	Method of choice for monitoring insulin; "pass-through" (ie, rapid color change and false negative) may occur over 2 g/dl—use 2-drop method if this occurs
Clinitest® 2-drop	Same as above	Add 2 drops of urine, then same as above	0–5 g/dl	Same as above, but less likely	Less accurate than other methods, but less susceptible to "pass-through"

a. From references 82-86 and product information.
b. Consult manufacturer's instructions for more detailed procedures.
c. Home blood glucose monitoring appears to be superior to urine glucose monitoring for evaluation of diabetic control and monitoring of insulin regimens; monitoring of hemoglobin A$_{1c}$ may be the best indicator of overall long-term glucose control.[84-86]

68:20.08 INSULINS

Insulins

Pharmacology. Insulin promotes cellular uptake of glucose, fatty acids and amino acids and their conversion to storage forms in most tissues.

Administration and Adult Dose. Dosing must be adjusted in response to improvement of clinical symptoms and blood and urine glucose levels. **For juvenile onset diabetes mellitus,** requirements may occasionally be as high as 200 units/day due to growth spurts. **Insulin resistance** is usually due to obesity and weight reduction will improve insulin response.[87,88] Occasionally, resistance is due to insulin destruction at the injection site, and these patients can use only IV insulin; other patients require large doses (up to 200 units/day) due to a decrease in insulin action at the receptor.[88,89] When switching from conventional or "single-peak" insulins to the "highly purified" insulins, dosage may need to be reduced; however, in many patients no change is necessary.[90] **For diabetic ketoacidosis,** low-dose regular insulin given continuously may decrease the risk of hypokalemia and prevent severe hypoglycemia,[91] dosing is started with 0.33 units/kg IV, followed by 7 units/hr SC, IM or IV; if no improvement occurs within 4 hr, large doses (200–400 units) should be used.[92] This method is effective regardless of the route of administration (SC, IM or IV), but IV is preferred in patients in shock.[93]

Dosage Individualization. Insulin requirements may be decreased in patients with renal or hepatic impairment, nausea and vomiting or hypothyroidism. Requirements may be increased during pregnancy, especially in the second and third trimesters, in those with high fever, hyperthyroidism, severe infections, and following trauma or surgery.

Dosage Forms. See Insulins Comparison Chart.

Patient Instructions. Patients should be instructed in the following areas: use of insulin syringes and needles, storage and handling of insulin, urine and/or blood glucose testing, adherence to proper diet and regular meals, personal hygiene (especially the feet), and recognition and treatment of hypoglycemia and hyperglycemia— see Sulfonylurea Agents.

Pharmacokinetics and Biopharmaceutics. *Onset and Duration.* See Insulins Comparison Chart.
Plasma Levels. Diabetics vary widely in their response to insulin; plasma levels are affected by obesity, diet, degree of activity, pancreatic beta cell activity, growth hormone and circulating antibodies.[94]
Fate. Insulin is primarily metabolized in the liver, although the kidneys appear to have a role in removal of about 18% of the daily insulin output.[95,96]
$t_{1/2}$. (Regular insulin) 4–5 min after IV administration.[91]

Adverse Reactions. Hypoglycemia is dose-related. Local allergic reactions, with an onset of 15 min–4 hr, are usually due to insulin impurities, and 70% of these patients have a history of interrupted treatment. Immune or non-immune insulin resistance occurs occasionally. Lipoatrophy at the injection site may occur, especially with repeated use of the same site; lipoatrophy may be less frequent with the highly purified insulins. Allergy, resistance and lipoatrophy may be overcome by switching to insulin from another animal source or to a more highly purified product (eg, single component pork). In general, pork insulin is less antigenic than beef-pork or pure beef insulin, because it is more structurally similar to human insulin.[89,90,92,97,98]

Contraindications.   Hypersensitivity, although desensitization procedures may be warranted in some patients.[99,100]

Precautions.   Use with caution in patients with renal or hepatic disease, or hypothyroidism. Insulin requirements may change when switching animal sources or to more purified products.

Parameters to Monitor.   Urine glucose should be monitored frequently as a routine; blood glucose should be measured frequently, at least initially, although methods are available for routine patient monitoring of blood glucose also[84]—see Glucose Testing Systems Comparison Chart. Long-term diabetic control may best be monitored using hemoglobin A_{1c}.[73,74] Subjective symptoms of hypoglycemia and hyperglycemia should be continually monitored by the patient. Observe for signs of lipoatrophy and allergic reactions.

Notes.   Insulin is stable for 6 months at constant room temperature and up to 24 months under refrigeration.[101] Insulin adsorbs to glass and plastic IV infusion equipment, with little difference between glass and plastic; maximal adsorption occurs within 15 seconds.[92,102,103] Adsorption may be minimized by the addition of small amounts (1–2%) of albumin to the infusion container,[102] however, this may be costly and unnecessary because patient response is generally adequate without addition of albumin. Variation can be minimized by flushing all new IV administration equipment with 50 ml of the insulin-containing solution (thereby saturating "binding sites") before it is used.[104]

Pump devices are available to deliver insulin dependently or independently of a measured serum glucose level. "Open-loop" devices can deliver insulin at a constant rate and can be manually controlled. "Closed-loop" devices (the "artificial pancreas") can deliver insulin at variable rates in response to serum glucose. Although these pump devices show some promising results, they are presently somewhat limited in clinical usefulness due to size, frequency of mechanical failure and cost.[105-107]

Biosynthetic "human" insulin has been produced by Eli Lilly using recombinant DNA technology. In one double-blind, crossover comparison, requirements of biosynthetic insulin were found to be approximately equal to bovine insulin. Slightly greater doses of biosynthetic insulin were required in patients who were previously stabilized on purified pork insulin. This difference is thought to be due to slightly faster absorption of the biosynthetic insulin from subcutaneous injection sites, resulting in a slightly more rapid onset and shorter duration than with purified pork. No differences in side effects or long-term control of diabetics have been identified between biosynthetic human insulin and highly purified animal insulins. (Clark AJL et al. Biosynthetic human insulin in the treatment of diabetes. Lancet 1982;2:354-7.) Now available as Humulin® R and Humulin® N.

Insulins Comparison Chart[a]

PRODUCT AND MANUFACTURER[f]	ANIMAL SOURCE AND STRENGTHS (UNITS/ML)	PURITY PRO-INSULIN[b] (PPM)	ONSET[c] (HOURS)	PEAK[c] (HOURS)	DURATION[c] (HOURS)	BUFFER[d]	MIXING COMPATIBILITIES[e]
RAPID-ACTING							
Insulin Injection (Regular)							
Actrapid® (Novo)	Pork-100	≤1	0.5–1	1–5	5–8	Acetate	NPH, lentes in all proportions; mixture with PZI is stable, but has no advantages
Actrapid® Human (Squibb-Novo)	Semisynthetic Human-100	≤1	g	g	g	None	
Humulin® R (Lilly)	Biosynthetic-100	—	g	g	g	None	
Insulin, Improved (Squibb)	Pork-40, 100	<25				None	
Insulin, Purified (Squibb)	Pork-100	<10				None	
Regular Iletin® (Lilly)	Beef/Pork-40, 100	<20				None	
Regular Iletin® II (Lilly)	Beef-100	<10				None	
	Pork-100, 500						
Velosulin® (Nordisk)	Pork-100	≤1				Phosphate	
Prompt Insulin Zinc Suspension (SemiLente)							
Semi-Lente Iletin® (Lilly)	Beef/Pork-40, 100	<20	0.5–3	2–10	12–16	Acetate	Regular, lentes; premixture with other lentes stable indefinitely
Semi-Lente Insulin, Improved (Squibb)	Beef-100	<25				Acetate	

Continued

Insulins Comparison Chart[a]

PRODUCT AND MANUFACTURER[f]	ANIMAL SOURCE AND STRENGTHS (UNITS/ML)	PURITY PRO-INSULIN[b] (PPM)	ONSET[c] (HOURS)	PEAK[c] (HOURS)	DURATION[c] (HOURS)	BUFFER[d]	MIXING COMPATIBILITIES[e]
Semitard® (Novo)	Pork-100	≤1				Acetate	
INTERMEDIATE-ACTING							
Isophane Insulin Suspension (NPH)							
Humulin® N (Lilly)	Biosynthetic-100	—	1–4 g	4–12 g	24–28 g	Phosphate	Regular in any proportion stable for 2–3 months
Insulatard® NPH (Nordisk)	Pork-100	≤1				Phosphate	
Isophane Insulin, Improved (Squibb)	Beef-40, 100	<25				Phosphate	
Isophane Insulin, Purified (Squibb)	Beef-100	<10				Phosphate	
NPH Iletin® (Lilly)	Beef/Pork-40, 100	<20				Phosphate	
NPH Iletin® II (Lilly)	Beef-100 Beef-100 Pork-100	<10				Phosphate	
Protaphane® (Novo)	Pork-100	≤1				Acetate	
Isophane Insulin Suspension/Insulin (70% NPH + 30% Regular)							
Mixtard® (Nordisk)	Pork-100	≤1	0.5	4–8	24	Phosphate	Regular, NPH in any proportion

Continued

Insulins Comparison Chart[a]

PRODUCT AND MANUFACTURER[f]	ANIMAL SOURCE AND STRENGTHS (UNITS/ML)	PURITY PRO-INSULIN[b] (PPM)	ONSET[c] (HOURS)	PEAK[c] (HOURS)	DURATION[c] (HOURS)	BUFFER[d]	MIXING COMPATIBILITIES[e]
Insulin Zinc Suspension (Lente; 70% Ultralente + 30% SemiLente)							
Lentard® (Novo)	Beef/Pork-100	≤1	1–3	6–15	22–28	None	Regular in all proportions stable for 2–3 months; lentes in all proportions stable indefinitely
Lente Iletin® (Lilly)	Beef/Pork-40, 100	<20				Acetate	
Lente Iletin® II (Lilly)	Beef-100	<10				Acetate	
	Pork-100	<25				Acetate	
Lente Insulin, Improved (Squibb)	Beef-40, 100	<10				Acetate	
Lente Insulin, Purified (Squibb)	Beef-100	≤1				Acetate	
Monotard® (Novo)	Pork-100	≤1	g	g	g	Acetate	
Monotard® Human (Squibb-Novo)	Semisynthetic Human-100						
LONG-ACTING							
Protamine Insulin Zinc Suspension (PZI)			1–6	14–24	≥36		
Protamine, Zinc & Iletin® (Lilly)	Beef/Pork-40, 100	<20				Phosphate	May mix with regular, but these mixtures offer no advantages
	Pork-100						
	Beef-100					Phosphate	
Protamine Zinc Insulin, Improved (Squibb)	Beef-100	<25					

Continued

Insulins Comparison Chart[a]

PRODUCT AND MANUFACTURER[f]	ANIMAL SOURCE AND STRENGTHS (UNITS/ML)	PURITY PRO-INSULIN[b] (PPM)	ONSET[c] (HOURS)	PEAK[c] (HOURS)	DURATION[c] (HOURS)	BUFFER[d]	MIXING COMPATIBILITIES[e]
Extended Insulin Zinc Suspension (Ultralente)							
Ultralente Iletin® (Lilly)	Beef/Pork-40, 100	<20	2-8	10-30	≥36		Regular in all proportions stable 2-3 months; lentes in all proportions stable indefinitely
Ultralente Insulin, Improved (Squibb)	Beef-100	<25				Acetate	
Ultratard® (Novo)	Beef-100	≤1				Acetate	
						Acetate	

a. From references 83,92 and product information.
b. Other contaminants such as glucagon-like substances, pancreatic polypeptide, somatostatin and vasoactive intestinal polypeptide may also be present; levels of these are very low in Novo and Nordisk products and Iletin® II products.
c. There may be variations within this range among manufacturers; onset and duration may be prolonged in long-standing diabetes and large doses may have prolonged durations of action.
d. All presently available insulins have an approximately neutral pH in the range of 7.0-7.8.
e. It is recommended that insulins from different manufacturers not be mixed; Humulin® products should not be mixed with other insulins.
f. Squibb and Novo products will be marketed as Squibb-Novo in the future.
g. Human insulins have a slightly more rapid onset and a shorter duration or action than other highly purified insulins.

68:32 PROGESTOGENS

General References: 108,109

Medroxyprogesterone Acetate

Depo-Provera®,
Provera®, Various

Pharmacology. A 17-α-acetoxy progesterone derivative. Progesterone transforms an estrogen-primed proliferative endometrium into a secretory endometrium. Progestogen-only contraceptives alter the cervical mucus, exert a progestational effect on the endometrium which interferes with implantation, and in some patients, suppresses ovulation.

Administration and Adult Dose. **PO for secondary amenorrhea, dysfunctional uterine bleeding and to induce withdrawal bleeding following postmenopausal estrogen replacement therapy** 5–10 mg/day, depending on degree of endometrial stimulation desired, administered for 5–10 days beginning on the presumed 16th–21st day of cycle (during 3rd week of estrogen administration). In cases of secondary amenorrhea, therapy can be started at any time. **PO for endometriosis** 10 mg tid for 6–9 months; **IM for endometriosis** 100 mg q 2 weeks for 4 doses, then 100 mg/week for 4 weeks. **IM for contraception** 150 mg q 3 months;[109,110] **IM for palliation of metastatic endometrial cancer** 400 mg–1 g/week initially, then maintenance dose of 400 mg q month.

Dosage Forms. **Tab** 2.5, 10 mg; **Inj** 100, 400 mg/ml.

Patient Instructions. See Class Instructions, 68:12.

Pharmacokinetics and Biopharmaceutics. *Onset and Duration.* Withdrawal bleeding (in estrogen-primed endometrium) occurs 2–7 days after last dose;[108,110] duration of 3 months or longer when given IM for contraception.[108,110]
  Fate. Metabolized by hydroxylation; 20–42% of dose is excreted as glucuronide and sulfate conjugates in urine; 5–13% of dose is excreted in feces.
  $t_{1/2}$. α phase 52 min; β phase 230 min; biological half-life 14.5 hr.[110]

Adverse Reactions. See Hormone Excess and Deficiency Symptomatology Comparison Chart. Menstrual irregularities and breakthrough bleeding are very frequent in the first 3 months after IM injection; amenorrhea, weight gain, malignant breast nodules in beagle dogs, masculinization of female fetus and congenital anomalies when taken during pregnancy occur.[110]

Contraindications. Pregnancy; presence or history of thrombophlebitis, thromboembolism or stroke; liver dysfunction; known or suspected malignancy of breast or genital organs; undiagnosed vaginal bleeding; missed abortion; as a diagnostic test for pregnancy.

Precautions. Use with caution in patients with a history of depression, diabetes or conditions worsened by fluid retention (eg, epilepsy, migraine, asthma and cardiac or renal dysfunction.)

Parameters to Monitor. Pretreatment physical examination with special reference to breast and pelvic organs and Pap smear.

Notes. Concurrent administration of estrogen with progestogen may be associated with less breakthrough bleeding than with progestogen alone for amenorrhea. IM administration is not approved in US, but may be a useful alternative contraceptive method for women who cannot use other methods.[109,111] There is inadequate evidence that progestogens are effective in preventing habitual abortion or treating threatened abortion; furthermore, progestogens may be harmful to the fetus during the first 4 months of pregnancy.

Norethindrone	Nor-Q.D.®, Micronor®, Norlutin®
Norethindrone Acetate	Norlutate®

Pharmacology.   Norethindrone and norethindrone acetate are 19-nortestosterone derivatives which share the actions of progestogens. See Medroxyprogesterone Acetate.

Administration and Adult Dose. **PO for contraception** (norethindrone) 0.35 mg/day continuously, starting on the first day of menses. **PO for dysfunctional uterine bleeding** (norethindrone) 5 mg (norethindrone acetate) 2.5 mg qid for 5 days to stop bleeding; on 5th day decrease dose to 5–20 mg/day of norethindrone or 2.5–10 mg/day of norethindrone acetate and maintain for 21 days to prevent recurrence. **PO for secondary amenorrhea or withdrawal bleeding following postmenopausal estrogen therapy** (norethindrone) 5–20 mg/day (norethindrone acetate) 2.5–10 mg/day starting on the 15th–20th day of the cycle and continued for 10 or 5 days respectively. In cases of secondary amenorrhea, therapy can be started at any time. **PO for endometriosis** (norethindrone) 10 mg/day (norethindrone acetate) 5 mg/day for 2 weeks, increased in 10 mg/day increments (norethindrone acetate—5 mg/day) q 2 weeks, until maintenance dose of 30 mg/day of norethindrone or 15 mg/day of norethindrone acetate is reached.

Dosage Forms. (Norethindrone) **Tab** 0.35 mg (Micronor®, Nor-Q.D.®); 5 mg (Norlutin®). (Norethindrone acetate) **Tab** 5 mg (Norlutate®).

Patient Instructions. See Class Instructions, 68:12.

Pharmacokinetics and Biopharmaceutics. *Onset and Duration.* Acute bleeding should decrease in 1–2 days and stop in 3–4 days. Withdrawal bleeding occurs in 2–7 days after last dose; onset of contraception after 1 week of therapy.
   Fate. Rapid and complete oral absorption, with peak concentration of norethindrone in 1 hr and unmeasurable concentrations in 48 hr. Less than 5% cleared as unchanged norethindrone; metabolites are excreted as glucuronide and sulfate conjugates in the urine and feces.[112]
   $t_{1/2}$. (Norethindrone and metabolites) 42–84 hr (average 70).[113]

Adverse Reactions. See Medroxyprogesterone Acetate.

Contraindications. See Medroxyprogesterone Acetate.

Precautions. See Medroxyprogesterone Acetate.

Parameters to Monitor. See Medroxyprogesterone Acetate.

Notes. Efficacy as a contraceptive is 2.54 pregnancies/100 woman years. Progestogen-only contraceptives are the drugs of choice for contraception during breast feeding or in patients with contraindications to estrogen therapy; see Oral Contraceptive Agents Comparison Chart. Norethindrone acetate differs from norethindrone only in potency; the acetate is twice as potent.

Progesterone
Hydroxyprogesterone Caproate

Lipo-Lutin®, Various
Delalutin®

Pharmacology. Progesterone is the natural hormone which induces secretory changes in the endometrium, relaxes uterine smooth muscle and maintains pregnancy. Esterification produces a more potent compound, hydroxyprogesterone caproate.

Administration and Adult Dose. IM for secondary amenorrhea and dysfunctional uterine bleeding (progesterone in oil) 50–200 mg (hydroxyprogesterone caproate) 125–250 mg. **IM for palliation of metastatic endometrial cancer** (hydroxyprogesterone caproate) 500 mg–1 g 2–3 times/week.

Dosage Forms. Inj (progesterone in oil) 25, 50, 100 mg/ml; (hydroxyprogesterone caproate in oil) 125, 250 mg/ml.

Patient Instructions. Bleeding should stop in a few days after injection; expect a normal period after a few days. The first 48 hr of menses may be excessive, but of normal duration. See also Class Instructions, 68:12.

Pharmacokinetics and Biopharmaceutics. *Onset and Duration.* Onset of withdrawal bleeding 2–6 days after IM progesterone and 2 weeks after IM hydroxyprogesterone caproate; duration 12–24 hr with progesterone, 9–17 days with hydroxyprogesterone caproate.
 Fate. Rapidly inactivated in the GI tract after PO administration; metabolized by liver and excreted 50–60% in urine as pregnanediol and isomers conjugated with glucuronide or sulfate; 5–10% is excreted in feces.

Adverse Reactions. Local reaction and swelling at site of progesterone injection. See Medroxyprogesterone Acetate.

Contraindications. See Medroxyprogesterone Acetate.

Precautions. See Medroxyprogesterone Acetate.

Parameters to Monitor. See Medroxyprogesterone Acetate.

68:36 THYROID AND ANTITHYROID

General References, Thyroid Replacement: 115,116
Antithyroid: 114,117

Class Instructions. Thyroid replacement. This medication must be taken regularly to maintain proper hormone levels in the body. Report immediately if chest pain (especially in elderly patients), palpitations, sweating, nervousness, or other signs of overdosage occur. Take any missed dose as soon as it is remembered, but if more than one is missed, do not double up doses.

Levothyroxine Sodium

Levothroid®, Synthroid®,
Various

Pharmacology. Synthetically prepared hormone identical to the thyroid hormone, T_4. Thyroid hormones are responsible for normal growth, development and energy metabolism.

Administration and Adult Dose. PO 100 mcg/day initially, increasing to maintenance dose of 100-200 mcg/day (2.25 ± 0.67 mcg/kg/day)[116] in 2-3 weeks, to maximum of 300 mcg/day. Poorly compliant young patients have been maintained on a once-a-week dosing regimen; however, this regimen may be dangerous in cardiac patients.[118] **IV for myxedema coma** 200-500 mcg; may follow with 100-300 mcg in 24 hr; use smaller doses in cardiovascular disease. **IM** indicated only for replacement therapy, if patient cannot take oral medication.

Dosage Individualization. In the elderly, those with cardiovascular disease and patients with severe, long-standing disease, start at 25 mcg/day and increase by 25 mcg/day increments at 3-4 week intervals.

Pediatric Dose. PO (under 6 months) 10 mcg/kg/day; (6-12 months) 8 mcg/kg/day; (1-5 yr) 6 mcg/kg/day; (5-10 yr) 4 mcg/kg/day.[15] Not less than 100 mcg/day under 1 yr old (cretinism).

Dosage Forms. **Tab** 25, 50, 100, 125, 150, 175, 200, 300, 400 mcg; **Inj** 100, 200, 500 mcg.

Patient Instructions. See Class Instructions.

Pharmacokinetics and Biopharmaceutics. *Onset and Duration.* PO onset 3-5 days; duration after cessation of therapy 7-10 days.[119] IV onset in myxedema coma 6-8 hr, maximum effect in 1 day.

Plasma Levels. T_4 = 6.5-9.5 mcg/dl (average 8.0); T_3 = 100-180 ng/dl.[116,120] Many drugs, pathological and physiological states affect binding and hence may affect results of some plasma level determinations.[15,119]

Fate. Oral absorption is 42-80% complete and is affected by many factors (eg, malabsorption, diet, cholestyramine).[124] Only 0.03% of total drug is unbound in plasma. About 85% is deiodinated in the body; half of this (43% of dose) forms T_3 which accounts for most, if not all, thyroid activity.[121,122] Other metabolites are formed in the liver, undergo an enterohepatic recirculation with reabsorption or excretion in the feces; 20-40% of a dose of thyroxine is eliminated in the feces.[15]

$t_{1/2}$. Euthyroid 6.5-7 days;[33,123] may increase to 9-10 days in hypothyroidism, decrease to 3-4 days in hyperthyroidism. Protein binding affects half-life (increased binding retards elimination and decreased binding increases elimination).[15]

Adverse Reactions. All are dose-related and can be avoided by slowly increasing the initial dose to the minimum effective maintenance dose. Signs of overdosage include headache, palpitations, chest pain, heat intolerance, sweating, leg cramps, weight loss, diarrhea, vomiting and nervousness. Physiologic doses of thyroid hormones in euthyroid patients are ineffective for weight reduction; larger doses may result in toxicity.

Contraindications. Thyrotoxicosis.

Precautions. Use with caution in acute myocardial infarction and uncorrected adrenal insufficiency. Initiate and increase dosage with caution in patients with cardiovascular disease, the elderly and in long-standing hypothyroidism. The status of other metabolic diseases, including diabetes, adrenal insufficiency, hyperadrenalism and panhypopituitarism may be affected by changes in thyroid status. See Drug Interactions chapter.

Parameters to Monitor. Free T_4, T_3, thyrotropin (TSH) and clinical status of the patient q 4-6 weeks initially. After stabilized, monitor free T_4 and clinical status at 6-12 month intervals;[21] in children, q 4 weeks initially and q 3-4 months after stabilization. Free T_4 should be monitored because TSH may remain elevated in children despite adequate replacement doses.[21]

Notes. Drug of choice for thyroid replacement because of purity, standardization, long half-life, large body pool and close simulation to normal physiologic hormone levels.[15,115,116,120] Protect from light. Significant bioinequivalence between brands has been reported.[136]

Liothyronine Sodium   Cytomel®, Various

Pharmacology. Synthetically prepared hormone identical to the thyroid hormone T_3. See Levothyroxine.

Administration and Adult Dose. PO for mild hypothyroidism 25 mcg/day initially, increasing by 12.5-25 mcg/day at 1-2 week intervals until desired response is obtained. PO for severe hypothyroidism 5 mcg/day initially, increasing by 5-10 mcg/day q 1-2 weeks until 25 mcg/day is reached, then increase by 12.5-25 mcg/day q 1-2 weeks until desired response is obtained. Usual maintenance dose ranges from 25-100 mcg/day. Dividing daily dosage into 2-3 doses may prevent wide plasma level fluctuations.[116,120] IV for myxedema coma 25 mcg q 6-12 hr or 100 mcg at once.[15] A way to prepare IV liothyronine from tablets has been published.[124] PO for T_3 suppression test 75-100 mcg/day for 7 days, then repeat ^{131}I thyroid uptake test.

Dosage Individualization. In the elderly and those with cardiovascular disease, start at 5 mcg/day and increase by 5 mcg/day increments q 2 weeks until desired response is obtained.

Pediatric Dose. PO (under 7 kg) 2.5 mcg/day initially; (over 7 kg) 5 mcg/day initially. Increase by 5 mcg/day at weekly intervals until desired effect is obtained. Usual maintenance dose is (under 1 yr) 15-20 mcg/day; (1-3 yr) 50 mcg/day; (over 3 yr) 25-50 mcg/day. Levothyroxine is the drug of choice in congenital hypothyroidism, however.

Dosage Forms. Tab 5, 25, 50 mcg; Inj (available by special request from manufacturer only) 114 mcg/ml.

Patient Instructions. See Class Instructions.

Pharmacokinetics and Biopharmaceutics. *Onset and Duration.* PO onset 1-3 days; duration after cessation of therapy 3-5 days.[119]
   Plasma Levels. During T_3 replacement, T_4 = 1 mcg/dl or less,[119] T_3 = peak of 450-700 ng/dl 1-2 hr after dose, returning to 100-180 ng/dl prior to the next dose 24 hr later.[120]
   Fate. Usually complete oral absorption, but may be decreased in congestive heart failure.[121] Excreted in the urine as deiodinated metabolites and their conjugates.[125]
   $t_{1/2}$. Euthyroid 1 day; may increase to 1.4 days in hypothyroidism, or decrease to 0.6 day in hyperthyroidism.[123]

Adverse Reactions. Dose-related (see Levothyroxine), but may appear more rapidly than with levothyroxine.

Contraindications. See Levothyroxine.

Precautions. See Levothyroxine.

Parameters to Monitor. See Levothyroxine, keeping T_3 plasma level data in mind.

Notes. May be the most useful drug in myxedema coma and other conditions where rapid onset of drug action is desirable.[15] Useful in diagnostic procedures where short duration of action is desirable.[115] Claimed by some to be useful in patients with cardiac disease because adverse effects will dissipate faster; however, adverse effects are more likely, because regulation of dosage is more difficult than with longer acting preparations.[115,119] Liothyronine and its mixtures (eg, thyroid, liotrix) cause "unphysiologic" peaks in plasma T_3 levels not found during levothyroxine replacement therapy.[120]

Thyroid Replacement Products Comparison Chart

DRUG	EQUIVALENT DOSE	DOSAGE FORMS	CONTENTS	RELATIVE ONSET & DURATION[a]	COMMENTS
Levothyroxine Levothroid® Synthroid® Various	100 mcg	Tab 25, 50, 100, 125, 150, 175, 200, 300, 400 mcg Inj 100, 200, 500 mcg	T_4	Long	Preparation of choice; bioinequivalence between brands reported[1,6]
Liothyronine Cytomel® Various	25 mcg	Tab 5, 25, 50 mcg Inj 114 mcg/ml	T_3	Short	Expensive
Thyroid Various	65 mg	Tab 16, 32, 65, 130, 150, 195, 260 mg	T_4 & T_3 in variable ratio	Intermediate	Cheapest product; rarely, allergy to animal protein occurs
Thyroglobulin Proloid® Various	65 mg	Tab 16, 32, 65, 100, 130, 200 mg	T_4 & T_3 in 2.5:1 ratio	Intermediate	Similar to thyroid, but more purified, standardized and costly
Liotrix Euthroid® Thyrolar®	#1 Tab[b]	Tab ¼, ½, 1, 2, 3[c]	T_4 & T_3 in 4:1 ratio	Intermediate	No advantages; more costly than others and confusing variation in tablet strengths exists

a. With equivalent doses.
b. 20% difference in hormone content between manufacturers; Euthroid®-1 contains T_4 60 mcg and T_3 15 mcg, Thyrolar®-1 contains T_4 50 mcg and T_3 12.5 mcg, other strengths are in same proportion.
c. Numbers represent equivalent dose of thyroid in grains.

Methimazole

Tapazole®

Methimazole is an antithyroid drug similar to propylthiouracil (PTU), but lacks the ability to decrease peripheral conversion of T_4 to T_3. Its half-life is 3 times that of PTU and is about 10 times more potent on a weight basis. Adverse effects differ little from PTU. Initial adult oral dose is 15 mg/day in mild hyperthyroidism, 30–40 mg/day in moderately severe hyperthyroidism or 60 mg/day in severe hyperthyroidism, given in three divided doses. Maintenance dose is 5–15 mg/day. Initial pediatric dose is 0.4 mg/kg/day given in three doses with a maintenance dose of one-half the initial dose. Methimazole is available as 5 and 10 mg tablets. When a parenteral thionamide is needed, methimazole tablets can be dissolved in saline solution and sterilized.[15,126]

Potassium Iodide

Various

Pharmacology. Iodide inhibits the synthesis and release of thyroid hormone. Large doses block the uptake of radioactive iodine by the thyroid gland.

Administration and Adult Dose. **PO for hyperthyroidism, prior to thyroidectomy or for thyrotoxic crisis** 50–100 mg (1–2 drops) q 8 hr diluted in a glass of water, milk or juice; doses as high as 500 mg/day have been used. Should be used with antithyroid drugs and propranolol in thyrotoxic crisis until euthyroid. Should be used for 7–10 days prior to thyroidectomy.[15] **PO for prophylaxis in a radiation emergency** 130 mg (100 mg iodine) immediately before or after exposure and daily for 3–7 days, to a maximum of 10 days after exposure.[127]

Pediatric Dose. **PO for thyrotoxicosis** 300 mg (6 drops) q 8 hr diluted as above. **PO for prophylaxis in a radiation emergency** (under 1 yr) 65 mg (50 mg iodine) immediately before or after exposure and daily for 3–7 days, to a maximum of 10 days after exposure; (over 1 yr) same as Adult Dose.

Dosage Forms. **Soln** (SSKI) 1 g/ml; **Syrup** 60 mg/ml; **Tab** 650 mg; **EC Tab** not recommended. See Notes.

Patient Instructions. Dilute solution in a glass of liquid before taking; may be taken with food, milk or an antacid to minimize stomach upset. Do not use if breast feeding; advise physician if pregnant. Do not use if solution turns brownish-yellow. If crystals form in the solution, they may be dissolved by warming the closed container in warm water. Dissolve tablets in 1/2 glass of water or milk before taking.

Pharmacokinetics and Biopharmaceutics. *Onset and Duration.* Onset 24–48 hr in hyperthyroidism with maximum effect in 10–15 days—see Notes.
   Plasma Levels. Iodide levels greater than 50 ng/ml inhibit iodide binding by thyroid in hyperthyroidism; greater than 200 ng/ml inhibit iodide uptake by normal thyroid.[119]
   Fate. Iodides are absorbed readily throughout GI tract; primarily excreted in urine.[128]

Adverse Reactions. Any adverse reactions warrant drug discontinuation. Hypersensitivity occurs occasionally and is manifested by angioedema, cutaneous hemorrhages, and symptoms resembling serum sickness. Iodism is indicated by metallic taste, GI upset, soreness of teeth and gums, coryza, frontal headache, painful swelling of salivary glands, diarrhea, acneiform skin eruptions and erythema of face and chest. Rarely, prolonged use can lead to goiter with hypothyroidism or hyperthyroidism.

Contraindications. Acute bronchitis; pulmonary edema; pregnancy is a relative contraindication due to possible development of fetal goiter; use as an expectorant in patients with hyperthyroidism.

Precautions. Use with caution in patients with pulmonary tuberculosis. Small bowel lesions are associated with enteric-coated potassium-containing tablets, which can cause obstruction, hemorrhage, perforation and possible death—this dosage form is not recommended. Iodides not recommended for use as expectorants due to their potential to induce acneiform eruptions, exacerbate existing lesions and adversely affect the thyroid.[129,130] See Drugs and Breast Feeding chapter.

Parameters to Monitor. Signs of iodism, hypothyroidism and parotitis should be checked occasionally during chronic use. Monitor serum potassium frequently in patients who are taking other drugs which may also affect serum potassium (eg, diuretics).

Notes. 1 drop of SSKI contains approximately 50 mg of potassium iodide. Most rapid onset of any treatment for hyperthyroidism; IV sodium iodide 1-2 g/day useful for rapid onset in thyrotoxicosis and thyroid storm.[114,119] Therapeutic effect dissipates after several weeks and thyrotoxicosis may be exacerbated by further iodide therapy.[15,109] Prevents uptake of ^{131}I for several weeks, and delays onset of thionamide therapy if given alone prior to a thionamide.[15,114] When used with a thionamide, it has been recommended to give iodides 1 hr after the thionamide dose.[114]

Propylthiouracil (PTU)   Various

Pharmacology. Antithyroid drug which interferes with the synthesis of thyroid hormones and decreases peripheral conversion of T_4 to T_3. An immunosuppressant effect on autoimmune antibodies has also been described.

Administration and Adult Dose. PO 100 mg q 8 hr initially; occasionally, initial doses of 900-1200 mg/day are required.[15] Many patients can be maintained on a once daily dosing regimen;[131] however, with larger doses and in resistant patients, giving the same dose in 4-6 divided doses may improve management.[15,124] After patient is euthyroid (usually 6-8 weeks), reduce dose to ⅓ over several weeks to maintenance dosage of 100-150 mg/day.[15,56,114] Traditional therapy has involved a year or more of antithyroid medication. Recent data, however, indicate that stopping therapy as soon as the euthyroid state is obtained is as effective as continuing therapy for a year or longer.[132]

Pediatric Dose. PO (6-10 yr) 50-150 mg/day initially; (10 yr and over) 150-300 mg/day initially. Maintenance dose is determined by patient response.

Dosage Forms. Tab 50 mg.

Patient Instructions. Sore throat, fever or oral lesions may be an early sign of a severe, but rare blood disorder and should be reported immediately to the physician or pharmacist. Also report any skin eruptions or yellowing of eyes and skin. Be sure to take at prescribed dosage intervals. If a dose is missed take it as soon as possible. If it is time for the next dose take both doses.[21] Tell any new physician or dentist that you are taking this medicine.

Pharmacokinetics and Biopharmaceutics. *Onset and Duration.*
Onset several days or weeks; severe cases respond the most rapidly.[56]

Fate. Rapidly absorbed (20–30 min) and clinical effects last only 2–3 hr.
Unchanged drug and metabolites are excreted in the urine.[15]

$t_{1/2}$. 1–1.6 hr in normal patients and hyperthyroidism after a single oral dose.[133-135]

Adverse Reactions. Skin rashes and urticaria occasionally occur; prevalence is dose-related.[117] Occasional arthralgia, paresthesias, GI disturbances, headache, dizziness or hypoprothrombinemia may occur. Dose-dependent agranulocytosis occurs rarely, usually in the first 2 months of therapy. Mild leukopenia may occur independently of agranulocytosis and is not always an indication for discontinuing the drug.[15,117] About 10% of patients with untreated hyperthyroidism have a WBC count below 4,000/cu mm.[21]

Precautions. PTU crosses the placenta and can cause fetal hypothyroidism and goiter; minimal doses (less than 300 mg/day) should be used in pregnancy. Thyroid dysfunction may diminish as pregnancy progresses, allowing a reduction in dosage and, in some cases, a withdrawal of therapy 2–3 weeks before delivery. Adjunctive therapy with thyroid hormone prevents maternal hypothyroidism, but because of minimal placental transfer, has little effect on the fetus.[21] See Drugs and Breast Feeding chapter. Obtain WBC and differential counts if patient reports signs of agranulocytosis such as fever, sore throat or malaise. Use with caution prior to surgery or during treatment with anticoagulants because of hypoprothrombinemic effect. See Drug Interactions chapter. A low prevalence of cross-sensitivity occurs between thionamide compounds for minor reactions, so if these occur another thionamide may be substituted; however, a 50% chance of reprecipitating agranulocytosis exists, so *do not* substitute another thionamide if this occurs.[15,56,117] Iodine, if used before PTU, may result in a delayed response to PTU.[15]

Parameters to Monitor. Clinical status of patient; plasma T_4, T_3 and TSH q month initially, then q 2–3 months.[21,117,119] Prothrombin time monitoring is advisable, particularly prior to surgery. Occasional liver function tests and CBC (but CBC may not be predictive of agranulocytosis because it may develop rapidly).[21]

Notes. Because PTU decreases peripheral conversion of T_4 to T_3, it is considered the thionamide of choice in treating thyrotoxic crisis.[15] Most patients eventually require surgery or treatment with radioactive iodine; however, a trial of PTU may be worthwhile in patients with minimal thyroid enlargement or very mild hyperthyroidism.[15]

References, 68:00 Hormones and Synthetic Substitutes

1. Azarnoff DL, ed. Steroid therapy. Philadelphia: WB Saunders, 1975.

2. Fauci AS, Dale DC, Balow JE. Glucocorticosteroid therapy: mechanisms of action and clinical considerations. Ann Intern Med 1976;84:304-15.

3. Axelrod L. Glucocorticoid therapy. Medicine 1976;55:39-65.

4. Mygind N, Hansen I, Pedersen CB et al. Intranasal beclomethasone dipropionate aerosol in allergic nasal diseases. Postgrad Med J 1975;51(Suppl 4):107-10.

5. Vilsvik JS, Jenssen AO, Walstad R. The effect of beclomethasone dipropionate aerosol on allergen induced nasal stenosis. Clin Allergy 1975;5:291-4.

6. Chatterjee SS, Nassar WY, Wilson O et al. Intranasal beclomethasone dipropionate and intranasal sodium cromoglycate: a comparative trial. Clin Allergy 1974;4:343-8.

7. Hendeles L, Weinberger M, Wong L. Medical management of noninfectious rhinitis. Am J Hosp Pharm 1980;37:1496-1504.

8. Godfrey S. The place of a new aerosol steroid, beclomethasone dipropionate, in the management of childhood asthma. Pediatr Clin North Am 1975;22:147-55.

9. Wyatt R, Waschek J, Weinberger M et al. Effects of inhaled beclomethasone dipropionate and oral alternate-day prednisone on pituitary-adrenal function in children with chronic asthma. N Engl J Med 1978;299:1387-92.

10. Nassif EG, Weinberger M, Thompson R et al. The value of maintenance theophylline in steroid-dependent asthma. N Engl J Med 1981;304:71-5.

11. Quinn S, Snader TC. Corticosteroid therapy for septic shock: review and analysis. Drug Intell Clin Pharm 1980;14:247-51.

12. Sheagren JN. Septic shock and corticosteroids. N Engl J Med 1981;305:456-8.

13. Carroll BJ. Clinical applications of the dexamethasone suppression test. Int Drug Ther Newsl 1981;16(1):1-4.

14. Pakes GE, Brogden RN, Heel RC et al. Flunisolide: a review of its pharmacological properties and therapeutic efficacy. Drugs 1980;19:397-411.

15. Gilman AG, Goodman LS, Gilman A, eds. Goodman and Gilman's the pharmacological basis of therapeutics. 6th ed New York: Macmillan, 1980.

16. Thorn GW. Clinical considerations in the use of corticosteroids. N Engl J Med 1966;274:775-81.

17. Harter JG, Reddy WJ, Thorn GW. Studies on an intermittent corticosteroid dosage regimen. N Engl J Med 1963;269:591-6.

18. Klinefelter HF, Winkenwerder WL, Bledsoe T. Single daily dose prednisone therapy. JAMA 1979;241:2721-3.

19. Byyny RL. Withdrawal from glucocorticoid therapy. N Engl J Med 1976;295:30-2.

20. Ahrens RC, Hendeles L, Weinberger M. The clinical pharmacology of drugs used in the treatment of asthma. In: Yaffe SJ, ed. Pediatric pharmacology: therapeutic principles in practice. New York: Grune & Stratton, 1980:233-80.

21. United States Pharmacopeial Convention Inc. United States Pharmacopia Dispensing Information 1980. Easton: Mack Publishing Co., 1980.

22. Liddle GW. Clinical pharmacology of the anti-inflammatory steroids. Clin Pharmacol Ther 1961;2:615-35.

23. Meikle AW, Tyler FH. Potency and duration of action of glucocorticoids. Am J Med 1977;63:200-7.

24. Sugita ET, Niebergal PJ. Bioavailability monograph: prednisone. J Am Pharm Assoc 1975;NS15:529-32.

25. Wilcox JB, Avery GS. Beclomethasone dipropionate corticosteroid inhaler. Drugs 1973;6:84-93.

26. Jenkins JS, Sampson PA. Conversion of cortisone to cortisol and prednisone to prednisolone. Br Med J 1967;2:205-7.

27. Gambertoglio JG, Amend WJC, Benet LZ. Pharmacokinetics and bioavailability of prednisone and prednisolone in healthy volunteers and patients: a review. J Pharmacokinet Biopharm 1980;8:1-52.

28. Uribe M, Go VLW. Corticosteroid pharmacokinetics in liver disease. Clin Pharmacokinet 1979;4:233-40.

29. Lewis GP, Jusko WJ, Burke CW et al. Prednisone side-effects' and serum-protein levels. Lancet 1971;2:778-81.

30. Conn HO, Blitzer BL. Nonassociation of adrenocorticosteroid therapy and peptic ulcer. N Engl J Med 1976;294:473-9.

31. The Boston Collaborative Drug Surveillance Program. Acute adverse reactions to prednisone in relation to dosage. Clin Pharmacol Ther 1972;13:694-8.

32. Anon. Oral corticosteroids. Med Lett Drugs Ther 1975;17:99-100.

33. Pagliaro LA, Benet LZ. Critical compilation of terminal half-lives, percent excreted unchanged, and changes of half-life in renal and hepatic dysfunction for studies in humans with references. J Pharmacokinet Biopharm 1975;3:333-83.

34. Melby JC. Clinical pharmacology of systemic corticosteroids. Annu Rev Pharmacol Toxicol 1977;17:511-27.

35. Tsuei SE, Moore RG, Ashley JJ et al. Disposition of synthetic glucocorticoids. I. Pharmacokinetics of dexamethasone in healthy adults. J Pharmacokinet Biopharm 1979;7:249-64.

36. Speroff L, Glass RH, Kase NG. Clinical Gynecologic Endocrinology and Infertility. 2nd Ed. Baltimore: Williams and Wilkins, 1978.

37. Rosenfield A. Oral and intrauterine contraception: a 1978 risk assessment. Am J Obstet Gynecol 1978;132:92-105.

38. Population Information Program. Oral contraceptives in the 1980's. Baltimore: The Johns Hopkins University. series A, number 6: 1982.

39. Brenner PF, Mishell DR. Contraception. In: Glass RH, ed. Office Gynecology. Baltimore: Williams and Wilkins, 1976:44-61.

40. Stadel BV. Oral contraceptives and cardiovascular disease (first of two parts). N Engl J Med 1981;305:612-18.

41. Stadel BV. idem (second of two parts). ibid:672-77.

42. Hendeles SM, Galand N, Schwers J. Metabolism of orally administered d-norgestrel in women. Acta Endocrinol 1972;71:557-68.

43. Kleinman RL, ed. Drug interactions with oral contraceptives. Int Planned Parenthood Fed Med Bull 1978;12:1.

44. Bacon JF, Shenfield GM. Pregnancy attributable to interaction between tetracycline and oral contraceptives. Br Med J 1980;2:293.

45. Patwardhan RV, Desmond PV, Johnson RF, et al. Impaired elimination of caffeine by oral contraceptives. J Lab Clin Med 1980;95:603-8.

46. Abernethy DR, Greenblatt DJ. Impairment of antipyrine metabolism by low-dose oral contraceptive steroids. Clin Pharmacol Ther 1981;29:106-10.

47. Dickey RP. Initial pill selection and managing the contraceptive pill patient. Int J Gynecol Obstet 1979;16:547-55.

48. Slone D, Shapiro S, Kaufman DW et al. Risk of myocardial infarction in relation to current and discontinued use of oral contraceptives. N Engl J Med 1981;305:420-4.

49. Quigley MM, Hammond CB. Estrogen replacement therapy—help or hazard? N Engl J Med 1979;301:646-8.

50. Greenblatt RB, Nezhat C, Karpas A. The menopausal syndrome hormone replacement therapy. In: Eskin BA, ed. The menopause. comprehensive management. New York: Masson Publishing, 1980:151-72.

51. Goldfarb JM, Little AB. Abnormal vaginal bleeding. N Engl J Med 1980;302:666-9.

52. Ortho Pharmaceutical Corporation. Ortho-Novum 10/11: a biphasic regimen (product monograph). Springfield, NJ: Omega Communications. 1982.

53. Catalona WJ, Scott WW. Carcinoma of the prostate: a review. J Urol 1978;119:1-8.

54. Ingle JN, Ahmann DL, Green SJ et al. Randomized clinical trial of diethylstilbestrol versus tamoxifen in postmenopausal women with advanced breast cancer. N Engl J Med 1981;304:16-21.

55. Kuchera LK. Postcoital contraception with diethylstilbestrol. Contraception 1974;10:47-54.

56. American Medical Association Department of Drugs. AMA drug evaluations. 4th ed. Littleton: Publishing Sciences Group, 1980.

57. Kepler JA, ed. American hospital formulary service. American Society of Hospital Pharmacists, Washington DC 1959-1982.

58. Yuzpe AA et al. A multicenter clinical investigation employing ethinyl estradiol combined with dl-norgestrel as a postcoital contraceptive agent. Fertil Steril 1982;37:508-13.

59. Keye WR, Jaffe RB. Hirsutism and dysfunctional uterine bleeding. In: Glass RH, ed. Office Gynecology. Baltimore: Williams and Wilkins, 1976:208-26.

60. Gordan GS. Drug treatment of the osteoporoses. Annu Rev Pharmacol Toxicol 1978;18:253-68.

61. Rigg LA, Hermann H, Yen SSC. Absorption of estrogens from vaginal creams. N Engl J Med 1978;298:195-7.

62. Antunes CMF, Stolley PD, Rosenshein NB et al. Endometrial cancer and estrogen use. N Engl J Med 1979;300:9-13.

63. Hoover R, Gray LA, Cole P et al. Menopausal estrogens and breast cancer. N Engl J Med 1976;295:401-5.

64. Weiss NS, Ure CL, Ballard JH et al. Decreased risk of fractures of the hip and lower forearm with postmenopausal use of estrogens. N Engl J Med 1980;303:1195-8.

65. Specht E. Hip fracture, skeletal fragility, osteoporosis and hormonal deprivation in elderly women. West J Med 1980;133:297-303.

66. Jackson JE, Bressler R. Clinical pharmacology of sulfonylurea hypoglycemic agents (two parts). Drugs 1981;22:211-45, 295-320.

67. Krall LP, Chabot VA. Oral hypoglycemic agent update. Med Clin North Am 1978;62:681-94.

68. Yu T-F, Berger L, Gutman AB. Hypoglycemia and uricosuric properties of acetohexamide and hydroxyhexamide. Metabolism 1968;17:309-15.

69. Cohen BD, Galloway JA, McMahon RE et al. Carbohydrate metabolism in uremia: blood glucose response to sulfonylurea. Am J Med Sci 1976;254:608-18.

70. Petitpierre B, Perrin L, Rudhardt M et al. Behavior of chlorpropamide in renal insufficiency and under the effect of associated drug therapy. Int J Clin Pharmacol Ther Toxicol 1972;6:120-4.

71. University Group Diabetes Program. A study of the effects of hypoglycemic agents on vascular complications in patients with adult-onset diabetes: II. Mortality results. Diabetes 1970;19(Suppl. 2):789-830.

72. Kilo C. The use of oral hypoglycemic agents. Hosp Prac 1979;14:103-10.

73. Bunn HF, Gabbay KH, Gallop, PM. The glycosylation of hemoglobin: relevance to diabetes mellitus. Science 1978;200:21-7.

74. Boden G, Master RW, Gordon SS et al. Monitoring metabolic control in diabetic outpatients with glycosylated hemoglobin. Ann Intern Med 1980;92:357-60.

75. Raptis S, Pfeiffer EF. Progress in oral therapy of diabetes mellitus with sulphonylurea of the second generation. Acta Diabetol Lat 1972;2:865-78.

76. Brogden RN, Heel RC, Pakes GE et al. Glipizide: a review of its pharmacological properties and therapeutic use. Drugs 1979;18:32-53.

77. Blohme G, Waldenstrom J. Glibenclamide and glipizide in maturity onset diabetes. Acta Med Scand 1979;206:263-7.

78. Anon. Which sulfonylurea in diabetes mellitus? Drug Ther Bull 1981;19:49-51.

79. Breidahl HD, Ennis GC, Martin FIR et al. Insulin and oral hypoglycaemic agents II: Clinical and therapeutic aspects. Drugs 1972;3:204-26.

80. Taylor JA. Pharmacokinetics and biotransformation of chlorpropamide in man. Clin Pharmacol Ther 1972;13:710-8.

81. Nelson E. Rate of metabolism of tolbutamide in test subjects with liver disease or with impaired renal function. Am J Med Sci 1964;248:657-9.

82. Nelson CJ. A guide to glucose urine testing systems for the pharmacist teaching the diabetic patient. Drug Intell Clin Pharm 1974;8:422-9.

83. Koda-Kimble MA. Diabetes mellitus. In: Koda-Kimble MA, Katcher BS, Young LY, eds. Applied therapeutics for clinical pharmacists. 2nd ed. San Francisco: Applied Therapeutics, 1978.

84. Christiansen C, Sachse M. Home blood glucose monitoring. Diab Educ 1980;6:13-21.

85. Shapiro B, Savage PJ, Lomatch D et al. A comparison of accuracy and estimated cost of methods for home blood glucose monitoring. Diabetes Care 1981;4:396-403.

86. Clements RS, Keane NA, Kirk KA et al. Comparison of various methods for rapid glucose estimation. Diabetes Care 1981;4:392-5.

87. Rearen GM, Olefsky JM. Role of insulin resistance in the pathogenesis of hyperglycemia. Adv Med Nutr 1978;2:229-264.

88. Savage PJ, Bennion LJ, Flock EV et al. Diet-induced improvement of abnormalities in insulin and glucagon secretion and in insulin receptor binding in diabetes mellitus. J Clin Endocrin Metab 1979;48:999-1007.

89. Galloway JA. When the patient is resistant or allergic to insulin. Med Times 1980;108:91-101.

90. Yue DK, Turtle JR. New forms of insulin and their use in the treatment of diabetes. Diabetes 1977;26:341-5.

91. Alberti KGMM, Nattrass M. Severe diabetic ketoacidosis. Med Clin North Am 1978;62:799-814.

92. Galloway JA, Bressler R. Insulin treatment in diabetes. Med Clin North Am 1978;62:663-80.

93. Fisher JN, Shahshahani MN, Kitabchi AE. Diabetic ketoacidosis: low-dose insulin therapy by various routes. N Engl J Med 1977;297:238-41.

94. Ginsberg S, Block MB, Mako ME et al. Serum insulin levels following administration of exogenous insulin. J Clin Endocrin Metab 1973;36:1175-9.

95. Rubenstein AH, Spitz I. Role of the kidney in insulin metabolism and excretion. Diabetes 1968;17:161-9.

96. Rabkin R, Simon NM, Steiner S et al. Effect of renal disease on renal uptake and excretion of insulin in man. N Engl J Med 1970;282:181-7.

97. Andreani D, Iavicoli M, Tamburrano G et al. Comparative trials with monocomponent (MC) and monospecies

(MS) pork insulins in the treatment of diabetes mellitus. Influence on antibody levels, on insulin requirement and on some complications. Horm Metab Res 1974;6:447-54.

98. Teuscher A. Treatment of insulin lipoatrophy with monocomponent insulin. Diabetologia 1974;10:211-4.

99. Mattson JR, Patterson R, Roberts M. Insulin therapy in patients with systemic insulin allergy. Arch Intern Med 1975;135:818-21.

100. Marble A. Allergy and diabetes in the treatment of diabetes mellitus. In: Joslin EP, Root HF, White P et al. eds. Diabetic Manual 10th ed. Philadelphia: Lea and Febiger, 1959:395-406.

101. Storvick WO, Henry HJ. Effect of storage temperature on stability of commercial insulin preparations. Diabetes 1968;17:499-502.

102. Petty C, Cunningham NL. Insulin adsorption by glass infusion bottles, polyvinylchloride infusion containers, and intravenous tubing. Anesthesiology 1979;36:330-7.

103. Whalen FJ, LeCain WK, Latiolais CJ. Availability of insulin from continuous low-dose insulin infusions. Am J Hosp Pharm 1979;36:330-7.

104. Peterson L, Caldwell J, Hoffman J. Insulin adsorbance to polyvinylchloride surfaces with implications for constant-infusion therapy. Diabetes 1976;25:72-4.

105. Albisser AM, Leibel BS, Ewart TG et al. Clinical control of diabetes by the artificial pancreas. Diabetes 1974;23:397-404.

106. Santiago JV, Clemens JM, Clarke WL et al. Closed-loop and open-loop devices for blood glucose control in normal and diabetic subjects. Diabetes 1979;28:71-81.

107. Rizza RA, Gerich JE, Haymond MW et al. Control of blood sugar in insulin-dependent diabetes: comparison of an artificial endocrine pancreas, continuous subcutaneous insulin infusion, and intensified conventional insulin therapy. N Engl J Med 1980;303:1313-8.

108. Nash HA. Depo-Provera. A review. Contraception 1975;12:377-93.

109. Kleinman RL. Injectable contraception. Int Planned Parenthood Fed Med Bull 1980;14:1-3.

110. Vecchio TJ. Long acting injectable contraceptives. In: Briggs MH, Christie GA, eds. Advances in steroid biochemistry and pharmacology, 1976;5:1-64.

111. Rosenfield AG. Injectable long-acting progestogen contraception: a neglected modality. Am J Obstet Gynecol 1974;120:537-48.

112. Fotherby K. Metabolism of synthetic steroids by animals and man. Acta Endocrinol 1974;185(Suppl):119-47.

113. Mills TM, Lin TJ, Braselton WE et al. Metabolism of oral contraceptive drugs. Am J Obstet Gynecol 1976;126:987-92.

114. Raber JH. The pharmacotherapy of thyroid storm. Drug Intell Clin Pharm 1980;14:344-52.

115. Refetoff S. Thyroid hormone therapy. Med Clin North Am 1975;59:1147-62.

116. Stock JM, Surks MI, Oppenheimer JH. Replacement dosage of l-thyroxine in hypothyroidism. A re-evaluation. N Engl J Med 1974;290:529-33.

117. Jackson I. Management of thyrotoxicosis. Am J Hosp Pharm 1975;32:933-9.

118. Sekadde CB, Slaunwhite WR, Aceto T, Murray K. Administration of thyroxine once a week. J Clin Endocrinol Metab 1974;39:759-64.

119. DeGroot LJ, Stanbury JB. The thyroid and its diseases. 4th ed. New York: J Wiley and Sons, 1975.

120. Surks MI, Schadlow AR, Oppenheimer JH. A new radioimmunoassay for plasma l-triiodothyronine: measurements in thyroid disease and in patients maintained on hormonal replacement. J Clin Invest 1972;51:3104-13.

121. Surks MI, Schadlow AR, Stock JM, Oppenheimer JH. Determination of iodothyronine absorption and conversion of l-thyroxine (T_4) to l-triiodothyronine (T_3) using turnover rate techniques. J Clin Invest 1973;52:805-11.

122. Inada M, Kasagi K, Kazama Y, et al. Estimation of thyroxine and triiodothyronine distribution and of the conversion rate of thyroxine to triiodothyronine in man. J Clin Invest 1975;55:1337-48.

123. Nicoloff JT, Low JC, Dussault JH, Fisher DA. Simultaneous measurement of thyroxine and triiodothyronine peripheral turnover kinetics in man. J Clin Invest 1972;51:473-83.

124. Brennan M.D. Clinical pharmacology. Series on pharmacology in practice 5. Thyroid hormones. Mayo Clin Proc 1980;55:33-44.

125. Pittman CS, Buck MW, Chambers JB. Urinary metabolites of ^{14}C-iabeled thyroxine in man. J Clin Invest 1972;51:1759-66.

126. Raber JH. The pharmacotherapy of thyroid storm. Drug Intell Clin Pharm 1980;14:344-52.

127. Kennedy D. Potassium iodide as a thyroid-blocking agent in a radiation emergency. Fed Reg 1978;43:58798-800.

128. Wade A, ed. Martindale, the extra pharmacopoeia. 27th ed. London: The Pharmaceutical Press, 1977.

129. American Academy of Pediatrics, Committee on Drugs: Adverse Reactions to Iodide Therapy of Asthma and Other Pulmonary Diseases. Pediatrics 1976;57:272-4.

130. Hendeles L, Weinberger M. A time to abandon the use of iodides in the management of pulmonary disease. Drug Intell Clin Pharm 1980;14:619-20.

131. Kammer H, Srinivasan K. The use of antithyroid drugs in a single daily dose. Treatment of diffuse toxic goiter. JAMA 1969;209:1325-7.

132. Greer MA, Kammer H, Bouma DJ. Short term antithyroid drug therapy for thyrotoxicosis of Graves' disease. N Engl J Med 1977;297:174-6.

133. Schyppan D, Riegelman S, Lehmann BV, Pilbrant A, Becker C. Preliminary pharmacokinetic studies of propylthiouracil in humans. J Pharmacokinet Biopharm 1973;1:307-18.

134. McMurray JF, Gilliland PF, Ratliff CF. Bourland PD. Pharmacodynamics of propylthiouracil in normal and hyperthyroid subjects after a single oral dose. J Endocrinol Metab 1975;41:362-4.

135. Sitar DS, Hunninghake DB. Pharmacokinetics of propylthiouracil in man after a single oral dose. J Clin Endocrinol Metab 1975;40:26-9.

136. Ramos-Gabatin A, Jacobson JM, Young RL. In vivo comparison of levothyroxine preparations. JAMA 1982;247:203-5.

137. Breitenfield RV, Hebert LA, Lemann J et al. Stability of renal transplant function with alternate-day corticosteroid therapy. JAMA 1980;244:151-6.

86:00 SPASMOLYTIC AGENTS

General References: 1-5

Theophylline   Theo-dur®, Slo-Phyllin®, Various

Pharmacology. Directly relaxes smooth muscle of bronchial airways and pulmonary blood vessels to act as a bronchodilator and pulmonary vasodilator; also is a diuretic, coronary vasodilator, cardiac stimulant and cerebral stimulant. It also improves diaphragmatic contractility and lessens diaphragmatic fatigue in normal subjects.[6] In addition to competitive inhibition of phosphodiesterase, it may inhibit prostaglandins or affect calcium transport.

Administration and Adult Dose. PO (theophylline), IV (aminophylline) **loading dose for acute asthma symptoms** 5 mg/kg (6 mg/kg aminophylline), if patient has taken no theophylline in previous 24 hr. In emergencies, 2.5 mg/kg (3 mg/kg aminophylline) may be given if an immediate plasma level cannot be obtained. Each 1 mg/kg (1.25 mg/kg aminophylline) results in about a 2 mcg/ml increase in plasma theophylline. Infuse IV aminophylline no faster than 25 mg/min. **Maintenance Dose**—see Maintenance Dose for Acute Symptoms Comparison Chart below. **PO for chronic asthma** (theophylline) initial dose 400 mg/day in divided doses, then increase if tolerated in approximately 25% increments at 3-day intervals to 13 mg/kg/day or 900 mg/day, whichever is less. Use plasma concentrations for subsequent dosage adjustment. For patients with CHF, liver dysfunction or cor pulmonale, initial dose must not exceed 400 mg/day unless plasma levels are measured. **IM, PR suppositories not recommended.**

Maintenance Dose for Acute Symptoms[a]

POPULATION GROUP	ORAL THEOPHYLLINE[b] (MG/KG/DAY)	IV AMINOPHYLLINE[c] (MG/KG/HR)
Newborn up to 24 days (for apnea/bradycardia)	2	0.1
Newborn 24 days and older (for apnea/bradycardia)	3	0.15
Infants 6 weeks–1 yr	0.2 × (age in weeks) + 5	0.05 × calculated daily theophylline
Children 1–9 yr	20	1
Children 9–12 yr, and adolescent daily smokers of cigarettes or marijuana, and otherwise healthy adult smokers under 50 yr	16	0.83
Adolescents 12–16 yr (nonsmokers)	13	0.68

Continued

Maintenance Dose for Acute Symptoms[a]

POPULATION GROUP	ORAL THEOPHYLLINE[b] (MG/KG/DAY)	IV AMINOPHYLLINE[c] (MG/KG/HR)
Otherwise healthy nonsmoking adults (including elderly patients)	10	0.52
Cardiac decompensation, cor pulmonale and/or liver dysfunction[d]	5	0.26

a. To maintain a plasma concentration of 10 mcg/ml, except 5 mcg/ml for newborn apnea/bradycardia.

b. In patients with less severe symptoms, a rapidly absorbed oral formulation may be used. The total daily dose is divided equally and administered q 4 hr in children, q 6 hr in infants and adults and q 12 hr in newborns.

c. Adjust infusion rate to maintain plasma concentration in the range of 10-20 mcg/ml.

d. Accumulation may occur over 5-7 days; do not exceed 400 mg/day unless plasma levels are measured.

Dosage Individualization. Plasma concentration monitoring is essential. If no doses have been missed or extra doses taken for previous 48 hr, and if peak plasma concentrations have been obtained (1-2 hr after liquid or plain uncoated tablet and 4 hr after most SR products), adjust dose using Theophylline Dosage Adjustment Guide which follows.

Theophylline Dosage Adjustment Guide

PLASMA CONCENTRATION[a] (MCG/ML)	ACTION
Therapeutic	
10-20	Maintain dose if tolerated; recheck plasma level at 6-12 month intervals
Too High	
20-25	Decrease doses by 10%.
25-30	Skip next dose and decrease subsequent doses by 25%; recheck level.
Over 30	Skip next 2 doses and decrease subsequent doses by 50%; recheck level
Too Low	
7.5-10	Increase dose by 25%.
5-7.5	Increase dose by 25%; recheck level

a. Appropriately measured peak—see Dosage Individualization.

Pediatric Dose. PO or IV for acute symptoms infuse over 20-30 min; same as Adult Dose. **PO for chronic asthma** (theophylline) initial dose (6-24 weeks) 8 mg/kg/day; (over 24 weeks) 16 mg/kg/day or 400 mg/day (whichever is less) in divided doses, then increase if tolerated, in approximately 25% increments at 3-day intervals to: (6 weeks-1 yr) (0.3) × (age in weeks) + 8 mg/kg/day; (1-9 yr) 24 mg/kg/day; (9-12 yr) 20 mg/kg/day; (12-16 yr) 18 mg/kg/day.[7,8] **IM, PR suppositories not recommended.**

Dosage Forms. See Theophylline Products Comparison Chart.

Patient Instructions. Do not chew or crush SR tablets or capsules. Take at equally spaced intervals around the clock. Report any nausea, vomiting, GI pain, headache or restlessness. Contents of Slo-Phyllin Gyrocaps® and Theo-dur® capsules may be mixed with a vehicle (applesauce or jam) and swallowed without chewing for patients who have difficulty swallowing capsules.

Pharmacokinetics and Biopharmaceutics. *Onset and Duration.* IV onset within 15 min with loading dose.[3]

Plasma Levels. Well correlated with clinical effects: therapeutic 10–20 mcg/ml;[9,10] toxicity increases over 20 mcg/ml—see Adverse Reactions. Saliva concentration is an unreliable predictor of plasma concentration.[11]

Fate. Plain uncoated tablets and solution well absorbed orally; enteric coated tablets and some SR dosage forms may be unreliably absorbed. Food may affect rate, but not extent of absorption. Rectal suppository absorption is slow and erratic and not recommended under any circumstances.[3,12] Rectal solutions may result in plasma concentrations comparable to oral solution. About 60% plasma protein bound (less in neonates); V_d 0.5 L/kg (greater in neonates).[9,13] Extensively metabolized in the liver to several inactive metabolites; 10% excreted unchanged in the urine.[3] Clearance decreased in elderly, patients with CHF, significant hepatic dysfunction, pulmonary edema, prolonged high fever and in patients receiving troleandomycin, erythromycin, cimetidine, high-dose allopurinol, propranolol or influenza A vaccine. Smoking increases theophylline metabolism; this effect may last for 3 months to 2 yr after cessation of smoking.[14]

$t_{1/2}$. 3–16 hr (average 8) in adult nonsmokers, 4.4 hr in adult smokers (1–2 packs per day) and 3–5 hr in children over 1 yr. Newborn infants, older patients with chronic obstructive pulmonary disease or cor pulmonale and patients with heart failure or liver disease may have a half-life greater than 24 hr. Dose-dependent kinetics in therapeutic range observed in children and rarely in adults.[15] Rate of metabolism progressively increases in infants during the first year of life.

Adverse Reactions. Local GI irritation may occur. Reactions occur more frequently at plasma concentrations over 20 mcg/ml and include anorexia, nausea, vomiting, epigastric pain, diarrhea, restlessness, irritability, insomnia and headache. Serious arrhythmias and convulsions (frequently leading to death or permanent brain damage) may occur at levels over 35 mcg/ml and are often *not* preceded by less serious toxicity; cardiovascular reactions include sinus tachycardia and life-threatening ventricular arrhythmias with PVCs. Rapid IV administration may be associated with hypotension, syncope, cardiac arrest (particularly if administered directly into CVP line) and death. IM is painful and offers no advantage. Serious toxicity and deaths have occurred with rectal suppositories due to erratic absorption.

Contraindications. Hypersensitivity to ethylenediamine (aminophylline).

Precautions. Use ideal body weight for dosage calculations in obese patients.[16,17] Use caution in severe cardiac disease, hypoxemia, hepatic disease, acute myocardial injury, cor pulmonale, CHF, peptic ulcer, underlying seizure disorder, migraine and neonates. The alcohol in oral liquid preparations is not needed for absorption and may cause side effects, especially in children. Do not give with other xanthine preparations. See Drug Interactions chapter.

Parameters to Monitor. Plasma theophylline concentrations before starting therapy, if patient previously taking theophylline,[18] then 1, 4, 12 and 24 hr after start of infusion,[4] and daily during continuous infusion.

Notes. The oral theophylline preparation of choice for chronic use, to achieve both sustained therapeutic concentrations and improved compliance, is a completely and slowly absorbed, SR formulation—see Theophylline Products Comparison Chart which follows. Combination products containing ephedrine increase CNS toxicity and have no therapeutic advantage over adequate plasma concentrations of theophylline alone.[19] Combination products with iodides are not recommended.[20] Dyphylline is chemically related to, but not a salt of, theophylline; the amount of dyphylline equivalent to theophylline is unknown. It is significantly less potent than theophylline, requiring larger doses; half-life of 2 hr requires more frequent dosing.[19]

Theophylline Products Comparison Chart[a]

PRODUCT	ANHYDROUS THEOPHYLLINE CONTENT	MEASURABLE DOSE INCREMENT[b] (MG)	COMMENTS
RAPIDLY ABSORBED (for acute therapy)			
Plain Uncoated Tablets			
Slo-Phyllin®	100 mg scored tablet	50	Plasma level fluctuation = 459%/117%[c]
	200 mg scored tablet	100	
Theophyl® Chewable	100 mg double scored	25	Microencapsulated; swallow rapidly and wash down to avoid bitter taste
Oral Liquids (Alcohol Free)			
Elixicon® Suspension	20 mg/ml	10	Shake vigorously before use; sugar and dye free
Slo-Phyllin GG® Syrup	10 mg/ml	5	Contains guaifenesin, an inert ingredient; dye free
Theolair® Liquid	5.3 mg/ml	2.5	
Rectal Solution			
Somophyllin®[d]	51 mg/ml	16	Only acceptable rectal dosage form; measure dose carefully
Intravenous Solution			
Aminophylline[d]	20 mg/ml	5	Use rubber stoppered vials to avoid glass particles from breaking ampules
Theophylline	800 mg/L	—	Available in large volume solutions only

Continued

Theophylline Products Comparison Chart[a]

PRODUCT	ANHYDROUS THEOPHYLLINE CONTENT	MEASURABLE DOSE INCREMENT[b] (MG)	COMMENTS
SLOW-RELEASE PRODUCTS[e] (for chronic asthma)			
Slo-Phyllin® Gyrocaps	60 mg capsule 125 mg capsule 250 mg capsule	30	Plasma level fluctuation = 225%/69%;[c] beads can be sprinkled on food for administration to infants; use one-half the contents of 60 mg capsule for 30 mg doses.
Sustaire®	100 mg scored tablet 300 mg scored tablet	50 150	Plasma level fluctuation = 87%/34%;[c] some rapid metabolizers may require 8 hr dosing intervals to avoid break-through of symptoms
Theo-dur®	100 mg scored tablet 200 mg scored tablet 300 mg scored tablet 50, 75, 125, 200 mg capsules	25 100 150	Some rapid metabolizers may require 8 hr dosing intervals to avoid break-through of symptoms; plasma level fluctuations = 38%/16% for 200 and 300 mg and 87%/34% for 100 mg tabs[c]

a. Only products with documented bioavailability and with dosage forms that permit incremental changes in dose are listed.
b. Accuracy of measurement decreases below 0.5 ml with suspensions and syrups because of viscosity; smaller amounts cannot be accurately measured. All liquid dosage forms should be measured with a syringe.
c. Predicted fluctuation between peak and trough (%) for 12-hr dosing interval; average child $t_{1/2}$ = 3.7 hr, average adult $t_{1/2}$ = 8.2 hr.[21]
d. The ethylenediamine portion of aminophylline causes urticaria or exfoliative dermatitis rarely.
e. Only Sustaire® and Theo-dur® have sufficiently slow and complete absorption to allow 12 hr dosing with minimal plasma concentration fluctuations in most patients.[21] Many products advertised for bid dosage (eg, LaBID®, Phyllocontin®) do not maintain plasma concentrations within the therapeutic range in many patients, especially children.[21]

References, 86:00 Spasmolytic Agents

1. Hendeles L, Weinberger M. Avoidance of adverse effects during chronic therapy with theophylline. Drug Intell Clin Pharm 1980;14:522-30.

2. Hendeles L, Weinberger M, Johnson G. Monitoring serum theophylline levels. Clin Pharmacokinet 1978;3:294-312.

3. Piafsky KM, Ogilvie RI. Dosage of theophylline in bronchial asthma. N Engl J Med 1975;292:1218-22.

4. Koup JR, Schentag JJ, Vance JW et al. System for clinical pharmacokinetic monitoring of theophylline therapy. Am J Hosp Pharm 1976;33:949-56.

5. Ahrens RC, Hendeles L, Weinberger M. The clinical pharmacology of drugs used in the treatment of asthma. In: Yaffe SJ, ed. Pediatric pharmacology: therapeutic principles in practice. New York: Grune & Stratton, Inc, 1980;233-80.

6. Aubier M, De Troyer A, Sampson M et al. Aminophylline improves diaphragmatic contractility. N Engl J Med 1981;305:249-52.

7. Hendeles L, Weinberger M, Wyatt R. Guide to oral theophylline therapy for the treatment of chronic asthma. Am J Dis Child 1978;132:876-80.

8. Nassif EG, Weinberger MM, Shannon D et al. Theophylline disposition in infancy. J Pediatr 1981;98:158-61.

9. Mitenko PA, Ogilvie RI. Rational intravenous doses of theophylline. N Engl J Med 1973;289:600-3.

10. Levy G. Pharmacokinetic control of theophylline therapy. In: Levy G ed. Clinical pharmacokinetics: a symposium. Washington, DC: American Pharmaceutical Association, Academy of Pharmaceutical Sciences, 1974;103-10.

11. Hendeles L, Burkey S, Bighley L et al. Unpredictability of theophylline saliva measurements in chronic obstructive pulmonary disease. J Allergy Clin Immunol 1977;60:335-8.

12. Weinberger M, Riegelman S. Rational use of theophylline for bronchodilatation. N Engl J Med 1974;291:151-3.

13. Jenne JW, Wyze MS, Rood FS et al. Pharmacokinetics of theophylline: application to adjustment of the clinical dose of aminophylline. Clin Pharmacol Ther 1972;13:349-60.

14. Powell JR, Thiercelin J-F, Vozeh S et al. The influence of cigarette smoking and sex on theophylline disposition. Am Rev Respir Dis 1977;116:17-23.

15. Weinberger M, Ginchansky E. Dose-dependent kinetics of theophylline disposition in asthmatic children. J Pediatr 1977;91:820-4.

16. Hendeles L, Weinberger M, Wyatt R. Guide to oral theophylline therapy for the treatment of chronic asthma. Am J Dis Child 1978;132:876-80.

17. Koup JR, Schentag JJ, Vance JW et al. System for clinical pharmacokinetic monitoring of theophylline therapy. Am J Hosp Pharm 1976;33:949-56.

18. Weinberger MW, Matthay RA, Ginchansky EJ et al. Intravenous aminophylline dosage: use of serum theophylline measurement for guidance. JAMA 1976;235:2110-3.

19. Weinberger M, Hendeles L. Pharmacotherapy of asthma. Am J Hosp Pharm 1976;33:1071-80.

20. Hendeles L, Weinberger M. A time to abandon the use of iodides in the management of pulmonary diseases. J Allergy Clin Immunol 1980;66:177-8.

21. Weinberger M, Hendeles L, Wong L. Relationship of formulation and dosing interval to fluctuation of serum theophylline concentration in children with chronic asthma. J Pediatr 1981;99:145-52.

88:00 VITAMINS

88:24 VITAMIN K ACTIVITY

Phytonadione

Aqua-Mephyton®,
Konakion®, Mephyton®

Pharmacology. A required cofactor for the hepatic microsomal enzyme system that carboxylates glutamyl residues in precursor proteins to γ-carboxyglutamyl residues. These proteins are present in vitamin K-dependent clotting factors (II, VII, IX and X), as well as noncollagen bone protein, some plasma proteins and the protein of several organs.[1]

Administration and Adult Dose. PO, SC or IM (Konakion® may only be given IM) 2.5-10 mg up to 25 mg initially. A single dose of 1-5 mg is usually sufficient to normalize PT during anticoagulant therapy, but in the presence of severe bleeding, 20-40 mg may be needed.[2-4] The initial dose may be repeated, based on PT and clinical response, after 12-48 hr if given PO and 6-8 hr if given parenterally. The smallest dose possible should be used to reverse anticoagulant effect, to obviate possible refractoriness to further anticoagulant therapy.[4,5] The normal daily nutritional requirement is about 30 ng/kg.[6] Aqua-Mephyton® should be used IV only if absolutely essential.

Pediatric Dose. **IM prophylaxis of hemorrhagic disease of the newborn** 0.5–1 mg. **SC or IM for treatment of hemorrhagic disease of the newborn** 1 mg; more if mother has been receiving an oral anticoagulant.

Dosage Forms. **Tab** (Mephyton®) 5 mg; **Inj** (Aqua-Mephyton®, Konakion®) 2, 10 mg/ml.

Pharmacokinetics and Biopharmaceutics. *Onset and Duration.* Reversal of anticoagulant effect is variable among individuals; parenteral onset often within 6 hr; peak and duration variable among individuals and with dose. A 5 mg dose IV usually returns PT to normal in 24–48 hr.[3] Large doses may cause prolonged refractoriness to oral anticoagulants.[4,5]

Fate. Absorbed from the GI tract via intestinal lymphatics only in the presence of bile; well absorbed after parenteral administration. Metabolized in the liver to hydroquinone form and epoxide form which are interconvertible with the quinone.[1] Little storage in the body occurs. In the absence of bile, hypoprothrombinemia develops over a period of several weeks.[4,5,7]

Adverse Reactions. The drug itself appears to be nontoxic; however, severe reactions (flushing, dyspnea, chest pain) and occasionally deaths have occurred after IV administration of Aqua-Mephyton®, possibly due to emulsifying agents.[4,8,9] This product should rarely be used IV, and only when other routes of administration are not feasible. A transient flushing sensation, peculiar taste and pain and swelling at the injection site have been reported. Large parenteral doses in neonates have caused hyperbilirubinemia.

Contraindications. Konakion® is contraindicated for other than IM use.

Precautions. Protect from the light at all times. Temporary resistance to oral anticoagulants may occur, especially with large doses. Reversal of anticoagulant activity may restore previous thromboembolic conditions. Either no effect or worsening of hypoprothrombinemia may occur in severe liver disease and repeated doses are not warranted if response to the initial dose is unsatisfactory.[4,8]

Parameters to Monitor. PT before, and at intervals after, administration of the drug. The testing interval depends on the route of administration, the condition being treated and the patient's status. See Administration and Adult Dose.

Notes. Drug of choice for reversal of oral anticoagulant therapy, but has no antagonist activity against heparin. Parenteral phytonadione and oral menadione and its derivatives are equally effective in treating hypoprothrombinemia caused by malabsorption.[2,8]

Vitamin K Activity Comparison Chart

DRUG	SYNONYMS	ORAL ABSORPTION	USES	SOURCES
Phytonadione Aqua-Mephyton® Konakion® Mephyton®	Vitamin K₁; phylloquinone	Via lymph; bile salts needed	1. Hypoprothrombinemia due to oral anticoagulants, antibacterials and salicylates 2. Hemorrhagic disease of the newborn 3. Malabsorption (parenteral or oral with bile salts)	Dietary & synthetic
Not commercially available	Vitamin K₂; menaquinone(s)	Via lymph; bile salts needed		Formed by bacteria in GI tract
Menadione	Vitamin K₃	Direct; bile salts not needed	1. Hypoprothrombinemia due to antibacterials and salicylates 2. Malabsorption due to lack of bile salts	Synthetic
Menadiol Sodium Diphosphate Kappadione® Synkayvite®	Vitamin K₄	Direct; bile salts not needed; converted to menadione in body; about half as potent as menadione	Same as menadione	Synthetic

References, 88:24 Vitamin K Activity

1. Suttie JW. The metabolic role of vitamin K. Fed Proc 1980;39:2730-5.
2. Gamble JR, Dennis EW, Coon WW et al. Clinical comparison of vitamin K_1 and water-soluble vitamin K. Arch Intern Med 1955;95:52-8.
3. Zieve PD, Solomon HM. Variation in the response of human beings to vitamin K_1. J Lab Clin Med 1969;73:103-10.
4. Mandel HG, Cohn VH. Fat-soluble vitamins; vitamins A, K, and E. In: Gilman AG, Goodman LS, Gilman A, eds. Goodman and Gilman's the pharmacological basis of therapeutics. 6th ed. New York: Macmillan, 1980:1583-601.
5. Koch-Weser J, Sellers EM. Drug interactions with coumarin anticoagulants (2 parts). N Engl J Med 1971;285:487-9, 547-58.
6. Frick PG, Riedler G, Brogli H. Dose response and minimal daily requirement for vitamin K in man. J Appl Physiol 1967;23:387-9.
7. Woolf IL, Babior BM. Vitamin K and warfarin. Am J Med 1972;53:261-7.
8. Finkel MJ. Vitamin K_1 and the vitamin K analogues. Clin Pharmacol Ther 1961;2:794-814.
9. Mattea EJ, Quinn K. Adverse reactions after intravenous phytonadione administration. Hosp Pharm 1981;16:224-35.

92:00 UNCLASSIFIED THERAPEUTIC AGENTS

ANTIGOUT AGENTS

(SEE ALSO URICOSURIC AGENTS 40:40)

General References: 1-5

Allopurinol

Lopurin®, Zyloprim®

Pharmacology. A structural analogue of the purine base hypoxanthine which competitively inhibits xanthine oxidase. This reduces both serum and urinary uric acid levels by blocking the conversion of hypoxanthine and xanthine to uric acid and by decreasing purine synthesis.[2]

Administration and Adult Dose. PO for gout 100 mg/day initially, then increase in 100 mg increments at weekly intervals until a serum uric acid level of 6 mg/dl or less is attained; dose within the following guidelines: PO 100 mg bid-tid (may give as a single daily dose) for maintenance of mild gout, and 400-600 mg/day for moderately severe tophaceous gout, to maximum of 800 mg-1 g/day for resistant cases.[3,4] Give dosages which exceed 300 mg/day in divided doses. Prophylactic maintenance doses of colchicine (500 mcg bid) should be given with allopurinol for several months due to an initial increased risk of gouty attacks. A fluid intake sufficient to yield a daily urinary output of at least 2 L and the maintenance of a neutral or slightly alkaline urine are desirable. Generally, normal serum urate levels are achieved in 1-3 weeks. In transferring from a uricosuric agent to allopurinol, reduce the uricosuric dosage over a period of several weeks, while gradually increasing the dose of allopurinol. **PO for secondary hyperuricemia associated with vigorous treatment of malignancies** 600-800 mg/day for 2-3 days is advisable with a high fluid intake; maintenance dose is 100-200 mg/day, to maximum of 800 mg/day.

Dosage Individualization. Reduce dosage in renal impairment as follows: 200 mg/day with a Cl_{cr} of 10-20 ml/min; to not greater than 100 mg/day with a Cl_{cr} of less than 10 ml/min, and also lengthen the dosing interval with a Cl_{cr} of less than 3 ml/min.

Pediatric Dose. PO for secondary hyperuricemia associated with malignancies (under 6 yr) 150 mg/day; (6-10 yr) 300 mg/day; evaluate response after 48 hr and adjust dosage as needed. Contraindicated in children for all other purposes.

Dosage Forms. Tab 100, 300 mg.

Patient Instructions. This drug may be taken with food, milk or an antacid to minimize stomach upset. Adults should drink at least 10–12 full glasses (240 ml each) of fluid each day.

Pharmacokinetics and Biopharmaceutics. *Onset and Duration.* A measurable decrease in uric acid occurs in 2–4 days; normal serum uric acid is achieved in 1–3 weeks.

Fate. Well absorbed from the GI tract and rapidly oxidized to oxipurinol, an active but less potent inhibitor of xanthine oxidase. 6–10% of a single dose is excreted in the urine as unchanged allopurinol and 45–65% as oxipurinol.[6,7]

$t_{1/2}$. (Allopurinol) less than 1 hr; (oxipurinol) 13.6 hr.[6-8]

Adverse Reactions. Most frequent is a maculopapular skin rash, but exfoliative, urticarial, purpuric and erythema multiforme lesions are also reported. Such reactions necessitate drug discontinuation as more severe hypersensitivity reactions such as vasculitis, toxic epidermal necrolysis, renal impairment and hepatic damage can occur. Hypersensitivity reactions usually begin approximately 4 weeks after start of therapy; fever and eosinophilia are frequently present.[9] Occasionally, nausea, vomiting and abdominal pain occur. Rarely, alopecia, cataract formation, bone marrow depression, leukopenia, leukocytosis or renal xanthine stones occur.

Contraindications. Children (except for hyperuricemia secondary to malignancy); lactation.

Precautions. Pregnancy. Should not be given to immediate relatives of patients with idiopathic hemochromatosis. Use with caution in renal impairment in reduced doses. See Drug Interactions chapter.

Parameters to Monitor. Serum uric acid levels; pretreatment 24-hour urinary uric acid excretion.[2] Periodic determination of liver function (particularly in patients with pre-existing liver disease). Renal function studies and CBC should be performed, especially during the first few months of therapy.

Notes. Drug of choice for patients with impaired renal function who respond poorly to uricosuric agents; however, these patients should be monitored closely because of an increased frequency of adverse reactions.[5,9] Uricosuric drugs enhance the renal clearance of oxipurinol and diminish the degree of xanthine oxidase suppression; however, in appropriate cases the net effect of combined treatment facilitates mobilization of uric acid deposits.[5,6] Concurrent use of salicylates, for their antirheumatic effect, does not compromise the action of allopurinol. Extemporaneously compounded allopurinol rectal suppositories may appear to be clinically effective; however, because of limited studies, this dosage form cannot be recommended.[10] IV drug is available from manufacturer for investigational use.

Colchicine   Various

Pharmacology. An anti-inflammatory agent relatively specific for gout, with activity probably due to the impairment of leukocyte chemotaxis and synovial cell phagocytosis of urate crystals present in the synovial fluid.

Administration and Adult Dose. **PO for acute gout** 0.5–1.2 mg initially, then 0.5 or 0.6 mg q 1–3 hr until pain is relieved or GI toxicity occurs (ie, nausea, vomiting or diarrhea), to maximum total dose of 8–10 mg. An interval of 3 days is advised if a second course is required. **PO for prophylaxis in chronic gout** 0.5–1.8 mg/day or every other day, depending on severity of the case. **Slow IV for acute gout** 1–2 mg diluted in 20 ml NS initially, then 0.5 mg q 6–12 hr prn, to maximum of 4 mg in 24 hr; extravasation must be avoided. **Do not administer by SC or IM routes.**

Dosage Individualization. During prolonged use, reduce both oral and IV doses in the presence of renal impairment.

Dosage Forms. **Granules** 500 mcg; **Tab** 500, 600 mcg; **Inj** 500 mcg/ml.

Patient Instructions. A supply of this drug should always be at hand and it should be taken promptly at the earliest symptoms of a gouty attack. Relief of gout pain or occurrence of nausea, vomiting or diarrhea indicate that the full therapeutic dose has been attained and no more drug should be taken. Black tarry stools or bright red blood in the stools may indicate gastrointestinal bleeding and should be reported immediately.

Pharmacokinetics and Biopharmaceutics. *Fate.* Well absorbed after oral administration, with partial hepatic deacetylation; V_d is 1–2 L/kg; 31% plasma protein bound.[11-14] Extensive leukocyte uptake with significant levels found up to 10 days. Both urinary (10–36%, in part unchanged) and fecal elimination occur.

$t_{1/2}$. 35–90 min (average 58) following a single 2 mg IV dose in normals; slightly shorter in patients with severe liver disease and longer in patients with gout or severe renal impairment.[12,13]

Adverse Reactions. Overdosage can cause hemorrhagic gastroenteritis, vascular damage leading to shock, nephrotoxicity and paralysis. As little as 7 mg has proved fatal, but much larger doses have been survived.[15] Nausea, vomiting and diarrhea are most frequent and may occur several hr after PO or IV drug administration; discontinue drug at first signs. Prolonged administration may cause bone marrow depression with agranulocytosis and aplastic anemia; peripheral neuritis and alopecia also reported.

Precautions. Use with great caution in elderly or debilitated patients, especially those with hepatic, renal, GI or heart disease.

Notes. Colchicine may be an effective anti-inflammatory agent in the therapy of the arthritis of pseudogout.[16] Continuous prophylactic colchicine therapy can be effective in suppressing the attacks of familial Mediterranean fever.[17]

ANTIPARKINSON AGENTS

(SEE ALSO BENZTROPINE AND TRIHEXYPHENIDYL 12:08 AND BROMOCRIPTINE 92:00)

General References: 18-20

Amantadine Hydrochloride   Symmetrel®

Pharmacology. An antiviral agent which possesses antiparkinson effect because of its ability to release dopamine. Used to treat both idiopathic and drug-induced parkinsonism.[18,21]

Administration and Adult Dose. **PO for parkinsonism** 100 mg bid, to maximum of 400 mg/day (with close supervision) in divided doses; initiate at 100 mg/day for at least one week in patients with serious associated illnesses or who are receiving other antiparkinson drugs. **PO for prophylaxis of influenza A illness** 200 mg/day in 1 or 2 doses. Begin prophylaxis as soon as possible after exposure and continue for 10 days after contact.

Dosage Individualization. Dosage must be reduced in renal impairment: give 200 mg loading dose on first day to all patients; then, for Cl_{cr} = 60 ml/min, dose is 150 mg/day; 40–50 ml/min, 100 mg/day; 30 ml/min, 200 mg twice/week; 20 ml/min, 100 mg three times/week; 10 ml/min or less, 150 mg/week. No additional doses needed with hemodialysis.[22]

Pediatric Dose. **PO for prophylaxis of influenza A illness** (1–9 yr) 4.4–8.8 mg/kg/day in 2–3 divided doses, to maximum of 150 mg/day; (9–12 yr) 100 mg bid.

Dosage Forms. **Cap** 100 mg; **Syrup** 10 mg/ml.

Patient Instructions. This drug may cause a confused state or other mental symptoms. Until the extent of this effect is known, caution should be used when driving, operating machinery, or performing other tasks requiring mental alertness.

Pharmacokinetics and Biopharmaceutics. *Onset and Duration.* Onset within 48 hr.
  Plasma Levels. Toxicity at levels above 1.5 mcg/ml.[22]
  Fate. Well absorbed from GI tract; 200 mg/day dosage produces a steady-state plasma level of 400–900 ng/ml in 4–7 days, with only a slight increase occurring thereafter. Over 90% of the drug is excreted unchanged in urine, with excretion more rapid in acidic urine.[23,24]
  $t_{1/2}$. 10–28.5 hr, pH-dependent;[23] 8.3 days in renal failure.[22]

Adverse Reactions. Occasionally, reversible and dose-related livedo reticularis, restlessness, confusion, hallucinations and other CNS and psychic disturbances. Rarely, congestive heart failure, orthostatic hypotension and convulsions occur.

Contraindications. Lactation.

Precautions. Pregnancy. Use with caution in patients receiving CNS drugs, and in those with the following conditions: liver disease, history of recurrent eczematoid rash, serious mental illness, seizures or epilepsy, congestive heart failure, peripheral edema, orthostatic hypotension, and particularly renal impairment and cerebrovascular disease in the elderly. Drug should not be abruptly discontinued in Parkinson's disease due to the potential of such actions for precipitating parkinsonian crises.

Parameters to Monitor. Carefully monitor for signs of toxicity at doses higher than 200 mg/day or in renal impairment.

Notes. Relatively few adverse reactions, but less effective than treatment with levodopa.[25] Therapeutic effectiveness is diminished after 1–2 months; either increasing dose, or gradual discontinuation of the drug for several weeks followed by reinitiation may be tried to regain effectiveness.[26] The combination of amantadine and levodopa is more effective than levodopa alone.[27] About 60% of patients respond to amantadine; those who respond also respond to levodopa, while nonresponders do not respond to levodopa.[18]

Levodopa

Bendopa®, Dopar®,
Larodopa®, Various

Pharmacology.   Levodopa, the precursor of dopamine, replenishes depleted stores of dopamine in the CNS of patients with parkinsonism.

Administration and Adult Dose.   PO for parkinsonism 250 mg bid-qid, then increase in 100–750 mg increments at 3–7 day intervals to a usual maintenance dose of 3–6 g/day in 3 or more divided doses, to maximum of 8 g/day in divided doses. Dose must be individualized by careful titration; significant therapeutic response may require up to 6 months of treatment.

Pediatric Dose.   Not recommended for children under 12 yr.

Dosage Forms.   **Cap** 100, 125, 250, 500 mg; **Tab** 100, 250, 500 mg.

Patient Instructions.   This drug may be taken with a small amount of food or antacid to minimize persistent stomach upset. Report any involuntary movements and consult physician or pharmacist before taking vitamin preparations.

Pharmacokinetics and Biopharmaceutics. *Onset and Duration.*
Onset about 2–3 weeks as the dosage reaches 2.5–3 g/day, although some patients require up to 6 months.[15]
   Fate. Rapidly absorbed from GI tract, but administration with food (particularly protein) results in slower absorption and a lower peak concentration. Less than 1% of absorbed levodopa penetrates into the CNS (the site of action) where it is converted to dopamine, the active drug. 95% of levodopa is decarboxylated peripherally to dopamine (which does not cross the blood-brain barrier), and it in turn is metabolized such that 85% of the dose is excreted as dopamine metabolites in the urine within 24 hr. Less than 1% is recovered as unchanged drug.[28]
   $t_{1/2}$. Approximately 1 hr.[29]

Adverse Reactions.   Generally reversible and dose-related. Anorexia, nausea, vomiting and involuntary movements occur most frequently. Orthostatic hypotension occurs especially frequently in elderly patients with a history of acute myocardial infarction or other cardiovascular disease.[30] Agitation, insomnia, depression and cardiac arrhythmias are observed occasionally; "on-off" phenomenon may occur with long-term therapy. Rarely, hemolytic anemia is reported.

Contraindications.   Children under 12 yr; narrow angle glaucoma; history of melanoma; lactation; MAO inhibitors (concurrent or two weeks prior to therapy); hemolytic anemia; G6PD deficiency.

Precautions.   Pregnancy. Use with caution in patients with psychosis, severe cardiovascular or pulmonary disease, bronchial asthma, renal, hepatic or endocrine disease, in patients with a history of active peptic ulcer, or myocardial infarction with residual arrhythmias (in this type of patient, the drug should be used in a facility with a coronary care unit), and in patients receiving antihypertensive drugs or having chronic wide angle glaucoma. Observe all patients for the development of depression with concomitant suicidal tendencies. Elevations of BUN, SGOT, SGPT, LDH, bilirubin, alkaline phosphatase, PBI, uric acid, and a positive Coombs' test have been reported, as have reductions in WBCs, hemoglobin and hematocrit. See Drug Interactions chapter.

Parameters to Monitor.   Periodically evaluate hepatic, hematopoietic, cardiovascular and renal function in all patients on extended therapy. In patients with glaucoma, monitor for changes in intraocular pressure.

Notes. Pyridoxine (vitamin B$_6$) in doses of 10–25 mg rapidly reverses the therapeutic and toxic effects of levodopa; vitamin preparations should be examined for content of this vitamin. Levodopa is considered the single most effective drug for Parkinson's disease, but long-term therapy is associated with fluctuations in effectiveness (including the "on-off" response) and increased adverse effects, which may necessitate frequent changes in dosages and dosing intervals.[31,32] Evidence suggests that levodopa therapy initiated early in the course of hepatic coma may be of some benefit.[33]

Carbidopa/Levodopa   Sinemet®

Pharmacology. See Levodopa; carbidopa is a peripheral decarboxylase inhibitor which prevents extracerebral metabolism of levodopa to dopamine. It has no other pharmacologic actions.

Administration and Adult Dose. PO for parkinsonism patients not now receiving levodopa, initiate with 10 mg carbidopa/100 mg levodopa or 25 mg carbidopa/100 mg levodopa tid, increasing by one tablet every day or every other day, up to 6 tablets/day. When patients have nausea or vomiting on low daily dosages of 10 mg carbidopa/100 mg levodopa, 25 mg carbidopa/100 mg levodopa may be substituted. If further titration is necessary, substitute with 25 mg carbidopa/250 mg levodopa tid, and if necessary increase by ½ or 1 tablet daily or every other day; PO maintenance dosage 3–6 tablets of 25 mg carbidopa/250 mg levodopa daily in divided doses, to maximum of 8 tablets of 25 mg/250 mg daily; if further titration is desired, levodopa alone should be added to the regimen. PO for patients receiving levodopa, discontinue levodopa for at least 8 hr before initiating treatment with a daily dosage that will provide approximately 25% of the previous levodopa daily dosage. It requires 75 to 150 mg of carbidopa daily to fully inhibit dopa decarboxylation. Therefore, patients receiving less than 75 mg of carbidopa and 750 mg of levodopa a day should receive additional carbidopa. For this reason, the manufacturer now makes a tablet containing 25 mg carbidopa only (Lodosyn®);[20,34,35] call MSD at (215) 699-5311 for information.

Pediatric Dose. Safety of use for children under 18 yr not established.

Dosage Forms. Tab 10 mg carbidopa/100 mg levodopa, 25 mg carbidopa/100 mg levodopa, 25 mg carbidopa/250 mg levodopa.

Patient Instructions. Report any involuntary movements which occur; do not take additional levodopa unless prescribed.

Pharmacokinetics and Biopharmaceutics. *Onset and Duration.* Onset may occur within days.[20]
    Fate. About 40–70% of an oral dose of carbidopa is absorbed. Carbidopa inhibits peripheral decarboxylation of levodopa, thereby increasing levodopa plasma levels and half-life and making more levodopa available for transport to the CNS. Metabolism of carbidopa is not extensive and about 30% is excreted unchanged in the urine.[36]
    $t_{1/2}$. (Levodopa) 1.2–2.3 hr when given with carbidopa.[37]

Adverse Reactions. See Levodopa. When compared with levodopa alone, many adverse effects are diminished, especially those related to GI upset; however, the frequency of orthostatic hypotension, psychic disturbances, and cardiac arrhythmias are unchanged, and dyskinesias may occur as frequently, with more severity, at a lower dose and sooner than with levodopa.[20,38,39]

Contraindications. See Levodopa.

Precautions. See Levodopa. Additionally, levodopa must be discontinued at least 8 hr before carbidopa/levodopa is started, and the dosage reduced about 75%, such that the carbidopa/levodopa dosage will provide 25% of the previous levodopa dosage. Be alert for dyskinesias, which may occur at lower doses and sooner than with levodopa alone.

Parameters to Monitor. See Levodopa.

Notes. Pyridoxine has little or no antagonistic effect when carbidopa and levodopa are given together.[40] Carbidopa/levodopa allows a smoother and more rapid therapeutic response than levodopa alone, and is superior to levodopa with respect to the number of patients showing improvement and in the amount of improvement shown. The optimal ratio of levodopa to carbidopa for their concurrent use is not the same for all patients.[20]

BROMOCRIPTINE

General References: 41,42

Bromocriptine Mesylate

Parlodel®

Pharmacology. An ergot alkaloid with dopamine agonist properties. It inhibits prolactin secretion, and in high doses, improves symptoms of Parkinson's disease.

Administration and Adult Dose. **PO for inhibition of lactation** (starting no sooner than 4 hr postpartum) 2.5 mg 1–3 times/day, usually 2.5 mg bid with meals for 14 days to maximum of 21 days. **PO for amenorrhea/galactorrhea** 2.5 mg bid-tid with meals for maximum of 6 months. **PO or Parkinson's disease** 1.25 mg initially bid with meals. Assess response at 2 week intervals and increase in 2.5 mg/day increments every 14–28 days until response obtained or intolerable side effects occur. Maintenance doses averaging 15 mg/day have been effective.[49] Safety of doses exceeding 100 mg/day has not been demonstrated. **PO for female infertility** 2.5 mg daily, increasing within 1 week to 2.5 mg bid-tid with meals.

Pediatric Dose. Safety and efficacy in children under 15 yr not established.

Dosage Forms. **Cap** 5 mg; **Tab** 2.5 mg.

Patient Instructions. This drug should be taken with food to minimize stomach upset. Drowsiness may occur, and caution should be taken when driving or operating machinery until the extent of this effect is known. Dizziness or faintness may occur, particularly with the first dose. Female patients should use some method of contraception during the use of this drug. Patients taking the drug for acromegaly should avoid or minimize the use of alcohol as they may become unusually sensitive to its effects.

Pharmacokinetics and Biopharmaceutics. *Onset and Duration.* Onset (milk secretion and breast engorgement) absent after 5 days postpartum;[43] (amenorrhea/galactorrhea) menses usually restored in 6–8 weeks and lactation usually 75% inhibited in 8–12 weeks.

Fate. About 28% oral absorption; 90–96% bound to albumin. Completely metabolized with metabolites primarily excreted in bile.

$t_{1/2}$. About 2 days.[44]

Adverse Reactions. Hypotension, dizziness, nausea and vomiting occur frequently; syncope occurs occasionally after the first dose; hypotension is most common in postpartum patients. Headache, dizziness, fatigue, abdominal cramps and GI disturbances may occur. Neuropsychiatric symptoms and alterations in awareness and behavior, sometimes accompanied by hallucinations occur rarely. In general, adverse reactions are more common in treatment of amenorrhea/galactorrhea and most common and severe in elderly Parkinson's patients.[41,43]

Precautions. In female infertility, use a mechanical contraceptive until drug treatment is completed. In amenorrhea/galactorrhea, fertility may return rapidly, so contraceptive measures should be used to prevent unwanted pregnancy. Discontinue drug as soon as pregnancy is detected. Use cautiously in renal or hepatic disease; history of mental disturbances; severe ischemic heart disease; or peripheral vascular disease.[41]

Notes. Investigational uses include male impotence, premenstrual syndrome, and long-term treatment of prolactin-secreting adenomas.[41,42]

CROMOLYN

General References: 45-47

Cromolyn Sodium

Intal®

Pharmacology. Inhibits release of histamine and SRS-A (slow-reacting substance of anaphylaxis) by preventing degranulation of mast cells; other mechanisms must also be involved, because it is equally effective in patients with exercise-induced bronchospasm and patients without allergies. It has no bronchodilator, antihistaminic or anti-inflammatory activity.[46]

Administration and Adult Dose. Inhal 20 mg tid-qid at regular intervals, using the inhaler supplied. A trial of 4 weeks is needed to determine patient response. Nebulizer solution should be administered using power-operated nebulizer.

Dosage Individualization. Some patients may be maintained on 20 mg tid during long-term use.[46-48]

Pediatric Dose. Inhal (5 yr and over) same as adult dose; for younger children, use 20 mg of nebulizer solution.

Dosage Forms. Inhal Cap 20 mg (not for oral use); Inhal Soln 10 mg/ml.

Patient Instructions. Do not stop therapy abruptly except on medical advice. Do not swallow capsule; capsules must be inhaled using the special inhaler and must be used regularly and continuously to be effective. Carefully follow directions for inhaler use included with the device. Do not use the drug to treat an acute asthmatic attack.

Pharmacokinetics and Biopharmaceutics. *Onset and Duration.* Onset within 1 min; duration at least 5 hr for most patients.[46]
   Fate. About 1% of inhaled dose is absorbed orally; about 8% is absorbed from the lung and peak plasma levels occur 15–20 min after inhalation.[46,47] Rapidly excreted unchanged in equal portions in the bile and urine;[46,47] remainder is either exhaled or swallowed and excreted in feces.
   $t_{1/2}$. 80–90 min after inhalation.[46,47]

Adverse Reactions. Bronchospasm and pharyngeal irritation occur occasionally. Use of a bronchodilator aerosol just prior to cromolyn may prevent bronchospasm.[46-48] Inhalation of gelatin capsule particles, inhaler or propeller have been reported rarely with capsule use.

Precautions. Not indicated for treatment of exacerbations of asthmatic symptoms. Caution in patients with lactose sensitivity (capsules only). Caution must be used when discontinuing the drug, particularly in patients whose oral corticosteroid dosage was reduced after cromolyn was started, because an acute exacerbation of asthma is possible. Cromolyn may be administered via aerosol in children younger than 5 yr, because inhalation may be difficult for this age group. Stop therapy if eosinophilic pneumonia (pulmonary infiltrates with eosinophilia) occurs.

Parameters to Monitor. Relief of asthmatic symptoms; proper dosing and use of inhaler should be monitored, as lack of compliance commonly contributes to treatment failures.[46,47]

Notes. Used in the prophylaxis of chronic asthma; however, a theophylline preparation in therapeutic doses is likely to be more effective.[45] Cromolyn is generally not useful when added to theophylline therapy. A trial of cromolyn may be indicated in asthmatic patients intolerant to theophylline or those with a history of migraine or seizure disorder. About 60–65% of pediatric patients respond to long-term cromolyn therapy alone and corticosteroid requirements may be reduced in others.[47,48] Before beginning therapy in patients with bronchodilator-unresponsive symptoms, give a short course of high-dose prednisone.

References, 92:00 Unclassified Therapeutic Agents

1. Rodnan GP, Robin JA, Tolchin SF et al. Allopurinol and gouty hyperuricemia: efficacy of a single daily dose. JAMA 1975;231:1143-7.
2. Boss GR, Seegmiller JE. Hyperuricemia and gout: classification, complications and management. N Engl J Med 1979;300:1459-68.
3. Simkin PA. Management of gout. Ann Intern Med 1979;90:812-6.
4. Mangini RJ. Drug therapy reviews: pathogenesis and clinical management of hyperuricemia and gout. Am J Hosp Pharm 1979;36:497-504.
5. Yu TF. Milestones in the treatment of gout. Am J Med 1974;56:676-85.
6. Elion GB, Yu TF, Gutman AB et al. Renal clearance of oxipurinol, the chief metabolite of allopurinol. Am J Med 1968;45:69-77.
7. Elion GB, Kovensky A, Hitchings GH. Metabolic studies of allopurinol, an inhibitor of xanthine oxidase. Biochem Pharmacol 1966;15:863-80.
8. Hande K, Reed E, Chabner B. Allopurinol kinetics. Clin Pharmacol Ther 1978;23:598-605.
9. Burkle WS. Allopurinol hypersensitivity. Drug Intell Clin Pharm 1979;13:218-23.
10. Chang SL, Kramer WG, Feldman S et al. Bioavailability of allopurinol oral and rectal dosage forms. Am J Hosp Pharm 1981;38:365-8.
11. Jusko WJ, Gretch M. Plasma and tissue protein binding of drugs in pharmacokinetics. Drug Metab Rev 1976;5:43-140.
12. Ertel NH, Mittler JC, Akgun S et al. Radioimmunoassay for colchicine in plasma and urine. Science 1976;193:233-5.
13. Wallace SL, Omokoku B, Ertel NH. Colchicine plasma levels: implications as to pharmacology and mechanism of action. Am J Med 1970;48:443-8.
14. Wallace SL. Colchicine. Semin Arthritis Rheum 1974;3:369-81.
15. Gilman AG, Goodman LS, Gilman A, eds. Goodman and Gilman's the pharmacological basis of therapeutics. 6th ed. New York: Macmillan, 1980.
16. Tabatabai MR, Cummings NA. Intravenous colchicine in the treatment of acute pseudogout. Arthritis Rheum 1980;23:370-4.
17. Lehman TJA, Peters RS, Schwabe AD. Long-term colchicine therapy of familial Mediterranean fever. J Pediatr 1978;93:876-8.
18. Cohen MM, Scheife RT. Pharmacotherapy of Parkinson's disease. Am J Hosp Pharm 1977;34:531-8.
19. Lieberman A, Goodgold M, Jonas S et al. Comparison of dopa decarboxylase inhibitor (carbidopa) combined with levodopa and levodopa alone in Parkinson's disease. Neurology 1975;25:911-6.
20. Boshes B. Sinemet and the treatment of parkinsonism. Ann Intern Med 1981;94:364-70.
21. Fann WE, Lake CR. Amantadine versus trihexyphenidyl in the treatment of neuroleptic-induced parkinsonism. Am J Psychiatry 1976;133:940-3.

22. Horadam VW, Sharp JG, Smilack JD et al. Pharmacokinetics of amantadine hydrochloride in subjects with normal and impaired renal function. Ann Intern Med 1981;94(part 1):454-8.

23. Pacifici GM, Nardini M, Ferrari P et al. Effect of amantadine on drug-induced parkinsonism: relationship between plasma levels and effect. Br J Clin Pharmacol 1976;3:883-9.

24. Bleindner WE, Harmon JB, Hewes WE et al. Absorption, distribution and excretion of amantadine hydrochloride. J Pharmacol Exp Ther 1965;150:484-90.

25. Mawdsley C, Williams IR, Pullar IA et al. Treatment of parkinsonism by amantadine and levodopa. Clin Pharmacol Ther 1972;13:575-83.

26. Schwab RS, Poskanzer DC, England AC et al. Amantadine in Parkinson's disease. JAMA 1972;222:792-5.

27. Walker JE, Potvin A, Tourtellotte W et al. Amantadine and levodopa in the treatment of Parkinson's disease. Clin Pharmacol Ther 1972;13:28-36.

28. Morgan JP, Bianchine JR, Spiegel HE et al. Metabolism of levodopa in patients with Parkinson's disease. Arch Neurol 1971;25:39-44.

29. Dunner DL, Brodie KH, Goodwin FK. Plasma DOPA respnse to levodopa administration in man: effects of a peripheral decarboxylase inhibitor. Clin Pharmacol Ther 1971;12:212-7.

30. Wener J, Rosenberg G, Grad B et al. Cardiovascular effects of levodopa in aged versus younger patients with Parkinson's disease. J Am Geriatr Soc 1976;24:185-8.

31. Anon. Drug therapy for Parkinson's disease. Med Lett Drugs Ther 1975;17:33-4.

32. Sweet RD, McDowell FH. Five year's treatment of Parkinson's disease with levodopa. Ann Intern Med 1975;83:456-63.

33. Fischer JE, Funovics JM, Falcao HA et al. L-Dopa in hepatic coma. Ann Surg 1976;183:386-91.

34. Hoehn MM. Increased dosage of carbidopa in patients with Parkinson's disease receiving low doses of levodopa. Arch Neurol 1980;37:146-9.

35. Tourtellotte WW, Syndulko K, Potvin AR et al. Increased ratio of carbidopa to levodopa in treatment of Parkinson's disease. Arch Neurol 1980;37:723-6.

36. Vickers S, Stuart EK, Bianchine JR et al. Metabolism of carbidopa L-(-)-α-hydrazino-3, 4-dihydroxy-α-methylhydrocinnamic acid monohydrate, an aromatic amino acid decarboxylase inhibitor, in the rat, dog, rhesus monkey, and man. Drug Metab Disp 1974;2:9-22.

37. Dunner DL, Brodie HKH, Goodwin FK. Plasma DOPA response to levodopa administration in man: effects of a peripheral decarboxylase inhibitor. Clin Pharmacol Ther 1971;12:212-7.

38. Celesia GG, Wanamaker WM. L-dopa-carbidopa: combined therapy for the treatment of Parkinson's disease. Dis Nerv Syst 1976;37:123-5.

39. Leibowitz M, Lieberman A. Comparison of dopa decarboxylase inhibitor (carbidopa) combined with levodopa and levodopa alone on the cardiovascular system of patients with Parkinson's disease. Neurology 1975;25:917-21.

40. Mars H. Levodopa, carbidopa, and pyridoxine in Parkinson disease. Arch Neurol 1974;30:444-7.

41. Parkes D. Bromocriptine. N Engl J Med 1979;301:873-8.

42. Avery GS ed. Focus on bromocriptine. Drugs 1979;17:313-88.

43. Duchesne C, Leke R. Bromocriptine mesylate for prevention of postpartum lactation. Obstet Gynecol 1981;57:464-7.

44. Friis ML, Gron U, Larsen N-E et al. Pharmacokinetics of bromocriptine during continuous oral treatment of Parkinson's disease. Eur J Clin Pharmacol 1979;15:275-80.

45. Weinberger M. Hendeles L. Pharmacotherapy of asthma. Am J Hosp Pharm 1976;33:1071-80.

46. Brogden RN, Speight TM, Avery GS. Sodium cromoglycate (cromolyn sodium): II. allergic rhinitis and other conditions. Drugs 1974;7:283-96.

47. Bierman CW, Soyka LF. The use of cromolyn sodium in the treatment of asthma in children. Pediatrics 1975;55:586-8.

48. Godfrey S, Balfour-Lynn L, Konig P. The place of cromolyn sodium in the long-term management of childhood asthma based on a 3- to 5-year follow-up. J Pediatr 1975;87:465-73.

49. Teychenne PF, Bergsrud D, Racy A et al. Bromocriptine: low-dose therapy in Parkinson disease. Neurology 1982;32:577-83.

INDEX

DRUGS IN THE INDEX are listed by nonproprietary name. Cross-references are provided for common brand names and for frequently used abbreviations. In addition, British Approved Names, where different from those used in the United States, are listed with the designation (BAN) following the name. For some large homogeneous drug groups (eg, thiazides, phenothiazines), each of the *individual* agents has page numbers listed even though only the drug *class* name appears in the text. This is to ensure that all information that is relevant to a particular agent is located easily. However, to gain maximum benefit from the index, the entries for both the specific agent and its drug class should be consulted.

Skin

NOTES

NOTES